Lippincott's
Illustrated Reviews:
Pharmacology

Lippincott's Illustrated Reviews: Pharmacology

editors
Richard A. Harvey, Ph.D.

Professor of Biochemistry
Department of Biochemistry
University of Medicine and Dentistry of New Jersey
Robert Wood Johnson Medical School
Piscataway, New Jersey

Pamela C. Champe, Ph.D.

Associate Professor of Biochemistry
Department of Biochemistry
University of Medicine and Dentistry of New Jersey
Robert Wood Johnson Medical School
Piscataway, New Jersey

contributing authors
Mary J. Mycek, Ph.D.

Adjunct Professor of Pharmacology
Department of Pharmacology
University of Medicine and Dentistry of New Jersey
New Jersey Medical School
Newark, New Jersey

Sheldon B. Gertner, Ph.D.

Interim Chairman
Department of Pharmacology
University of Medicine and Dentistry of New Jersey
New Jersey Medical School
Newark, New Jersey

Maria Menna Perper, Ph.D.

Adjunct Assistant Professor of Psychiatry
Department of Psychiatry
University of Medicine and Dentistry of New Jersey
Robert Wood Johnson Medical School
Piscataway, New Jersey

J. B. LIPPINCOTT COMPANY
Philadelphia   New York   London   Hagerstown

Acquisitions Editor: Richard Winters
Production Manager: Janet Greenwood
Production Service: Charles Field
Compositor: TCSystems, Inc.
Printer/Binder: Malloy Lithographing Inc.

3   5   6   4   2

Library of Congress Cataloging-in-Publication Data

Pharmacology.

(Lippincott's illustrated reviews)
Includes index.
1. Pharmacology—Outlines, syllabi, etc.   2. Pharmacology—Examinations, questions, etc.   [DNLM: 1. Pharmacology—examination questions.   2. Pharmacology—outlines.   QV 17 P536]   I. Harvey, Richard A.   II. Champe, Pamela C.   III. Mycek, Mary Julia.   IV. Gertner, Sheldon B.   V. Perpner, Maria Menna.   VI. Series.
RM301.14.P47   1992   615'.1'076   91-62109
ISBN 0-397-51039-X

The authors and publisher have exerted every effort to ensure that drug selection and dosage set forth in this text are in accord with current recommendations and practice at the time of publication. However, in view of ongoing research, changes in government regulations, and the constant flow of information relating to drug therapy and drug reactions, the reader is urged to check the package insert for each drug for any change in indications and dosage and for added warnings and precautions. This is particularly important when the recommended agent is a new or infrequently employed drug.

Preface

WHO WILL FIND THIS BOOK USEFUL

Lippincott's Illustrated Reviews: Pharmacology integrates and summarizes the essentials of medical pharmacology for (1) students in the health-related professions who are preparing for licensure examination USMLE Step 1 (National Board Examination Part I, FLEX), ECFMG, FMGEM, and (2) professionals who wish to review or update their knowledge in this rapidly expanding area of biomedical science. The *Illustrated Review* uses an information-intensive, outline format along with summary figures and practice questions to teach this complex material.

HOW TO USE THIS BOOK

OUTLINE TEXT *Lippincott's Illustrated Reviews: Pharmacology* uses a unique expanded outline format which allows the rapid review and assimilation of facts and concepts. The current knowledge in the field of medical pharmacology has been "predigested" and the relevant information has been recast in a hierarchical organization. Important topics are shown in bold print, whereas the names of drugs are featured in an italic typeface. This organization enables the reader to readily scan a page to locate specific information or to find a particular drug. A phonetic pronunciation guide for drug names assures that the reader will have a conversational familiarity with the therapeutic agents described in the book. Each chapter starts with a chart that lists and classifies the drugs to be discussed in that chapter. This permits the reader to immediately understand and remember the significant relationships among the facts and concepts.

ILLUSTRATIONS *Lippincott's Illustrated Reviews: Pharmacology* contains more than 400 original illustrations, each carefully crafted to compliment and amplify the text. This volume features a new kind of diagram in which pharmacological processes are illustrated with a blend of graphics and explanations. This marriage of words and art allows the reader to integrate a body of knowledge without the distraction of constantly shifting from text to illustrations. For example, to sort out the intricacies of neurotransmitter synthesis and release in an ordinary textbook would require repeated skipping from text to figures. By contrast, the *Illustrated Review* (see for example, Figure 4.3, p.37) reveals the major steps and their significance at a glance.

CROSS-REFERENCES WITHIN THIS BOOK *Lippincott's Illustrated Review: Pharmacology* not only permits the easy assimilation of pharmacological facts and concepts but also provides an extensive network of more than 300 cross-references to other relevant information in the volume. Thus, when readers encounter a new block of information, they are immediately directed to related material that reinforces and expands the original information. This elaborate matrix of references provides a cross fertilization that increases learning and retention. The student ends up with the "the big picture."

CROSS-REFERENCES TO OTHER BOOKS IN THE SERIES   A unique feature of this volume is the large number of references to *Lippincott's Illustrated Reviews: Biochemistry,* which is the biochemistry volume in the Lippincott series. Designated as **InfoLink** references, they are located at the end of each chapter. This permits a reader with an interest in learning additional information related to a particular topic to readily locate relevant material covered in *Lippincott's Illustrated Review: Biochemistry.* **InfoLink** also emphasizes the interrelationships between these biomedical disciplines—a skill that is increasingly being tested by the USMLE Step 1 (National Board Examination, Part I).

QUESTIONS AND ANSWERS   A total of more than 250 practice questions (of the types used by the National Board of Medical Examiners and other standardized test writers) are included at the end of each chapter to enable readers to check their progress in mastering the material. Answers with explanations are provided to ensure that the reader knows both the correct answer and also why the distractors in the multiple choice questions are incorrect. These answers and their explanations are juxtaposed with the original questions in a special section at the end of the book. Thus, readers can confirm the correct answers to a group of study questions without the disorientation of flipping from page to page.

FINDING INFORMATION   An extensive index of more than 3,000 entries permits the reader to instantly locate specific information. The index includes a citation of the page where the pronunciation guide for each major drug can be found and also includes commonly used trade-names of drugs. A separate glossary provides easy access to definitions of over 250 specialized medical terms that are used in *Lippincott's Illustrated Review: Pharmacology.*

Acknowledgments

We are grateful for the generous input and encouragement of our friends and colleagues at the University of Medicine and Dentistry of New Jersey, particularly Drs. Margaret Brostrom, Richard Howland, Rajendra Kapila, Zigmund Kaminski, Ronald Morris, Betty Pancake, Dennis Quinlan, Marilyn Saunders, and Don Wolff. In addition, Drs. Joseph Cohen, Sonya Sobrian, and William West of Howard University College of Medicine, and Mr. Robert Horowitz, made valuable contributions to the project.

We wish to thank Tristin Harvey for her contribution of computer graphics. We also received outstanding artistic support from Ms. Jo Gershman, Mr. Michael Cooper, and Mr. Robert Glessman, and constant positive encouragement (and exhortations to get the book finished) from our editor, Mr. Richard Winters of Lippincott. Final editing and assembly of the book has been greatly enhanced through the efforts of Ms. Janet Greenwood, Mr. Charles Field, and Ms. Joan Powers. Lastly, but far from least, we want to thank Drs. Marilyn Schorin and Sewell Champe for their unfailing contributions to and support of this project.

Brief Contents

UNIT VII: Anti-Inflammatory Drugs and Autacoids

Expanded Contents

UNIT IV: Drugs Affecting the Cardiovascular System

UNIT VII: *Anti-inflammatory Drugs and Autacoids*

Lippincott's
Illustrated Reviews:
Pharmacology

Absorption, Distribution, and Elimination of Drugs

1

I. OVERVIEW

The aim of drug therapy is to rapidly deliver and maintain therapeutic, yet nontoxic, levels of drug in the target tissues. To achieve this goal, the clinician must recognize that the speed of onset of drug action, the intensity of the drug's effect, and the duration of the drug action are controlled by three fundamental pathways of drug movement in the body (Figure 1.1). First, drug absorption from the site of administration permits entry of the therapeutic agent (either directly or indirectly) into plasma (input). Second, the drug may then leave the blood stream and distribute into the interstitial and intracellular fluids (distribution). Third, a process consisting primarily of urinary excretion and/or hepatic metabolism causes the drug and its metabolites to be eliminated from the body (output). This chapter and Chapter 2 describe how knowledge of these processes influences the clinician's decision as to the route of administration, drug loading, and dosing interval.

II. ROUTES OF DRUG ADMINISTRATION

The route of administration is determined primarily by the properties of the drug to be employed and by the therapeutic objectives, for example, the desirability of a rapid onset of action or the need for long-term administration. There are two major routes of drug administration, enteral and parenteral (Figure 1.2 illustrates the subcategories of these routes as well as other methods of drug administration).

A. Enteral

1. **Oral:** Giving a drug by mouth is the most common route of administration, but it uses the most complicated pathway to the tissues. Some drugs are absorbed from the stomach; however, the duodenum is often the major site of entry to the systemic circulation, since it provides a larger absorptive surface. [Note: Most

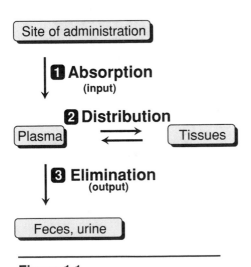

Figure 1.1
Schematic representation of drug absorption, distribution, and elimination.

1

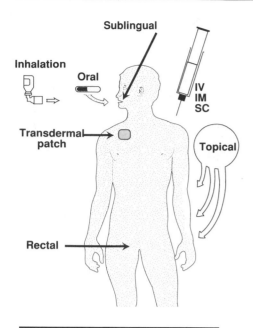

Figure 1.2
Commonly used routes of drug
administration. (IV=intravenous;
IM=intramuscular; SC=
subcutaneous).

Enteral – oral, subling, rectal
Parenteral – IV, IM, SC
other – inhalation, topical, transdermal

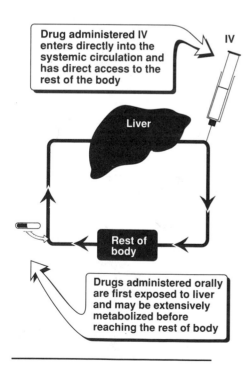

Drug administered IV
enters directly into the
systemic circulation and
has direct access to the
rest of the body

Drugs administered orally
are first exposed to liver
and may be extensively
metabolized before
reaching the rest of body

Figure 1.3
First-pass metabolism can occur
with orally administered drugs. (IV =
intravenous).

drugs absorbed from the gastrointestinal (GI) tract enter the hepatic portal circulation and encounter the liver before they are distributed in the general circulation (Figure 1.3).]

2. **Sublingual:** Placement under the tongue allows the drug to diffuse into the capillary network and therefore to enter the systemic circulation directly. Administration of an agent by this route has the advantage that the drug bypasses the liver and is not inactivated by hepatic metabolism. [Note: First-pass metabolism by the liver limits the efficacy of many drugs when taken orally. For example, more than 90% of *nitroglycerin* is cleared during a single passage through the liver.]

3. **Rectal:** Fifty percent of the drainage of the rectal region bypasses the hepatic portal circulation; thus the biotransformation of drugs that are metabolized by the liver is minimized. Both the sublingual and the rectal routes of administration have the additional advantage that they prevent the destruction of the drug by intestinal enzymes or by low pH in the stomach. [Note: The rectal and sublingual routes are also useful if the drug induces vomiting when given orally or if the patient is already vomiting.]

B. Parenteral

Parenteral administration is used for drugs that are poorly absorbed from the gastrointestinal tract and for agents, such as *insulin,* that are unstable in the GI tract. Parenteral administration is also used for treatment of unconscious patients and with drugs that require a rapid onset of action. Parenteral administration provides the most control over the actual dose of drug delivered to the body. The three major parenteral routes are intravenous, intramuscular, and subcutaneous (see Figure 1.2).

1. **Intravenous (IV):** This is the most common parenteral route. For drugs that are not absorbed orally, there is often no other choice. With IV administration, the drug is not absorbed by the GI tract; therefore, first-pass metabolism by the liver is avoided. This route permits a rapid effect and a maximal degree of control over the circulating levels of the drug. Intravenous injection of some drugs may induce hemolysis or other adverse reactions caused by the rapid delivery of high concentrations of drug to the plasma and tissues.

2. **Intramuscular (IM):** Drugs administered intramuscularly can be specialized depot preparations—often a suspension of drug in a nonaqueous vehicle, such as ethylene glycol or peanut oil. As the vehicle diffuses out of the muscle, the drug precipitates at the site of injection. The drug then dissolves slowly, providing a sustained dose over an extended period of time. The classic example is sustained-release *protamine zinc insulin* (p.239) whose slow diffusion from the muscle produces an extended hypoglycemic effect. Intramuscular administration is also used for rapid onset of action, such as *epinephrine* in anaphylaxis.

3. **Subcutaneous (SC):** This route of administration, like that of IM injection, provides absorption that is somewhat slower than the *IV*

IV route. SC injection minimizes the risks associated with intravascular injection.

C. Other

1. **Inhalation:** This route of administration is used for drugs that can be dispersed in an aerosol or that vaporize easily. Inhalation provides the rapid delivery of a drug across the large surface area of the alveolar membrane and can produce actions almost as rapidly as intravenous injection.

2. **Topical:** Topical application is used when a local effect of the drug is desired. For example, in the treatment of dermatophytosis, *clotrimazole* (p.312) is applied as a cream directly to the skin.

3. **Transdermal:** This route of administration achieves systemic effects by application of drugs to the skin, usually via a transdermal patch. This route is most often used for the sustained delivery of drugs, such as the antimotion sickness agent *scopolamine* (p.48) or the antianginal drug *nitroglycerin* (p.171).

III. ABSORPTION OF DRUGS

Absorption is the transfer of a drug from its site of administration to the blood stream. The rate and efficiency of absorption depend on the route of administration. For intravenous administration, absorption is complete, that is, the total dose of drug reaches the systemic circulation. Drug administration by other routes may result in only partial absorption. For example, oral administration requires that a drug dissolve in the gastrointestinal fluid and then penetrate the epithelial cells of the intestinal mucosa.

A. Transport of drug from the GI tract

Drugs may be absorbed from the GI tract by either passive diffusion or active transport.

1. **Passive diffusion:** The driving force for passive absorption of a drug is the concentration gradient across a membrane separating two body compartments, that is, the drug moves from a region of high concentration to a region of low concentration. Passive diffusion does not involve a carrier, is not saturable, and shows a low structural specificity. The vast majority of drugs gain access to the body by this mechanism. Lipid-soluble drugs readily move across most biological membranes, whereas water-soluble drugs penetrate the cell membrane through aqueous channels (Figure 1.4).

2. **Active transport:** This mode of drug entry involves specific carrier proteins and shows saturation kinetics, much in the same way that an enzyme-catalyzed reaction shows a maximum velocity at high substrate levels.[1] Active transport is energy dependent and is driven by the hydrolysis of ATP (Figure 1.4). It is capable of moving drugs against a concentration gradient, that is, from a region of low drug concentration to a region of high drug con-

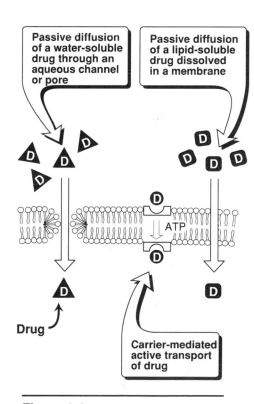

Figure 1.4
Schematic representation of drugs crossing cell membrane of epithelial cell of gastrointestinal tract.

centration. A few drugs that closely resemble the structure of a naturally occurring metabolite are actively transported across cell membranes using these specific carrier proteins.

B. Effect of pH on drug absorption

Many drugs are either weak acids or weak bases. Acidic drugs (HA) release a H^+ causing a charged anion (A^-) to form.[2]

$$HA \rightleftarrows H^+ + A^-$$

Weak bases (BH^+) can also release a H^+; however the protonated form of basic drugs is usually charged, and loss of a proton produces the uncharged base (B).

$$BH^+ \rightleftarrows B + H^+$$

A drug tends to pass through membranes if it is uncharged (Figure 1.5). Thus, for a weak acid, the uncharged HA can permeate through membranes, and A^- cannot. For a weak base, the uncharged form, B, penetrates through the cell membrane, and BH^+ does not. Therefore, the effective concentration of the permeable form of each drug at its absorption site is determined by relative concentrations of the charged and uncharged forms. The ratio between the two forms is, in turn, determined by the pH at the site of absorption and by the strength of the weak acid or base, which is represented by the pK_a (Figure 1.6). [Note: The pK_a is a measure of the strength of the interaction of a compound with a proton. The lower the pK_a, the stronger the acid.]

C. Physical factors influencing absorption

1. **Blood flow to the absorption site:** Blood flow to the intestine is much greater than the flow to the stomach; thus absorption from the intestine is favored over that from the stomach.

2. **Total surface area available for absorption:** Because the intestine has a surface rich in microvilli, it has a far greater surface area than that of the stomach; thus absorption of the drug across the intestine is more efficient.

3. **Contact time at the absorption surface:** If a drug moves through the GI tract very quickly, as in severe diarrhea, it is not well absorbed. Conversely, anything that delays the transport of the drug from the stomach to the intestine delays the rate of absorption of the drug. [Note: Parasympathetic input increases the rate of gastric emptying, whereas sympathetic input (prompted, for example, by exercise or stressful emotions) prolongs gastric emptying. Also, the presence of food in the stomach both dilutes the drug and slows gastric emptying. Therefore, a drug taken with a meal is absorbed more slowly.]

IV. BIOAVAILABILITY

Bioavailability is the extent of absorption of a drug following its administration by routes other than intravenous injection. Bioavailability

A. Weak acid

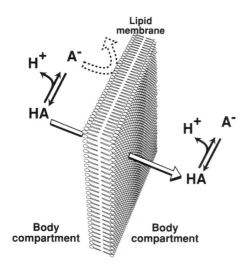

B. Weak base

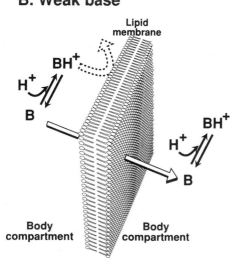

Figure 1.5
A. Diffusion of non-ionized form of a weak acid through lipid membrane;
B. Diffusion of non-ionized form of a weak base through lipid membrane.

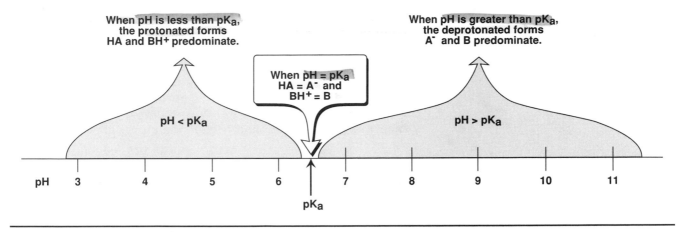

Figure 1.6
The distribution of a drug between its ionized and un-ionized form depends on the ambient pH and pK_a of the drug. For illustrative purposes, the drug has been assigned a pK_a of 6.5.

is expressed as the fraction of administered drug that gains access to the systemic circulation in a chemically unchanged form. For example, if 100 mg of a drug is administered orally and 70 mg of this drug is absorbed unchanged, the bioavailability is 70%.

A. Determination of bioavailability

Bioavailability is determined by comparing plasma levels of a drug after a particular route of administration (for example, oral administration) with plasma drug levels achieved by intravenous administration which enables all of the agent to enter the circulation. When the drug is given orally, only part of the administered dose appears in the plasma. By plotting plasma concentrations of the drug versus time, one can measure the area under the curve. This curve reflects the extent of absorption of the drug. [Note: By definition this is 100% for drugs administered intravenously.] Bioavailability of a drug administered orally is the ratio of the area calculated for oral administration compared with the area calculated for IV injection (Figure 1.7).

B. Factors that influence bioavailability

1. **First pass hepatic metabolism:** When a drug is absorbed across the GI tract, it must traverse the portal system before entering the systemic circulation (see Figure 1.3). If the drug is rapidly metabolized by the liver, the amount of unchanged drug that gains access to the systemic circulation is decreased. Many drugs, such as *propranolol,* undergo a significant biotransformation during a single passage through the liver.

2. **Solubility of drug:** Drugs that are very hydrophilic are poorly absorbed because of their inability to cross the lipid-rich cell membranes. Paradoxically, drugs that are extremely hydrophobic are also poorly absorbed, because they are totally insoluble in the aqueous body fluids and, therefore, cannot gain access to the surface of cells. For a drug to be readily absorbed it must be largely hydrophobic yet have some solubility in aqueous solutions.

$$\text{Bioavailability} = \frac{\text{AUC oral}}{\text{AUC injected}} \times 100$$

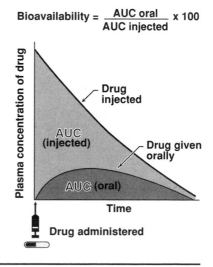

Figure 1.7
Determination of the bioavailability of a drug. (AUC = area under curve).

3. **Chemical instability:** Some drugs, such as *penicillin G,* are unstable to the pH of gastric juice contents.

4. **Nature of the drug formulation:** Drug absorption may be altered by factors unrelated to the chemistry of the drug. For example, particle size, salt form, crystal polymorphism, and the presence of excipients (such as binders and dispersing agents) can influence the ease of dissolution and, therefore, alter the rate of absorption.

C. Bioequivalence

Two related drugs are bioequivalent if they show comparable bioavailability. Two related drugs with a significant difference in bioavailability are said to be bioinequivalent.

D. Therapeutic equivalence

Two similar drugs are therapeutically equivalent if they have comparable efficacy and safety. [Note: Clinical effectiveness often depends both on maximum serum drug concentrations and the time after administration required to reach peak concentration. Therefore, two drugs that are bioequivalent may not be therapeutically equivalent.]

V. DRUG DISTRIBUTION

Drug distribution is the process by which a drug leaves the blood stream and enters the interstitium (extracellular fluid) or the cells of the tissues. The delivery of a drug from the plasma to the interstitium primarily depends on blood flow, capillary permeability, and the degree of binding of the drug to plasma and tissue proteins.

A. Blood flow

The rate of blood flow to the tissue capillaries varies widely as a result of the unequal distribution of cardiac output to the various organs. Blood flow to the brain, liver, and kidney is greater than that to the skeletal muscles, whereas adipose tissue has a still lower rate of blood flow.

B. Capillary permeability

Capillary permeability is determined by capillary structure and by the chemical nature of the drug.

1. **Capillary structure:** Capillary structure varies widely in terms of the fraction of the basement membrane that is exposed by slit junctions between endothelial cells. In the brain, the capillary structure is continuous, and there are no slit junctions (Figure 1.8). This contrasts with the liver and spleen, where a large part of the basement membrane is exposed by large discontinuous capillaries. Large plasma proteins can cross this basement membrane.

A. Structure of brain capillary

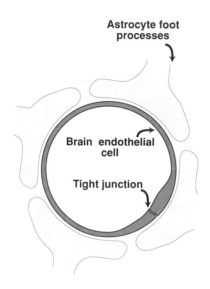

Astrocyte foot processes

Brain endothelial cell

Tight junction

B. Permeability of brain capillary

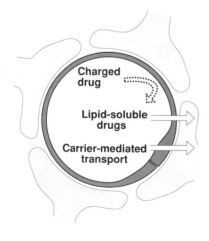

Charged drug

Lipid-soluble drugs

Carrier-mediated transport

Figure 1.8
Cross section of brain capillary.

a. **Blood-brain barrier:** In order to enter the brain, drugs must pass through the endothelial cells of the capillaries of the CNS. Lipid-soluble drugs readily penetrate into the CNS, since they can dissolve in the membrane of the endothelial cells. Ionized or polar drugs generally fail to enter the CNS, since they are unable to pass through the endothelial cells of the CNS, which have no slit junctions. These tightly juxtaposed cells form tight junctions that constitute the so-called blood-brain barrier (Figure 1.8).

2. **Drug structure:** The chemical nature of the drug strongly influences its ability to cross cell membranes. Hydrophobic drugs, which have a uniform distribution of electrons and no net charge, readily move across most biological membranes. These drugs can dissolve in the lipid membranes and are therefore permeable to the entire cell's surface. The major factor influencing the hydrophobic drug's distribution is the blood flow to the area. By contrast, hydrophilic drugs, which have either a nonuniform distribution of electrons or a positive or negative charge, do not readily penetrate cell membranes. These drugs must go through the slit junctions.

C. Binding of drugs to proteins

Reversible binding to plasma proteins sequesters drugs in a non-diffusable form and slows their transfer out of the vascular compartment. As the concentration of the free drug decreases due to elimination by metabolism or excretion, the bound drug dissociates from the protein. This maintains the free drug concentration as a constant fraction of the total drug in the plasma (see p.10 for a further discussion of drug binding by proteins).

VI. VOLUME OF DISTRIBUTION

The volume of distribution is a hypothetical volume of fluid into which the drug is disseminated. Although the volume of distribution has no physiological or physical basis, it is sometimes useful to compare the distribution of a drug with the volumes of the water compartments in the body (Figure 1.9).

A. Water compartments in the body

Once a drug enters the body, from whatever route of administration, it has the potential to distribute into any one of three functionally distinct compartments of body water.

1. **Plasma compartment:** If a drug has a very large molecular weight or binds extensively to plasma proteins, it is too large to move out through the endothelial slit junctions of the capillaries and thus is effectively trapped within the plasma (vascular) compartment. As a consequence, the drug distributes in a volume (the plasma) that is about 4% of the body weight or, in a 70-kg individual, about 3 L of body fluid.

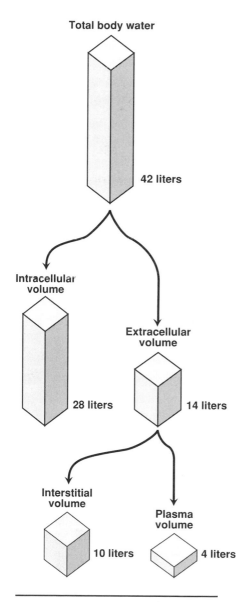

Figure 1.9
Relative size of various distribution volumes within a 70 kg individual.

2. **Extracellular fluid:** If the drug has a low molecular weight, but is hydrophilic, it can move through the endothelial slit junctions of the capillaries into the interstitial fluid. However, hydrophilic drugs cannot move across the membranes of cells to enter the water phase inside the cell. These drugs distribute into a volume which is the sum of the plasma water and the interstitial fluid, which together constitute the extracellular fluid. This is about 20% of the body weight, or about 14 L in a 70-kg individual.

3. **Total body water:** If the drug has a low molecular weight and is hydrophobic, it can not only move into the interstitium through the slit junctions but can also move through the cell membranes into the intracellular fluid. The drug therefore distributes into a volume of about 60% of body weight, or about 42 L in a 70-kg individual.

B. The apparent volume of distribution (Vd)

A drug rarely associates exclusively with one of the water compartments of the body. Instead, the vast majority of drugs distribute into several compartments, often avidly binding cellular components, for example, lipids (abundant in adipocytes and cell membranes), proteins (abundant in plasma and within cells), or nucleic acids (abundant in the nuclei of cells). Therefore, the volume into which drugs distribute is called the apparent volume of distribution or V_d.

1. Determination of V_d

a. The apparent volume into which a drug distributes, V_d, is determined by injection of a standard dose of drug. The drug is initially contained entirely in the vascular system. The agent may then move from the plasma into the interstitium and into cells, causing the plasma concentration to decrease with time (Figure 1.10). Assume for simplicity that the drug is not eliminated from the body. The drug then achieves a uniform concentration that is sustained with time. The concentration within the vascular compartment is the total amount of drug administered divided by the volume into which it distributes, V_d:

$$C = D/V_d \text{ or } V_d = D/C$$

C = plasma concentration of drug
D = Total amount of drug in the body

For example, if 25 mg of a drug (D = 25 mg) is administered and the plasma concentration is 1.0 mg/L, the V_d = 25 mg/1.0 mg/L = 25 L.

b. In reality, drugs are eliminated from the body, and a plot of plasma concentration versus time shows two phases. The initial decrease in plasma concentration is due to a rapid distribution phase in which the drug is transferred from the plasma into the interstitium and the intracellular water. This is followed by a slower elimination phase during which the drug

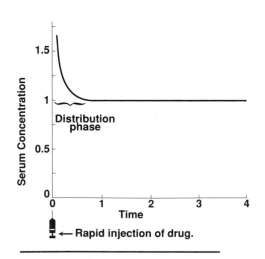

Figure 1.10
Drug concentrations in serum after a single injection of drug at time = 0. Assume that drug distributes but is not eliminated.

leaves the plasma compartment and is lost from the body, for example, by renal elimination or hepatic biotransformation (Figure 1.11). The rate at which the drug is eliminated is usually proportional to the concentration of drug, that is, the rate with most drugs is first order and shows a linear relationship with time if $\log_{10}C$ (rather than C) is plotted versus time (Figure 1.12).

c. Assume that the elimination process began at the time of injection and continued throughout the distribution phase. Then the concentration of drug in the plasma, C, can be extrapolated back to zero time (the time of administration) to determine C_0, which is the concentration of drug that would have been achieved had the distribution phase been achieved instantly.

For example, if 10 mg of drug is injected into a patient and the plasma concentration extrapolated to zero time concentration is $C_0 = 1.0$ mg/L (from graph shown in Figure 1.12), then $V_d = 10$ mg/1.0 mg/L = 10 L.

d. The apparent volume of distribution assumes that the drug distributes uniformly in a single compartment. However, most drugs distribute unevenly in several compartments and the volume of distribution does not describe a real, physical volume but rather reflects the ratio of drug in the extraplasmic spaces relative to the plasma space. Nonetheless, V_d is useful since it can be used to calculate the amount of drug needed to achieve a desired plasma concentration.

For example, assume the arrhythmia of a cardiac patient is not well controlled due to inadequate plasma levels of *digitalis*. Suppose the concentration of the drug in the plasma is C_1 and the desired level of digitalis (known from clinical studies) is a higher concentration, C_2. The clinician needs to know how much additional drug should be administered to bring the circulating level of drug from C_1 to C_2.

$V_d \cdot C_1$ = amount of drug initially in body

$V_d \cdot C_2$ = amount of drug in the body needed to achieve the desired plasma concentration

The difference between the two values is the additional dosage needed which equals $V_d(C_2-C_1)$

2. A large V_d has an important influence on the half-life of a drug, since drug elimination depends on the amount of drug delivered to the liver or kidney per unit of time. Delivery of drug to the organs of elimination depends not only on blood flow but also on the fraction of the drug in the plasma. If the V_d for a drug is large, most of the drug is in the extraplasmic space and is unavailable to the excretory organs. Therefore, any factor that increases the volume of distribution can lead to an increase in the half-life and extend the duration of action of the drug. [Note: An exceptionally large V_d indicates considerable sequestration of the drug in some organ or compartment.]

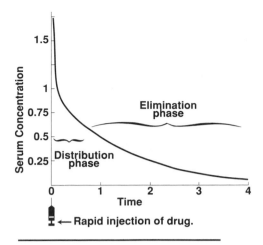

Figure 1.11
Drug concentrations in serum after a single injection of drug at time = 0. Assume that drug distributes and is subsequently eliminated.

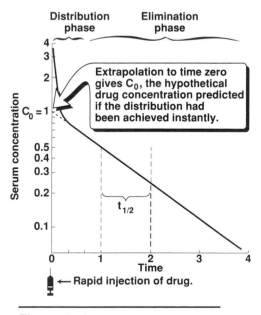

Figure 1.12
Drug concentrations in serum after a single injection of drug at time = 0. Data plotted on log scale.

VII. BINDING OF DRUGS TO PLASMA PROTEINS

Drug molecules may bind to plasma protein, usually albumin. Drug molecules bound to plasma proteins are pharmacologically inactive; only the free, unbound drug can act on target sites in the tissues and elicit a biological response. By binding to plasma proteins, drugs become "trapped" and in effect, inactive.

A. Class I drugs: Dose less than available binding sites

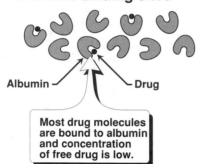

Albumin ⎯ ⎯ Drug

Most drug molecules are bound to albumin and concentration of free drug is low.

B. Class II drugs: Dose greater than available binding sites

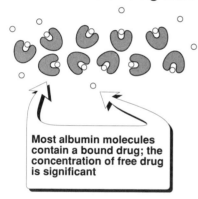

Most albumin molecules contain a bound drug; the concentration of free drug is significant

C. Administration of a Class I and a Class II drug.

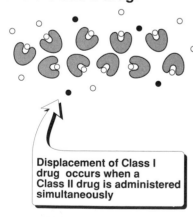

Displacement of Class I drug occurs when a Class II drug is administered simultaneously

Figure 1.13
Binding of Class I and Class II drugs to albumin when drugs are administered alone (A,B), or together (C).

A. Binding capacity of albumin

The binding of drugs to albumin is reversible and may show low capacity (one drug molecule per albumin molecule) or high capacity (a number of drug molecules binding to a single albumin molecule). Drugs can also bind with varying affinities. Albumin has the strongest affinity for anionic drugs (weak acids) and hydrophobic drugs. Most hydrophilic drugs and neutral drugs do not bind to albumin. [Note: Many drugs are hydrophobic, since this property permits absorption after oral administration.]

B. Competition for binding between drugs

When two drugs are given, each with high affinity for albumin, they compete for the available binding sites. The drugs with high affinity for albumin can be divided into two classes, depending on whether the dose of drug (the amount of drug found in the body under conditions used clinically) is greater than or less than the binding capacity of albumin (the number of millimoles of albumin multiplied by the number of binding sites Figure 1.13).

1. **Class I drugs:** If the dose of drug is less than the binding capacity of albumin, then the dose/capacity ratio is low. The binding sites are in excess of the available drug, and the drug fraction bound is high. This is the case for Class I drugs.

2. **Class II drugs:** These drugs are given in doses that greatly exceed the number of albumin binding sites. The dose/capacity ratio is high, and a relatively high proportion of the drug exists in the free state, not bound to albumin.

3. **Clinical importance of drug displacement:** This assignment of drug classification assumes importance when a patient who is taking a Class I drug, such as *tolbutamide,* is given a Class II drug, such as a sulfonamide. The *tolbutamide* is normally 95% bound, and only 5% is free. This means that most of the drug is sequestered on albumin and is inert in terms of exerting pharmacological actions. If a sulfonamide is administered, it displaces *tolbutamide* from albumin, leading to a rapid increase in the concentration of free *tolbutamide* in plasma, because almost 100% is now free compared with the initial 5%. The *tolbutamide* concentration does not remain elevated since the drug moves out of the plasma into the interstitial fluid and achieves a new equilibrium.

C. Conclusions

If the V_d is large, the drug displaced from the albumin moves to sites in the periphery, where it is unavailable to the elimination organs. The V_d thus increases, and the half-life of the drug is prolonged. If the V_d is small, the newly displaced drug does not move into the tissues as much, and the increase in free drug in the plasma is more profound. If the therapeutic index (p.20) of the drug is small, this increase in drug concentration may have significant clinical consequences. Thus, the impact of drug displacement from albumin depends on both V_d and the therapeutic index of the drug.

VIII. DRUG METABOLISM

Drugs are most often eliminated by biotransformation and/or excretion into the urine or bile. The liver is the major site for drug metabolism, but specific drugs may undergo biotransformation in other tissues.

A. Kinetics of metabolism:

1. **First-order kinetics:** The metabolic transformation of drugs is catalyzed by enzymes, and most of the reactions obey Michaelis-Menten kinetics.[3]

$$v = \text{rate of drug metabolism} = \frac{V_{max}[C]}{K_m + [C]}$$

In most clinical situations the concentration of the drug, [C], is much less than the Michaelis constant, K_m, and the Michaelis-Menten equation reduces to

$$v = \text{rate of drug metabolism} = V_{max}[C]/K_m$$

that is, the rate of drug metabolism is directly proportional to the concentration of free drug, and first-order kinetics are observed (Figure 1.14). This means that a constant percent of drug is metabolized per unit time.

2. **Zero order kinetics:** With a few drugs, such as *aspirin, ethanol,* and *phenytoin,* the doses are very large; thus, the [C] is much greater than K_m, and the velocity equation becomes:

$$v = \text{rate of drug metabolism} = V_{max}[C]/[C] = V_{max}$$

The enzyme is saturated by a high free-drug concentration, and the rate of metabolism remains constant over time. This is called zero-order kinetics, and a constant amount of drug is metabolized per unit time.

B. Reactions of drug metabolism

The kidney cannot efficiently eliminate lipophilic drugs that readily cross cell membranes and are reabsorbed in the distal tubules (see

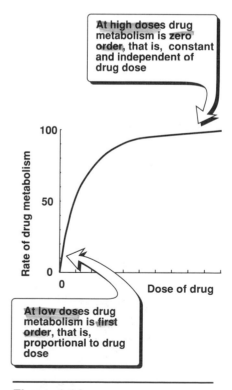

At high doses drug metabolism is zero order, that is, constant and independent of drug dose

At low doses drug metabolism is first order, that is, proportional to drug dose

Figure 1.14
Effect of drug dose on the rate of metabolism.

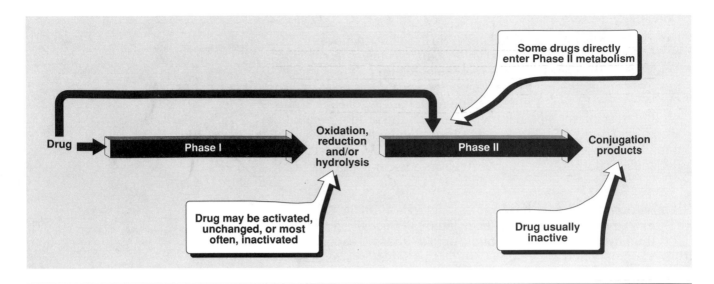

Figure 1.15
The biotransformations of drugs.

p.21). Therefore, lipid-soluble agents must first be metabolized in the liver using two general sets of reactions, called Phase I and Phase II (Figure 1.15).

1. **Phase I**

   a. Phase I reactions function to convert lipophilic molecules into more polar molecules by introducing or unmasking a polar functional group, such as -OH, or $-NH_2$. Phase I metabolism may increase, decrease, or leave unaltered the drug's pharmacological activity. The Phase I reactions most frequently involved are catalyzed by the cytochrome P-450 system, also called, microsomal mixed function oxidase.

   $$\text{Drug} + O_2 + \text{NADPH} \rightarrow \text{Drug}_{\text{modified}} + H_2O + \text{NADP}^+$$

   b. The P-450 system is a family of enzymes that occur in most cells, but that are particularly abundant in the liver. Each of the enzymes has a broad and, therefore, sometimes overlapping specificity. Many drugs are able to induce elevated levels of cytochrome P-450, resulting in an increased rate of metabolism of the drug, as well as other drugs biotransformed by the P-450 system. This enzyme induction is indicated in Figure 1.16.

   c. Other Phase I reactions, not involving the P-450 system, include amine oxidation (e.g., oxidation of catecholamines, histamine), alcohol dehydrogenation (e.g., ethanol oxidation), and hydrolysis (e.g., hydrolysis of *procainamide*).

2. **Phase II**

   a. Phase II consists of conjugation reactions. If the metabolite from Phase I metabolism is sufficiently polar, it can be ex-

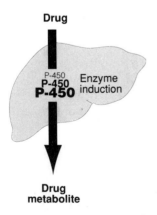

Figure 1.16
Schematic representation of drug-induced elevation of hepatic cytochrome P-450.

creted by the kidneys. However, many metabolites are sufficiently lipophilic to be reabsorbed and undergo a subsequent conjugation reaction with an endogenous substrate, such as glucuronic acid, sulfuric acid, acetic acid, or an amino acid. These conjugates are polar, usually more water-soluble and most often inactive. Glucuronidation is the most common and the most important conjugation reaction. Neonates are deficient in this conjugating system. [Note: Drugs already possessing an -OH, -HN_2, or -COOH group many be conjugated without prior Phase I metabolism.] The highly polar drug conjugates may then be excreted by the kidney.

b. Not all drugs undergo Phase I and II reactions in that order. For example, *isoniazid* is first acetylated (a Phase II reaction) and then hydrolyzed to isonicotinic acid (a Phase I reaction).

Study Questions (see p. 403 for answers).

Choose the ONE best answer.

1.1 Which one of the following statements is correct?

A. Weak bases are absorbed efficiently across the epithelial cells of the stomach.
B. Coadministration of atropine speeds the absorption of a second drug.
C. Drugs showing large V_d can be efficiently removed by dialysis of the plasma.
D. Stressful emotions can lead to a slowing of drug absorption.
E. If the V_d for a drug is small, most of the drug is in the extraplasmic space.

1.2 Which one of the following is true for a drug whose elimination from plasma shows first-order kinetics?

A. The half-life of the drug is proportional to the drug concentration in plasma.
B. The amount eliminated per unit time is constant.
C. The rate of elimination is proportional to the plasma concentration.
D. Elimination involves a rate-limiting enzymic reaction operating at its maximal velocity.
E. A plot of drug concentration versus time is a straight line.

1.3 All of the following statements are true EXCEPT:

A. Aspirin (pK_a = 3.5) is 90% in its lipid-soluble, protonated form at pH = 2.5.
B. The basic drug promethazine (pK_a = 9.1) is more ionized at pH = 7.4 than at pH = 2.

C. Absorption of a weakly basic drug is likely to occur faster from the intestine than from the stomach.
D. Acidification of the urine accelerates the secretion of a weak base, pK_a = 8.
E. Uncharged molecules more readily cross cell membranes than charged molecules.

1.4 A patient is treated with drug A, which has a high affinity for albumin and is administered in amounts that do not exceed the binding capacity of albumin. A second drug, B, is added to the treatment regimen. Drug B also has a high affinity for albumin but is administered in amounts that are 100 times the binding capacity of albumin. Which of the following occurs after administration of drug B?

A. An increase in tissue concentrations of drug A.
B. A decrease in tissue concentrations of drug A.
C. A decrease in volume of distribution of drug A.
D. A decrease in the half-life of drug A.
E. Addition of more drug A significantly alters the serum concentration of unbound drug B.

1.5 The addition of glucuronic acid to a drug

A. decreases its water solubility.
B. usually leads to inactivation of the drug.
C. is an example of a Phase I reaction.
D. is an important pathway in the newborn.
E. involves cytochrome P-450.

1.6 Drugs showing zero-order kinetics of elimination

    A. are more common that those showing first-order kinetics.
    B. decrease in concentration exponentially with time.
    C. have a half-life independent of dose.
    D. show a plot of drug concentration versus time that is linear.
    E. show a constant fraction of the drug eliminated per unit time.

1.7 A drug, given as a 100-mg single dose, results in a peak plasma concentration of 20 μg/ml. The apparent volume of distribution is (assume a rapid distribution and negligible elimination prior to measuring the peak plasma level):

    A. 0.5 L.
    B. 1 L.
    C. 2 L.
    D. 5 L.
    E. 10 L.

1.8 Which one of the following statements is correct?

    A. A drug given intravenously has more potential for first-pass hepatic metabolism than the same drug given orally.
    B. Inhalation has the disadvantage of very slow absorption.
    C. Passive diffusion typically involves a specific carrier protein and shows saturation kinetics.
    D. Bioavailability of a drugs administered intravenously is 100%.
    E. An exceptionally large K_d indicates that the drug is rapidly metabolized.

Chapter 1

[1]See enzymes, V_m in **Biochemistry** for concept of maximal velocity as the limiting rate of reaction observed at substrate concentrations high compared to K_m (see index).

[3]See enzymes, Michaelis-Menten equation in **Biochemistry** for a more complete discussion of enzyme kinetics.

[2]See K_a (acid dissociation constant) in **Biochemistry** for a more complete discussion of ionization of weak acids and bases.

Pharmacokinetics and Drug Receptors

2

I. OVERVIEW

Pharmacokinetics describe the time-dependent changes of plasma drug concentration and the time-dependent changes of the total amount of drug in the body following various routes of administration. The two most common routes of drug administration are intravenous infusion and a fixed-dose, fixed-time interval regimen, for example, "two tablets every four hours."

II. KINETICS OF INTRAVENOUS INFUSION

A. Steady-state drug levels in blood

With a continuous intravenous infusion, the rate of drug entry into the body is constant. The rate of drug exit from the body increases proportionately as the plasma concentration increases and at every point in time is proportional to the plasma concentration of drug. This is described by the equation:

$$\text{Rate of drug exit} = k_e C$$

C = the plasma concentration of drug
k_e = first-order rate constant for drug removal by the body

Therefore, following the initiation of an intravenous infusion, the plasma concentration of drug rises until the rate of drug eliminated from the body (which is plasma concentration-dependent) precisely balances the input rate. Thereafter the plasma concentration of drug remains constant at a steady-state value (Figure 2.1). Two principal questions can be asked about this process. First, what is the relationship between the rate of drug infusion and the plasma concentration of drug achieved at the plateau, or steady state? Second, what length of time is required to achieve the steady-state drug concentration?

B. Influence of the rate of drug infusion

A steady-state plasma concentration of drug occurs when the rate of drug elimination is equal to the rate of administration (Figure 2.1). It can be shown that

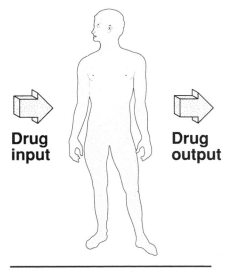

Figure 2.1
At steady state, input (rate of infusion) equals output (rate of elimination).

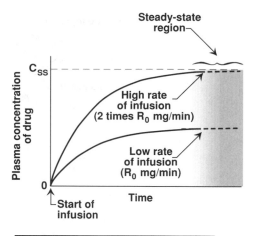

Figure 2.2
Effect of infusion rate on the steady-state concentration of drug in plasma. (R_0 = rate of infusion of drug).

$$C_{ss} = R_o/k_eV_d = R_o/CL_t$$

where C_{ss} = the steady state concentration of drug
R_0 = the infusion rate (e.g., mg/min)
k_e = first order rate constant for drug elimination from the total body
V_d = volume of distribution
CL_t = total body clearance (p.22)

Since k_e, CL_t, and V_d are constant for a given drug, C_{ss} is directly proportional to R_o, that is, the steady-state plasma concentration is directly proportional to the infusion rate. For example, if the infusion rate is doubled, the plasma concentration ultimately achieved at the steady state is doubled (see Figure 2.2). Furthermore, the steady-state concentration is inversely proportional to the clearance of the drug, CL_t. Thus, any factor that decreases clearance, such as liver or kidney disease, increases the steady-state concentration of an infused drug.

C. Time required to reach the steady state

1. **Exponential approach to steady state:** The concentration of drug rises from zero at the start of the infusion to its ultimate steady-state level C_{ss}. The fractional rate of approach to a steady state is achieved by a first-order process. The rate constant for attainment of steady state is the rate constant for total body elimination of the drug, k_e. Thus, 50% of the final steady-state concentration of drug is observed after t equals $t_{1/2}$, where $t_{1/2}$ (or

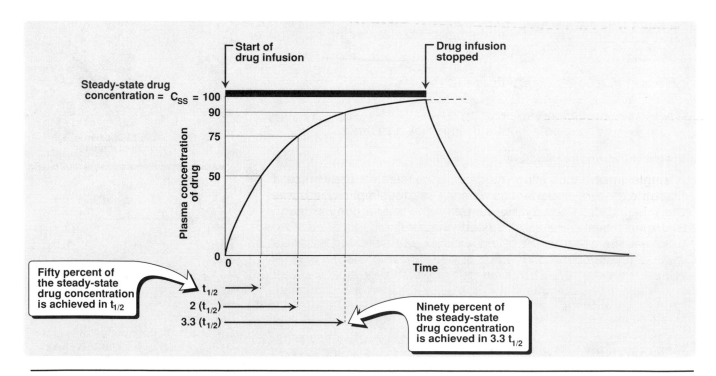

Figure 2.3
Rate of attainment of steady-state concentration of drug in plasma.

half-life) is the time required for the drug concentration to change by 50%. Waiting another half-life allows the drug concentration to approach 75% of C_{ss} (Figure 2.3). The drug concentration is 90% of the final steady-state concentration in 3.3 times $t_{1/2}$.

2. **Effect of the rate of drug infusion:** The sole determinant of the rate of approach to steady state is the $t_{1/2}$ or k_e for the drugs, and the steady state is influenced only by the factors that affect the half-life; it is not affected by the rate of drug infusion. Although increasing the rate of infusion of drug increases the rate at which any given concentration of drug in plasma is achieved, it does not influence the time required to reach the ultimate steady-state concentration. This is because the steady-state concentration of drug rises directly with the infusion rate.

3. **Rate of drug decline:** When the infusion is stopped, the plasma concentration of drug declines to zero with the same time course observed in approaching the steady state.

4. **Loading dose:** A delay in achieving the desired plasma levels of drug may be clinically unacceptable. Therefore, a "loading dose" of drug can be injected as a single dose to achieve the desired plasma level rapidly, followed by an infusion to maintain the steady state (maintenance dose). In general, the loading dose can be calculated as:

$$\text{Loading dose} = (V_d) \text{ (desired steady-state plasma concentration)}$$

III. KINETICS OF FIXED-DOSE, FIXED-TIME INTERVAL REGIMENS

Administration of a drug is often more convenient by fixed doses than by continuous infusion, but fixed doses result in time-dependent fluctuations in the circulating level of drug.

A. Single intravenous injection

A single intravenous drug injection is considered first, since it illustrates several important concepts. First, for simplicity, assume the injected drug rapidly distributes into a single compartment. Since the rate of elimination is usually first order in drug concentration, the circulating level of drug decreases exponentially with time (Figure 2.4). [Note: The $t_{1/2}$ does not depend on the dose of drug administered.]

B. Multiple intravenous injections

1. When a drug is given repeatedly at regular intervals, the plasma concentration increases until a steady state is reached (Figure 2.5). Since most drugs are eliminated exponentially with time, some drug from the first dose remains in the body at the time that the second dose is taken, and some from the second dose at the

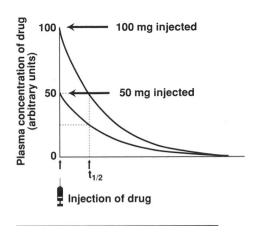

Figure 2.4
Effect of dose of single intravenous injection of drug on plasma levels.

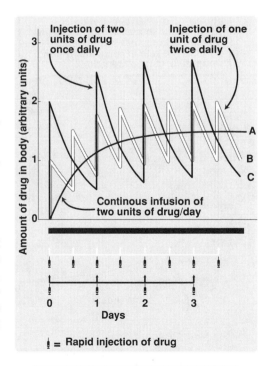

Figure 2.5
Predicted plasma concentrations of a drug given by infusion (A), twice daily injection (B), or once daily injection (C). Model assumes rapid mixing in a single body compartment and a $t_{1/2}$ of 12 hours.

time that the third dose is taken, and so forth. Therefore, the drug accumulates until within the given dosing interval the rate of drug loss (driven by elevated plasma concentration) exactly balances the rate of drug administration, that is, a steady state is achieved.

2. The plasma concentration of the drug oscillates about a mean. Using smaller doses at shorter intervals reduces the amplitude of the swings in drug concentration. However, the steady-state concentration of the drug and the rate at which the steady state is approached are not affected by the frequency of dosing.

For example, the white curve of Figure 2.5 shows the amount of drug in the body when one gram of drug is administered intravenously to a patient, and the dose is repeated at a time interval that corresponds to the half-life of the drug. At the end of the first dosing interval, 0.50 g of drug remains from the first dose when the second dose is administered. At the end of the second dosing interval, 0.75 g is present when the third dose is taken. The minimal amount of drug during the dosing interval progressively increases and approaches a value of 1.00 g, whereas the maximal values immediately following drug administration progressively approaches 2.00 g. Therefore, at the steady state, 1.00 g of drug is lost during the dosing interval, which is exactly matched by the rate at which the drug is administered, that is, the "rate in" equals the "rate out." As in the case for intravenous infusion (p.16), 90% of the steady-state value is achieved in 3.3 times $t_{1/2}$.

C. Orally administered drugs

Most drugs that are administered on an outpatient basis are taken orally on a fixed-dose, fixed-time interval regimen, usually a specific dose, one, two or three times daily. In contrast to intravenous injection, orally administered drugs may be absorbed slowly, and the plasma concentration of the drug is influenced by both the rate of absorption and the rate of drug elimination (Figure 2.6).

D. Pharmacokinetics in man

The above discussions assume that the drug distributes into a single compartment. In actuality, most drugs equilibrate between two or three compartments and, thus, display complex kinetic behavior.

IV. DOSE-RESPONSE QUANTITATION

A. Drug receptors

A drug receptor is a specialized target macromolecule that binds a drug and mediates its pharmacological actions. Drugs may interact with enzymes (e.g., inhibition of dihydrofolate reductase by *trimethoprim,* p.267), nucleic acids (e.g., blockade of transcription by *dactinomycin,* p.346) or membrane-bound receptors (e.g., alteration of membrane permeability by *epinephrine,* p.33). In each case,

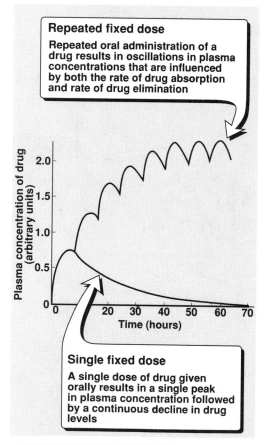

Repeated fixed dose

Repeated oral administration of a drug results in oscillations in plasma concentrations that are influenced by both the rate of drug absorption and rate of drug elimination

Single fixed dose

A single dose of drug given orally results in a single peak in plasma concentration followed by a continuous decline in drug levels

Figure 2.6
Predicted plasma concentrations of a drug given by repeated oral administrations.

the formation of the drug-receptor complex leads to a biological response, and the magnitude of the response is proportional to the number of drug-receptor complexes:

Drug + Receptor → Drug-receptor complex → Effect

For some drugs, the nature of the target molecule is unknown. The actions of a few drugs are not mediated by specific receptors, but depend on nonspecific chemical or physical interactions. For example, anesthetic gases (p.111) are thought to alter the structure of the membrane.

B. Graded dose-response curve

The magnitude of the drug effect depends on its concentration at the receptor site, which in turn is determined by the dose of drug administered (and by factors characteristic of the drug, such as rate of absorption, distribution, and metabolism). The effect of a drug is most easily analyzed by plotting the magnitude of the response versus the log of the drug dose, giving the graded dose-response curve (Figure 2.7).

1. **Efficacy:** Efficacy is the maximal response produced by a drug and depends on the number of drug-receptor complexes formed and the efficiency with which the activated receptor produces a cellular action (Figure 2.7). Efficacy is analogous to maximal velocity for an enzyme catalyzed reaction.[1]

2. **Potency:** Potency is a measure of how much drug is required to elicit a response. The lower the dose required for a given response, the more potent the drug. Potency is most often expressed as the dose of drug that gives 50% of the maximal response, ED_{50} (Figure 2.7). A drug with a low ED_{50} is more potent than a drug with a larger ED_{50}. The affinity of the receptor for a drug is an important factor in determining the potency.

3. **Slope of dose-response curve:** The slope of the midportion of the dose-response curve varies from drug to drug. A steep slope indicates that a small increase in drug dosage produces a large change in response.

C. Reversible antagonists

1. **Competitive:** These agents interact with receptors at the same site as the agonist and, thus, compete for binding of the agonist (Figure 2.8). A competitive antagonist shifts the dose-response curve to the right, causing the drug to behave as if it were less potent. This behavior is analogous to a competitive inhibitor for an enzyme-catalyzed reaction.[2]

2. **Noncompetitive:** These agents bind to the receptor at a site different from the agonist binding site and either prevent the binding of the agonist or prevent the agonist from activating the receptor. A noncompetitive antagonist decreases the maximal response and is analogous to a noncompetitive inhibitor for an enzyme-catalyzed reaction.

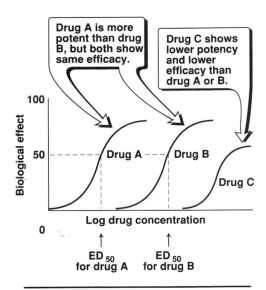

Figure 2.7
Typical dose response curve for drugs showing differences in potency and efficacy. ED_{50} = drug dose that shows 50% of maximal response.

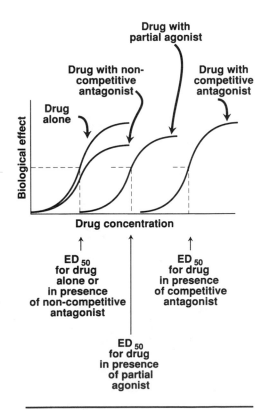

Figure 2.8
Effects of drug antagonists.

3. **Partial agonist:** These agents cause less response than a full agonist. A partial agonist may have an increased, decreased, or equivalent affinity for the receptor as an agonist.

V. THERAPEUTIC INDEX

A. Definition

The therapeutic index of a drug is the ratio of the dose that produces toxicity to the dose which produces a clinically desired or effective response. The therapeutic index is thus a measure of the drug's safety, since a large value indicates that there is a wide margin between doses that are effective and doses that are toxic.

$$\text{Therapeutic index} = \text{toxic dose/effective dose}$$

B. Determination of therapeutic index

1. The therapeutic index is determined by measuring the frequency of direct response and toxic response at various doses of drug. For example, Figure 2.9 shows the response to *warfarin,* an oral anticoagulant with a narrow therapeutic index, and *penicillin,* an antimicrobial drug with a large therapeutic index. As the dose of *warfarin* is increased, a greater fraction of the patients respond (in this case the desired response is two-fold increases in prothrombin time) until eventually all patients respond.

2. At higher doses of *warfarin,* a toxic response occurs, in this case a high degree of anticoagulation that results in hemorrhage. Note that when the therapeutic index is low, it is possible to have a range of concentrations where the effective and toxic responses overlap, that is, some patients hemorrhage while others achieve the desired two-fold prolongation of prothrombin time.

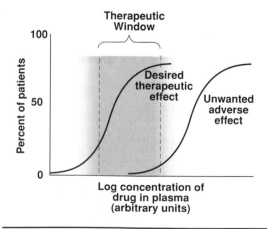

A. Warfarin: Small therapeutic index

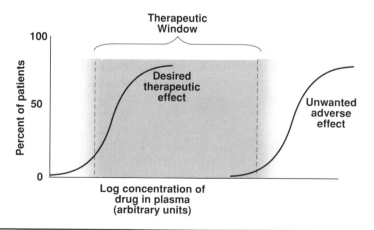

B. Penicillin: Large therapeutic index

Figure 2.9
Cumulative percent of patients responding to plasma levels of drug.

Agents with low therapeutic index are those drugs where bio-inequivalence is likely to result in a therapeutic consequence (p.6)

3. For drugs with a large therapeutic index, such as *penicillin* (Figure 2.9), it is safe and common to give doses in excess (often about ten-fold excess) of that which is minimally required to achieve a desired response. In this case, the bioavailability does not critically alter the therapeutic effects.

4. Variation in patient response is most likely to occur with a drug showing a narrow therapeutic index, since the effective and toxic concentrations are similar.

VI. DRUG ELIMINATION

A. Renal elimination of a drug

1. **Glomerular filtration:** Drugs enter the kidney through renal arteries, which divide to form a glomerular capillary plexus. Free drug (not bound to albumin) flows through the capillary slits into Bowman's space as part of the glomerular filtrate (Figure 2.10). The glomerular filtration rate (GFR = 125 ml/min) is normally about 20% of the renal plasma flow (RPF = 600 ml/min). Lipid solubility and pH do not influence the passage of drug into the glomerular filtrate.

2. **Proximal tubular secretion:** Drug that was not transferred into the glomerular filtrate leaves the glomeruli through efferent arterioles, which divide to form a capillary plexus surrounding the nephric lumen. Secretion primarily occurs in the proximal tubules by two energy-requiring active transport systems, one for anions (for example, deprotonated forms of weak acids) and one for cations (protonated form of weak bases). Each of these transport systems shows a low specificity and can transport many compounds; thus, competition between drugs for the carrier can occur within each transport system.

3. **Distal tubular reabsorption:** As a drug moves toward the distal convoluted tubule, its concentration increases and exceeds that of the perivascular space. The drug, if uncharged, may diffuse out of the nephric lumen. Manipulating the pH of the urine may be used to minimize the amount of back diffusion and hence increase the clearance of an undesirable drug. For example, a patient presenting with a phenobarbitol overdose can be given bicarbonate, which alkalinizes the urine and keeps the drug ionized; thus its reabsorption is decreased. If the drug is a weak base, acidification of the urine with NH_4Cl leads to protonation of the drug and an increase in its clearance. This is called "ion trapping."

4. **Role of drug metabolism:** Most drugs are lipid soluble and diffuse out of the kidney's tubular lumen when the drug concentration in the filtrate becomes greater than that in the perivascular space.

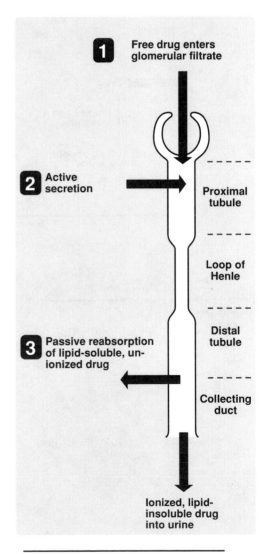

Figure 2.10
Drug elimination by the kidney.

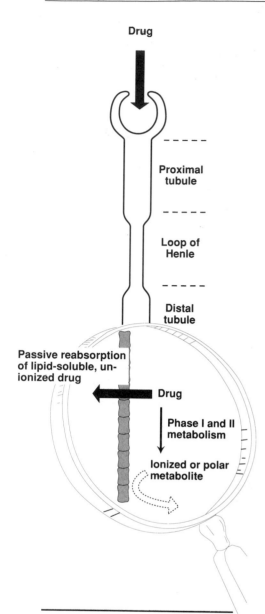

Figure 2.11
Effect of drug metabolism on reabsorption in the distal tubule.

In order to minimize this reabsorption, drugs are modified by the body to be more polar using two types of reactions: The first, or Phase I reaction (p.12), involves either the addition of hydroxyl groups or the removal of blocking groups from hydroxyl or amino groups. The second, or Phase II reaction, uses conjugation with sulfate, glycine, and glucuronic acid to increase polarity. These conjugates are ionized, and the charged molecules cannot back-diffuse out of the kidney lumen (Figure 2.11).

B. Quantitative aspects of renal drug elimination

1. **Clearance (of plasma):** Clearance is expressed as the volume of plasma from which all drug is removed in a given time, for example, as ml/min. Clearance equals the amount of renal plasma flow multiplied by the extraction ratio, and since these are normally invariant over time, clearance is constant.

2. **Extraction ratio:** This ratio is the decline of drug concentration in the plasma from the arterial to the venous side of the kidney. The drugs enter the kidneys at concentration C_1 and exit the kidneys at concentration C_2.

3. **Excretion rate:**

$$\text{Excretion rate} = (\text{clearance}) \cdot (\text{plasma concentration})$$
$$\text{mg/min} \qquad \text{ml/min} \qquad \text{mg/ml}$$

The elimination of a drug follows first-order kinetics, and the concentration of drug in plasma drops exponentially with time. This may be used to determine the half-life of the drug. [Note: The half-life is the time during which the concentration of the drug decreases from C to 1/2C.]

$$t_{1/2} = 0.693/k_e$$

C. Total body clearance

The kidney is often the major organ of excretion; however, the liver also contributes to drug loss through metabolism and/or excretion into the bile. The drug may then either be excreted into the feces or reabsorbed through enterohepatic circulation. The total body clearance (CL_{total}) is the sum of the clearances from the various drug-metabolizing and drug-eliminating organs.

$$\text{Clearance}_{total} = \text{Clearance}_{hepatic} + \text{Clearance}_{renal} +$$
$$\text{Clearance}_{pulmonary} + \text{Clearance}_{other}$$

D. Volume of distribution and the half-life of a drug

The half-life of a drug is inversely related to its clearance and directly proportional to its volume of distribution.

$$t_{1/2} = 0.693\, V_d/\text{total body clearance}$$

This equation shows that as the volume of distribution increases, the half-life of a drug becomes longer. The larger the volume of distribution, the more drug is outside the plasma compartment and is unavailable for excretion by the kidney.

E. Clinical situations resulting in increased drug half-life

When a patient has an abnormality that alters the half-life of a drug, adjustment in dosage is required. It is important to be able to predict in which patients a drug is likely to have a longer half-life. The half-life of a drug is increased:

1. with diminished renal plasma flow, for example, in cardiogenic shock, heart failure, or hemorrhage.

2. with addition of a second drug which displaces the first from albumin and, hence, increases volume of distribution of the drug.

3. with decreased extraction ratio, for example, as seen in renal disease.

4. with decreased metabolism, for example, when another drug inhibits its biotransformation.

Study Questions (see p.404 for answers).

Choose the ONE best answer.

2.1 A drug with a half-life of 12 hours is administered by continuous intravenous infusion. How long will it take for the drug to reach 90% of its final steady-state level?

A. 18 hours.
B. 24 hours.
C. 30 hours.
D. 40 hours.
E. 48 hours.

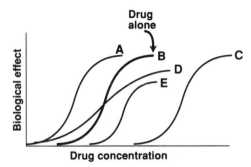

2.2 Which of the following results in a doubling of the steady-state concentration of a drug?

A. Doubling the rate of infusion.
B. Maintaining the infusion rate, but doubling the loading dose.
C. Doubling the rate of infusion and doubling the concentration of the infused drug.
D. Tripling the rate of infusion.
E. Quadrupling the rate of infusion.

2.3 The graded dose-response curve for a drug is shown as curve B in the above graph. Which curve best describes the response expected in the presence of a competitive antagonist?

A. Curve A.
B. Curve B.
C. Curve C.
D. Curve D.
E. Curve E.

2.4 Which of the following statements is correct?

  A. If 10 mg of drug A produces the same response as 100 mg of drug B, drug A is more efficacious than drug B.
  B. The greater the efficacy, the greater the potency of a drug.
  C. In selecting a drug, potency is usually more important than efficacy.
  D. In the presence of a full agonist, a partial agonist acts like a competitive inhibitor.
  E. Variation in response to a drug among different individuals is most likely to occur with a drug showing a large therapeutic index.

2.5 Which of following most closely describes the clearance rate of a drug that is infused at a rate of 4 mg/min and produces a steady-state concentration of 6 mg/L in the plasma?

  A. 67 ml/min.
  B. 132 ml/min.
  C. 300 ml/min.
  D. 667 ml min.
  E. 1,200 ml/min.

2.6 The antimicrobial drug, tetracycline, is found to be therapeutically effective when 250 mg of drug are present in the body. The $t_{1/2}$ of tetracycline is 8 hours. What is the correct rate of infusion?

  A. 7 mg/min.
  B. 12 mg/min.
  C. 22 mg/min.
  D. 37 mg/min.
  E. 45 mg/min.

2.7 A drug has a V_d of 30 L and a clearance rate of 20 L/hr, with 50% being eliminated by the liver and 50% excreted by the kidney. A maintenance regimen is 200 mg every 12 hours. Which of the following most closely produces the same steady-state concentration in a patient with 50% renal function?

  A. 25 mg every 3 hours.
  B. 100 mg every 6 hours.
  C. 150 mg every 12 hours.
  D. 150 mg every 6 hours.
  E. 200 mg every 6 hours.

2.8 Which of the following is least likely to influence the response to a drug?

  A. Affinity of receptor for drug.
  B. Efficacy.
  C. Bioavailability.
  D. Therapeutic index.
  E. Route of administration.

[1]See *enzymes, V_m* in **Biochemistry** for concept of maximal velocity as the limiting rate of reaction observed at substrate concentrations high compared to K_m (see index.

[2]See *enzymes, inhibition* in **Biochemistry** for concept of inhibitor molecules competing with substrate for binding at the active site of an enzyme.

The Autonomic Nervous System

3

I. OVERVIEW

The autonomic nervous system, along with the endocrine system, coordinates the regulation and integration of body functions. The endocrine system sends signals to target tissues by varying the levels of blood-borne hormones. By contrast, the nervous system exerts its influence by the rapid transmission of electrical impulses over nerve fibers. Drugs that produce their primary therapeutic effect by altering the functions of the autonomic nervous system are called autonomic drugs and are discussed in the following four chapters. These autonomic agents act either by stimulating portions of the autonomic nervous system or by blocking the action of the autonomic nerves. This chapter outlines the fundamental physiology of the autonomic nervous system and describes the role of neurotransmitters in the communication between extracellular events and chemical changes within the cell.

II. INTRODUCTION TO THE NERVOUS SYSTEM

A. Organization of the nervous system

1. **Anatomical divisions within the nervous system:** The nervous system is divided into two anatomical divisions, the central nervous system (CNS), which is composed of the brain and spinal cord, and the peripheral nervous system, which includes neurons located outside the brain and spinal cord, that is, any nerves that enter or leave the CNS (Figure 3.1). The peripheral nervous system can be further divided into the efferent division, whose neurons carry signals away from the brain and spinal cord to the peripheral tissues, and the afferent division, whose neurons bring information from the periphery to the CNS.

2. **Functional divisions within the nervous system:** The efferent portion of the peripheral nervous system can be further divided into two major functional subdivisions, the somatic and autonomic systems (Figure 3.1). The somatic efferents are involved in voluntary activity such as contraction of the skeletal muscles. The autonomic system is an involuntary system that functions to control the everyday needs and requirements of the body without the

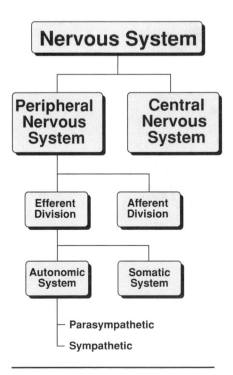

Figure 3.1
Organization of the nervous system.

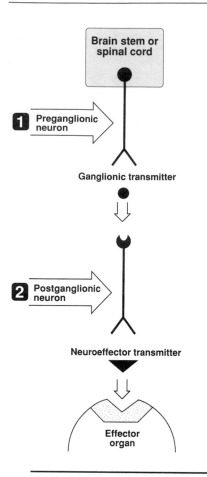

Figure 3.2
Efferent neurons of the
autonomic nervous system.

conscious participation of the mind. It is composed primarily of visceral motor (efferent) neurons which innervate smooth muscle of the viscera, cardiac muscle, and the exocrine glands.

B. Anatomy of the autonomic nervous system

1. **Preganglionic and postganglionic neurons:** The autonomic nervous system carries nerve impulses from the CNS to the effector organs by way of two types of efferent neurons (Figure 3.2). The first nerve cell is called a preganglionic neuron and its cell body is contained within the CNS. Preganglionic neurons emerge from the brain stem or spinal cord and make a synaptic connection in a ganglion (an aggregation of nerve cell bodies located in the peripheral nervous system). These ganglia function as relay stations between the preganglionic neuron and a second nerve cell, the postganglionic neuron. The latter neuron has a cell body originating in the ganglion. It sends efferent fibers that terminate on smooth muscles of the viscera, cardiac muscle, and the exocrine glands (Figure 3.2). The involuntary tissues that are innervated by the autonomic system are referred to as effector organs.

2. **Sympathetic:** The efferent autonomic nervous system can be divided into the sympathetic and the parasympathetic nervous systems (see Figure 3.1). The preganglionic neurons of the sympathetic system come from thoracic and lumbar regions of the spinal cord and synapse in two cord-like chains of ganglia that run in parallel on each side of the spinal cord. Axons of the postganglionic neuron extend from these ganglia to the glands and viscera. [Note: The adrenal medulla, like the sympathetic ganglia, receives preganglionic fibers from the sympathetic system. Lacking axons, the adrenal medulla, in response to stimulation by neurotransmitters, influences other organs by secreting the hormone *epinephrine* (and lesser amounts of *norepinephrine*) into the blood.]

3. **Parasympathetic:** The parasympathetic preganglionic fibers arise from the cranial and sacral areas of the spinal cord and synapse in ganglia near or on the effector organs. In both the sympathetic and parasympathetic systems, postganglionic fibers extend from the ganglia to effector organs.

C. Functions of the autonomic nervous system

1. **Sympathetic:**

   a. The sympathetic division is activated in response to stressful situations, such as trauma, fear, hypoglycemia, cold, or exercise. The effect of sympathetic output is to increase heart rate and blood pressure, to mobilize energy stores of the body, and to increase blood flow to skeletal muscles and heart while diverting flow from the skin and internal organs. Sympathetic stimulation also results in dilation of the pupils and the bronchioles (Figure 3.3).

   b. The changes experienced by the body during emergencies has been referred to as the "fight or flight" response (Figure 3.4). These reactions are triggered both by direct sympathetic

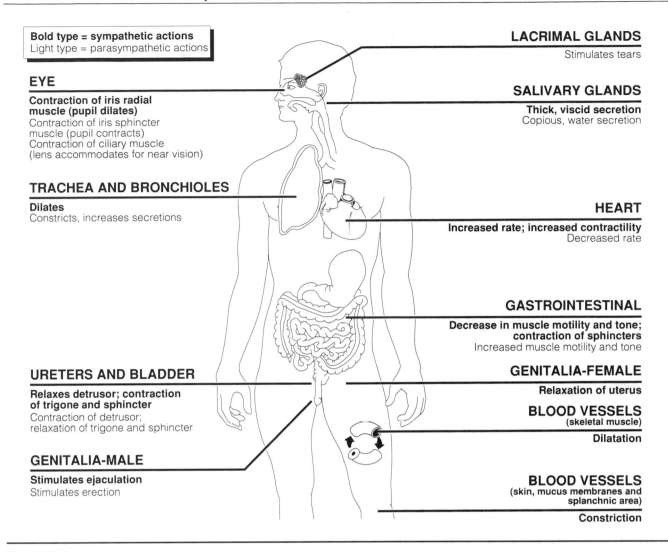

Figure 3.3
Action of sympathetic **(bold type)** and parasympathetic (light type) nervous systems on effector organs.

activation of the effector organs and by stimulation of the adrenal medulla to release *epinephrine* and lesser amounts of *norepinephrine.* These hormones enter the blood stream and promote responses in effector organs that contain adrenergic receptors (see p. 61). The sympathetic nervous system tends to function as a unit and often discharges as a complete system, for example, during severe exercise or in reactions to fear (Figure 3.4). This system with its diffuse distribution of postganglionic fibers is involved in a wide array of physiological activities, but it is not essential for life.

2. **Parasympathetic:**

a. The parasympathetic division usually acts to oppose or balance the actions of the sympathetic division. The parasympathetic system is not a functional entity as such and never discharges as a complete system. If it did, it would produce massive, undesirable, and unpleasant symptoms. Instead, discrete parasympathetic fibers are activated separately, and the

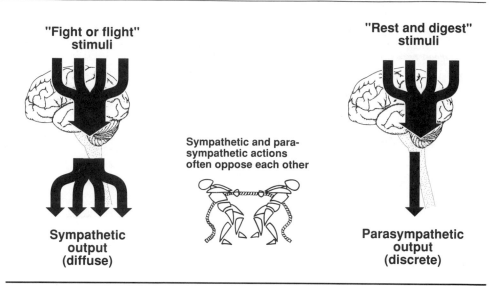

Figure 3.4
Sympathetic and parasympathetic actions are elicited by different stimuli.

system functions to affect specific organs, such as the stomach or eye.

b. The parasympathetic division is involved in such activities as accommodation of near vision, movement of food, and urination (Figure 3.3) and is essential for life. The parasympathetic system is generally dominant over the sympathetic system in "rest or digest" situations (Figure 3.4).

D. Role of CNS in autonomic control of viscera

Although the autonomic nervous system is a motor system, it does require sensory input from peripheral structures to provide information on the state of affairs in the body.

1. **Reflex arcs:** Streams of afferent impulses, arising in the viscera and other autonomically innervated structures, travel to integrating centers in the hypothalamus, medulla oblongata, and spinal cord. These centers in the CNS respond to the stimuli by sending out efferent reflex impulses via the autonomic nervous system (Figure 3.5).

a. Most of the afferent impulses are translated into reflex responses without involving consciousness. For example, a fall in blood pressure causes pressure-sensitive neurons (baroreceptors in the heart, vena cava, aortic arch, and carotid sinuses) to send fewer impulses to cardiovascular centers in the brain. This prompts a reflex response of increased sympathetic output to the heart and vasculature, and decreased parasympathetic output to the heart, which results in a compensatory rise in blood pressure and tachycardia (Figure 3.5).

2. **Emotions and the autonomic nervous system:** Stimuli that evoke feelings of strong emotion, such as rage, fear, or pleasure, can modify the activity of the autonomic nervous system. This interaction is probably the basis of psychosomatic disease. For example, stress and worry have long been known to be involved in the etiology of peptic ulcer and hypertension.

E. Dual innervation by the autonomic nervous system

1. **Dual innervation:** Most organs in the body are innervated by both divisions of the autonomic nervous system. Thus, the heart has vagal parasympathetic innervation that slows contraction, and sympathetic innervation that speeds contraction. Despite this dual innervation, one system usually predominates in controlling the activity of a given organ. For example, in the heart, the vagus is the predominant controlling factor for rate.

2. **Organs receiving only sympathetic innervation:** Although most tissues receive dual innervation, some effector organs, such as the adrenal medulla, kidney, pilomotor muscles, and sweat glands, receive innervation only from the sympathetic system. The control of blood pressure is also mainly a sympathetic activity, with essentially no participation by the parasympathetic system.

F. Somatic nervous system

The efferent somatic nervous system differs from the autonomic system in that a single motor neuron, originating in the CNS, travels directly to skeletal muscle without the mediation of ganglia. As noted earlier, the somatic nervous system is under voluntary control, whereas the autonomic is an involuntary system.

III. CHEMICAL SIGNALING BETWEEN CELLS

Neurotransmission in the autonomic nervous system is an example of the more general process of chemical signaling between cells. In addition to neurotransmission, other types of chemical signaling are the release of local mediators and the secretion of hormones.

A. Local mediators

Most cells in the body secrete chemicals that act locally, that is, they act on cells in their immediate environment. These chemical signals are rapidly destroyed or removed; thus, they do not enter the blood and are not distributed throughout the body. Histamine (p.388) and prostaglandins (p.361) are examples of local mediators.

B. Hormones

Specialized endocrine cells secrete hormones into the blood stream, where they travel throughout the body exerting effects on target cells distributed in the body. These are described in Chapters 25-27.

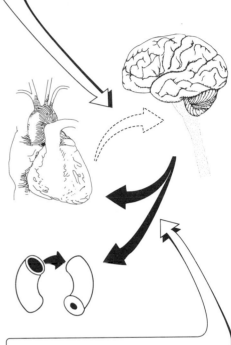

1 AFFERENT INFORMATION

● Drop in blood pressure

● Reduced stretch of baro-receptors in aortic arch

● Reduced frequency of afferent impulses to medulla (brain stem)

2 REFLEX RESPONSE

Efferent reflex impulses via the autonomic nervous system cause:

● Inhibition of parasympathetic and activation of sympathetic division

● Increased peripheral resistance and cardiac output

● Increased blood pressure

Figure 3.5
Baroreceptor reflex arc responds to a decrease in blood pressure.

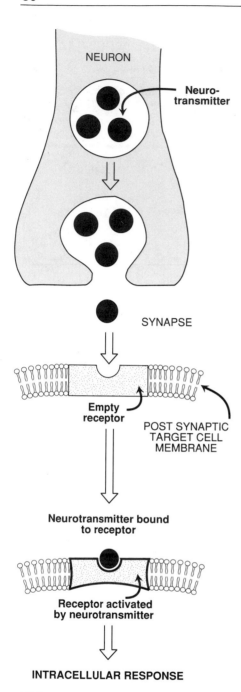

Figure 3.6
Neurotransmitter binding triggers
an intracellular response.

C. Neurotransmitters

1. **Role of neurotransmitters:** Each neuron is a distinct anatomic unit, and no structural continuity exists between most neurons. Communication between nerve cells—and between nerve cells and effector organs—occurs through the release of specific chemical signals, called neurotransmitters, from the nerve terminals. These substances rapidly diffuse across the gap (synapse) between nerve endings and combine with specific receptors on the postsynaptic (target) cell (Figure 3.6).

2. **Membrane receptors:** All neurotransmitters and most hormones and local mediators are too hydrophilic to penetrate the lipid bilayer of target-cell plasma membranes; instead, their signal is mediated by binding to specific receptors on the cell surface.

3. **Types of neurotransmitters:** Although over 50 chemical signal molecules in the nervous system have tentatively been identified, 6 signal compounds—norepinephrine (and the closely related epinephrine), acetylcholine, dopamine, serotonin, histamine and γ-aminobutyric acid—are most commonly involved in the actions of therapeutically useful drugs. Each of these chemical signals binds to a specific family of receptors that are schematically shown in Figure 3.7. [Note: The shapes of each model neurotransmitter and its receptor are used consistently in the following chapters.] Cholinergic and adrenergic neurotransmitters are the primary chemical signals in the autonomic nervous system, whereas a wide variety of neurotransmitters function in the central nervous system (Figure 3.7).

   a. **Acetylcholine:** The autonomic nerve fibers can be classified into two groups based on the chemical nature of the neurotransmitter released. If transmission is mediated by acetylcholine, the neuron is termed cholinergic. Acetylcholine mediates the transmission of nerve impulses across autonomic ganglia in both the sympathetic and parasympathetic nervous systems (Figure 3.8). Transmission from the autonomic postganglionic nerves to the effector organs in the parasympathetic system also involves the release of acetylcholine. In the somatic nervous system, transmission at the neuromuscular junction (that is, between nerve fibers and voluntary muscles) is also cholinergic.

   b. **Norepinephrine and epinephrine:** If *norepinephrine* or *epinephrine* is the transmitter, the fiber is called adrenergic (*adrenaline* being another name for *epinephrine*). In the sympathetic system, *norepinephrine* mediates the transmission of nerve impulses from autonomic postganglionic nerves to effector organs. *Norepinephrine* and adrenergic receptors are discussed in Chapters 6 and 7. A summary of the neuromediators released and the type of receptors within the peripheral nervous system is shown in Figure 3.8. [Note: A few sympathetic fibers, such as those involved in sweating, are cholinergic; for simplicity, they are not shown on Figure 3.8.]

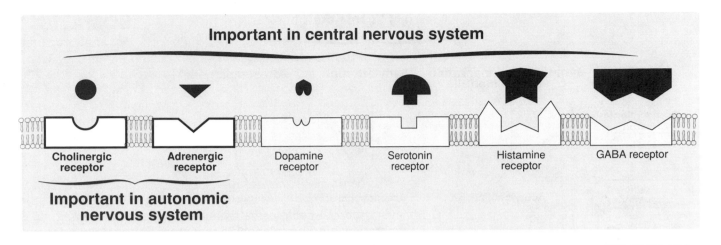

Figure 3.7
Schematic representation of several important neurotransmitters approaching their specific receptors.

4. **Intracellular response:** The binding of chemical signals to receptors causes proteins within the cell membrane to be activated, ultimately resulting in a cellular response such as the phosphorylation of intracellular proteins or changes in the conductivity of ion channels. The mechanism whereby neurotransmitter binding evokes a response is detailed in the following section.

IV. SECOND MESSENGER SYSTEMS

A neurotransmitter can be thought of as a signal, and a receptor as a signal detector and transducer. "Second messenger" molecules, produced in response to neurotransmitter binding to receptor, translate the extracellular signal into a response within the cell. Each component serves as a link in the communication between extracellular events and chemical changes within the cell.

A. Actions of membrane receptors

1. **Direct regulation of ionic permeability:** Neurotransmitter receptors are membrane proteins that provide a binding site that recognizes and responds to neurotransmitter molecules. Some receptors, such as the postsynaptic receptors of nerve or muscle, are directly linked to membrane ion channels; thus, binding of the neurotransmitter occurs rapidly (within fractions of a millisecond) and directly affects ion permeability (Figure 3.9A). The effect of neurotransmitters on these chemically gated ion channels is discussed on p.84 and 93.

2. **Regulation involving second messenger molecules:** Some receptors are not directly coupled to ion gates. Rather, the receptor signals its recognition of a bound neurotransmitter by initiating a series

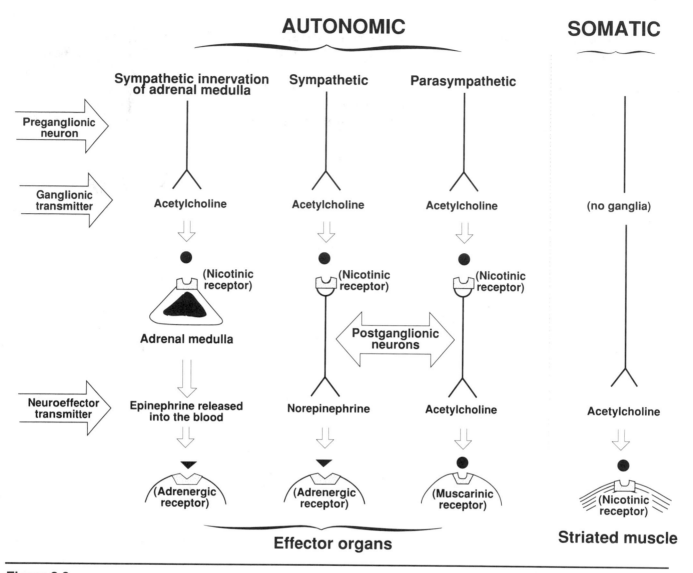

Figure 3.8
Summary of the neurotransmitters released and the types of receptors found within the autonomic and somatic nervous systems. [Note: This schematic diagram does not show that the parasympathetic ganglia are close to or on the surface of the effector organs and that the post ganglionic fibers are usually shorter than the preganglionic fibers.]

of reactions, which ultimately results in a specific intracellular response. "Second messenger" molecules—so named because they intervene between the original message (the neurotransmitter or hormone) and the ultimate effect on the cell—are part of the cascade of events that translates neurotransmitter binding into a cellular response. The two most widely recognized second messengers are the adenyl cyclase system and the calcium/polyphosphatidylinositol system.

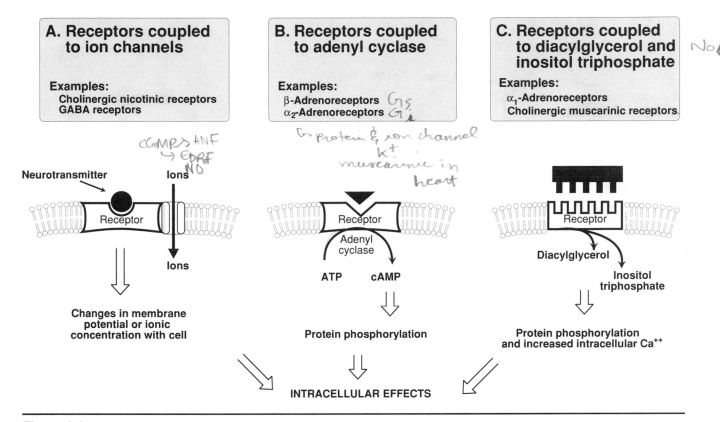

Figure 3.9
Three mechanisms whereby binding of a neurotransmitter leads to a cellular effect.

Study Questions   (see p.406 for answers).

Answer A if 1,2, and 3 are correct.
B if 1 and 3 are correct.
C if 2 and 4 are correct.
D if only 4 is correct.
E if 1,2,3 and 4 are all correct.

3.1 Which of the following statements concerning the autonomic nervous system is/are correct?

1. The autonomic nervous system is composed entirely of efferent neurons.
2. The sympathetic division is activated in response to stressful situations.
3. The parasympathetic division originates from cell bodies in the central nervous system.
4. The control of blood pressure is mainly a sympathetic activity, with essentially no participation by the parasympathetic system.

3.2 Which of the following statements concerning the parasympathetic nervous system is/are correct?

1. The actions of the parasympathetic division usually oppose the effects of the sympathetic division.
2. The parasympathetic system often discharges as a single, functional system.
3. The parasympathetic division is involved in accommodation of near vision, movement of food, and urination.
4. The postganglionic fibers of the parasympathetic division are long, compared to those of the sympathetic nervous system.

3.3 Which of the following compounds function(s) as second messengers?

    1. cAMP.
    2. Inositol 1,4,5-triphosphate.
    3. Diacylglycerol.
    4. GTP.

3.4 Which of the following is/are characteristic of parasympathetic stimulations?

    1. Increase in intestinal motility.
    2. Inhibition of bronchial secretion.
    3. Contraction of sphincter muscle in the iris of the eye (miosis).
    4. Contraction of sphincter of urinary bladder.

Choose the ONE best answer.

3.5 Administration of a drug that acts to dilate arterioles would cause which one of the following?

    A. Increased output from the parasympathetic neurons.
    B. Bradycardia (decreased heart rate).
    C. Increased contractility of the heart.
    D. No change in arterial blood pressure.
    E. Activation of the sympathetic and parasympathetic output to the heart.

Questions 3.6-3.7: For the following two questions use the diagram shown below, which represents the parasympathetic, sympathetic and somatic nervous systems.

3.6 Norepinephrine acts as a neurotransmitter at which of the following sites?

    A. Site A.
    B. Site B.
    C. Sites C and D.
    D. Site D.
    E. Sites D and E.

3.7 Acetylcholine acts as a neurotransmitter at which of the following sites?

    A. Site A only.
    B. Site B only.
    C. Sites C and D only.
    D. Sites D and B only.
    E. Sites A, C, D and E only.

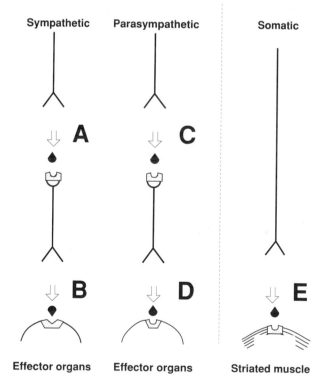

Sympathetic   **Parasympathetic**   **Somatic**

A   C

B   D   E

Effector organs   **Effector organs**   **Striated muscle**

Cholinergic Agonists

4

I. OVERVIEW

Drugs affecting the autonomic nervous system are divided into two subgroups according to the type of neuron involved in their mechanism of action. The cholinergic drugs, which are described in this and the following chapter, act on receptors that are activated by acetylcholine. The second group—the adrenergic drugs (discussed in Chapters 6 and 7)—act on receptors that are stimulated by *norepinephrine* or *epinephrine.* Both the cholinergic and adrenergic drugs act either by stimulating or blocking neurons of the autonomic nervous system. Figure 4.1 summarizes the cholinergic agonists discussed in this chapter.

II. THE CHOLINERGIC NEURON

The preganglionic fibers terminating in the adrenal medulla, the autonomic ganglia (both parasympathetic and sympathetic), and the postganglionic fibers of the parasympathetic division use acetylcholine as a neurotransmitter (Figure 4.2). Cholinergic neurons innervate voluntary muscles of the somatic system and are also found in the CNS.

A. Neurotransmission at cholinergic neurons

Neurotransmission in cholinergic neurons involves six steps. The first four, synthesis, storage, release and binding of the acetylcholine to a receptor, are followed by the fifth step, degradation of the neurotransmitter in the synaptic gap (that is, the space between the nerve endings and adjacent receptors located on nerves or effector organs), and the sixth step, the recycling of choline (Figure 4.3).

1. **Synthesis of acetylcholine:** Choline is transported from the extracellular fluid into the cytoplasm of the cholinergic neuron by a carrier system that cotransports sodium and is inhibited by the drug *hemicholinium.* Choline reacts enzymically with acetyl CoA to form acetylcholine.

2. **Storage of acetylcholine in vesicles:** Once synthesized, acetylcholine is transported into synaptic vesicles where it is stored in granules.

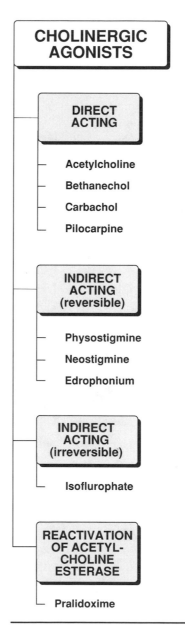

CHOLINERGIC AGONISTS

DIRECT ACTING
- Acetylcholine
- Bethanechol
- Carbachol
- Pilocarpine

INDIRECT ACTING (reversible)
- Physostigmine
- Neostigmine
- Edrophonium

INDIRECT ACTING (irreversible)
- Isoflurophate

REACTIVATION OF ACETYLCHOLINE ESTERASE
- Pralidoxime

Figure 4.1
Summary of cholinergic agonists.

3. **Release of acetylcholine:** When an action potential arrives at a nerve ending, voltage-sensitive calcium channels in the presynaptic membrane open, causing an increase in the concentration of intracellular calcium. Elevated calcium levels promote the fusion of synaptic vesicles with the cell membrane and release of acetylcholine into the synapse. This release is blocked by botulinum toxin. By contrast, black widow spider venom causes all of the cellular acetylcholine stored in synaptic vesicles to spill into the synaptic gap.

4. **Binding to receptor:** Acetylcholine released from the synaptic vesicles diffuses across the synaptic space and binds to either postsynaptic receptors on the target cell or to presynaptic receptors in the membrane of the neuron that released the acetylcholine (see p.58 for a discussion of the presynaptic receptor).

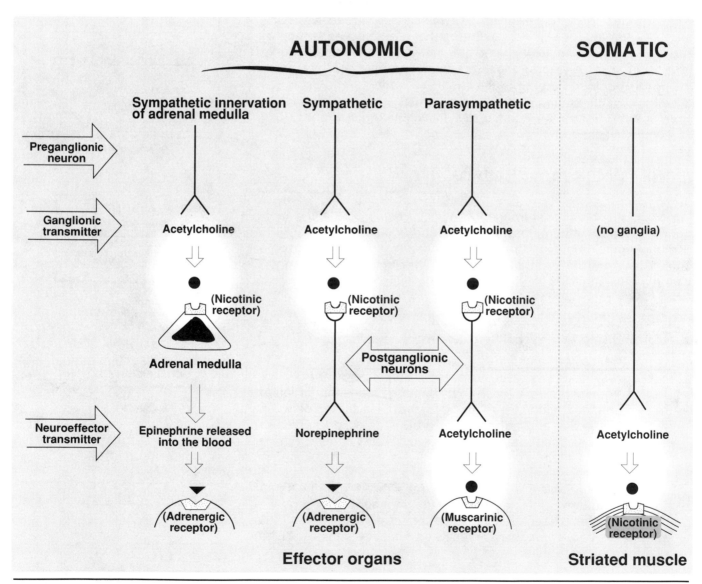

Figure 4.2
Sites of actions of cholinergic agonists in the autonomic and somatic nervous systems.

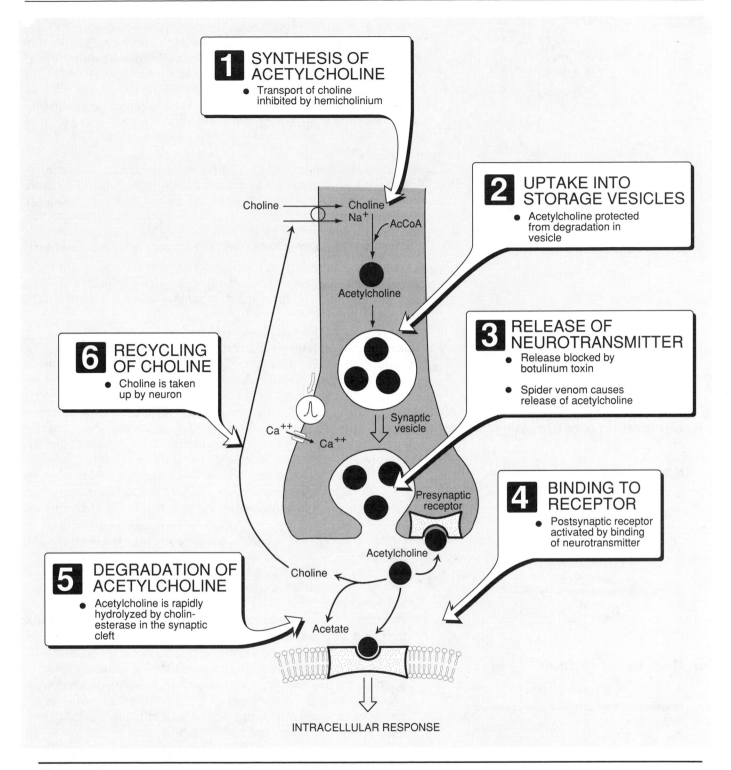

Figure 4.3
Synthesis and release of acetylcholine from the cholinergic neuron.

This leads to a biological response within the cell (nerve impulse initiation in postganglionic fiber or activation of specific enzymes in effector cells) as mediated by second messenger molecules, which were discussed in on p.32.

5. **Degradation of acetylcholine:** Acetylcholine is rapidly cleaved into choline and acetate by the enzyme acetylcholinesterase (Figure 4.3).

6. **Recycling of choline:** Choline may be recaptured by a high affinity transport system that pulls the molecule back into the neuron, where it is acetylated and stored until release by the subsequent action potential.

B. Cholinergic receptors (cholinoceptors)

Two families of cholinoceptors, designated muscarinic and nicotinic receptors, can be distinguished from each other on the basis of their different affinities for agents that mimic the action of acetylcholine (cholinomimetic agents).

1. **Muscarinic receptors:** These receptors, in addition to binding acetylcholine, also recognize muscarine, an alkaloid that is present in certain poisonous mushrooms. By contrast, the muscarinic receptors show only a weak affinity for nicotine (Figure 4.4). Muscarinic receptors are found mainly on the autonomic effector organs, that is, heart, smooth muscle, and exocrine glands (see Figure 4.2). Thus, drugs with muscarinic actions preferentially stimulate muscarinic receptors on these tissues, but at high concentration may show some activity at nicotinic receptors. Muscarinic receptors have recently been shown to consist of at least five different subtypes: M_1, M_2, M_3 M_4, and M_5.

   a. Although all five subtypes have been found on neurons, M_1 receptors are also found on gastric parietal cells; M_2 receptors, on cardiac cells and smooth muscle; and M_3 receptors, on exocrine glands and smooth muscle.

   b. Attempts are currently underway to develop muscarinic agonists and antagonists that are directed against specific receptor subtypes. For example, *pirenzepine,* a tricyclic anticholinergic drug, selectively inhibits M_1 muscarinic receptors, such as in the gastric mucosa. At therapeutic doses, *pirenzepine* does not cause many of the side effects seen with the non–subtype-specific drug *atropine.* Therefore, *pirenzepine* can be useful in the treatment of gastric and duodenal ulcers (see p.225).

2. **Nicotinic receptors:** These receptors, in addition to binding acetylcholine, also recognize nicotine but show only a weak affinity for muscarine (Figure 4.4). Nicotine initially stimulates and then blocks the receptor. Nicotinic receptors are located in the CNS, adrenal medulla, autonomic ganglia, and the neuromuscular junction (see Figure 4.2). Drugs with nicotinic action stimulate the nicotinic receptors located on these tissues. The nicotinic receptors of autonomic ganglia differ from those of the neuro-

A. Muscarinic receptors

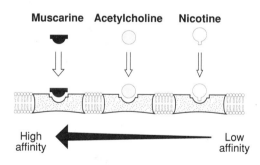

B. Nicotinic receptors

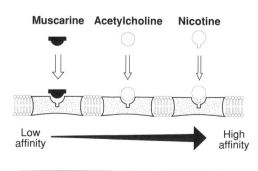

Figure 4.4
Types of cholinergic receptors.

muscular junction. For example, ganglionic receptors are selectively blocked by *hexamethonium,* whereas neuromuscular junction receptors are specifically blocked by *tubocurarine* (see p.49).

III. DIRECT-ACTING CHOLINERGIC AGONISTS

Cholinergic agonists mimic the effects of acetylcholine by binding directly to cholinoceptors. These agents are synthetic esters of choline, such as *carbachol* and *bethanechol,* or naturally occurring alkaloids, such as *pilocarpine* (see Figure 4.5). All of the direct-acting cholinergic drugs have longer durations of action than acetylcholine. Some of the more therapeutically useful drugs (*pilocarpine* and *bethanechol*) preferentially bind to muscarinic receptors and are sometimes referred to as muscarinic agents. [Note: Muscarinic receptors are located primarily, but not exclusively, at the neuroeffector junction of the parasympathetic nervous system.] However, as a group, the direct-acting agonists show little specificity in their actions, a fact which limits their clinical usefulness.

A. Acetylcholine

Acetylcholine [a se teel KOE leen], which is the neurotransmitter of parasympathetic and cholinergic nerves, is therapeutically of little importance, both because of its multiplicity of actions and its rapid inactivation by acetylcholinesterase. Acetylcholine has both muscarinic and nicotinic activity.

1. **Actions**

   a. **Decrease in heart rate and cardiac output:** The actions of acetylcholine on the heart mimic the effects of vagal stimulation. For example, acetylcholine, if injected intravenously, produces a brief decrease in cardiac rate and stroke volume as a result of a reduction in the rate of firing at the sinoatrial (SA) node. [Note: It should be remembered that normal vagal activity is regulated by the release of acetylcholine at the SA node.]

   b. **Decrease in blood pressure:** Injection of acetylcholine causes vasodilation and the lowering of blood pressure. Although no significant innervation of the vasculature by the parasympathetic system exists, there are cholinergic receptors on the blood vessels which respond by causing vasodilation. In the absence of administered drugs, these receptors have no known function, since acetylcholine is never released into the vasculature in any significant quantities. *Atropine* blocks these muscarinic receptors and prevents acetylcholine from producing vasodilation.

   c. **Other actions:** Acetylcholine stimulates the gut to increase motility and stimulates increased secretions there and in the bronchioles. It also stimulates secretions from salivary glands and increases motility of smooth muscle in the genitourinary tract. In the eye, acetylcholine is involved in stimulating ciliary

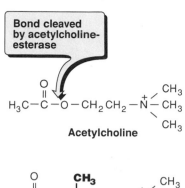

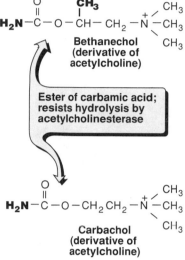

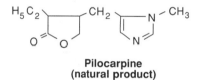

Figure 4.5
Comparisons of the structures of some cholinergic agonists.

muscle contraction for near vision and constriction of the pupillae sphincter muscle, causing miosis (marked constriction of the pupil).

2. **Therapeutic uses:** There are no therapeutic uses.

B. Bethanechol

Bethanechol [be THAN e kole] is a carbamic ester and, hence, is not rapidly hydrolyzed by acetylcholinesterase, although it is hydrolyzed by other esterases. It has little or no nicotinic actions but does have strong muscarinic activity. Its major actions are on the smooth musculature of the bladder and GI tract. It has a duration of action of about 1 hour.

1. **Actions:** *Bethanechol* directly stimulates muscarinic receptors, causing increased intestinal motility and tone, and it also stimulates the detrusor muscles of the bladder, causing expulsion of urine.

2. **Therapeutic applications:** In urological treatment, *bethanechol* is often used to stimulate the atonic bladder, particularly in postpartum or postoperative urinary retention.

3. **Adverse effects:** *Bethanechol* causes the actions of generalized cholinergic stimulation, including sweating, salivation, flushing, decreased blood pressure, nausea, abdominal pain, diarrhea, and bronchospasm.

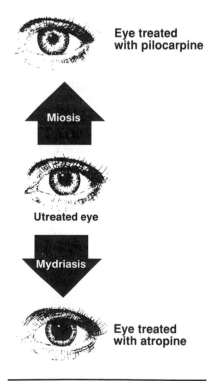

Eye treated with pilocarpine

Miosis

Utreated eye

Mydriasis

Eye treated with atropine

Figure 4.6
Actions of pilocarpine and atropine on the iris and ciliary muscle of the eye.

C. Carbachol (Carbamylcholine)

Carbachol [KAR ba kole] has both muscarinic as well as nicotinic actions. Since it is an ester of carbamic acid (like *bethanechol*) rather than acetic acid, *carbachol* is a poor substrate for acetylcholinesterase and therefore is not readily hydrolyzed. It is biotransformed by other esterases but at a much slower rate. A single administration can last as long as one hour.

1. **Actions:** *Carbachol* has profound effects on both the cardiovascular system and the gastrointestinal system because of its ganglion-stimulating activity and may first stimulate and then depress these systems. It can cause release of *epinephrine* from the adrenal medulla by its nicotinic action.

2. **Therapeutic uses:** Because of its high potency and relatively long duration of action, *carbachol* is rarely used therapeutically, except in the eye as a miotic agent, to cause contraction of the pupil.

3. **Adverse effects:** The adverse effects are similar to those of *bethanechol.*

D. Pilocarpine

The alkaloid *pilocarpine* [pye loe KAR peen] is a useful cholinergic agonist. Compared with acetylcholine and its derivatives, it is far less potent. It is unaffected by acetylcholinesterase. *Pilocarpine* exhibits mainly muscarinic activity.

1. **Actions:** Applied topically to the cornea, *pilocarpine* produces a rapid miosis and contraction of the ciliary muscle. The eye undergoes a spasm of accommodation, and vision is fixed at some particular distance, making it impossible to focus (Figure 4.6). Note the opposing effects of *atropine,* a muscarinic blocker, on the eye (see p. 45).

2. **Therapeutic use in glaucoma:** *Pilocarpine* is extremely effective in opening the trabecular meshwork around Schlemm's canal, causing an immediate drop in intraocular pressure as a result of the escape of aqueous humor. *Pilocarpine* is the drug of choice in the acute lowering of intraocular pressure of both narrow-angle (also called closed-angle) and open-angle (also called wide-angle) glaucoma. This action lasts a few hours and can be repeated. Cholinesterase inhibitors, such as *isoflurophate,* have longer durations of action. [Note: Carbonic anhydrase inhibitors, such as *acetazolamide* (see p.215), *epinephrine* (p.62), and the β adrenergeric blocker, *timolol* (see p.76), are also used in treating glaucoma but are not used for the emergency lowering of intraocular pressure.]

3. **Adverse effects:** *Pilocarpine* can enter the brain and cause CNS disturbances. It stimulates sweat secretion.

IV. ANTICHOLINESTERASES (REVERSIBLE)

These compounds indirectly provide a cholinergic action by binding to acetylcholinesterase and thereby reversibly inhibiting the hydrolysis of acetylcholine produced endogenously at the cholinergic nerve endings. This results in the accumulation of acetylcholine in the synaptic space (Figure 4.7). These drugs thus provoke a response at all cholinoceptors in the body, including both muscarinic and nicotinic receptors of the autonomic nervous system as well as the neuromuscular junction and the brain.

A. Physostigmine

Physostigmine [fi zoe STIG meen] is an alkaloid (i.e., a nitrogenous compound found in plants) that reversibly inactivates acetylcholinesterase. The result is potentiation of cholinergic activity throughout the body.

1. **Actions:** *Physostigmine* stimulates not only muscarinic and nicotinic sites of the autonomic nervous system but also the nicotinic receptors of the neuromuscular junction. *Physostigmine* can enter the CNS.

2. **Therapeutic uses:**

   a. The drug increases intestinal and bladder motility, which serve as its therapeutic action in atony of either organ.

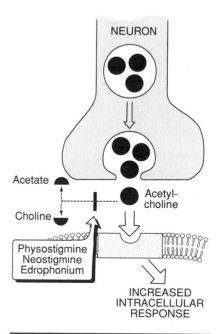

Figure 4.7
Mechanisms of action of indirect (reversible) cholinergic agonists.

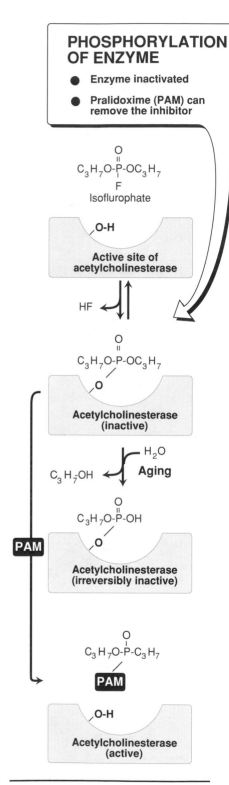

PHOSPHORYLATION OF ENZYME

- Enzyme inactivated
- Pralidoxime (PAM) can remove the inhibitor

$$C_3H_7O\text{-}\overset{\overset{O}{\|}}{\underset{\underset{F}{|}}{P}}\text{-}OC_3H_7$$

Isoflurophate

O-H

Active site of acetylcholinesterase

HF

$$C_3H_7O\text{-}\overset{\overset{O}{\|}}{P}\text{-}OC_3H_7$$

O

Acetylcholinesterase (inactive)

H_2O

C_3H_7OH **Aging**

$$C_3H_7O\text{-}\overset{\overset{O}{\|}}{P}\text{-}OH$$

O

PAM

Acetylcholinesterase (irreversibly inactive)

$$C_3H_7O\text{-}\overset{\overset{O}{\|}}{P}\text{-}C_3H_7$$

PAM

O-H

Acetylcholinesterase (active)

Figure 4.8
Covalent modification of acetylcholinesterase by isoflurophate.

b. Placed topically in the eye, it produces miosis and spasm of accommodation and a lowering of intraocular pressure. It is used to treat glaucoma, but *pilocarpine* is more effective.

c. *Physostigmine* is also used in the treatment of overdoses of *atropine, phenothiazines,* and tricyclic antidepressants.

3. **Adverse effects:**

a. The effects of *physostigmine* on the central nervous system may lead to convulsions when high doses are used. The inhibition of acetylcholinesterase at the skeletal neuromuscular junction causes the accumulation of acetylcholine and ultimately results in paralysis of skeletal muscle.

b. In general, when the drug is used therapeutically to stimulate parasympathetic muscarinic sites, such low doses are used that they cause little change in skeletal muscle or CNS function.

B. Neostigmine

Neostigmine [nee oh STIG meen] is a synthetic compound that reversibly inhibits acetylcholinesterase. However, it differs from *physostigmine* in being more polar and therefore does not enter the CNS. It has a greater effect than that of *physostigmine* on skeletal muscle and can stimulate contractility before it paralyzes. *Neostigmine* has a long duration of action, usually 2-4 hours. *Neostigmine* is used to stimulate the bladder and GI tract. *Neostigmine* is also used as an antidote for *tubocurarine* and other competitive neuromuscular blocking agents (see p.49). *Neostigmine* has found use in symptomatic treatment of myasthenia gravis, an autoimmune disease caused by antibodies that damage the acetylcholine receptors of neuromuscular junctions. Adverse effects include actions of generalized cholinergic stimulation, such as salivation, flushing, decreased blood pressure, nausea, abdominal pain, diarrhea, and bronchospasm.

C. Edrophonium

The actions of *edrophonium* [ed roe FOE nee um] are similar to *neostigmine,* except that it is more rapidly absorbed and has a shorter duration of action (10-20 minutes). *Edrophonium* is useful in the diagnosis of myasthenia gravis. Intravenous injection of *edrophonium* leads to a rapid increase in muscle strength.

V. ANTICHOLINESTERASES (IRREVERSIBLE)

A number of synthetic compounds have the capacity to covalently bind to acetylcholinesterase. The result is a long lasting increase in acetylcholine at all sites where it is released. Many of these drugs are extremely toxic and have been called nerve gases. Related compounds such as parathion are employed as insecticides.

A. Isoflurophate

1. **Mechanism of action:** *Isoflurophate* [eye soe FLURE oh fate] (di-isopropylfluorophosphate, DFP) is an organic phosphate that covalently binds to acetylcholinesterase (Figure 4.8). Once this occurs, the enzyme is permanently inactivated, and restoration of acetylcholinesterase activity requires the synthesis of new enzyme molecules. Following covalent modification of acetyl-cholinesterase, the phosphorylated enzyme slowly releases one of its isopropyl groups (Figure 4.8). This loss of an alkyl group, which is called aging, makes it impossible for chemical reactivators, such as *pralidoxime* (see later), to break the bond between the remaining drug and the enzyme. Newer nerve gases that are stored by the military, age in minutes or seconds. DFP ages in 6-8 hours.

2. **Actions:** Actions include generalized cholinergic stimulation, paralysis of motor function (causing breathing difficulties), and convulsions.

3. **Therapeutic uses:** Very weak solutions of the drug are used topically in the eye for the chronic treatment of glaucoma. The effects may last for up to one week after a single administration. *Atropine* in high dosage can reverse many of the central effects of *isoflurophate.*

4. **Reactivation of acetylcholinesterase:** *Pralidoxime* (PAM) is a synthetic compound that can reactivate inhibited acetylcholinesterase. It was designed to bind tenaciously with the acetylcholinesterase inhibitor and to pull it off the inhibited enzyme. If given soon enough, before aging of the alkylated enzyme occurs, it can reverse the effects of *isoflurophate.* With the newer nerve gases, which produce aging of the enzyme complex within seconds, *pralidoxime* is less effective.

Figure 4.9 summarizes some of the adverse effects of the cholinergic agonists. Figure 4.10 shows the therapeutic uses of these agents.

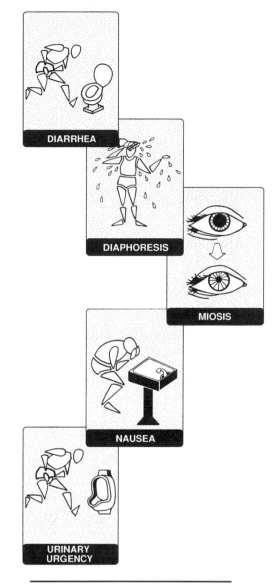

Figure 4.9
Some adverse effects observed with cholinergic drugs.

Study Questions   (see p.407 for answers).

Answer A if 1,2 and 3 are correct.
    B if 1 and 3 are correct.
    C if 2 and 4 are correct.
    D if only 4 is correct.
    E if 1,2,3 and 4 are all correct.

4.1 Which of the following is/are expected symptoms of poisoning with isoflurophate?

    1. Paralysis of skeletal muscle.
    2. Increased bronchial secretions.
    3. Miosis.
    4. Tachycardia.

4.2 Which of the following correctly match a cholinergic agonist with its pharmacological actions?

    1. Bethanechol: Stimulates atonic bladder.
    2. Carbachol: Induces release of epinephrine from the adrenal medulla.
    3. Acetylcholine: Decreases heart rate and cardiac output.
    4. Pilocarpine: Reduces intraocular pressure.

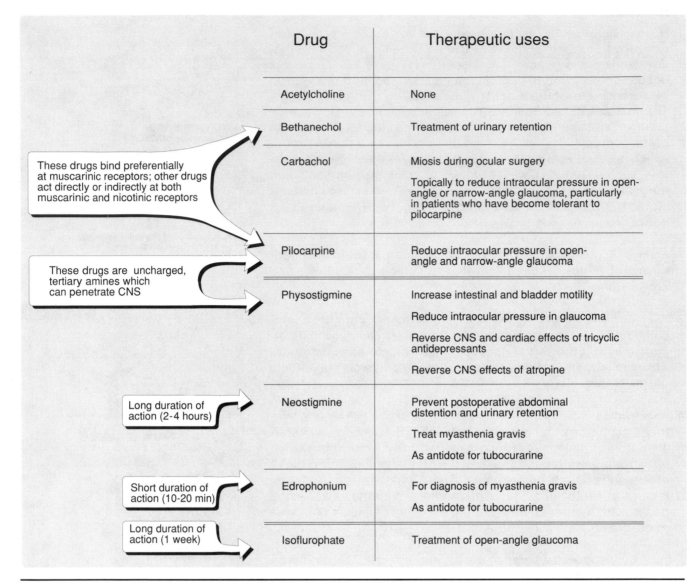

Figure 4.10
Summary of actions of cholinergic agonists.

4.3 Pilocarpine:

1. is used to lower intraocular pressure in glaucoma.
2. selectively binds to nicotine receptors.
3. is not cleaved by acetylcholinesterase.
4. causes profuse sweating.

4.4 Physostigmine:

1. acts at peripheral muscarinic and nicotinic receptors.
2. produces CNS effects.
3. can be used to treat an overdose of atropine.
4. is hydrolyzed by acetylcholinesterase.

4.5 An overdose of neostigmine:

1. may result in bowel hypermotility, salivation, and sweating.
2. has a shorter duration of action than edrophonium.
3. increases the acetylcholine concentration at the neuromuscular junction.
4. is contraindicated in glaucoma.

Cholinergic Antagonists

5

I. OVERVIEW

The cholinergic antagonists (also called cholinergic blockers or anti-cholinergic drugs) bind to cholinoceptors but do not trigger the usual receptor-mediated intracellular effects. The most useful of these agents selectively block the muscarinic synapses of the parasympathetic nerves. The effects of parasympathetic innervation are thus blocked, and the actions of sympathetic stimulation are left unopposed. A second group of drugs, the ganglionic blockers, show a preference for the nicotinic receptors of the sympathetic and parasympathetic ganglia. A third family of compounds, the neuromuscular blocking agents, interfere with transmission of efferent impulses to skeletal muscles. Figure 5.1 summarizes the cholinergic antagonists discussed in this chapter.

II. ANTIMUSCARINIC AGENTS

These compounds block muscarinic receptors (Figure 5.2) causing inhibition of all parasympathetic functions. In addition, these drugs block the few exceptional sympathetic neurons that are cholinergic, such as those innervating sweat glands. In contrast to the cholinergic agonists, which have limited usefulness therapeutically, the cholinergic blockers are beneficial in a variety of clinical situations. Because they do not block nicotinic receptors, the antimuscarinic drugs have little or no action at skeletal neuromuscular junctions or autonomic ganglia.

A. Atropine

Atropine [A troh peen], a belladonna alkaloid, does not resemble acetylcholine chemically, yet it has a high affinity for muscarinic receptors, where it binds competitively (Figure 5.3). *Atropine* is both a central and peripheral muscarinic blocker. Its general actions last about 4 hours except when placed topically in the eye, where the action may last for days.

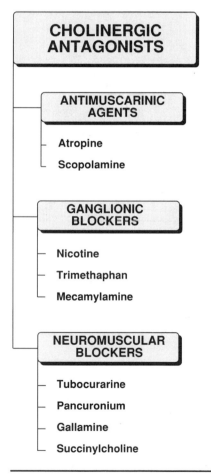

Figure 5.1
Summary of cholinergic antagonists.

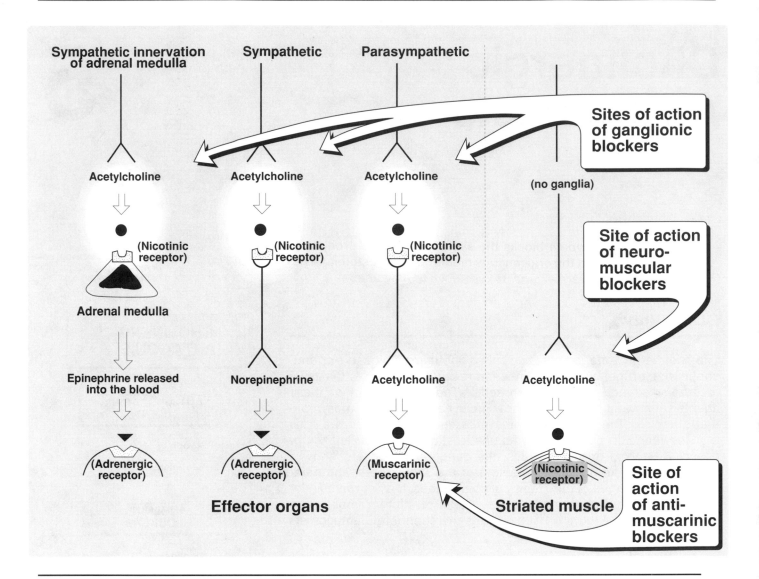

Figure 5.2
Sites of actions of cholinergic antagonists.

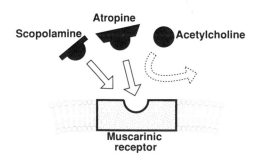

Figure 5.3
Competition of atropine and scopolamine with acetylcholine for the muscarinic receptor.

1. **Actions:**

   a. **Eye:** *Atropine* blocks all cholinergic activity on the eye, resulting in mydriasis (dilation of the pupil) and cycloplegia (inability to focus for near vision).

   b. **Gastrointestinal (GI):** *Atropine* is often used as an antispasmodic to reduce activity of the GI tract. *Atropine* and *scopolamine* (which is discussed in the next section) are probably the most potent drugs available that produce this effect. Although gastric motility is reduced, hydrochloric acid production is not significantly reduced. Thus, the drug is not very effective in promoting healing of a peptic ulcer. However, *pirenzepine* (p.38), an M₁-muscarinic antagonist, is effective in reducing gastric acid secretion.

c. **Urinary system:** *Atropine* is also employed to reduce hypermotility states of the urinary bladder. It is still occasionally used in enuresis (involuntary voiding of urine) among children but α-adrenergic agonists may be more effective.

d. **Cardiovascular:** *Atropine* produces divergent effects on the cardiovascular system, depending on the dose (Figure 5.4). In doses lower than approximately 0.5 mg the predominant effect is a decreased cardiac rate. This is due to central activation of vagal efferent outflow. With higher doses of *atropine,* the cardiac muscarinic receptor is blocked, and the cardiac rate increases. This generally requires at least 1 mg of *atropine,* which is a higher dose than ordinarily given.

e. **Secretions:** *Atropine* blocks the salivary glands to produce a drying effect on the oral mucous membrane (xerostomia). The salivary glands are exquisitely sensitive to *atropine.*

2. **Therapeutic uses:**

a. In the eye, *atropine* exerts a cycloplegic effect and permits the measurement of refractive errors without interference by the accommodative capacity of the lens. Individuals 40 years of age and older have decreased ability to accommodate, and drugs are not necessary for an accurate refraction. Moreover, *atropine* may induce a glaucoma attack in susceptible individuals.

b. *Atropine* is used as an antispasmodic agent to relax the gastrointestinal tract and bladder.

c. *Atropine* is used for the treatment of overdoses of organophosphate (contained in certain insecticides) and some types of mushroom poisoning (mushrooms contain cholinergic substances). *Atropine* blocks the effects of excess acetylcholine that results from inhibition of acetylcholinesterase by drugs such as *physostigmine* (p.41).

d. The drug is also used as an antisecretory agent to block secretions in the upper and lower respiratory tracts prior to surgery.

3. **Pharmacology:** *Atropine* has a half-life of about 2 hours and is eliminated primarily in the urine.

4. **Adverse effects:**

a. *Atropine* may cause dry mouth, blurring of vision, tachycardia, and constipation. Effects on the CNS include restlessness, confusion, hallucinations, and delirium.

b. In older individuals, the use of *atropine* to induce mydriasis and cycloplegia is considered too risky since it may induce an attack of glaucoma in someone with a latent condition. [Note: *Atropine* is found in a large number of over-the-counter products that contain more than one ingredient.]

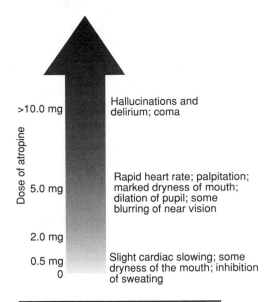

Figure 5.4
Dose-dependent effects of atropine.

Dose of atropine

>10.0 mg — Hallucinations and delirium; coma

5.0 mg — Rapid heart rate; palpitation; marked dryness of mouth; dilation of pupil; some blurring of near vision

2.0 mg

0.5 mg — Slight cardiac slowing; some dryness of the mouth; inhibition
0 — of sweating

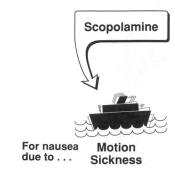

For nausea   Motion
due to . . .   Sickness

Figure 5.5
Scopolamine is an effective anti-motion sickness agent.

B. Scopolamine

Scopolamine [skoe POL a meen], another belladonna alkaloid, produces peripheral effects similar to those of *atropine*. However, *scopolamine* has greater action on the CNS and a longer duration of action in comparison to those of *atropine*. It has some special actions indicated below.

1. **Actions:**

   a. *Scopolamine,* is one of the most effective anti-motion sickness drugs available (Figure 5.5). It is often administered via a transdermal patch placed behind the ear.

   b. *Scopolamine* has the unusual effect of blocking short-term memory. The mechanism is totally unknown.

   c. *Scopolamine* also produces sedation in contrast to *atropine*.

2. **Therapeutic uses:** Its therapeutic uses are similar to those of *atropine*.

   a. *Scopolamine* is particularly effective in the prevention of motion sickness. As with all such drugs used for this condition, it is much more effective prophylactically than for treating the condition after it occurs.

   b. The amnesic action of *scopolamine* is often made use of in anesthetic procedures, particularly during childbirth.

3. **Pharmacology and adverse effects:** These aspects are similar to those of *atropine*.

III. GANGLIONIC BLOCKERS

Ganglionic blockers act at the nicotinic receptors in the autonomic ganglia (see Figure 5.2). These drugs are not effective as neuromuscular antagonists (p.49). No ganglionic blocker is currently available that selectively blocks only parasympathetic or sympathetic ganglia. Thus, these drugs block the entire output of the autonomic nervous system at the nicotinic receptor. The effects observed are complex and widespread, making it impossible to achieve selective actions. Therefore, ganglionic blockade is rarely used therapeutically today.

A. Nicotine

Nicotine depolarizes ganglia, resulting first in stimulation of and followed by paralysis of all ganglia. The effects are complex, including an increase in blood pressure and cardiac rate, and increased peristalsis and secretions. At higher doses, the blood pressure falls because of ganglionic blockade, and activity both in the GI tract and bladder musculature ceases. See p.102 for a full discussion of *nicotine*.

B. Trimethaphan

Trimethaphan [trye METH a fan] is a short-acting, competitive nicotinic ganglionic blocker that must be given by intravenous infusion. A single injection lasts no longer than 1-2 minutes. Today, the drug is used for the emergency lowering of blood pressure, for example, in hypertension caused by pulmonary edema. When it is given by continuous intravenous infusion, it lowers blood pressure instantly. The blood pressure level can be controlled by the infusion rate.

C. Mecamylamine

Mecamylamine [mek a MILL a meen] produces a competitive nicotinic block of the ganglia. The duration of action is about 10 hours after a single administration. The uptake of the drug via oral absorption is good in contrast to *trimethaphan.*

IV. NEUROMUSCULAR BLOCKING DRUGS

The previous sections of this chapter have described drugs that interfere with cholinergic transmission in the autonomic nervous system; thus, these drugs affect neurotransmission at either the ganglia or the effector organs. This section presents drugs that block cholinergic transmission between motor nerve endings and the nicotinic receptors on the neuromuscular end-plate of skeletal muscle (see Figure 5.2). These neuromuscular blockers are structural analogs of acetylcholine and act either as antagonists (nondepolarizing type) or agonists (depolarizing type) at the receptors on the end-plate of skeletal muscle. The neuromuscular blockers are clinically useful during surgery to produce complete muscle relaxation, without the depressant effects of deep anesthesia. A second group of muscle relaxants, the central muscle relaxants, are used to control spastic muscle tone. These drugs include *diazepam* (p.93), *dantrolene* (which acts directly on muscles by interfering with the release of calcium from the sarcoplasmic reticulum), and *baclofen* (which probably acts at GABA receptors in the central nervous system).

A. Nondepolarizing (competitive) blockers

The first drug that was found capable of blocking the skeletal neuromuscular junction was curare, which was used by the natives of the Amazon in South America to paralyze game during hunting expeditions. The drug *tubocurarine* [too boe kyoo AR een] was ultimately purified and introduced into clinical practice in the early 1940s. *Tubocurarine* and its synthetic derivatives have significantly increased the safety of anesthesia, since less anesthetic is required to produce muscle relaxation.

1. Mechanism of action

   a. At low doses, nondepolarizing neuromuscular blocking drugs, such as *tubocurarine, gallamine* [GAL a meen], and *pancu-*

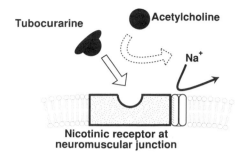

Figure 5.6
Mechanism of action of
competitive neuromuscular
blocking drugs.

ronium [pan kyoo ROE nee um] combine with the nicotinic receptor and prevent the binding of acetylcholine (Figure 5.6). These drugs thus prevent depolarization of the muscle cell membrane and inhibit muscle contraction. Because these agents compete with acetylcholine at the receptor, they are called competitive blockers. Their action can be overcome by increasing the concentration of acetylcholine in the synaptic gap, for example, by administration of cholinesterase inhibitors such as *neostigmine* or *edrophonium* (p.42).

b. At high doses, the nondepolarizing blockers block the ion channels of the end-plate. This leads to further weakening of neuromuscular transmission and reduces the ability of acetylcholinesterase inhibitors to reverse the actions of nondepolarizing muscle relaxants.

2. **Actions**

   a. **Tubocurarine**

      1) **Paralysis:** Not all muscles are equally sensitive to blockade by competitive blockers. Small, rapidly contracting muscles of the face and eye are most susceptible and are paralyzed first, followed by the fingers. Thereafter the limbs, neck, and trunk muscles are paralyzed. Then the intercostal muscles are affected, and lastly, the diaphragm muscles are paralyzed. Neuromuscular blockade by *tubocurarine* lasts from 20 minutes to as long as 1-2 hours after a single administration, depending on the dosage.

      2) **Other effects:** *Tubocurarine* can produce a small degree of ganglionic blockade by blocking nicotinic receptors at autonomic ganglia. The adrenal medulla may also be blocked. *Tubocurarine* causes a fall in blood pressure by releasing histamine from mast cells. Histamine release may be in sufficient amount to produce bronchospasm and skin wheals.

   b. **Pancuronium**: This drug has a mechanism of action similar to that of *tubocurarine* but does not release histamine; therefore, it has little ability to lower blood pressure. Its duration of action is similar to *tubocurarine* but *pancuronium* is five times more potent and has largely replaced *tubocurarine.*

   c. **Gallamine**: This drug does not cause histamine release or decrease blood pressure. Its duration of action is similar to *tubocurarine. Gallamine* blocks the cardiac vagus at the muscarinic site causing sinus tachycardia.

3. **Therapeutic uses:** These blockers are used therapeutically as adjuvant drugs in surgical anesthesia.

4. **Pharmacology:** All neuromuscular blocking agents have to be given parenterally by injection, since their uptake via oral absorption is very poor. They penetrate membranes very poorly and do not enter cells or pass across the blood-brain barrier. Many of the drugs are not metabolized and are excreted in the urine

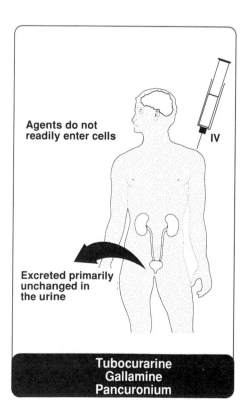

Agents do not
readily enter cells

IV

Excreted primarily
unchanged in
the urine

Tubocurarine
Gallamine
Pancuronium

unchanged. Most of the nondepolarizing drugs have a relatively long duration of action, ranging from 30 minutes to 1-2 hours.

5. **Adverse effects:** *Tubocurarine* may cause bronchospasm and skin wheals because of the release of histamine.

6. **Drug Interactions**

   a. Anticholinesterases, like *neostigmine, physostigmine,* and *edrophonium* can overcome the action of nondepolarizing neuromuscular blockers, but with increased dosage, they can cause a depolarizing block as a result of enhanced acetylcholine concentrations.

   b. Halogenated hydrocarbon anesthetics like *halothane* act to enhance neuromuscular blockade by exerting a stabilizing action at the neuromuscular junction.

   c. Aminoglycoside antibiotics like *streptomycin* inhibit acetylcholine release from cholinergic nerves by competing with calcium ion. They synergize with *tubocurarine* and other competitive blockers, enhancing the block.

   d. Calcium channel blockers increase the neuromuscular block of *tubocurarine* and other competitive blockers as well as depolarizing blockers.

B. Depolarizing agents

1. **Mechanism of action:** Depolarizing neuromuscular blocking drugs, such as *succinylcholine* [suk sin ill KOE leen], attach to the nicotinic receptor and act like acetylcholine to depolarize the junction (Figure 5.7). Unlike acetylcholine, which is instantly destroyed by acetylcholinesterase, the depolarizing agents persist at high concentrations in the synaptic cleft. They remain attached to the receptor for a relatively longer time, providing a constant stimulation of the receptor. The depolarizing agents first cause the sodium channel associated with the nicotinic receptors to open, which results in depolarization of the receptor (Phase I). This causes a transient twitching of the muscle (fasciculations). The continued binding of the depolarizing agent renders the receptor incapable of transmitting further impulses. With time, the continuous depolarization gives way to gradual repolarization as the sodium channel closes or is blocked. This causes a resistance to depolarization (Phase II) and a flaccid paralysis.

2. **Actions:** These drugs cause muscular fasciculations that last a few minutes. The sequence of paralysis may be slightly different, but as with the competitive blockers, the respiratory muscles are paralyzed last. *Succinylcholine* initially produces muscle fasciculations, followed within a few minutes by paralysis. The drug does not produce ganglionic block, except in high doses; although it does have weak histamine-releasing action. Duration of action of *succinylcholine* is extremely short, since this drug is rapidly broken down by plasma cholinesterase.

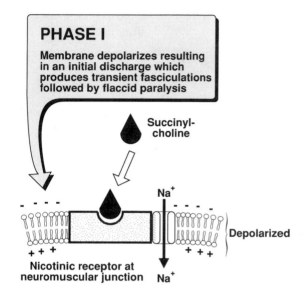

PHASE I

Membrane depolarizes resulting in an initial discharge which produces transient fasciculations followed by flaccid paralysis

Succinylcholine

Na⁺

Depolarized

Nicotinic receptor at neuromuscular junction   Na⁺

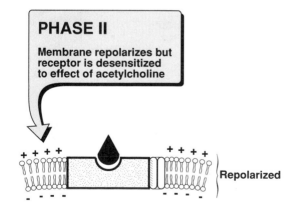

PHASE II

Membrane repolarizes but receptor is desensitized to effect of acetylcholine

Repolarized

Figure 5.7
Mechanism of action of depolarizing neuromuscular blocking drugs.

Drug	Therapeutic uses
Atropine	In ophthalmology to produce mydriasis and cycloplegia prior to refraction
	To treat spastic disorders of GI and lower urinary tract
	To treat organophosphate poisoning
	To supress respiratory secretions prior to surgery
Scopolamine	In obstetrics with morphine to produce amnesia and sedation
	To prevent motion sickness
Nicotine	None
Trimethaphan	Short-term treatment of hypertension
Mecamylamine	Treatment of moderately severe to severe hypertension
Tubocurarine Pancuronium Gallamine	As skeletal muscle relaxant in general anesthesia
	To facilitate mechanical ventilation
Succinylcholine	As skeletal muscle relaxant in general anesthesia
	To facilitate intubation

Contraindicated in narrow-angle glaucoma

Adverse effects commonly observed with cholinergic antagonists

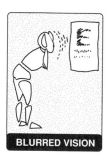 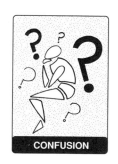 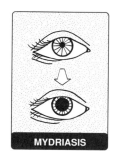 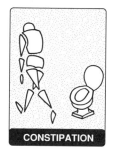 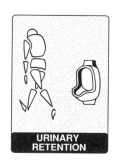

BLURRED VISION **CONFUSION** **MYDRIASIS** **CONSTIPATION** **URINARY RETENTION**

Figure 5.8
Summary of cholinergic antagonists.

3. **Therapeutic uses:** Because of its rapid onset and short duration of action, *succinylcholine* is useful when rapid endotracheal intubation is required.

4. **Pharmacology:** *Succinylcholine* is rapidly hydrolyzed by plasma cholinesterase and is only effective for several minutes. It is therefore usually given by continuous infusion.

5. **Adverse effects:** *Succinylcholine* has more side effects than the nonpolarizing blockers, but it has the advantage of short duration of action and rapid onset. When *halothane* is used as an anesthetic, administration of *succinylcholine* has occasionally caused malignant hyperthermia in genetically susceptible people (with muscular rigidity and hyperpyrexia). This is treated by rapid cooling and by administration of *dantrolene* which blocks release of Ca^{++} from the sarcoplasmic reticulum of muscle cells. *Dantrolene* reduces heat production and muscle tone.

Important characteristics of the muscarinic antagonists are summarized in Figure 5.8.

Study Questions   (see p.408 for answers).

Answer A if 1,2 and 3 are correct.
   B if 1 and 3 are correct.
   C if 2 and 4 are correct.
   D if only 4 is correct.
   E if 1,2,3 and 4 are all correct.

5.1 Which of the following correctly describe(s) the pharmacological actions of atropine?

   1. Acts at peripheral and central muscarinic cholinergic receptors.
   2. Acts to decrease the motility of gut.
   3. Useful in treating poisoning by organophosphate insecticides.
   4. Shows less CNS depressant action than scopolamine.

5.2 Which of the following are useful in treating poisoning with an organophosphate poison, such as parathion?

   1. Atropine and pralidoxime, when administered within hours of exposure to poison.
   2. Neostigmine.
   3. Scopolamine.
   4. Carbachol.

5.3 Which of the following are correctly paired?

   1. Succinylcholine: Depolarizes neuromuscular end-plate.
   2. Neostigmine: Reverses the effects of nondepolarizing blockers, such as tubocurarine.
   3. Tubocurarine: May cause the release of histamine.
   4. Gallamine: Acts only at neuromuscular junction.

Choose the ONE best answer.

5.4 Which ONE of the following drugs most closely resembles atropine in its pharmacological actions?

   A. Scopolamine.
   B. Trimethaphan.
   C. Physostigmine.
   D. Acetylcholine.
   E. Carbachol.

5.5 Which one of the following drugs does NOT produce miosis (marked constriction of the pupil)?

   A. Carbachol.
   B. Isoflurophate.
   C. Atropine.
   D. Pilocarpine.
   E. Neostigmine.

5.6 Which one of the following drugs would be useful in the long-term treatment of myasthenia gravis?

   A. Edrophonium.
   B. Atropine.
   C. Neostigmine.
   D. Scopolamine.
   E. Bethanechol.

Adrenergic Agonists

6

I. OVERVIEW

The adrenergic drugs affect receptors that are stimulated by *norepinephrine* or *epinephrine*. Some adrenergic drugs act directly on the adrenergic receptor (adrenoceptor) either by activating the receptor or by blocking the action of *norepinephrine* and *epinephrine*. Other drugs of this group act by altering the release of *norepinephrine* by the adrenergic neuron. This chapter describes drugs that either directly or indirectly stimulate the adrenoceptor (Figure 6.1).

II. THE ADRENERGIC NEURON

The adrenergic neuron releases *norepinephrine* as a neurotransmitter. These neurons are found in the central nervous system (CNS) and are also part of the sympathetic nervous system where they serve as links between preganglionic neurons and the effector organs. The adrenergic neuron and the receptor located on the effector organ are the sites of action of the adrenergic drugs (Figure 6.2).

A. Neurotransmission at adrenergic neurons

Neurotransmission in adrenergic neurons closely resembles that already described for the cholinergic neurons (p.35), except that *norepinephrine* is the neurotransmitter instead of acetylcholine. Neurotransmission involves five steps: the synthesis, storage, release, and receptor binding of the *norepinephrine,* followed by removal of the neurotransmitter from the synaptic gap (Figure 6.3).

1. **Synthesis of norepinephrine:** Tyrosine is transported into the cytoplasm of the adrenergic neuron, where the amino acid is hydroxylated to Dopa by tyrosine hydroxylase. This is the rate-limiting step in the formation of *norepinephrine.* Dopa is decarboxylated to form *dopamine*[1].

2. **Storage of norepinephrine in vesicles:** Once synthesized, *dopamine* is transported into synaptic vesicles using an amine transporter system that is also involved in the re-uptake of preformed *norepinephrine* (see section II.A.5, later). This carrier system is blocked by *reserpine* (see p.79). *Dopamine* is hydroxylated to form *nor-*

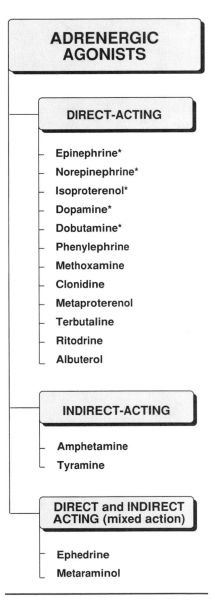

Figure 6.1
Summary of adrenergic agonists. Agents marked with asterisk (*) are catecholamines.

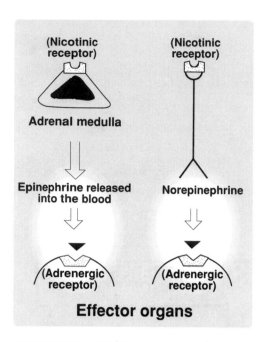

Figure 6.2
Sites of actions of adrenergic agonists.

epinephrine. In the adrenal medulla, *norepinephrine* is methylated to yield *epinephrine.* The adrenal medulla releases about 85% *epinephrine* and 15% *norepinephrine* on stimulation.

3. **Release of norepinephrine:** An action potential arriving at the nerve ending triggers an influx of calcium ions from the extracellular fluid into the cytoplasm of the neuron. This increase in calcium causes vesicles inside the neuron to fuse with the cell membrane and release their contents into the synapse. This release is blocked by drugs such as *guanethidine* and *bretylium* (see p.79).

4. **Binding by receptor:** *Norepinephrine* released from the synaptic vesicles diffuses across the synaptic space and binds to either postsynaptic receptors on the effector organs or to presynaptic receptors on the nerve ending (Figure 6.3). The recognition of *norepinephrine* by the membrane receptors triggers a cascade of events within the cell, resulting in the formation of intracellular second messengers that act as a link (transducer) in the communication between the neurotransmitter and the action generated within the effector cell. Adrenergic neurons use both the cyclic AMP second messenger system and the phosphoinositide cycle, described on p.33.

5. **Removal of norepinephrine:** *Norepinephrine* may diffuse out of the synaptic space and enter the general circulation, or it may be recaptured by an uptake system that pulls the *norepinephrine* back into the neuron. The uptake by the plasma membrane involves a sodium-potassium activated ATPase that can be inhibited by tricyclic antidepressants, such as *imipramine* (see p.119), or by *cocaine* (Figure 6.3).

   a. Once *norepinephrine* enters the cytoplasm of the adrenergic neuron it may reenter the adrenergic vesicle via the amine transporter system and be stored for further release by another action potential.

   b. *Norepinephrine* can also be oxidized by monoamine oxidase (MAO) present in neuronal mitochondria, or it may be converted to O-methylated derivatives by catechol-O-methyltransferase (COMT), which is associated with the membranes of postsynaptic cells. The metabolic products of these reactions are excreted in the urine as VMA (vanillylmandelic acid), metanephrine, and normetanephrine.

B. Adrenergic receptors (adrenoceptors)

1. **α and β adrenoceptors:** In the sympathetic nervous system, several classes of adrenoceptors can be distinguished. Two families of receptors, designated "α" and "β", were initially identified on the basis of their responses to the adrenergic agonists, *epinephrine, norepinephrine,* and *isoproterenol.*

   a. For example, α receptors show a weak response to the synthetic agonist, *isoproterenol,* but are responsive to the natu-

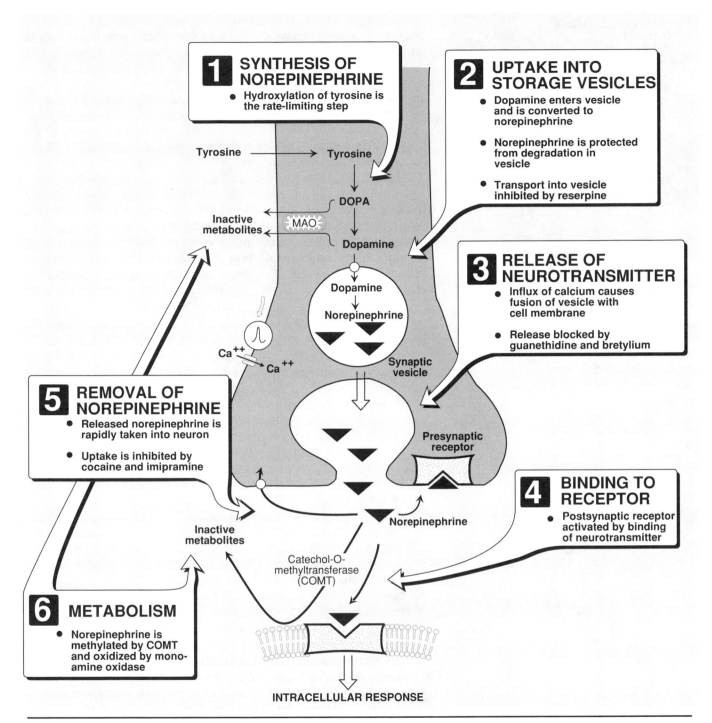

Figure 6.3
Synthesis and release of norepinephrine from the adrenergic neuron.

A. α Adrenoceptors

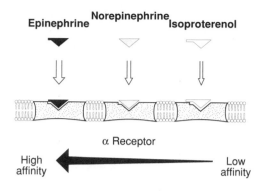

B. β Adrenoceptors

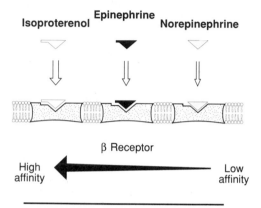

Figure 6.4
Types of adrenergic receptors.

rally occurring catecholamines, *epinephrine*, and *norepinephrine* (Figure 6.4). For α receptors the rank order of potency is:

epinephrine ≥ *norepinephrine* >> *isoproterenol*

b. By contrast, β receptors exhibit a different set of responses, characterized by a strong response to *isoproterenol*, with less sensitivity to *epinephrine* and *norepinephrine* (Figure 6.4). For β receptors, the rank order of potency is:

isoproterenol > *epinephrine* ≥ *norepinephrine*

2. **α_1 and α_2 receptors:** The α adrenoceptors are subdivided into two groups, α_1 and α_2, based on their affinities for α agonists and blocking drugs. For example, the α_1 receptors have a higher affinity for *phenylephrine* (see p.66) than do the α_2 receptors. Conversely, the drug *clonidine* (see p.67) selectively binds to α_2 receptors, and has less effect on α_1 receptors.

a. **α_1 receptors:** These receptors are present on the postsynaptic membrane of the effector organs and mediate many of the classic effects originally designated as α-adrenergic effects involving constriction of smooth muscle (Figure 6.5). Activation of α_1 receptors leads to a rise in cytosolic calcium ions as well as to the activation of calcium-dependent protein kinases (see p.33). In many cells, activation of the α_1 receptor results in the hydrolysis of polyphosphoinositides, producing diacylglycerol and inositol triphosphate (IP_3, p.33).

b. **α_2 receptors:** These receptors, located primarily on presynaptic nerve endings, function to control adrenergic neuromediator output. When a sympathetic adrenergic nerve is stimulated, it releases *norepinephrine*, which traverses the synaptic cleft and reaches the α_1 receptor that it stimulates. Some of the *norepinephrine* released from the presynaptic neuron "circles back" and reacts with the α_2 receptor on the neuronal membrane (Figure 6.5). The stimulation of the α_2 receptor causes feedback inhibition of the ongoing release of *norepinephrine* from the stimulated adrenergic neuron. This inhibitory action decreases further output from the adrenergic neuron and serves as a local modulating mechanism for reducing sympathetic neuromediator output when there is high sympathetic activity. In contrast to α_1 receptors, the effects of binding at α_2 receptors are mediated by inhibition of adenylate cyclase and a fall in the levels of intracellular cAMP.

3. **β_1 and β_2 receptors:** The β adrenoceptors can be subdivided into two groups, β_1 and β_2, based on their affinities for adrenergic agonists and antagonists. β_1 receptors have approximately equal affinities for *epinephrine* and *norepinephrine*, whereas β_2 receptors have a higher affinity for *epinephrine* than for *norepinephrine*. Thus, tissues with a predominance of β_2 receptors (such as the vasculature of skeletal muscle) are particularly responsive to the hormonal effects of circulating *epinephrine* released by the adrenal medulla. Binding of a neurotransmitter at the β_1 or β_2 receptor results in activation of adenylate cyclase and therefore increased concentrations of cAMP within the cell (see p.33).

4. **Distribution of receptors:** Adrenergically innervated organs and tissues have, in many instances, a predominance of one type of receptor. For example, tissues such as the vasculature to skeletal muscle have both α_1 and β_2 receptors, but the β_2 receptors predominate. Other tissues may have one type of receptor exclusively, with practically no significant numbers of other types of adrenergic receptors. For example, the heart contains predominantly β_1 receptors.

5. **Characteristic responses mediated by adrenoceptors:** It is useful to organize the physiological responses to adrenergic stimulation according to receptor type, since many drugs preferentially stimulate or block one type of receptor. Figure 6.6 summarizes the most prominent effects mediated by the adrenoceptors. As a generalization, stimulation of α receptors characteristically produces vasoconstriction (particularly in skin and abdominal viscera) and an increase in total peripheral resistance and blood pressure. Conversely, stimulation of β receptors characteristically causes cardiac stimulation, vasodilation (in skeletal vascular beds), and bronchiolar relaxation (Figure 6.6).

III. CHARACTERISTICS OF ADRENERGIC AGONISTS

A. Structure-activity relationship of adrenergic agonists

Most of the adrenergic drugs are derivatives of β-phenylethylamine (Figure 6.7). Substitution of chemical groups on the benzene ring or on the ethylamine side chains produces a great variety of compounds with varying abilities to differentiate between α and β receptors and to penetrate the CNS. Two important structural features of these drugs are the number and location of OH substitutions on the benzene ring and the nature of the substituent on the amino nitrogen.

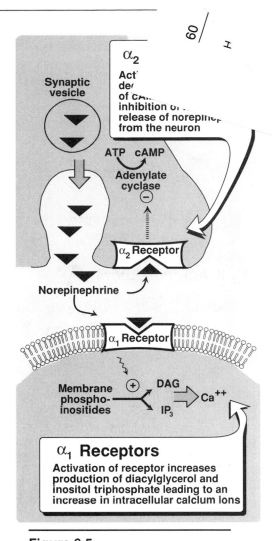

Figure 6.5
Second messengers mediate the effects of α receptors. DAG = diacylglcerol; IP$_3$ = inositol triphosphate.

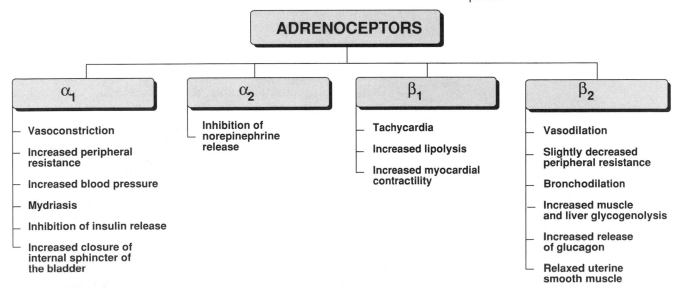

Figure 6.6
Major effects mediated by α– and β–adrenoceptors.

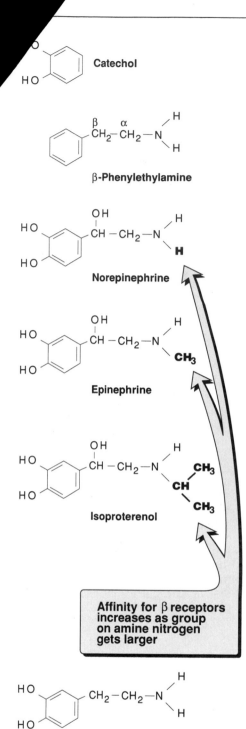

Figure 6.7
Structures of several important adrenergic agonists.

1. **Catecholamines:** Sympathomimetic amines that contain the 3,4-dihydroxybenzene group (such as, *epinephrine, norepinephrine, isoproterenol,* and *dopamine*) are called catecholamines, since 3,4-dihydroxybenzene is known as catechol (Figure 6.7). These compounds share the following properties:

   a. **High potency:** Drugs with OH groups in the 3 and 4 positions on the benzene ring show the highest potency in activating α or β receptors.

   b. **Rapid inactivation:** The catecholamines are rapidly metabolized in the gut wall by catechol-O-methyltransferase (COMT) and in the liver and gut wall by monoamine oxidase (MAO). Thus catecholamines have only a brief period of action when given parenterally and are ineffective when administered orally because of poor absorption.

   c. **Poor penetration into the CNS:** Catecholamines are polar and therefore do not readily penetrate into the CNS. Nevertheless, most of these drugs have some clinical effects (anxiety, tremor, headaches) that are attributable to action on the CNS.

2. **Non-catecholamines:** Compounds lacking the catechol hydroxyl groups have longer half-lives, since they are not metabolized by COMT. Drugs with a substitution at the α-carbon, such as *ephedrine* (see p. 68), which contains an α-methyl group, are poor substrates for MAO. These compounds thus show a prolonged duration of action, since MAO is an important route of detoxification. Increased lipid solubility of many of the non-catecholamines permits greater access to the CNS. These compounds may act indirectly by causing the release of stored catecholamines (see p.68).

3. **Substitution on amine nitrogen:** The nature and bulk of the substituent on the amine nitrogen is important in determining the β selectivity of the adrenergic agonist. For example, *epinephrine* with a -CH$_3$ substituent on the amine nitrogen is more potent at β receptors than *norepinephrine*, which has no substituent. Similarly, *isoproterenol* with an isopropyl substituent -CH(CH$_3$)$_2$ on nitrogen (Figure 6.7), is a strong β agonist with little α activity (see Figure 6.4).

B. Mechanism of action of adrenergic agonists

1. **Direct-acting agonists:** These drugs act directly on α or β receptors, producing effects similar to those that occur following stimulation of sympathetic nerves or release of the hormone *epinephrine* from the adrenal medulla (Figure 6.8). Examples of direct-acting agonists include *epinephrine, norepinephrine, isoproterenol,* and *phenylephrine.*

2. **Indirect-acting agonists:** These agents cause the release of *norepinephrine* from the cytoplasm or vesicles of the adrenergic neuron (Figure 6.8). The *norepinephrine* released from the adrenergic neuron then traverses the synapse and stimulates the α or β

receptors. Indirect-acting agonists include *amphetamine* and *tyramine.*

3. **Mixed-action mechanism:** Some agonists, such as *ephedrine* and *metaraminol,* have the capacity both to directly stimulate adrenoceptors and to cause the release of *norepinephrine* from the adrenergic neuron (Figure 6.8).

IV. DIRECT-ACTING ADRENERGIC AGONISTS

A. Epinephrine

Epinephrine [ep i NEF rin] is one of five catecholamines—*epinephrine, norepinephrine, dopamine, dobutamine,* and *isoproterenol*—commonly used in therapy. The first three catecholamines occur naturally, the latter two are synthetic compounds (see Figure 6.7). *Epinephrine* is synthesized from tyrosine in the adrenal medulla and released, along with small quantities of *norepinephrine,* into the blood stream. *Epinephrine* interacts with both α and β receptors. At low doses, β effects on the vascular system predominate, whereas at high doses, α effects are strongest.

1. **Actions:**

   a. **Cardiovascular:** The major actions of *epinephrine* are on the cardiovascular system. Epinephrine stimulates the strength of myocardium contraction (positive inotropic: β_1 action) and increases its rate of contraction (positive chronotropic: β_1 action). Cardiac output therefore increases. With these effects comes increased oxygen demands on the myocardium. *Epinephrine* constricts arterioles in the skin, mucous membranes, and viscera (α effects) and dilates vessels going to skeletal muscle (β_2 effects). The cumulative effect, therefore, is an increase in systolic blood pressure, coupled with a slight decrease in diastolic pressure (Figure 6.9).

   b. **Respiratory:** *Epinephrine* causes powerful bronchodilation by acting directly on bronchial smooth muscle (β_2 action). This action relieves all known allergic- or histamine-induced bronchoconstriction. In the case of anaphylactic shock, this can be lifesaving. In individuals suffering from an acute asthmatic attack, *epinephrine* rapidly relieves the dyspnea (labored breathing) and increases the tidal volume (volume of gases inspired and expired).

   c. **Hyperglycemia:** *Epinephrine* has a significant hyperglycemic effect because of increased glycogenolysis (β_2 effect), increased release of glucagon (β_2 effect), and a decreased release of insulin (α effect).[2]

   d. **Lipolysis:** *Epinephrine* initiates lipolysis through its β_1-agonist activity. There are β_1 receptors on adipose tissue, which when stimulated, result in activation of adenyl cyclase to increase production of cyclic AMP. Cyclic AMP stimulates a hormone-

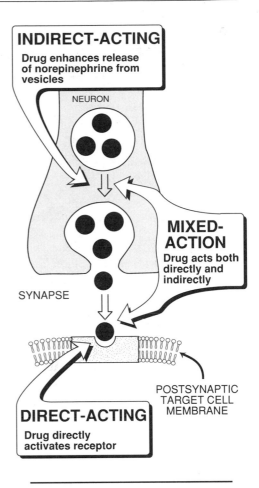

INDIRECT-ACTING
Drug enhances release of norepinephrine from vesicles

NEURON

MIXED-ACTION
Drug acts both directly and indirectly

SYNAPSE

POSTSYNAPTIC TARGET CELL MEMBRANE

DIRECT-ACTING
Drug directly activates receptor

Figure 6.8
Site of action of direct-, indirect- and mixed-acting adreneric agonists.

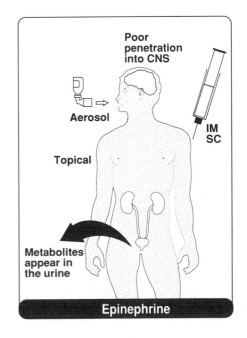

Poor penetration into CNS

Aerosol

IM
SC

Topical

Metabolites appear in the urine

Epinephrine

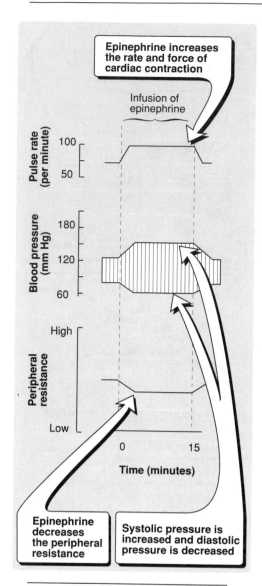

Figure 6.9
Cardiovascular effects of intravenous infusion of low doses of epinephrine.

sensitive lipase, which initiates the hydrolysis of the tria-cylglycerol to free fatty acids and glycerol.

2. **Biotransformations:** *Epinephrine,* like the other catecholamines, is metabolized by two enzymatic pathways: one involves catechol-O-methyl transferase (COMT), and the other involves monoamine oxidase (MAO) (Figure 6.3). The final metabolites found in the urine are metanephrine and vanillylmandelic acid. [Note: Urine also contains normetanephrine, a product of *norepinephrine* metabolism.]

3. **Therapeutic uses**

   a. **Bronchospasm:** *Epinephrine* is probably the primary drug used to treat any condition of the respiratory tract where the presence of bronchoconstriction has resulted in diminished respiratory exchange. Thus, in treatment of acute asthma and anaphylactic shock, *epinephrine* is the drug of choice; within a few minutes after subcutaneous administration, greatly improved respiratory exchange is observed. Administration may be repeated after a few hours. However, selective β_2 agonists, such as *terbutaline,* are presently favored in the chronic treatment of asthma because of a longer duration of action.

   b. **Glaucoma:** In ophthalmology, a 2% *epinephrine* solution may be used topically to reduce intraocular pressure in open-angle glaucoma. It reduces the production of aqueous humor by vasoconstriction of the ciliary body blood vessels.

   c. **Anaphylactic shock:** *Epinephrine* is the drug of choice for the treatment of acute hypersensitivity reactions in response to allergens.

   d. **In anesthetics:** Local anesthetic solutions usually contain 1:100,000 parts *epinephrine* (p.116). The effect of the drug is to greatly increase the duration of the local anesthesia. It does this by producing vasoconstriction at the site of injection, thereby allowing the local anesthetic to remain longer at the site before being absorbed into the circulation and metabolized. Very weak solutions of *epinephrine* 1:100,000 can also be used topically to vasoconstrict mucous membranes to control oozing of capillary blood.

4. **Pharmacology:** *Epinephrine* has a rapid onset but brief duration of action. The drug is administered subcutaneously, by inhalation, or topically to the eye. Oral administration is ineffective, since *epinephrine* and the other catecholamines are inactivated by the intestine.

5. **Adverse effects:**

   a. **CNS disturbances:** *Epinephrine* can produce adverse CNS effects that include anxiety, fear, tension, headache, and tremor.

b. **Hemorrhage:** The drug may induce cerebral hemorrhages as a result of the vasopressor effects, causing a marked elevation of blood pressure.

c. **Cardiac arrhythmias:** *Epinephrine* can trigger cardiac arrhythmias, particularly if the patient is receiving *digitalis.*

d. **Pulmonary edema:** *Epinephrine* can induce pulmonary edema.

6. **Interactions**

a. **Hyperthyroidism:** *Epinephrine* may show enhanced cardiovascular actions in patients with hyperthyroidism. If *epinephrine* is required in such an individual, the dose must be reduced. The mechanism appears to involve increased production of adrenergic receptors in the hyperthyroid individual.

b. **Cocaine:** In the presence of *cocaine, epinephrine* produces exaggerated cardiovascular actions. This is due to the ability of *cocaine* to prevent re-uptake of catecholamines into the adrenergic neuron; thus, like *norepinephrine, epinephrine* remains at the receptor site for longer periods of time (see Figure 6.3).

B. Norepinephrine

Since *norepinephrine* [nor ep i NEF rin] is the neuromediator of adrenergic nerves, it should theoretically stimulate all types of adrenergic receptors. In practice, when the drug is given in therapeutic doses to humans, the α-adrenergic receptor is most affected.

1. **Cardiovascular Actions**

a. **Vasoconstriction:** *Norepinephrine* produces intense vasoconstriction and thereby increases peripheral resistance (an α_1-receptor effect). Both systolic and diastolic blood pressures increase.

b. **Baroreceptor reflex:** In isolated cardiac tissue *norepinephrine* stimulates cardiac contractility; however, in vivo, little if any cardiac stimulation is noted. This is due to the fact that *norepinephrine* induces a reflex increase in vagal activity by enhancing baroreceptor activity. This bradycardia is sufficient to counteract the local actions of *norepinephrine* on the heart (Figure 6.10).

c. **Effect of atropine pretreatment:** If *atropine* (which blocks the transmission of vagal effects, see p.28) is given before *norepinephrine*, then *norepinephrine* stimulates the heart and produces tachycardia.

2. **Therapeutic uses:** *Norepinephrine* is used to treat shock; however, *dopamine* (see p.64) is better, because it does not

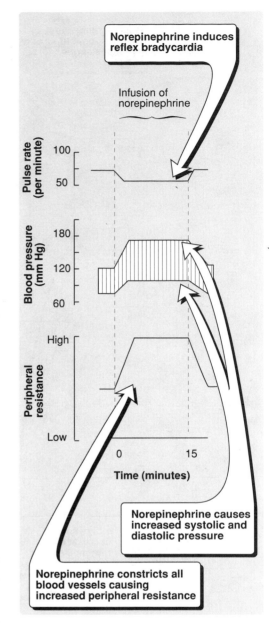

Figure 6.10
Cardiovascular effects of intravenous infusion of norepinephrine.

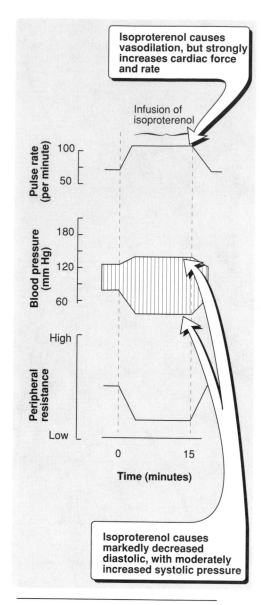

Isoproterenol causes vasodilation, but strongly increases cardiac force and rate

Infusion of isoproterenol

Isoproterenol causes markedly decreased diastolic, with moderately increased systolic pressure

Figure 6.11
Cardiovascular effects of intravenous infusion of isoproterenol.

reduce blood flow to the kidney as does *norepinephrine*. Other actions of the drug are not considered clinically significant. It is never used for asthma. [Note: When *norepinephrine* is used as a drug, it is sometimes called *levarterenol*.]

C. Isoproterenol

Isoproterenol [eye soe proe TER a nole] is a direct-acting synthetic catecholamine that predominantly stimulates both β_1 and β_2 adrenergic receptors. The actions on α receptors are considered insignificant. Its chemical structure is given in Figure 6.7.

1. **Actions:**

   a. **Cardiovascular:** *Isoproterenol* produces intense stimulation of the heart to increase its rate and force of contraction, causing increased cardiac output (Figure 6.11). It is as active as *epinephrine* in this action and is therefore useful in the treatment of atrioventricular block or cardiac arrest. *Isoproterenol* also dilates the arterioles of skeletal muscle (β_2), resulting in a decrease in peripheral resistance. Because of its cardiac stimulatory action, it may increase systolic blood pressure slightly, but it greatly reduces mean arterial and diastolic blood pressure (Figure 6.11).

   b. **Pulmonary:** A profound and rapid bronchodilation is produced by the drug (β_2 action, Figure 6.12). *Isoproterenol* is as active as *epinephrine* and rapidly alleviates an acute attack of asthma, when taken by inhalation (which is the recommended route). This action lasts about one hour and may be repeated by subsequent doses.

   c. **Other effects:** Other actions on β receptors, such as increases in blood sugar and increased lipolysis can be demonstrated, but are not clinically significant.

2. **Therapeutic uses:** *Isoproterenol* is used as a bronchodilator in asthma and to stimulate the heart.

3. **Administration:** *Isoproterenol* can be absorbed systemically by the sublingual mucosa but is more reliably absorbed when given parenterally or as an inhaled aerosol.

4. **Adverse effects:** *Isoproterenol's* adverse effect are similar to those of *epinephrine.*

D. Dopamine

Dopamine [DOE pa meen], the immediate metabolic precursor to *norepinephrine*, occurs naturally in the CNS in the basal ganglia, where it functions as a neurotransmitter (see p.85). *Dopamine* can activate α- and β- adrenergic receptors. In addition, dopaminergic receptors, distinct from the α- and β-adrenergic receptors, occur in the peripheral mesenteric and renal vascular beds.

1. **Actions:**

   a. **Cardiovascular actions:** *Dopamine* exerts a stimulatory effect on the β_1 receptors of the heart, having both inotropic and chronotropic effects (Figure 6.12). At very high doses, *dopamine* activates α receptors on the vasculature, resulting in vasoconstriction.

   b. **Renal and visceral actions:** Dopamine dilates renal and splanchnic arterioles by activating dopaminergic receptors, thus increasing blood flow to the kidneys and other viscera (Figure 6.12). These receptors are not affected by α- or β-blocking drugs. Therefore, *dopamine* is clinically useful in the treatment of shock, in which significant increases in sympathetic activity might compromise renal function. [Note: Similar *dopamine* receptors are found in the autonomic ganglia and in the CNS.]

2. **Therapeutic uses:**

   a. **Shock:** *Dopamine* is the drug of choice for shock and is given by continuous infusion. It raises the blood pressure by stimulating the heart (β_1 action). In addition, it enhances perfusion to the kidney and splanchnic areas, as described earlier. An increased blood flow to the kidney enhances the glomerular filtration rate and causes sodium diuresis. In this regard, *dopamine* is far superior to *norepinephrine*, which diminishes the blood supply to the kidney and may cause kidney shutdown.

   b. **Congestive heart failure:** *Dopamine* is useful in treating refractory congestive heart failure (see p.158).

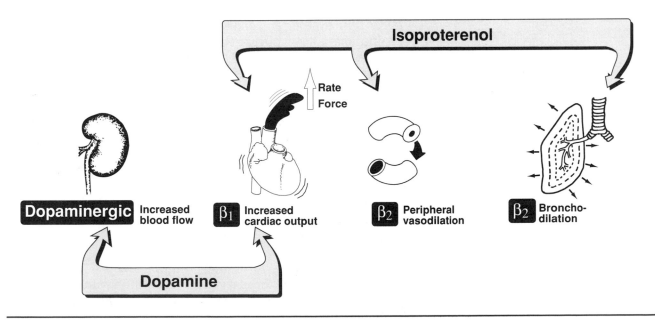

Figure 6.12
Clinically important actions of isoproterenol and dopamine.

3. **Adverse effects:** An overdose of *dopamine* produces the same effects as sympathetic stimulation. *Dopamine* is rapidly metabolized to homovanillic acid, and its adverse effects (nausea, hypertension, arrhythmias) are therefore short-lived.

E. Dobutamine

1. **Actions:** *Dobutamine* [doe BYOO ta meen] is a synthetic, direct-acting catecholamine that is a β_1-receptor agonist. It increases cardiac contractility and output with few vascular effects.

2. **Therapeutic uses:** *Dobutamine* is used to increase cardiac output in congestive heart failure (p.158). The drug increases cardiac output with little change in the heart rate and does not significantly elevate oxygen demands of the myocardium—a major advantage over other sympathomimetic drugs.

3. **Adverse effects:**

   a. **Cardiovascular:** *Dobutamine* should be used with caution in atrial fibrillation, since the drug increases atrioventricular conduction.

   b. **Other:** Other adverse effects are the same as those for *epinephrine.*

F. Phenylephrine

Phenylephrine [fen ill EF rin] is a direct-acting, synthetic adrenergic drug that binds primarily to α receptors and favors α_1 receptors over α_2 receptors.

1. **Cardiovascular effects:** *Phenylephrine* is a vasoconstrictor that raises both systolic and diastolic blood pressures. It has no effect on the heart itself but induces reflex bradycardia when given parenterally. It is often used topically on the nasal mucous membranes and in ophthalmic solutions for mydriasis.

2. **Therapeutic uses:** As a nasal decongestant, *phenylephrine* produces prolonged vasoconstriction. The drug is used to raise blood pressure and to terminate episodes of supraventricular tachycardia (rapid heart action arising both from the atrioventricular junction and atria).

3. **Adverse effects:** Large doses can cause hypertensive headache and cardiac irregularities.

G. Methoxamine

Methoxamine [meth OX a meen] is a direct-acting synthetic adrenergic drug that binds primarily to α receptors, with α_1 receptors favored over α_2 receptors. *Methoxamine* raises blood pressure by stimulating α_1 receptors in the arterioles, causing vasoconstriction. This causes an increase in total peripheral resistance. *Methoxamine* is used clinically to relieve attacks of paroxysmal supraventricular tachycardia. It is also used to overcome hypotension during surgery involving *cyclopropane* or *halothane* anesthetics (see p.112). In contrast to most other adrenergic drugs, *methoxamine* does not tend to trigger cardiac arrhythmias in the heart that is sensitized by these general anesthetics. Adverse effects include hypertensive headache and vomiting.

H. Clonidine

Clonidine [KLOE ni deen] is an α_2 agonist that is used in essential hypertension to lower blood pressure because of its action on the CNS (see p.182). It can be used to minimize the symptoms that accompany withdrawal from opiates or benzodiazepines. *Clonidine* acts centrally to produce inhibition of sympathetic vasomotor centers.

I. Metaproterenol

Metaproterenol [met a proe TER e nole], although chemically similar to *isoproterenol*, is not a catecholamine and is resistant to methylation by COMT. It can be administered orally or by inhalation. The drug acts primarily at β_2 receptors, producing little effect on the heart. *Metaproterenol* produces dilation of the bronchioles and improves airway function. The drug is useful as a bronchodilator in the treatment of asthma and to reverse bronchospasm.

J. Terbutaline

Terbutaline [ter BYOO te leen] is a β_2 agonist with more selective properties than *metaproterenol* and with a longer duration of action. It is used as a bronchodilator and to reduce uterine contractions in premature labor.

K. Ritodrine

Ritodrine [RI toe dreen] is a selective β_2 agonist that is used to relax the uterine contractions of premature labor.

L. Albuterol

Albuterol [al BYOO ter ole] is a selective β_2 agonist with properties similar to those of *terbutaline*. The drug is used to relieve bronchospasm.

V. INDIRECT-ACTING ADRENERGIC AGONISTS

A. Amphetamine

Amphetamine's [am FET a meen] marked central stimulatory action is often mistaken by drug abusers as its only action. However, the drug can increase blood pressure significantly by α-agonist action on the vasculature as well as β-stimulatory effects on the heart. Its peripheral actions are mediated primarily through the cellular release of stored catecholamines; thus, *amphetamine* is an indirect-acting adrenergic drug. The actions and uses of amphetamines are discussed under stimulants of the CNS (see p.105)

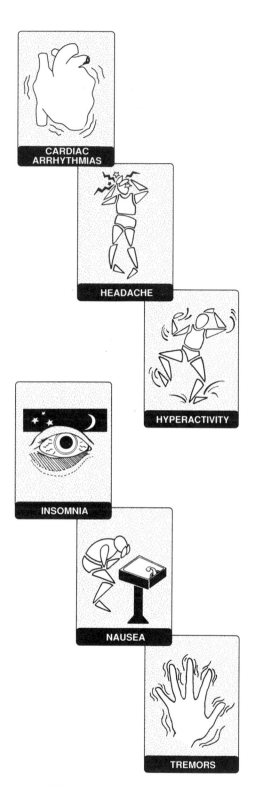

Figure 6.13
Some adverse effects observed with adrenergic agonists.

B. Tyramine

Tyramine [teer a meen] is not a clinically useful drug, but it is found in fermented foods, such as ripe cheese and Chianti wine (see MAO inhibitors, p.125). It is a normal by-product of tyrosine metabolism. Like *amphetamine*, *tyramine* can enter the nerve terminal and displace stored norepinephrine. The released catecholamine acts on adrenoceptors.

VI. MIXED-ACTION ADRENERGIC AGONISTS

A. Ephedrine

Ephedrine [e FED rin], a plant alkaloid, is now made synthetically. The drug is a mixed-action adrenergic agent. It not only releases stored *norepinephrine* from nerve endings (Figure 6.8) but also directly stimulates both α and β receptors. Thus, a wide variety of adrenergic actions ensue that are similar to those of *epinephrine*, although less potent. *Ephedrine* is not a catechol and is a poor substrate for COMT and MAO; thus, the drug has a long duration of action. *Ephedrine* has excellent absorption orally and penetrates into the central nervous system.

1. **Actions:**

   a. **Cardiovascular:** *Ephedrine* raises systolic and diastolic blood pressures by vasoconstriction and cardiac stimulation.

   b. **Pulmonary:** *Ephedrine* produces bronchodilation, but it is less potent than *epinephrine* or *isoproterenol* in this regard and produces its action more slowly. It is therefore used prophylactically in chronic treatment of asthma to prevent attacks, rather than to treat the acute attack.

   c. **Skeletal muscle:** *Ephedrine* enhances contractility and improves motor function in myasthenia gravis, particularly when used in conjunction with anticholinesterases (see p.42).

   d. **Central nervous system:** *Ephedrine* produces a mild stimulation of the central nervous system. This increases alertness, decreases fatigue, and prevents sleep. It also improves athletic performance.

2. **Therapeutic uses:** *Ephedrine* is used to treat asthma, as a nasal decongestant (due to its local vasoconstrictor action), and to raise blood pressure.

B. Metaraminol

Metaraminol [met a RAM i nole] is a mixed-acting adrenergic drug with actions similar to *norepinephrine.* This agent has been used in the treatment of shock (when an infusion of *norepinephrine* or *dopamine* is not possible) and to treat acute hypotension. It is given

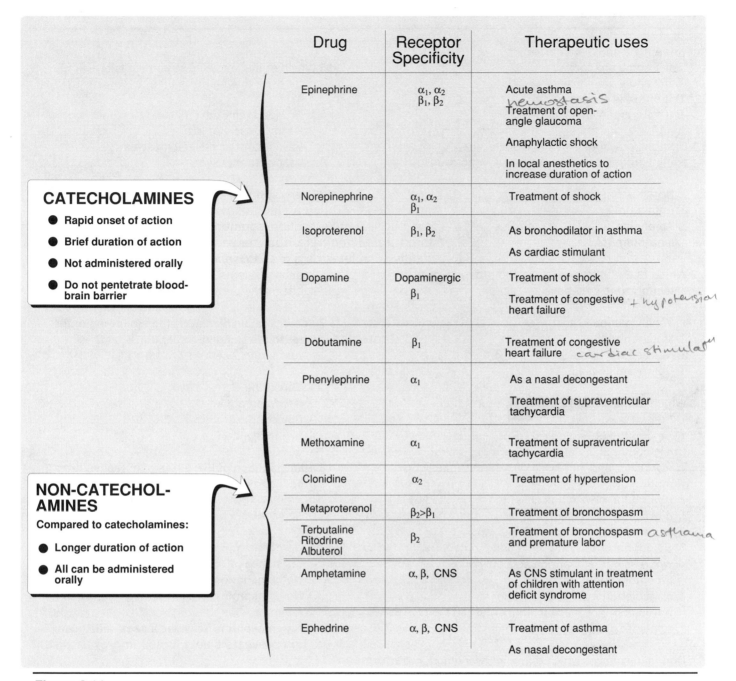

Drug	Receptor Specificity	Therapeutic uses
Epinephrine	α_1, α_2 β_1, β_2	Acute asthma *hemostasis* Treatment of open-angle glaucoma Anaphylactic shock In local anesthetics to increase duration of action
Norepinephrine	α_1, α_2 β_1	Treatment of shock
Isoproterenol	β_1, β_2	As bronchodilator in asthma As cardiac stimulant
Dopamine	Dopaminergic β_1	Treatment of shock Treatment of congestive heart failure *+ hypotension*
Dobutamine	β_1	Treatment of congestive heart failure *cardiac stimulant*
Phenylephrine	α_1	As a nasal decongestant Treatment of supraventricular tachycardia
Methoxamine	α_1	Treatment of supraventricular tachycardia
Clonidine	α_2	Treatment of hypertension
Metaproterenol	$\beta_2 > \beta_1$	Treatment of bronchospasm
Terbutaline Ritodrine Albuterol	β_2	Treatment of bronchospasm *asthma* and premature labor
Amphetamine	α, β, CNS	As CNS stimulant in treatment of children with attention deficit syndrome
Ephedrine	α, β, CNS	Treatment of asthma As nasal decongestant

CATECHOLAMINES
- Rapid onset of action
- Brief duration of action
- Not administered orally
- Do not pentetrate blood-brain barrier

NON-CATECHOL-AMINES

Compared to catecholamines:
- Longer duration of action
- All can be administered orally

Figure 6.14
Summary of the adrenergic agonists.

parenterally as a single injection. It enhances cardiac activity and produces mild vasoconstriction.

The important characteristics of the adrenergic agonists are summarized in Figures 6.13 and 6.14.

Study Questions   (see p.409 for answers).

Answer A if 1,2 and 3 are correct.
  B if 1 and 3 are correct.
  C if 2 and 4 are correct.
  D if only 4 is correct.
  E if 1,2,3 and 4 are all correct.

6.1 Diastolic pressure is increased after the administration of which of the following drugs?

1. Norepinephrine.
2. Epinephrine.
3. Amphetamine.
4. Isoproterenol.

6.2 Which of the following is/are end products of catecholamine metabolism?

1. Vanillylmandelic acid.
2. Metanephrine.
3. Normetanephrine.
4. Homovanillic acid.

6.3 Which of the following is/are correct statements?

1. Among the physiological responses caused by α-receptor stimulation are vasoconstriction, mydriasis, and increased gastrointestinal motility.
2. Among the physiological responses caused by β-receptor stimulation are vasodilation, cardiac stimulation, and bronchial relaxation.
3. Epinephrine acts on both α and β receptors, whereas norepinephrine acts only on α receptors and β_1 receptors.
4. Administration of atropine prior to norepinephrine leads to an increase in heart rate after norepinephrine administration.

6.4 Dopamine causes which of the following actions:

1. Increases cardiac output.
2. Dilates renal vasculature.
3. Increases production of urine.
4. Increases blood pressure.

6.5 Which of the following structures is/are more responsive to β agonists than to α agonists?

1. Bronchial smooth muscle.
2. Radial muscle of iris.
3. Vasculature of skeletal muscle.
4. Vasculature of skin.

6.6 Phenylephrine

1. is an α agonist that causes vasoconstriction.
2. is a cardioselective β agonist.
3. is often found in over-the-counter nasal decongestants.
4. affects the parasympathetic nervous system.

6.7 Administration of which of the following drugs leads to the stimulation of both α- and β-adrenergic receptors?

1. Ephedrine.
2. Isoproterenol.
3. Epinephrine.
4. Methoxamine.

6.8 Administration of low doses of norepinephrine produces a decrease in heart rate. Which one of the following statements best explains this observation?

1. Norepinephrine decreases the peripheral resistance.
2. Norepinephrine activates β_2 receptors.
3. Norepinephrine directly decreases the heart rate.
4. Norepinephrine activates a vagal reflex that decreases the heart rate.

[1]See *catecholamines* in **Biochemistry** for further information on the synthesis of dopamine and its conversion to norepinephrine and epinephrine (see index).

[2]See *epinephrine, and glycogen metabolism; epinephrine, effect on insulin secretion* in **Biochemistry** for discussion of effects of epinephrine on metabolism.

Adrenergic Antagonists

7

I. OVERVIEW

The adrenergic antagonists (also called blockers) bind to adrenoceptors but do not trigger the usual receptor-mediated intracellular effects. These drugs act by either reversibly or irreversibly binding to the receptor, thus preventing their activation by endogenous catecholamines. Like the agonists, the adrenergic antagonists are classified according to their relative affinity for α or β receptors. The receptor-blocking drugs discussed in this chapter are summarized in Figure 7.1.

II. α-ADRENERGIC BLOCKING AGENTS

Drugs that block α adrenoceptors have profound effects on blood pressure. Since normal sympathetic control of the vasculature occurs in large part through α-adrenergic receptor agonist action, blockade of these receptors reduces the sympathetic tone of the blood vessels, resulting in decreased peripheral vascular resistance. This induces a reflex tachycardia resulting from the decrease in blood pressure. [Note: β receptors, including β_1 adrenoceptors on the heart, are not affected by α blockade.] The α-receptor blocking agents, with the exception of *prazosin* and *labetalol,* have only limited clinical applications.

A. Phenoxybenzamine

Phenoxybenzamine [fen ox ee BEN za meen], a drug related to the nitrogen mustards, forms a covalent linkage to the α_1-postsynaptic and α_2-presynaptic receptors (Figure 7.2). The block is irreversible and noncompetitive; the only mechanism the body has to overcome the block is the ability to synthesize new α_1 adrenoceptors. This synthesis occurs in approximately one day. Therefore, the actions of *phenoxybenzamine* last at least 24 hours after a single administration. When the drug is injected, a delay of a few hours occurs before α blockade develops, since the molecule must undergo metabolic transformation to the active form.

1. **Actions:**

   a. **Cardiovascular effects:** *Phenoxybenzamine* blocks α receptors and prevents vasoconstriction of peripheral blood vessels by

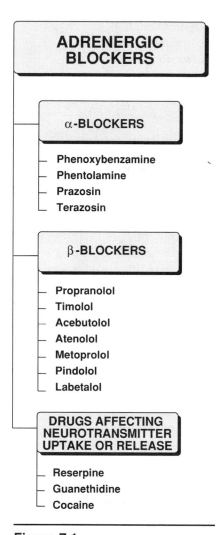

Figure 7.1
Summary of blocking agents and drugs affecting neurotransmitter uptake or release.

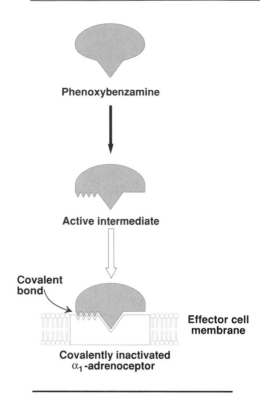

Figure 7.2
Covalent inactivation of α_1 adrenoceptor by phenoxybenzamine.

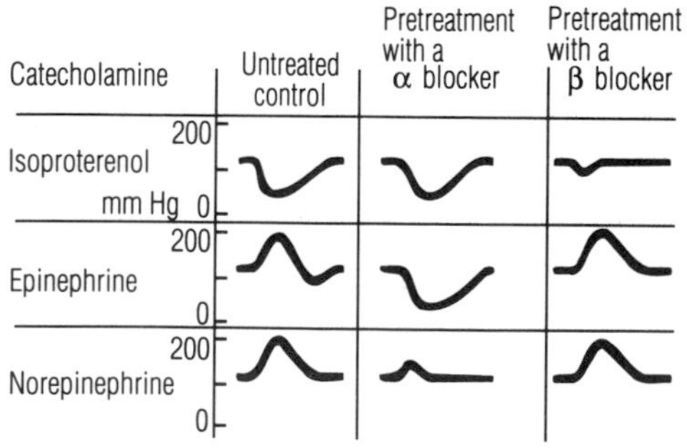

endogenous catecholamines. This leads to a decrease in blood pressure and peripheral resistance that causes a reflex tachycardia. The drug has not been successful in maintaining lowered blood pressure among hypertensive patients and thus has been discontinued clinically for this purpose.

b. **Postural hypotension:** *Phenoxybenzamine* induces postural (orthostatic) hypotension because of its blockade of the α_1- receptors. When the individual stands rapidly, blood pools in the lower extremities causing faintness.

c. **Epinephrine reversal:** All α-adrenergic blockers reverse the α-agonist actions of *epinephrine*. For example, the ability of *epinephrine* to produce vasoconstriction is blocked, but vasodilation of other vascular beds occurring by β-agonist action is not blocked. Therefore, the systemic blood pressure decreases in response to *epinephrine* given in the presence of *phenoxybenzamine* (Figure 7.3). [Note: The actions of *norepinephrine* are not reversed but diminished, since *norepinephrine* has no significant β-agonist action on the vasculature.] *Phenoxybenzamine* has no effect on the actions of *isoproterenol,* which is a pure β agonist (Figure 7.3).

d. **Sexual function:** *Phenoxybenzamine,* like all α blockers, adversely affects male sexual function. Ejaculation of semen is inhibited, with the possibility of retrograde ejaculation when it does occur. This is due to inability of the internal sphincter of the bladder to close during ejaculation.

2. **Therapeutic uses**

a. **Urinary system:** *Phenoxybenzamine* treatment results in the inability of the internal sphincter of the bladder to close completely. In patients with neurogenic vesicular dysfunction, in which the internal sphincter closes spontaneously during micturition, urine stagnates in the bladder because of incomplete voiding. In such patients, *phenoxybenzamine* is of inestimable value in allowing all the urine held in the bladder to be expressed.

b. **Paraplegics:** All paraplegics suffer from autonomic hyperreflexia. In this condition, the mere process of micturition sets up reflexes that result in increased sympathetic activity to the blood vessels and causes enhanced blood pressure. This predisposes paraplegics to strokes. *Phenoxybenzamine* blunts this effect and aids in normalizing the paraplegic patient's blood pressure.

c. **Benign prostatic hypertrophy:** *Phenoxybenzamine* is of value in reducing the size of the prostate in benign hypertrophy. This allows more normal urination by reducing the obstruction of the prostate around the urethra.

d. **Treatment of pheochromocytoma-induced hypertension:** Pheochromocytoma, a catecholamine-secreting tumor of cells derived from the adrenal medulla, is most often diagnosed by

Figure 7.3
Summary of effects of adrenergic blockers on the changes in blood pressure induced by isoproterenol, epinephrine, and norepinephrine.

chemical measurement of circulating catecholamines and urinary excretion of catechol metabolites. *Phenoxybenzamine* and *phentolamine* (see later) are used in the management of these tumors, particularly in cases where the catecholamine-secreting cells are diffuse and therefore inoperable.

3. **Adverse effects:**

   a. *Phenoxybenzamine* can cause postural hypotension, inhibit ejaculation, cause nasal stuffiness, and may induce nausea and vomiting.

   b. The drug also may cause tachycardia, mediated by the baroreceptor reflex.

B. Phentolamine

1. **Actions:** In contrast to *phenoxybenzamine, phentolamine* [fen TOLE a meen] produces a competitive block of α_1 and α_2 receptors. The drug's action lasts for approximately 4 hours after a single administration. Like *phenoxybenzamine,* it produces postural hypotension and causes *epinephrine* reversal.

2. **Therapeutic uses:**

   a. **Pheochromocytoma:** *Phentolamine* is used in the diagnosis of pheochromocytoma and in other clinical situations associated with excess release of catecholamines.

   b. **Frostbite:** Occasionally, *phentolamine* is used for rapid α_1 blockade in cases of frostbite; the object is to increase blood flow to the digits by dilation of the arterioles.

3. **Adverse effects:**

   a. **Cardiac:** *Phentolamine*-induced reflex cardiac stimulation and tachycardia are mediated by the baroreceptor reflex. The drug can also trigger arrhythmias and anginal pain.

   b. **Postural hypotension:** Like *phenoxybenzamine,* it may cause postural hypotension.

   c. **Gastrointestinal (GI):** The drug may produce GI stimulation, leading to aggravation of peptic ulcers.

C. Prazosin and terazosin

Prazosin [PRA zoe sin) and *terazosin* [ter AY zoe sin] produce a competitive block of the α_1 receptor without blocking the α_2 receptor. In contrast to *phenoxybenzamine* and *phentolamine, prazosin* and *terazosin* are effective in the treatment of hypertension.

1. **Cardiovascular effects:** *Prazosin* and *terazosin* decrease peripheral vascular resistance and lower arterial blood pressure by causing the relaxation of both arterial and venous smooth mus-

cle. These drugs cause only minimal changes in cardiac output, renal blood flow, and glomerular filtration rate.

2. **Therapeutic uses:** Individuals with elevated blood pressure have been treated with *prazosin* or *terazosin* for moderate periods of time and do not become tolerant to its action (p.182). However, the first dose of *prazosin* produces an exaggerated hypotensive response that has resulted in syncope (fainting) in some patients. This action has been termed a "first-pass" effect and may be minimized by adjusting the first dose to one third or one fourth of the normal dose.

3. **Adverse effects:**

   a. *Prazosin* may cause nasal congestion, GI hypermotility, fluid retention, and orthostatic hypotension (although to a lesser degree than that observed with *phenoxybenzamine* and *phentolamine*).

   b. Male sexual function is not as severely affected by *prazosin* as it is by *phenoxybenzamine* and *phentolamine*.

III. β-ADRENERGIC BLOCKING AGENTS

All the clinically available β blockers are competitive antagonists. Nonselective β blockers block both β_1 and β_2 receptors, whereas cardioselective β blockers primarily block β_1 receptors. These drugs also show differences in intrinsic sympathomimetic activity, in central nervous system (CNS) effects, and in pharmacokinetics. Although all β blockers lower blood pressure in hypertension, they do not induce postural hypotension because the α adrenoceptor is not blocked; therefore, normal sympathetic control of the vasculature is maintained. The β blockers are also effective in treating angina, cardiac arrhythmias, myocardial infarction, and glaucoma, as well as serving in the prophylaxis of migraine headaches.

A. Propranolol

Propranolol [proe PRAN oh lole] is the prototype β-adrenergic blocker and blocks both β_1 and β_2 receptors.

1. **Actions** (summarized in Figure 7.4):

   a. **Cardiovascular:** *Propranolol* diminishes cardiac output, having both negative inotropic and chronotropic effects. The resulting bradycardia usually limits the dose of the drug. Cardiac output, work, and oxygen consumption are decreased by blockade of β_1 receptors; these effects are useful in improving cardiac function in the treatment of angina (p.174).

   b. **Peripheral vasoconstriction:** Blockade of β receptors prevents β_2-mediated vasodilation. The decrease in cardiac output leads to decreased blood pressure. This hypotension triggers a reflex peripheral vasoconstriction, which is reflected in reduced blood flow to the fingers and toes. In balance, there is a

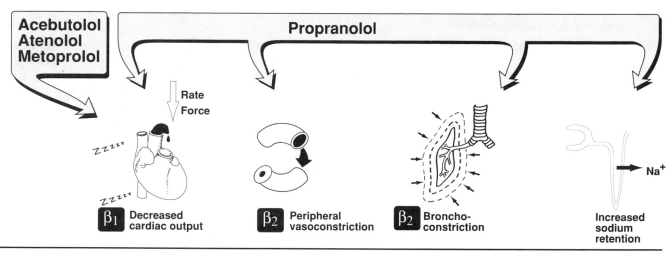

Figure 7.4
Actions of propranolol and β₁ blockers.

gradual reduction of both systolic and diastolic blood pressures in hypertensive patients. No postural hypotension occurs, since the α-adrenergic receptor that controls vascular resistance is unaffected.

c. **Bronchoconstriction:** Blocking β₂ receptors in the lungs of susceptible patients causes contraction of the smooth muscle in the bronchioles. This can precipitate a respiratory crisis in patients with chronic obstructive pulmonary disease, such as asthma, and can cause death by suffocation.

d. **Increased Na+ retention:** Reduced blood pressure causes a fall in renal perfusion that results in an increase in Na⁺ retention and plasma volume. This compensatory response in some cases tends to elevate the blood pressure. For these patients, β blockers are often combined with a diuretic to prevent Na⁺ retention.

e. **Disturbances in glucose metabolism:** β blockade leads to decreased glycogenolysis and decreased glucagon secretion. Therefore, if a diabetic is to be given *propranolol,* very careful monitoring of blood sugar is essential, since pronounced hypoglycemia may occur after *insulin* injection.

f. **Blocks action of isoproterenol:** All β blockers, including *propranolol,* have the ability to block the actions of *isoproterenol* on the cardiovascular system. Thus, in the presence of a β blocker, *isoproterenol* does not produce the typical decrease in mean arterial pressure, the decrease in diastolic pressure, nor cardiac stimulation (see Figure 7.3). [Note: In the presence of a β blocker, *epinephrine* no longer lowers diastolic blood pressure nor stimulates the heart, but its vasoconstrictive action (mediated by α receptors) remains unimpaired. The actions of *norepinephrine* on the cardiovascular system are primarily mediated by α receptors and are, therefore, unaffected.]

CHRONIC OPEN-ANGLE GLAUCOMA

- Most common form of glaucoma

- Leads to a gradual, painless, but inevitable loss of vision due to damage to optic nerve

- Treatment with β–adrenergic blocker (e.g., timolol) is effective

- Long-term treatment with miotic agents (e.g., pilocarpine) is also effective

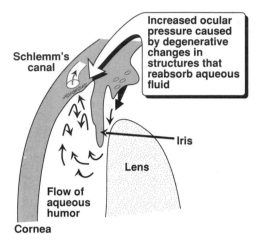

Increased ocular pressure caused by degenerative changes in structures that reabsorb aqueous fluid

Schlemm's canal

Iris

Lens

Flow of aqueous humor

Cornea

ACUTE CLOSED-ANGLE GLAUCOMA

- Onset is often rapid (several hours) and accompanied by pain

- A common cause is dilation of the pupil set off by an emotional crisis, which results in sympathetic discharge of norepinephrine and increased circulating epinephrine

- Prompt treatment with a miotic agent (e.g., pilocarpine) is essential to prevent loss of vision

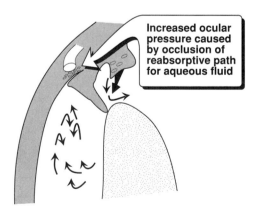

Increased ocular pressure caused by occlusion of reabsorptive path for aqueous fluid

Figure 7.5
Summary of glaucoma.

2. Therapeutic effects

a. **Hypertension:** *Propranolol* lowers blood pressure in hypertension by decreasing cardiac output (p. 179).

b. **Glaucoma:** *Propranolol* and other β blockers, particularly *timolol* (p.77), are useful in diminishing intraocular pressure in glaucoma. This occurs by decreasing the secretion of aqueous humor by the ciliary body. Treatment for many glaucoma patients has been maintained for years with such drugs. When the drugs are used in glaucoma, they neither affect the ability of the eye to focus for near vision, nor change pupil size, as do the cholinergic drugs. However, in an acute attack of glaucoma, *pilocarpine* is still the drug of choice, and the β blockers are only used to treat this disease chronically (Figure 7.5).

c. **Migraine:** *Propranolol* has also been found to be effective in reducing migraine episodes. Once the attack has occurred, then the usual therapy with ergot preparations (p.387) or other drugs are used. The value of the β blockers is in the treatment of chronic migraine in which the drug decreases the incidence and severity of the attacks. The mechanism may be an ability of β blockers to block catecholamine-induced vasodilation in the brain vasculature.

d. **Hyperthyroidism:** *Propranolol* and other β blockers are effective in blunting the widespread sympathetic stimulation that occurs in hyperthyroidism. In acute hyperthyroidism (thyroid storm), β blockers may be lifesaving in protecting against serious cardiac arrhythmias.

e. **Angina pectoris:** *Propranolol* reduces the oxygen requirement of heart muscle and therefore is effective in reducing the chest pain on exertion that is common in angina (p.174). Tolerance to moderate exercise is increased and this is noticeable by improvement in the electrocardiogram. However, treatment with *propranolol* does not allow strenuous physical exercise, such as tennis.

f. **Myocardial infarction:** *Propranolol* and other β blockers have a protective effect on the myocardium. Thus, patients who have had one myocardial infarction appear to be protected against a second heart attack by prophylactic use of β blockers. In addition, administration of a β-blocker immediately following a myocardial infarction reduces infarct size and quickens recovery. The mechanism for these effects may be blocking of the actions of released catecholamines coming from damaged cardiac tissue, which would stimulate an already damaged heart. *Propranolol* also reduces the incidence of sudden arrhythmic death after myocardial infarction (p.167).

3. Adverse effects:

a. **Bronchoconstriction:** *Propranolol* has serious and potentially lethal side effect when administered to an asthmatic (Figure

7.6). An immediate contraction of the bronchiolar smooth muscle prevents air from being carried into the lungs. Deaths by asphyxiation have been reported among a number of asthmatics who were inadvertently administered the drug. Therefore, *propranolol* must never be used in treating any individual with obstructive lung disease.

b. **Arrhythmias:** Treatment with the β blockers must never be stopped quickly. Rapid withdrawal may precipitate cardiac arrhythmias, which may be severe. The β blockers must be tapered off gradually during 1 week.

c. **Sexual impairment:** Since sexual function in the male occurs through α-adrenergic activation, β blockers do not block normal ejaculation nor affect the internal bladder sphincter. On the other hand, a small number of men do complain of impaired sexual activity. The reasons for this are not clear and may not depend on blockade of β receptors.

d. **Disturbances in glucose metabolism:** β blockade leads to decreased glycogenolysis and decreased glucagon secretion. Fasting hypoglycemia may occur.

e. **Other:** Triacylglycerol levels are increased.

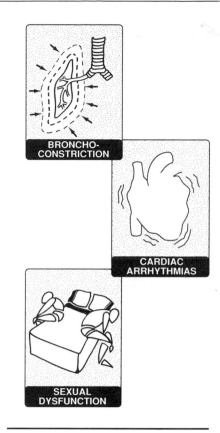

Figure 7.6
Adverse effects commonly observed in individuals treated with propranolol.

B. Timolol

Timolol [TYE moe lole] is a nonselective β blocker that is more potent than *propranolol*. It reduces the production of aqueous humor in the eye and is used topically in the treatment of glaucoma and systemically for treating hypertension (Figure 7.5).

C. Acebutolol, atenolol, and metoprolol

Drugs that preferentially block the β_1 receptors have been developed to eliminate the unwanted bronchoconstrictor effect (β_2) of *propranolol* seen among asthmatic patients. Cardioselective β blockers, such as *acebutolol* [a se BYOO toe lole], *atenolol* [a TEN oh lole], and *metoprolol* [me TOE proe lole], antagonize β_1 receptors at doses 50 to 100 times less than that required to block β_2 receptors. This cardioselectivity is thus most pronounced at low doses and is lost at high drug doses. [Note: *Acebutolol* has some intrinsic agonist activity (see next section).]

1. **Actions:** These drugs are effective in lowering blood pressure in hypertension and in increasing exercise tolerance in angina (see Figure 7.4). In contrast to *propranolol,* these cardiospecific blockers have relatively little effect on pulmonary function, peripheral resistance, and carbohydrate metabolism. Nevertheless, one must carefully monitor asthmatics to make certain that respiratory activity is not reduced.

2. **Therapeutic use in hypertension:** The cardioselective β blockers are useful in hypertensive patients with impaired pulmonary function that is caused by asthma or cigarette smoking. Since these drugs have less effect on peripheral vascular β_2 receptors,

A. Agonists
(e.g., epinephrine)

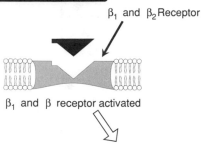

β_1 and β_2 Receptor

β_1 and β receptor activated

CELLULAR EFFECTS

B. Antagonists
(e.g., propranolol)

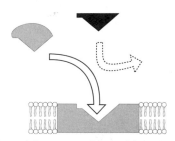

β_1 and β_2 receptor blocked, but not activated

C. Partial agonists
(e.g., pindolol and acebutolol)

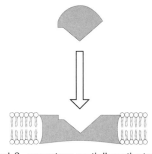

β_1 and β_2 receptors partially activated but unable to respond to more potent catecholamines

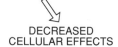

DECREASED CELLULAR EFFECTS

Figure 7.7
Comparison of agonists, antagonists, and partial agonists of β adrenoceptors.

coldness of extremities, a common side effect of β-blocker therapy, is less frequent. Cardioselective β blockers are useful in diabetic hypertensive patients who are receiving *insulin* or oral hypoglycemic agents.

D. Pindolol and acebutolol

1. **Actions:**

   a. **Cardiovascular:** *Acebutolol* and *pindolol* [PIN doe lole] are not true blockers; instead they have the ability to weakly stimulate both β_1 and β_2 receptors (Figure 7.7) and are said to have intrinsic sympathomimetic activity (ISA). These partial agonists stimulate the β receptor to which they are bound, yet they inhibit stimulation by the more potent endogenous catecholamines, *epinephrine* and *norepinephrine.* The result of these opposing actions is a much diminished effect on cardiac rate and cardiac output, compared to β blockers without ISA.

   b. **Decreased metabolic effects:** Blockers with ISA minimize the disturbances of lipid and carbohydrate metabolism seen with other β blockers.

2. **Therapeutic use in hypertension:** β Blockers with ISA are effective in hypertensive patients with moderate bradycardia, since a further decrease in heart rate is less pronounced with these drugs. Carbohydrate metabolism is less affected with *acebutolol* and *pindolol* than it is with *propranolol,* making them valuable in the treatment of diabetics. In addition, these agents are used effectively in hypertensive athletes; these partial agonists do not diminish stamina and performance as do other β-blockers.

E. Labetalol

1. **Actions:** *Labetalol* [la BET a lole] is a reversible β blocker with concurrent α_1-blocking actions. α_1-blockade produces peripheral vasodilation and thereby reduces blood pressure. *Labetalol* thus contrasts with the other β blockers that produce peripheral vasoconstriction and is useful in treating hypertensive patients for whom increased peripheral vascular resistance is undesirable. Labetalol does not alter serum lipid or blood glucose levels.

2. **Therapeutic use in hypertension:** *Labetalol* is useful for treating the elderly or black hypertensive patient in whom increased peripheral vascular resistance is undesirable.

3. **Adverse affects:** Orthostatic hypotension and dizziness are associated with α_1 blockade.

IV. DRUGS AFFECTING NEUROTRANSMITTER RELEASE OR UPTAKE

As was noted on p.67, some agonists, such as *amphetamine* and *tyramine,* do not act directly on the adrenoceptor but rather exert their effects indirectly on the adrenergic neuron by causing the release of neurotransmitter from storage vesicles. Similarly, some adrenergic blocking agents act on the adrenergic neuron, either blocking neurotransmitter release or altering the uptake of the neurotransmitter into the adrenergic nerve.

A. Reserpine

Reserpine [re SER peen], a plant alkaloid, blocks the ability of adrenergic neurons to transport norepinephrine from the cytoplasm into storage vesicles (p.55). This causes an ultimate depletion of *norepinephrine* levels in the adrenergic neuron, since monoamine oxidase can degrade the *norepinephrine.* Sympathetic function, in general, is impaired because of decreased release of *norepinephrine.*

1. **Cardiovascular actions:** Hypertensive patients taking the drug show a gradual decline in blood pressure. *Reserpine* slows the cardiac rate simultaneously with the decline in blood pressure. The drug has a slow onset of action and a long duration of action. When one stops taking the drug, the actions persist for many days.

2. **Other actions:** Although it lowers blood pressure, *reserpine* does not produce significant orthostatic hypotension. It does interfere with normal sexual function and ejaculation of semen in the male patient. In addition, by blocking sympathetic function, the drug appears to accentuate parasympathetic activity, particularly in the GI tract. The most noticeable action is enhanced gastric acid secretion. The drug should never be given to anyone with a history of peptic ulcer.

3. **Therapeutic uses:** *Reserpine* is used in the treatment of hypertension.

4. **Adverse effects:** After months of therapy, difficulty in sleeping and nighttime hallucinations have occurred among a number of patients. In addition, a very small number of patients have become depressed and have had suicidal tendencies. Since *reserpine* has a major tranquilizing effect on the central nervous system, CNS monoamines are depleted, which may be the cause of the depression seen with the drug.

B. Guanethidine

1. **Actions:** *Guanethidine* [gwahn ETH i deen] inhibits the response of the adrenergic nerve to stimulation or to indirectly-acting sympathomimetic amines. *Guanethidine* acts by blocking the release of stored *norepinephrine.* This results in a gradual lowering of

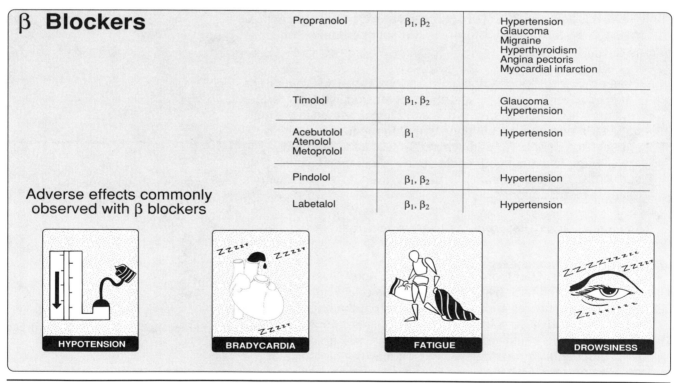

Drug	Receptor Specificity	Therapeutic uses
α Blockers		
Phenoxy-benzamine	α_1, α_2	Incomplete urinary voiding Autonomic hyperreflexia Benign prostatic hypertrophy Treatment of pheochromocytoma-induced hypertension
Phentolamine	α_1, α_2	Diagnosis of pheochromocytoma Treatment of frostbite
Prazosin	α_1	Hypertension
Terazosin	α_1	Hypertension

Adverse effects commonly observed with α blockers

ORTHOSTATIC HYPOTENSION   TACHYCARDIA   VERTIGO   SEXUAL DYSFUNCTION

Drug	Receptor Specificity	Therapeutic uses
β Blockers		
Propranolol	β_1, β_2	Hypertension Glaucoma Migraine Hyperthyroidism Angina pectoris Myocardial infarction
Timolol	β_1, β_2	Glaucoma Hypertension
Acebutolol Atenolol Metoprolol	β_1	Hypertension
Pindolol	β_1, β_2	Hypertension
Labetalol	β_1, β_2	Hypertension

Adverse effects commonly observed with β blockers

HYPOTENSION   BRADYCARDIA   FATIGUE   DROWSINESS

Figure 7.8
Summary of α- and β- adrenergic antagonists.

blood pressure in hypertensives, and a decrease in cardiac rate. [Note: There is also an accentuation of parasympathetic tone of the gastrointestinal tract.] *Guanethidine* also displaces norepinephrine from storage vesicles (thus producing a transient increase in blood pressure). This leads to gradual depletion of norepinephrine in the nerve ending.

2. **Therapeutic uses:** *Guanethidine* is used in the treatment of hypertension.

3. **Adverse effects:** *Guanethidine* commonly causes orthostatic hypotension and interferes with male sexual function.

C. Cocaine

Cocaine [koe KANE] is unique among local anesthetics (p.116) in having the ability to block the Na^+-K^+-activated ATPase (required for cellular uptake of norepinephrine) in the cell membrane of the adrenergic neuron (p.56). This block leads to accumulation of *norepinephrine* in the synaptic space, resulting in enhancement of sympathetic activity and potentiation of the actions of *epinephrine* and *norepinephrine.* Therefore, small doses of the catecholamines produce greatly magnified effects in an individual taking *cocaine* as compared to one who is not. In addition, the duration of action of *epinephrine* and *norepinephrine* is increased. *Cocaine* as a CNS stimulant and drug of abuse is discussed on p.104.

Figure 7.8 summarizes the α-and β-adrenergic agonists

Study Questions   (see p.410 for answers).

Answer A if 1,2 and 3 are correct.
    B if 1 and 3 are correct.
    C if 2 and 4 are correct.
    D if only 4 is correct.
    E if 1,2,3 and 4 are all correct.

7.1 Which of the following drugs decrease(s) airway resistance?

1. Epinephrine.
2. Prazosin.
3. Terbutaline.
4. Propranolol.

7.2 Systolic pressure is decreased after the injection of which of the following drugs?

1. Phenylephrine.
2. Dopamine.
3. Ephedrine.
4. Reserpine.

7.3 Which of the following no longer causes an increase in blood pressure after the chronic administration of reserpine?

1. Tyramine.
2. Ephedrine.
3. Amphetamine.
4. Norepinephrine.

7.4 In a cocaine abuser, which of the following drugs is ineffective in causing vascular actions?

1. Reserpine.
2. Tyramine.
3. Clonidine.
4. Guanethidine.

7.5 Which of the following drugs interferes with micturition in the elderly male?

1. Atropine.
2. Cocaine.
3. Ephedrine.
4. Amphetamine.

7.6 Which of the following dilate the pupil and decrease intraocular pressure?

1. Atropine.
2. Timolol.
3. Pilocarpine.
4. Phenylephrine.

7.7 Reflex bradycardia occurs by the use of which of the following drugs?

1. Phentolamine.
2. Phenylephrine.
3. Phenoxybenzamine.
4. Norepinephrine.

7.8 Which of the following drugs antagonize(s) the bronchodilating effects of isoproterenol?

1. Labetalol.
2. Phentolamine.
4. Propranolol.
3. Phenylephrine.

7.9 Which of the following groups of drugs is/are in correct order of DECREASING affinity for β receptors

1. Epinephrine > norepinephrine > isoproterenol.
2. Isoproterenol > epinephrine > norepinephrine.
3. Phenylephrine > epinephrine > terbutaline.
4. Propranolol > prazosin = phentolamine.

7.10 Which of the following drugs is useful in treating tachycardia?

1. Phenoxybenzamine.
2. Isoproterenol.
3. Phentolamine.
4. Propranolol.

7.11 Which of the following statements are true?

1. The administration of epinephrine after pretreatment with phenoxybenzamine causes vasodilation.
2. Blockage of α receptors with phentolamine can be overcome by increasing the concentration of agonist.
3. Atropine causes mydriasis by blocking the parasympathetic impulses to the sphincter muscle of the iris.
4. Guanethidine decreases the blood pressure response to amphetamine.

Treatment of Parkinson's Disease

8

I. OVERVIEW OF THE CNS

Most drugs that affect the central nervous system (CNS) act by altering some step in the neurotransmission process. Drugs affecting the CNS may act presynaptically by influencing the production, storage, or termination of action of neurotransmitters. Other agents may activate or block postsynaptic receptors. This chapter provides an overview of the CNS with a focus on those neurotransmitters that are involved in the actions of the clinically useful CNS drugs. These concepts are useful in understanding the etiology of and the treatment strategies for Parkinson's disease--a disorder caused by the death of a group of brain cells whose actions are mediated by the neurotransmitter dopamine. Figure 8.1 shows the drugs used in the treatment of Parkinson's disease.

II. NEUROTRANSMISSION IN THE CNS

A. Similarities to the autonomic nervous system

In many ways, the basic functioning of neurons in the CNS is similar to that of the autonomic nervous system described in Chapter 3. For example, transmission of information in the CNS and in the periphery both involve the release of neurotransmitters that diffuse across the synaptic space to bind to specific receptors on the postsynaptic neuron. In both systems, the recognition of the neurotransmitter by the membrane receptor of the postsynaptic neuron triggers intracellular changes (p.31).

B. Differences from the autonomic nervous system

Several major differences exist between neurons in the peripheral autonomic nervous system and those of the CNS. The circuitry of the CNS is much more complex than the autonomic nervous system, and the number of synapses in the CNS is far greater. The CNS, unlike the peripheral autonomic nervous system, contains powerful networks of inhibitory neurons that are constantly active in modulating the rate of neuronal transmission. In addition, the CNS communicates through the use of more than 10 (and perhaps as

---

ANTIPARKINSON'S DRUGS

- Levodopa
- Carbidopa
- Bromocriptine
- Amantadine
- Deprenyl
- Antimuscarinic agents

Figure 8.1
Summary of agents used in the treatment of Parkinson's disease.

CNS uses
many as 50) different neurotransmitters. In contrast, the autonomic
ANS system uses only two primary neurotransmitters, *acetylcholine* and
norepinephrine.

III. SYNAPTIC POTENTIALS

In the CNS, receptors at most synapses are coupled to ion channels, that is, binding of the neurotransmitter to the postsynaptic membrane receptors results in a rapid but transient opening of ion channels. Open channels allow ions inside and outside the cell membrane to flow down their concentration gradients. The resulting change in the ionic composition across the membrane of the neuron alters the post-synaptic potential, producing either depolarization or hyperpolarization of the postsynaptic membrane, depending on the specific ions that move and the direction of their movement.

A. Excitatory pathways

Neurotransmitters can be classified as excitatory or inhibitory, depending on the nature of the action they elicit. Stimulation of excitatory neurons causes a movement of ions that results in a depolarization of the postsynaptic membrane. These excitatory postsynaptic potentials (EPSP) are generated by several processes:

1. Stimulation of an excitatory neuron releases neurotransmitter molecules, such as norepinephrine or acetylcholine, which bind to receptors on the postsynaptic cell membrane. This causes a transient increase in the permeability of Na^+ ions.

2. The influx of sodium causes a weak depolarization or excitatory postsynaptic potential (EPSP).

3. If the number of excitatory fibers stimulated increases, more excitatory neurotransmitter is released, finally causing the EPSP depolarization of the postsynaptic cell to pass threshold, and an all-or-none action potential is generated. The generation of a nerve impulse typically reflects the activation of synaptic receptors by thousands of excitatory neurotransmitter molecules released from many nerve fibers. (See Figure 8.2 for an example of an excitatory pathway.)

B. Inhibitory pathways

Stimulation of inhibitory neurons causes movement of ions that results in a hyperpolarization of the postsynaptic membrane. These inhibitory postsynaptic potentials (IPSP) are generated by several processes:

1. Stimulation of inhibitory neurons releases neurotransmitter molecules, such as γ-aminobutyric acid (GABA) or glycine, which bind to receptors on the postsynaptic cell membrane. This causes a transient increase in the permeability of specific ions, such as, potassium and chloride ions.

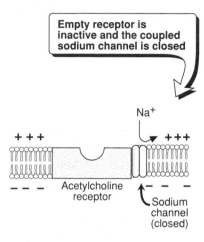

A. Receptor empty (no agonists)

Empty receptor is inactive and the coupled sodium channel is closed

Na^+

+ + +   + + +

– – – Acetylcholine
receptor
Sodium
channel
(closed)

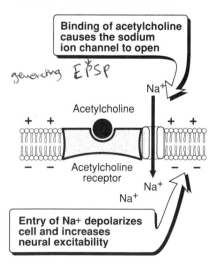

B. Receptor binding of excitatory neurotransmitter

Binding of acetylcholine causes the sodium ion channel to open

generating EPSP

Na^+

Acetylcholine

+ +   + +

– – Acetylcholine
receptor
Na^+

Na^+

Entry of Na+ depolarizes cell and increases neural excitability

Figure 8.2
Binding of excitatory neuro-transmitter, acetylcholine, causes depolarization of neuron.

2. The influx of chloride ions and efflux of potassium ions cause a weak hyperpolarization or inhibitory postsynaptic potential (IPSP), which moves the postsynaptic potential away from its firing threshold. This diminishes the generation of action potentials.

3. Most neurons in the CNS receive both EPSP and IPSP input. Thus, several different types of neurotransmitters may act on the same neuron, but each binds to its own specific receptor. The overall resultant action is due to the summation of the individual actions of the various neurotransmitters on the neuron. The neurotransmitters are not uniformly distributed in the CNS but are localized in specific clusters of neurons whose axons may synapse with specific regions of the brain. Many neuronal tracts thus seem to be chemically coded, and this may offer greater opportunity for selective modulation of certain neuronal pathways. (See Figure 8.3 for an example of an inhibitory pathway.)

IV. OVERVIEW OF PARKINSON'S DISEASE

Parkinsonism is a progressive disorder of muscle movement, characterized by tremors, muscular rigidity, bradykinesia (slowness in initiating and carrying out voluntary movements), and postural and gait abnormalities. Parkinson's disease is the fourth most common neurologic disorder among the elderly, affecting 500,000 people in the United States alone. Most cases involve people over the age of 65 among whom the incidence is about 1:100 individuals.

A. Etiology

The cause of Parkinson's disease is unknown for most patients. The disease is correlated with a reduction in the activity of inhibitory dopaminergic neurons in the substantia nigra and corpus striatum—parts of the brain's basal ganglia system, which is responsible for motor control. Genetic factors do not play a dominant role in the etiology of Parkinson's disease, although they may exert some influence on an individual's susceptibility to the disease. It appears increasingly likely that an unidentified environmental factor may be responsible for the loss of dopaminergic neurons.

1. **Substantia nigra:** The substantia nigra, part of the extrapyramidal system, is the source of dopaminergic neurons that terminate in the striatum (Figure 8.4). Each dopaminergic neuron makes thousands of synaptic contacts within the striatum and therefore modulates the activity of a large number of cells. These dopaminergic projections from the substantia nigra fire tonically, rather than in response to specific muscular movements or sensory input. Thus, the dopaminergic system appears to serve as a tonic, sustaining influence on motor activity, rather than participating in specific movements.

2. **Striatum:** Normally, the striatum is connected to the substantia nigra by neurons that secrete the inhibitory transmitter GABA at their termini in the substantia nigra. In turn, cells of the substantia nigra send neurons back to the striatum, secreting the inhibi-

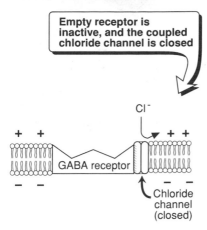

A. Receptor empty (no agonists)

Empty receptor is inactive, and the coupled chloride channel is closed

Cl⁻

GABA receptor

Chloride channel (closed)

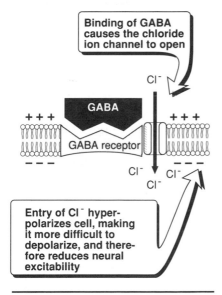

B. Receptor binding of inhibitory neurotransmitter

Binding of GABA causes the chloride ion channel to open

Cl⁻

GABA

GABA receptor

Cl⁻ Cl⁻ Cl⁻

Entry of Cl⁻ hyperpolarizes cell, making it more difficult to depolarize, and therefore reduces neural excitability

Figure 8.3
Binding of inhibitory neurotransmitter, γ=aminobutyric acid (GABA), causes hyperpolarization of neuron.

Sites of inhibition (-) or excitation (+) in the striatum and substantia nigra

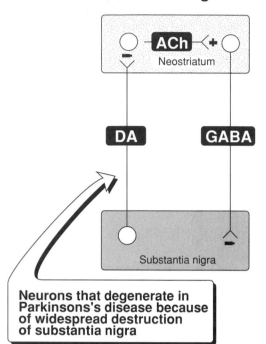

Neurons that degenerate in Parkinsons's disease because of widespread destruction of substantia nigra

Figure 8.4
Location of dopaminergic neurons deficient in Parkinson's disease. DA=dopamine; GABA= γ-amino-butyric acid; ACh=Acetylcholine.

tory transmitter dopamine at their termini. This mutual inhibitory pathway normally maintains a degree of inhibition of the two separate areas. Nerve fibers from the cerebral cortex and thalamus secrete acetylcholine in the neostriatum, causing excitatory effects that initiate and regulate gross intentional movements of the body.

3. **Secondary parkinsonism:** Parkinsonian symptoms infrequently follow viral encephalitis or multiple small vascular lesions. Drugs such as the phenothiazines and *haloperidol* (p.130), whose major pharmacologic action is blockade of dopamine receptors in the brain, may also produce parkinsonian symptoms. These drugs should not be used in parkinsonian patients.

B. Strategy of treatment

In addition to an abundance of inhibitory dopaminergic neurons, the neostriatum is also rich in excitatory cholinergic neurons, which oppose the action of dopamine (Figure 8.4). Many of the symptoms of parkinsonism reflect an imbalance between the excitatory cholinergic neurons and the greatly diminished number of inhibitory dopaminergic neurons. Therapy is aimed at restoring dopamine in the basal ganglia and antagonizing the excitatory effect of cholinergic neurons, thus reestablishing the correct dopamine/acetylcholine balance.

V. DRUGS USED IN PARKINSON'S DISEASE

Currently available drugs offer temporary relief from the symptoms of the disorder, but do not arrest or reverse the neuronal degeneration caused by the disease.

A. Levodopa (L-dopa) and carbidopa

Levodopa is a metabolic precursor of dopamine. It restores dopamine levels in the extrapyramidal centers (substantia nigra) that atrophy during parkinsonism. Relief provided by *levodopa* is only symptomatic and lasts only while the drug is present in the body.

1. **Mechanism of action:**

   a. **Levodopa:** Since parkinsonism results from insufficient dopamine in specific regions of the brain, attempts have been made to replenish the dopamine deficiency. Dopamine itself does not cross the blood-brain barrier, but its immediate precursor *levodopa* [lee voe DOE pa] is readily transported into the CNS and is converted to dopamine in the brain (Figure 8.5). Large doses of *levodopa* are required because much of the drug is decarboxylated to dopamine in the periphery (Figure 8.5) resulting in peripheral side effects (nausea, vomiting, cardiac arrhythmias, hypotension).

   b. **Carbidopa:** The effects of *levodopa* on the CNS can be greatly enhanced by coadministering *carbidopa* [kar bi DOE pa], a dopamine decarboxylase inhibitor that does not cross the blood-brain barrier. *Carbidopa* diminishes the metabolism of levodopa in the GI tract and peripheral tissues; thus, it increases the availability of *levodopa* to the CNS. The addition of *carbidopa* lowers the dose of *levodopa* needed by 4- to 5-fold and consequently decreases the severity of the side effects of peripherally formed dopamine.

2. **Actions:** *Levodopa* decreases the rigidity, tremors, and other symptoms of parkinsonism.

3. **Therapeutic uses:** *Levodopa* in combination with *carbidopa* is a potent and efficacious drug regimen currently available to treat Parkinson's disease. In approximately two thirds of patients with Parkinson's disease, *levodopa/carbidopa* treatment substantially reduces the severity of the disease for the first few years of treatment. Patients then typically experience a decline in response during the third to fifth year of therapy.

4. **Absorption and metabolism:** The drug is absorbed rapidly from the small intestine when empty of food. *Levodopa* has an extremely short half-life (1-2 hours), which causes fluctuations in plasma

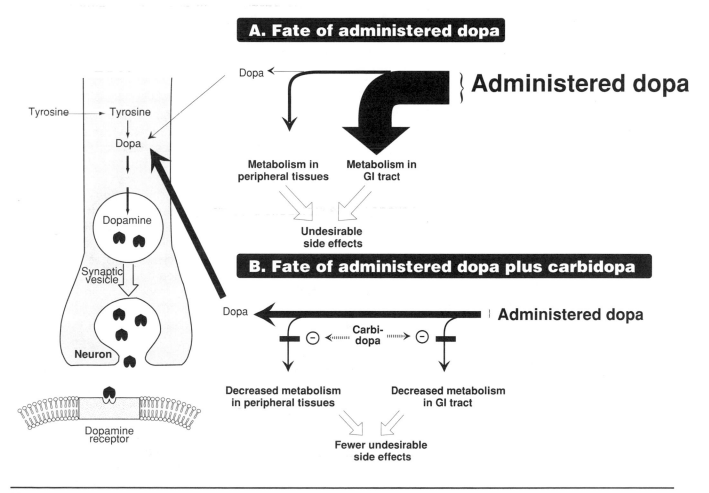

Figure 8.5
Synthesis of dopamine in the absence and presence of carbidopa, an inhibitor of dopamine decarboxlylase in the peripheral tissues.

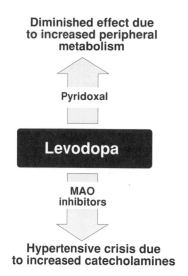

Figure 8.6
Some drug interactions observed with levodopa.

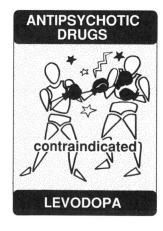

concentration. This may produce fluctuations in motor response ("on-off" phenomenon) which may cause the patient to suddenly lose normal mobility and experience tremors, cramps, and immobility. Ingestion of meals, particularly if high in protein content, interferes with the transport of *levodopa* into the CNS. Large, neutral amino acids (e.g., leucine and isoleucine) compete with *levodopa* for absorption from the gut and for transport across the blood-brain barrier. Withdrawal from the drug must be gradual.

5. **Adverse effects:**

   a. **Peripheral effects:** Anorexia, nausea, and vomiting occur because of stimulation of the emetic center. Tachycardia and ventricular extrasystoles result from dopaminergic action on the heart. Hypotension may also develop. Adrenergic action on the iris causes mydriasis, and in some individuals, blood dyscrasias and a positive reaction to Coombs' test are seen. Saliva and urine are a brownish color because of the melanin pigment produced from catecholamine oxidation.

   b. **CNS effects:** Visual and auditory hallucinations and abnormal involuntary movements (dyskinesia) may occur. These CNS effects are the opposite of parkinsonian symptoms and reflect the overactivity of dopamine at receptors in the basal ganglia. *Levodopa* can also cause mood changes, depression, and anxiety.

6. **Interactions:** The vitamin pyridoxine (B_6) increases the peripheral breakdown of *levodopa* and diminishes its effectiveness (Figure 8.7). Concomitant administration of *levodopa* and monoamine oxidase (MAO) inhibitors, such as *deprenyl* (p. 89) produce a hypertensive crisis caused by enhanced catecholamine production; therefore, caution is required when they are used simultaneously. In many psychotic patients, *levodopa* exacerbates symptoms, possibly through the buildup of central amines. In patients with glaucoma, the drug can cause an increase in intraocular pressure. Cardiac patients should be carefully monitored, because of the possible development of cardiac arrhythmias. Antipsychotic drugs are contraindicated in parkinsonian patients, since these block dopamine receptors and produce a parkinsonian syndrome themselves.

B. Bromocriptine

Bromocriptine [broh moh KRIP teen], an ergotamine derivative, acts as a dopamine receptor agonist. The drug produces little response in patients that do not react to *levodopa*. It is often used with *levodopa* in patients responding to drug therapy. The dose is increased gradually during a period of 2-3 months. Side effects severely limit the utility of the dopamine agonists. The actions of *bromocriptine* are similar to those of *levodopa*, except that hallucination, confusion, delirium, nausea, and orthostatic hypotension are more common, whereas dyskinesia is less prominent. In psychiatric illness, *bromocriptine* causes the mental condition to worsen. Serious cardiac problems may develop, particularly in patients with a history of myocardial infarction. In patients with peripheral vascular disease, a worsening of the vasospasm occurs, and in patients with peptic ulcer, there is also a worsening of the ulcer.

C. Amantadine

It was accidentally discovered that the antiviral drug, *amantadine* [a MAN ta deen], effective in the treatment of influenza (p.329), has antiparkinsonism action. It appears to enhance the synthesis, release, or re-uptake of dopamine from the surviving nigral neurons. [Note: If dopamine release is already at a maximum, *amantadine* has no effect.] The drug may cause restlessness, agitation, confusion, and hallucination, and at high doses, it may induce acute toxic psychosis. Orthostatic hypotension, urinary retention, peripheral edema, and dry mouth may also occur. *Amantadine* is less efficacious than *levodopa,* but it has fewer side effects. The drug has little effect on tremor but is more effective than the anticholinergics against rigidity and bradykinesia.

D. Deprenyl

Deprenyl [de PREN al] selectively inhibits monoamine oxidase B which metabolizes dopamine, but does not inhibit monoamine oxidase A which metabolizes *norepinephrine* and serotonin. By thus decreasing the metabolism of dopamine, *deprenyl* has been found to increase dopamine levels in the brain (Figure 8.7). Therefore, it enhances the actions of *levodopa,* and when these drugs are administered together, *deprenyl* substantially reduces the required dose of *levodopa.* However, combined use of these agent must be avoided because hypertensive crisis may arise. Recent data suggest that early use of *deprenyl* may actually prolong the period before severe symptoms set in by as much as 50%.

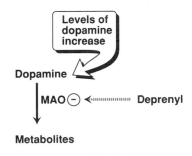

Figure 8.7
Action of deprenyl in dopamine metabolism.

E. Antimuscarinic agents

The antimuscarinic agents are much less efficacious than *levodopa,* and these drugs play only an adjuvant role in antiparkinsonism therapy. The actions of *atropine, scopolamine, benztropine, trihexyphenidyl,* and *biperiden* are similar, although individual patients may respond more favorably to one drug. All these drugs can induce mood changes. They produce xerostomia (dryness of the mouth) and visual problems as do all muscarinic blockers. They interfere with gastrointestinal peristalsis and cannot be used in patients with glaucoma, prostatic hypertrophy, or pyloric stenosis. Blockage of cholinergic transmission produces effects similar to augmentation of dopaminergic transmission (again, because of the creation of an imbalance in the dopamine/acetylcholine ratio). Adverse effects are similar to those caused by high doses of *atropine* (p.45), e.g., pupillary dilation, confusion, hallucination, urinary retention, and dry mouth.

Study Questions   (see p.412 for answers).

Choose the ONE best answer.

8.1 Which of the following statements is correct?

  A. Chlorpromazine is indicated in treating the
     nausea of levodopa treatment.
  B. Vitamin B$_6$ increases the effectiveness of
     levodopa.
  C. Administration of dopamine is an effective
     treatment of Parkinson's disease.
  D. Levodopa-induced nausea is reduced by
     carbidopa.
  E. Nonspecific MAO-inhibitors, such as
     phenelzine, are a useful adjunct to levodopa
     therapy.

8.2 Which of the following statements is INCORRECT?

  A. Parkinsonian patients are characterized by
     increased ratio of dopaminergic/cholinergic
     activity in the neostriatum.
  B. Overtreatment of Parkinson's disease can result
     in the symptoms of psychosis.
  C. Diets rich in protein may decrease the effects of
     L-dopa.
  D. Dyskinesia is the most important side effect of
     L-dopa.
  E. Treatment with deprenyl can delay the onset of
     parkinsonian symptoms.

8.3 All of the following statements are correct EXCEPT

  A. Atropine blocks cholinergic pathway in the
     neostriatum.
  B. Deprenyl inhibits monoamine oxidase B and
     increases dopamine levels in the brain.
  C. Bromocriptine directly activates dopaminergic
     receptors.
  D. Amantadine inhibits the metabolism of
     levodopa.
  E. Antimuscarinic agents are generally less
     efficacious then levodopa in the treatment of
     Parkinson's disease.

Anxiolytic and Hypnotic Drugs

I. OVERVIEW

Anxiety is an unpleasant state of tension, apprehension, or uneasiness—a fear that seems to arise from an unknown source. Disorders involving anxiety are the most common mental disturbances. The symptoms of severe anxiety are similar to those of fear (such as tachycardia, sweating, trembling, palpitations) and involve sympathetic activation. Episodes of mild anxiety are common life experiences and do not warrant treatment. However, the symptoms of severe, chronic, debilitating anxiety may be treated with antianxiety drugs (sometimes called anxiolytic or minor tranquilizers), and/or some form of psycho- or behavioral therapy.

Since all the antianxiety drugs also cause some sedation, the same drugs often function clinically as both anxiolytic and hypnotic (sleep-inducing) agents. Until recently, the barbiturates and related compounds were used at low doses for anxiolytic effects and at higher doses to promote sleep. Overdoses of these agents cause unconsciousness and often death from respiratory depression. The introduction of the benzodiazepines in 1961 provided a group of anxiolytic drugs without the graded depression of the CNS caused by barbiturates. The benzodiazepines have quickly replaced many of the early anxiolytic and hypnotic agents. Figure 9.1 summarizes the anxiolytic and hypnotic agents.

II. BENZODIAZEPINES

Benzodiazepines are the most widely used anxiolytic drugs. They have largely replaced barbiturates and *meprobamate* (p.98) in the treatment of anxiety, since the benzodiazepines are more effective and safer (Figure 9.2). All the benzodiazepines share the same unusual structure, that is, a 7-membered ring containing two nitrogens that are sandwiched between two aromatic rings (Figure 9.3). Approximately 20 benzodiazepine derivatives that have different substituent groups are currently clinically useful.

A. Mode of action

1. **Inhibitory action of γ-aminobutyric acid (GABA):** Benzodiazepines bind to specific, high affinity sites on the cell membrane, which

---

ANXIOLYTIC AND HYPNOTIC DRUGS

BENZODIAZEPINES

- Clorazepate
- Chlordiazepoxide
- Diazepam
- Flurazepam
- Quazepam
- Alprazolam
- Lorazepam
- Temazepam
- Oxazepam
- Triazolam

OTHER ANXIOLYTIC DRUGS

- Buspirone
- Hydroxyzine
- Ethanol

BARBITURATES

- Phenobarbital
- Pentobarbital
- Secobarbital
- Amobarbital
- Thiopental

NONBARBITURATE SEDATIVES

- Chloral hydrate
- Glutethimide
- Meprobamate
- Antihistamine

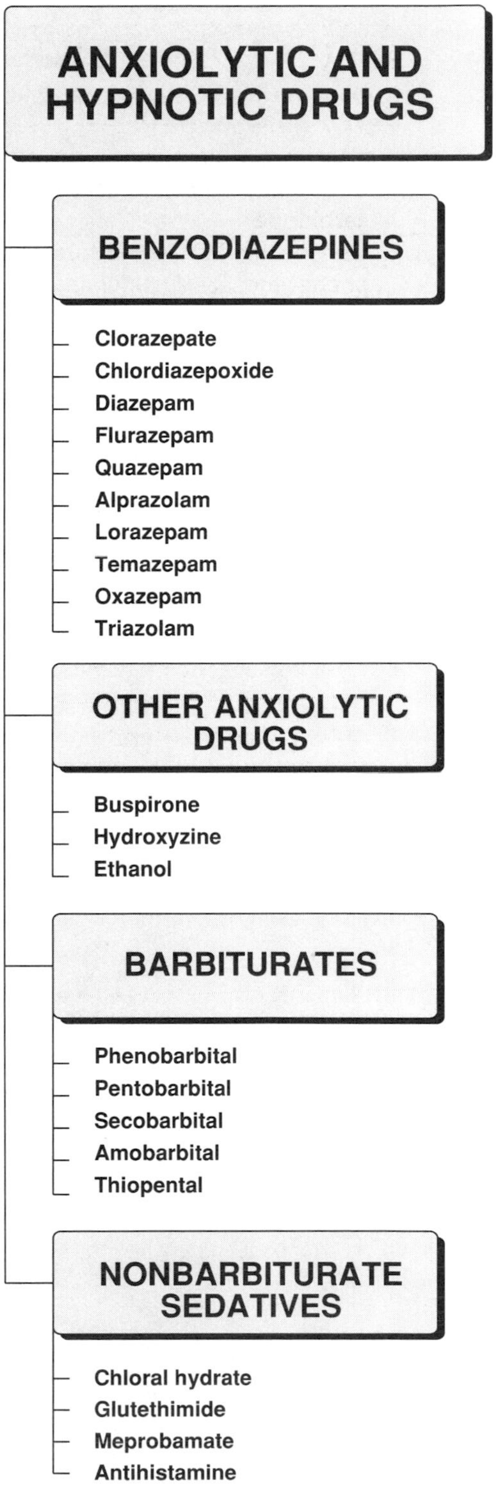

Figure 9.1
Summary of anxiolytic and hypnotic drugs.

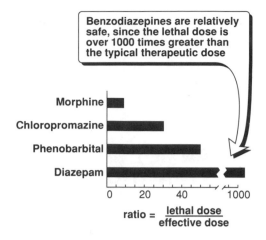

Figure 9.2
Ratio of lethal dose to effective dose for morphine (an opioid, Chapter 14), chlorpromazine (a neuroleptic, Chapter 13), and the anxiolytic, hypnotic drugs, phenobarbital and diazepam.

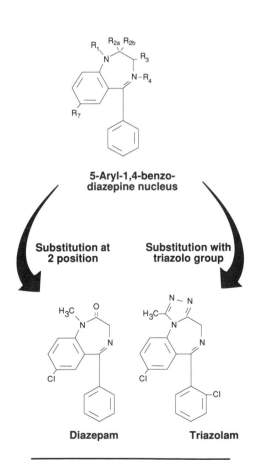

Figure 9.3
Structural formulas of two clinically useful benzodiazepines.

are separate from but adjacent to the receptor for GABA. Binding of GABA to its receptor triggers an opening of a chloride channel, which leads to an increase in chloride conductance (Figure 9.4). The influx of chloride ions causes a small hyperpolarization that moves the postsynaptic potential away from its firing threshold and thus inhibits the formation of action potentials (p.84).

2. **Effects of benzodiazepines on GABA:** The binding of benzodiazepines enhances the affinity of GABA receptors for this neurotransmitter, resulting in a more frequent opening of adjacent chloride channels (Figure 9.4). This in turn results in enhanced hyperpolarization and further inhibition of neuronal firing.

3. **The benzodiazepine receptor:** These receptors are found only in the CNS, and their location parallels that of the GABA neurons. Benzodiazepines and GABA mutually increase the affinity of their binding sites without actually changing the total number of sites. The clinical effects of the various benzodiazepines correlate well with each drug's binding affinity for the GABA receptor-chloride ion channel complex.

B. Actions

The benzodiazepines have no antipsychotic activity nor any analgesic action and do not affect the autonomic nervous system. All the benzodiazepines exhibit the following actions to a greater or lesser extent:

1. **Reduction of anxiety:** At low doses, the benzodiazepines are anxiolytic. They are thought to reduce anxiety by selectively inhibiting neuronal circuits in the limbic system of the brain.

2. **Sedative and hypnotic actions:** All the benzodiazepines used to treat anxiety have some sedative properties. At higher doses, certain benzodiazepines produce hypnosis.

3. **Anticonvulsant:** Several of the benzodiazepines have anticonvulsant activity and are used to treat epilepsy.

4. **Muscle relaxant:** The benzodiazepines relax the spasticity of skeletal muscle, probably by increasing presynaptic inhibition in the spinal cord.

C. Therapeutic uses

The individual benzodiazepines show small differences in their relative anxiolytic, anticonvulsant, and sedative properties. However, the duration of action varies widely among this group, and pharmacokinetics are often important in selecting the drug of choice.

1. **Anxiety disorders:** The benzodiazepines are useful in treating the anxiety that accompanies some forms of depression and schizophrenia. These drugs should not be used to alleviate the normal

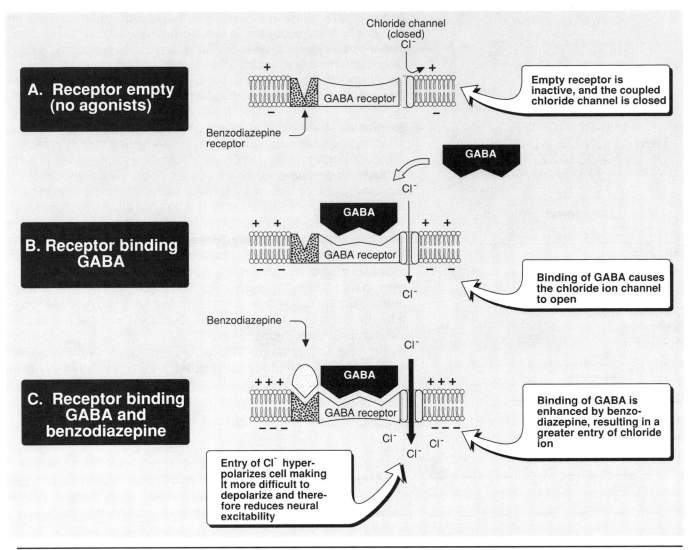

Figure 9.4
Schematic diagram of benzodiazepine-GABA-chloride ion channel complex. GABA= γ–aminobutyric acid.

stress of everyday life, but should be reserved for continued severe anxiety, and then should only be used for short periods of time because of addiction liability. The longer acting agents such as *diazepam* [dye AZ e pam], are often preferred since anxiety may require treatment for prolonged periods of time. The antianxiety effects of the benzodiazepines are less subject to tolerance than the sedative and hypnotic effects. For panic disorders, *alprazolam* [al PRAY zoe lam] is effective for short- and long-term treatment, although it may cause withdrawal reactions in about 30% of sufferers.

2. **Muscular disorder:** *Diazepam* is useful in the treatment of skeletal muscle spasms such as occur in muscle strain, and in treating spasticity from degenerative disorders, such as multiple sclerosis and cerebral palsy.

3. **Seizures:** *Clonazepam* is useful in the chronic treatment of epilepsy, whereas *diazepam* is the drug of choice in terminating grand mal epileptic seizures and status epilepticus (p.150). *Chlordiazepoxide* [klor di az e POX ide], *clorazepate* [klor AZ e pate], *diazepam*, and *oxazepam* [ox A ze pam] are useful in the acute treatment of alcohol withdrawal.

4. **Sleep disorders:** Not all the benzodiazepines are useful as hypnotic agents, although all have sedative or calming effects. *Lorazepam* [lor A ze pam], *temazepam* [tem AZ e pam], and *triazolam* [trye AY zoe lam] have relatively short durations of action and are therefore used to induce sleep in patients with recurring insomnia. *Temazepam* is useful for insomnia caused by the inability to stay asleep, whereas *triazolam* is effective in treating individuals who have difficulty in going to sleep. Tolerance often develops within a few days. Withdrawal of the drug often results in rebound insomnia (particularly with *triazolam*), leading the patient to demand another prescription. These drugs are best used intermittently, rather than daily. *Flurazepam* [flure AZ e pam] significantly reduces both sleep-induction time and the number of awakenings, and increases the duration of sleep. *Flurazepam* has a long-acting effect (Figure 9.5) and causes little rebound insomnia. With continued use, the drug has been shown to maintain its effectiveness for up to 4 weeks.

D. Pharmacology

1. **Absorption and distribution:** The lipophilic benzodiazepines are rapidly and completely absorbed after oral administration and are distributed throughout the body.

2. **Duration of actions:** The half-lives of the benzodiazepines are very important clinically, since the duration of action may determine the therapeutic usefulness. The benzodiazepines can be roughly divided into short-, intermediate- and long-acting groups (Figure 9.5). The longer acting agents form active metabolites with long half-lives.

3. **Fate:** Most benzodiazepines, including *chlordiazepoxide* and *diazepam*, are metabolized by the hepatic microsomal metabolizing system (p. 12) to compounds that are also active. For these benzodiazepines, the apparent half-life of the drug represents the combined actions of the parent drug and its metabolites. The benzodiazepines are excreted in urine as glucuronides or oxidized metabolites.

E. Dependence

Psychological and physical dependence on benzodiazepines can develop if high doses of the drug are given over a prolonged period. Abrupt discontinuation of the benzodiazepines results in withdrawal symptoms, including confusion, anxiety, agitation, restlessness, insomnia, and tension. Because of the long half-lives of some of the benzodiazepines, withdrawal symptoms may not occur until a number of days after discontinuation of therapy. Ben-

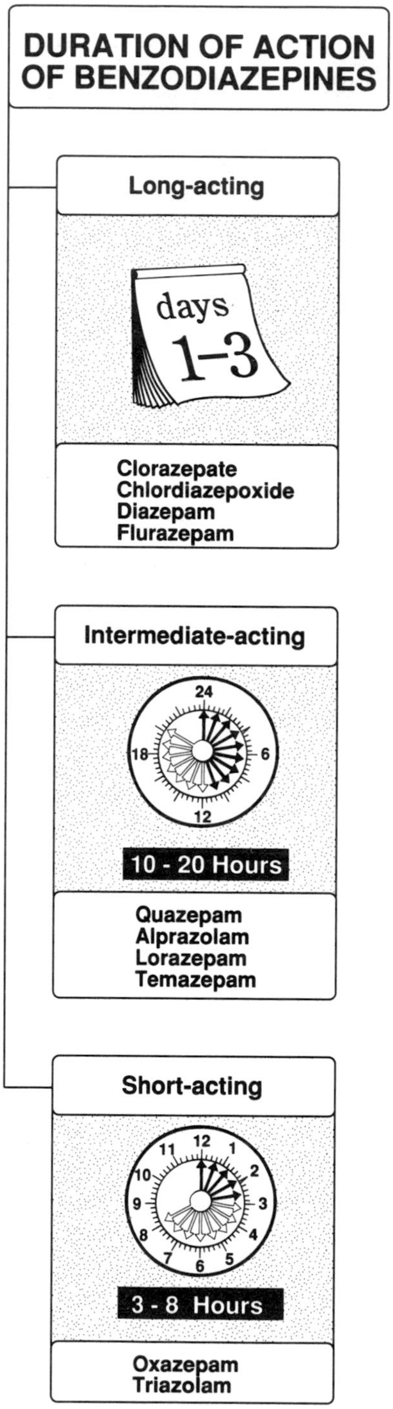

DURATION OF ACTION OF BENZODIAZEPINES

Long-acting

days 1-3

Clorazepate
Chlordiazepoxide
Diazepam
Flurazepam

Intermediate-acting

10 - 20 Hours

Quazepam
Alprazolam
Lorazepam
Temazepam

Short-acting

3 - 8 Hours

Oxazepam
Triazolam

Figure 9.5
Comparison of the durations of action of the benzodiazepines.

zodiazepines with a short elimination half-life, such as *triazolam* and *temazepam*, induce more abrupt and severe withdrawal reactions than those seen with drugs that are slowly eliminated, such as *flurazepam* (Figure 9.6).

F. Adverse effects

1. **Drowsiness and confusion:** These effects are the two most common side effects of the benzodiazepines. Ataxia occurs at high doses and precludes activities that require fine motor coordination, such as driving an automobile. Cognitive impairment (decreased long-term recall and acquisition of new knowledge) can occur with use of benzodiazepines. *Triazolam*, the benzodiazepine with the most rapid elimination, often shows a rapid development of tolerance, early morning insomnia and daytime anxiety along with amnesia and confusion.

2. **Precautions:** Use benzodiazepines cautiously in treating patients with liver disease. They potentiate alcohol and other CNS depressants. Benzodiazepines are, however, considerably less dangerous than other anxiolytic and hypnotic drugs. As a result, drug overdose is seldom lethal, unless other central depressants, such as alcohol, are taken concurrently.

III. OTHER ANXIOLYTIC AGENTS

A. Buspirone

Buspirone [byoo SPYE rone] is useful in the treatment of generalized anxiety disorders and has an efficacy comparable to the benzodiazepines. The actions of *buspirone* appear to be mediated by serotonin (5-HT$_{1A}$) receptors, although other receptors could be involved, since *buspirone* displays some affinity for DA$_2$ dopamine receptors and 5-HT$_2$ serotonin receptors. The mode of action thus differs from that of the benzodiazepines. Further, *buspirone* lacks anticonvulsant and muscle-relaxant properties of the benzodiazepines and causes only minimal sedation. The frequency of adverse effects is low, and the most common effects are headaches, dizziness, nervousness, and lightheadness. Sedation and psychomotor and cognitive dysfunction are minimal, and dependence is unlikely. *Buspirone* has the disadvantage of a slow onset of action. The drug has lower interactive effects with other CNS depressants.

B. Hydroxyzine

Hydroxyzine [hye DROX i zeen] is an antihistamine with antiemetic activity. It has a low tendency for habituation; thus it is useful for patients with anxiety, who have a history of drug abuse. It is also often used for sedation in dental patients.

C. Ethanol

Ethanol (ethyl alcohol) has antianxiety and sedative effects, but its toxic potential outweighs its benefits. Ethanol [ETH an ol] is a CNS

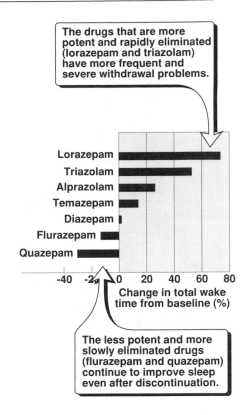

Figure 9.6
Frequency of rebound insomnia resulting from discontinuation of benzodiazepine therapy.

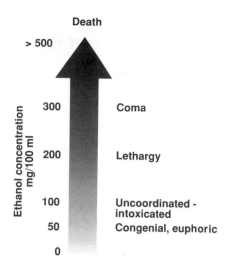

Figure 9.7
Effects of various levels of alcohol in the blood.

depressant, producing sedation and ultimately hypnosis with increasing dosage. Ethanol has a shallow dose-response curve; therefore, sedation occurs over a wide dosage range. Coma and death occur at blood concentrations of above 100 mM or 460 mg/100 ml (Figure 9.7). The effects of acute ethanol intoxication include the loss of inhibitions, increased self-confidence, slurred speech, and euphoria. At higher dosage, intellectual and motor performances are impaired. Chronic ingestion of ethanol results in fatty liver, jaundice, and cirrhosis, which is a common cause of death in alcoholics. Alcohol synergizes with many other sedative agents and can produce severe CNS depression with antihistamines or barbiturates.

1. **Disulfiram:** Ethanol is metabolized primarily in the liver, first to acetaldehyde by alcohol dehydrogenase, and then to acetate by aldehyde dehydrogenase. *Disulfiram* [dye SUL fi ram] blocks the oxidation of acetaldehyde to acetic acid by inhibiting aldehyde dehydrogenase (Figure 9.8). This results in the accumulation of acetaldehyde in the blood, causing flushing, tachycardia, hyperventilation, and nausea. *Disulfiram* has found some use in the patient seriously desiring to stop alcohol ingestion. A conditioned avoidance response is induced so that the patient abstains from alcohol to prevent the unpleasant effects of *disulfiram*-induced acetaldehyde accumulation.

IV. BARBITURATES

The barbiturates were formerly the mainstay of treatment used to sedate the nervous system or to induce and maintain sleep. Today, they have been largely replaced by the benzodiazepines, mainly because barbiturates induce tolerance, drug-metabolizing enzymes, physical dependence, and very severe withdrawal symptoms. Foremost is their ability to cause coma in toxic doses. Certain barbiturates, such as *thiopental,* are still used to induce anesthesia (p.114).

A. Mode of action

Barbiturates are thought to interfere with sodium and potassium transport across cell membranes. This leads to inhibition of the mesencephalic reticular activating system. Polysynaptic transmission is inhibited in all areas of the CNS. Barbiturates also potentiate GABA action on chloride entry into the neuron, although they do not bind at the benzodiazepine receptor.

B. Actions

Barbiturates are classified according to their duration of action (Figure 9.9). For example, *thiopental* [thye oh PEN tal], which acts within seconds and has a duration of action of about 30 minutes, is used in the intravenous induction of anesthesia (p.114). By contrast, *phenobarbital* [fee noe BAR bi tal], which has a duration of action greater than a day, is useful in the treatment of seizures (p.148). *Pentobarbital* [pen toe BAR bi tal], *secobarbital* [see koe BAR bi tal] and *amobarbital* [am oh BAR bi tal] are short-acting barbiturates, which are effective as sedative and hypnotic (but not antianxiety) agents.

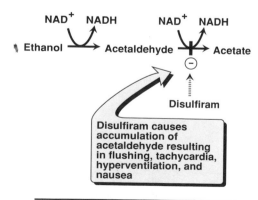

Figure 9.8
Metabolism of ethanol.

1. **Depression of CNS:** At low doses, the barbiturates produce sedation (calming effect, reducing excitement). At higher doses, the drug causes hypnosis (artificially-produced sleep), followed by anesthesia (loss of feeling or sensation), and finally coma and death. Thus, any degree of depression of the CNS is possible, depending on the dose. Barbiturates do not raise the pain threshold and have no analgesic properties. They may even exacerbate pain.

2. **Respiratory depression:** Barbiturates suppress the hypoxic and chemoreceptor response to CO_2, and overdosage is followed by respiratory depression and death.

3. **Enzyme induction:** Barbiturates induce P-450 microsomal enzymes in the liver (p.12). Therefore, chronic barbiturate administration diminishes the action of many drugs that are dependent on P-450 metabolism to reduce their concentration.

C. Therapeutic uses

1. **Anesthesia:** Selection of a barbiturate is strongly influenced by the desired duration of action. The ultra–short-acting barbiturates, such as *thiopental,* are used intravenously to induce surgical anesthesia.

2. **Anticonvulsant:** *Phenobarbital* is used in long-term management of tonic-clonic seizures, status epilepticus, and eclampsia. *Phenobarbital* has been regarded as the drug of choice for treatment of young children with febrile seizures. However, *phenobarbital* can depress cognitive performance in children treated for febrile seizures, and the drug should be used cautiously. *Phenobarbital* has specific anticonvulsant activity that is distinguished from the nonspecific CNS depression.

3. **Anxiety:** Barbiturates have been used as mild sedatives to relieve anxiety, nervous tension, and insomnia. Most have been replaced by the benzodiazepines.

D. Pharmacology

1. **Absorption and distribution:** Barbiturates are absorbed orally and distributed widely throughout the body. All barbiturates redistribute in the body from the brain to the splanchnic areas, to skeletal muscle, and finally to adipose tissue. This movement is important in causing the short duration of action of *thiopental* and similar short-acting derivatives (p.114).

2. **Fate:** Barbiturates are metabolized in the liver and inactive metabolites are excreted in the urine.

E. Adverse effects

1. **CNS:** Barbiturates cause drowsiness, impaired concentration, and mental and physical sluggishness.

2. **Drug hangover:** Hypnotic doses of barbiturates produce a feeling of tiredness well after the patient awakes. This drug hangover

---

DURATION OF ACTION OF BARBITURATES

Long-acting

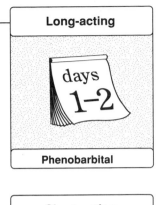

days 1-2

Phenobarbital

Short-acting

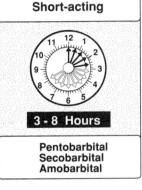

3 - 8 Hours

Pentobarbital
Secobarbital
Amobarbital

Ultra-short-acting

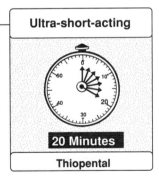

20 Minutes

Thiopental

Figure 9.9
Barbiturates classified according to their duration of actions.

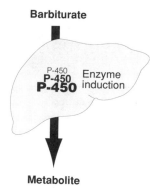

Barbiturate

P-450 Enzyme induction

Metabolite

leads to impaired ability to function normally for many hours after waking. Occasionally, nausea and dizziness occur.

3. **Precautions:** Barbiturates induce the P-450 system, increase porphyrin synthesis, and are contraindicated in patients with acute intermittent porphyria.

4. **Addiction:** Abrupt withdrawal from barbiturates may cause tremors, anxiety, weakness, restlessness, nausea and vomiting, seizures, delirium, and cardiac arrest. Withdrawal is much more severe than that associated with opiates and can result in death.

5. **Poisoning:** Barbiturate poisoning has been a leading cause of death among suicides for many decades. Severe depression of respiration is coupled with central cardiovascular depression, and results in a shock-like condition with shallow, infrequent breathing. Treatment includes artificial respiration and purging the stomach of its contents if the drug has been taken recently. Hemodialysis may be necessary if large quantities have been taken. Alkalinization of the urine often aids in the elimination of *phenobarbital.*

V. NONBARBITURATE SEDATIVES

A. Chloral hydrate

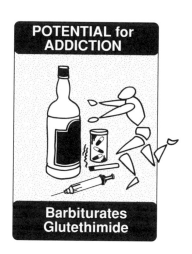

POTENTIAL for ADDICTION

Barbiturates Glutethimide

Chloral hydrate [KLOR al HYE drate] is a trichlorinated derivative of acetaldehyde that is converted to trichloroethanol in the body. The drug is an effective sedative and hypnotic that induces sleep in about 30 minutes and lasts about 6 hours. *Chloral hydrate* is irritating to the gastrointestinal tract and causes epigastric distress. It also produces an unusual, unpleasant taste sensation.

B. Glutethimide

Glutethimide [gloo TETH i mide] produces an effect ranging from sedation to hypnosis, depending on the dose. It has addiction liability and severe withdrawal symptoms. Like the barbiturates, tolerance develops. The drug has strong anticholinergic activity manifested by xerostomia, inhibition of gastrointestinal motility, and mydriasis.

C. Meprobamate

Meprobamate [me proe BA mate] was the first of the modern antianxiety drugs. It is less effective than the benzodiazepines in the treatment of anxiety. It rarely causes hypnosis even at high doses. It depresses polysynaptic reflexes in the spinal cord, causing skeletal muscle relaxation and weak analgesia in musculo-skeletal disorders.

D. Antihistamines

Nonprescription antihistamines such as *diphenhydramine, doxylamine,* and *pyrilamine* are effective in treating some types of in-

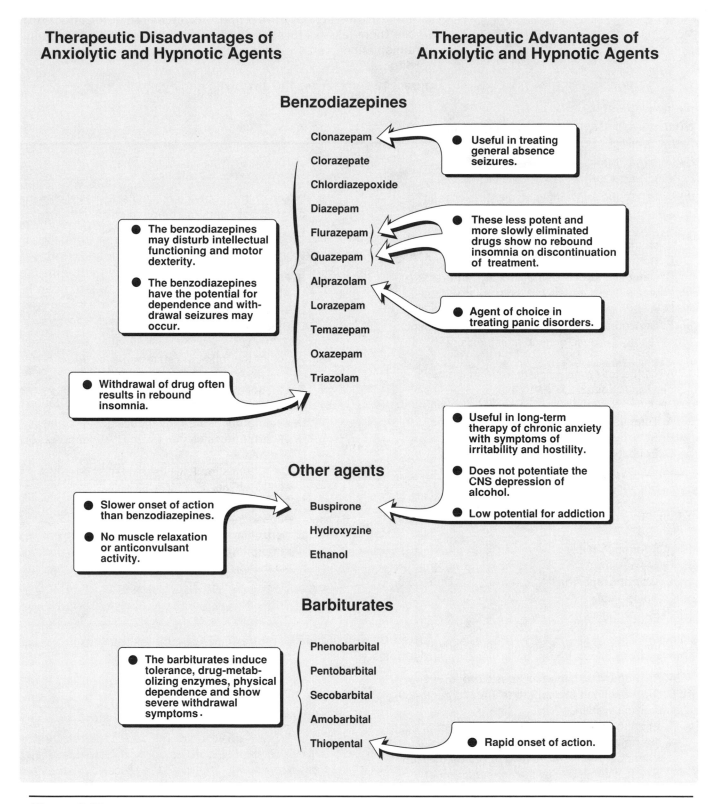

Figure 9.10
Therapeutic disadvantages and advantages of some anxiolytic and hypnotic agents.

somnia. However, they have numerous undesirable side effects that make them less useful than the benzodiazepines. These sedative antihistamines are marketed in numerous over-the-counter products.

Figure 9.10 summarizes the anxiolytic and hypnotic drugs.

Study Questions   (see p. 412 for answers).

Choose the ONE best answer.

9.1 Which of the following statements is correct?

A. Benzodiazepines directly open chloride channels.
B. Benzodiazepines show analgesic actions.
C. Clinical improvement of anxiety requires 2-4 weeks of treatment with benzodiazepines.
D. All benzodiazepines have some sedative effects.
E. Benzodiazepines, like other CNS depressants, readily produce general anesthesia.

9.2 All of the following respond to treatment with benzodiazepines EXCEPT:

A. Tetanus.
B. Schizophrenia.
C. Epileptic seizure.
D. Insomnia.
E. Anxiety.

9.3 Which of the following is a short-acting hypnotic?

A. Phenobarbital.
B. Diazepam.
C. Chlordiazepoxide.
D. Thiopental.
E. Flurazepam.

9.4 Which of the following statements is correct?

A. Phenobarbital shows analgesic properties.
B. Diazepam and phenobarbital induce the P-450 enzyme system.
C. Phenobarbital is useful in the treatment of acute intermittent porphyria.
D. Phenobarbital induces respiratory depression, which is enhanced by the consumption of ethanol.
E. Buspirone has actions similar to the benzodiazepines.

9.5 Which of the following benzodiazepines shows the greatest potential for "rebound insomnia" after discontinuance of long-term treatment?

A. Triazolam.
B. Flurazepam.
C. Alprazolam.
D. Temazepam.
E. Diazepam.

9.6 Which of the following statements is correct?

A. Ethanol at intoxicating levels shows first-order metabolism.
B. Respiratory depression induced by high doses of barbiturates can be treated by administration of ethanol.
C. Disulfiram stimulates the oxidation of acetaldehyde.
D. Benzodiazepines do not cause physical dependence.
E. Benzodiazepines can be used to treat the symptoms of withdrawal in the chronic alcoholic.

CNS Stimulants

10

I. OVERVIEW

Drugs that primarily stimulate the central nervous system (CNS) can be divided into three broad groups (Figure 10.1). Psychomotor stimulants cause excitement and euphoria, decrease feelings of fatigue, and increase motor activity. The second category, convulsants and respiratory stimulants, have minimal effect on mental function but produce exaggerated reflex responses, increased activity in the respiratory and vasomotor centers, and convulsions at high doses. The third group, hallucinogens, produce profound changes in thought patterns and mood, with little effect on the brainstem and spinal cord. Many of the CNS stimulants can cause mood-altering states when taken in high doses for nonmedical purposes. As a group, the psychomotor stimulants have few clinical uses, but they are important as drugs of abuse, along with the CNS depressants described in Chapter 9, and the narcotics described in Chapter 14 (Figure 10.2).

II. PSYCHOMOTOR STIMULANTS

A. Methylxanthines

Methylxanthines include *theophylline* [thee OFF i lin] found in tea, *theobromine* [thee o BRO min] found in cocoa, and *caffeine* [kaf EEN]. *Caffeine*, the most widely consumed stimulant in the world, is found in highest concentration in coffee but is also present in tea, cola drinks, chocolate candy, and cocoa.

1. **Mechanism of action:** The methylxanthines may act by several mechanisms, including translocation of extracellular calcium, increase in cyclic AMP and cyclic GMP caused by inhibition of phosphodiesterase, and blockade of adenosine receptors.

2. **Actions:**

   a. **Central nervous system:** The spinal cord is stimulated only by very high doses (2-5 g) of *caffeine*. The *caffeine* contained in

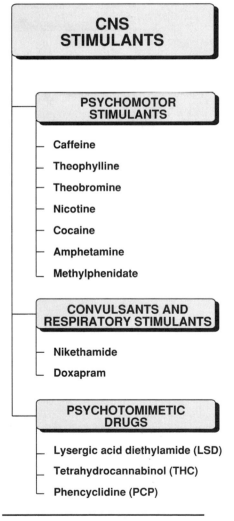

CNS STIMULANTS

PSYCHOMOTOR STIMULANTS
- Caffeine
- Theophylline
- Theobromine
- Nicotine
- Cocaine
- Amphetamine
- Methylphenidate

CONVULSANTS AND RESPIRATORY STIMULANTS
- Nikethamide
- Doxapram

PSYCHOTOMIMETIC DRUGS
- Lysergic acid diethylamide (LSD)
- Tetrahydrocannabinol (THC)
- Phencyclidine (PCP)

Figure 10.1
Summary of CNS stimulants.

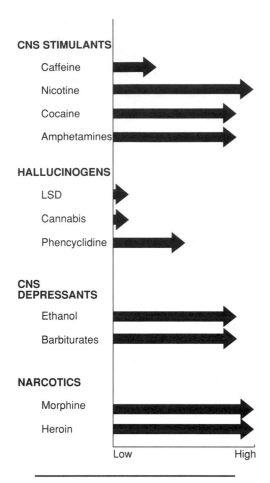

CNS STIMULANTS
- Caffeine
- Nicotine
- Cocaine
- Amphetamines

HALLUCINOGENS
- LSD
- Cannabis
- Phencyclidine

CNS DEPRESSANTS
- Ethanol
- Barbiturates

NARCOTICS
- Morphine
- Heroin

Low   High

Figure 10.2
Relative potential for dependence for commonly abused substances.

one to two cups of coffee (100-200 mg) causes a decrease in fatigue and increased mental alertness as a result of stimulating the cortex and other areas of the brain. Consumption of 1.5 grams of *caffeine* (12-15 cups of coffee) produces anxiety and tremors.

b. **Cardiovascular:** *Caffeine* increases heart rate and output at high doses. *Caffeine* may induce arrhythmias, such as premature contractions in sensitive individuals.

c. **Smooth muscle:** *Caffeine* and its derivatives relax the smooth muscles of the bronchioles.

d. **Diuretic action:** *Caffeine* has a weak diuretic action, resulting in increased output of sodium, chloride, and potassium in the urine.

e. **Gastric mucosa:** All methylxanthines stimulate secretion of HCl from the gastric mucosa. Individuals with peptic ulcers should avoid beverages containing methylxanthines. [Note: HCl secretion is blocked by H_2-histamine blockers (p.393).]

3. **Therapeutic uses:** *Theophylline* is still the most popular treatment for chronic asthma. The drug relaxes the bronchioles, but its blood concentration has to be carefully controlled to prevent toxicity. In status asthmaticus, *theophylline* has been used particularly when the patient has not responded well to β_2-adrenergic agonists. (See p.208 for a more complete description of *theophylline*.)

4. **Pharmacology:** The methylxanthines are well absorbed orally. *Caffeine* distributes throughout the body, including the brain. The drugs cross the placenta to the fetus and are secreted into the mothers's milk. All the methylxanthines are metabolized in the liver, and the metabolites are then excreted in the urine.

5. **Adverse effects:**

a. Moderate doses of *caffeine* cause insomnia, anxiety, and agitation. A high dosage is required to show toxicity, which is manifested by emesis and convulsions. The lethal dose is about 10 g for *caffeine* (about 100 cups of coffee), which induces cardiac arrhythmias; death from *caffeine* is thus highly unlikely.

b. **Withdrawal syndrome:** Lethargy, irritability, and headache occur in users who have consumed more than 600 mg of *caffeine* per day (roughly 6 cups of coffee/day) and then suddenly stop.

B. Nicotine

Nicotine [NIC o teen], the active ingredient in tobacco, is second only to *caffeine* as the most widely used CNS stimulant, and second only to alcohol as the most abused drug. *Nicotine* is a toxic and addictive drug, and in combination with the tars and carbon monoxide found in cigarette smoke, it is a serious risk factor for lung disease, various cancers, heart disease, and other illnesses.

1. **Mechanism of action:** In low doses, *nicotine* causes ganglionic stimulation by depolarization. At high doses, *nicotine* causes ganglionic blockade (p.48). Nicotine receptors exist in the CNS where similar actions occur. (See nicotinic receptors, p.38,48.)

2. **Actions:**

   a. **CNS:** *Nicotine* is highly lipid-soluble and freely penetrates into the CNS where it stimulates and then depresses the vital medullary and respiratory centers. Cigarette smoking or administration of low doses of nicotine produces arousal and relaxation and promotes improvement in attention, learning, reaction time, and problem solving, as well as some degree of euphoria. High doses of *nicotine* result in central respiratory paralysis and severe hypotension caused by medullary paralysis (Figure 10.3).

   b. **Peripheral effects:** The effects of *nicotine* are complex and include rises in blood pressure and cardiac rate and increased peristalsis and secretions. At higher doses, the blood pressure falls as a result of ganglionic blockade, and activity ceases both in the gastrointestinal tract and bladder musculature. In small doses, *nicotine* constricts the blood vessels to the digits and impairs flow. Patients with peripheral vascular disease have their condition exacerbated. In addition, coronary blood flow may diminish because of vasoconstriction, resulting in severe problems for the patient with angina. Hypertensive patients should not smoke because *nicotine* has the potential to cause increased blood pressure.

3. **Therapeutic uses:** *Nicotine* has no therapeutic uses, but the toxicology of the substance is of great significance because it is ingested by all who smoke.

4. **Pharmacology:** Absorption of *nicotine* occurs by oral mucosa, lungs, gastrointestinal mucosa, and skin. Most cigarettes contain 6-8 mg of *nicotine*, whereas the acute lethal dose is 60 mg. Over 90% of *nicotine* inhaled in smoke is absorbed. Tolerance to the toxic effects of *nicotine* develops rapidly, often within days.

   a. **Nicotine-substitution therapy:** Recently, chewing gum containing 2 mg of *nicotine* has been shown to reduce nicotine-withdrawal symptoms and to help smokers stop smoking. The blood concentration of *nicotine* obtained from chewing gum is typically about one half of the level observed with smoking (Figure 10.4). Cessation programs that combine pharmacological and behavioral therapy are the most successful.

5. **Adverse effects:**

   a. **CNS:** The CNS effects of *nicotine* include irritability and tremors.

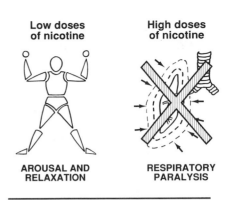

Figure 10.3
Actions of nicotine on the central nervous system.

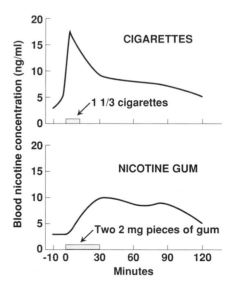

Figure 10.4
Blood concentrations of nicotine in individuals who smoked cigarettes or chewed nicotine gum.

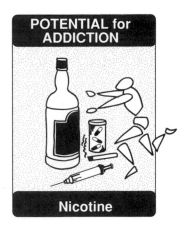

b. **Peripheral:** *Nicotine* may cause intestinal cramps, diarrhea, and increased heart rate and blood pressure.

c. **Accelerated drug metabolism:** Cigarette smoking increases the rate of metabolism of a number of drugs. It is not known which of the over 3,000 components of cigarette smoke are responsible for these changes, although the benzopyrenes have been implicated.

d.**Withdrawal syndrome:** Physical dependence on *nicotine* develops rapidly and is severe. A craving for tobacco is accompanied by irritability, anxiety, restlessness, difficulty in concentrating, headaches, and insomnia. Appetite is often affected, and gastrointestinal pain often occurs.

C. Cocaine

Cocaine [koe KANE] is a cheap, widely available, and highly addictive drug that is currently abused daily by over 3 million people in the United States, more than 5 times the number addicted to heroin.

1. **Mechanism of action:** *Cocaine* blocks the neuronal re-uptake of *norepinephrine*, *serotonin*, and *dopamine* by the presynaptic fibers (Figure 10.5). This block potentiates the actions of natural catecholamines and results in enhancement of CNS and sympathetic actions. In particular, the prolongation of dopaminergic effects in the brain's pleasure system (limbic system), causes the intense euphoria that *cocaine* initially stimulates. Chronic administration of cocaine leads to depletion of dopamine, causing the chronic user to become severely depressed and to crave cocaine.

2. **Actions:**

a. **Central nervous system:** *Cocaine* is a powerful stimulant of the cortex and the brainstem. The drug increases mental awareness and produces a feeling of well-being and euphoria that is similar to that caused by *amphetamine*. Like *amphetamines*, *cocaine* can produce hallucinations, delusions, and paranoia. *Cocaine* increases motor activity, and at high doses it causes tremors and convulsions, followed by respiratory and vasomotor depression.

b. **Sympathetic nervous systems:** *Cocaine* potentiates the action of *norepinephrine* and produces the "fight or flight" syndrome, characteristic of adrenergic stimulation, that is, tachycardia, hypertension, pupillary dilation, and peripheral vasoconstriction (p.26). Cardiac arrhythmias, which may be fatal, often occur.

3. **Therapeutic uses:** *Cocaine* is used topically as a local anesthetic in ear, nose, and throat surgery. [Note: *Cocaine* is unique in that it is the only local anesthetic possessing vasoconstrictor action.]

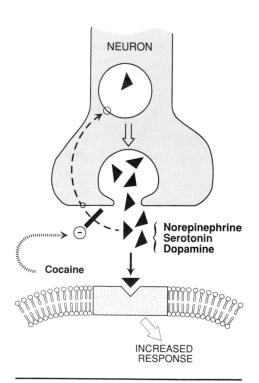

Figure 10.5
Mechanism of action of cocaine.

4. **Pharmacology:** *Cocaine* is self-administered by chewing, intranasal snorting, smoking and intravenous (IV) injection. An IV injection leads to a rapid onset of euphoric effects, which last for just a few minutes. The potential for overdosage is greatest with IV injection. Intranasal use takes 15-20 minutes to peak, and the high disappears in 1.0-1.5 hours. Cocaine-induced seizures are treated with intravenous administration of *diazepam* (p.94), and *propranolol* (p.76) may be required to treat life-threatening cardiac arrhythmias.

5. **Adverse effects:**

a. **Anxiety:** The drug may precipitate acute anxiety reactions, including increased blood pressure and heart rate, sweating, and paranoia. Administration of benzodiazepines or *phenothiazines* is useful in controlling severe agitation experienced during withdrawal.

b. **Depression:** Like all stimulant drugs, cocaine stimulation of the CNS is followed by a period of mental depression. After prolonged use, withdrawal from *cocaine* is followed by severe physical and emotional depression.

c. **Perforation of nasal septum:** *Cocaine* inhalation causes constriction of the vessels in the nose and may cause ischemia of the nasal tissue. The prolonged vasoconstriction accompanying chronic inhalation of *cocaine* can lead to necrosis and perforation of the nasal septum.

D. Amphetamine

Amphetamine shows neurochemical and clinical effects that are quite similar to those of *cocaine*.

1. **Mechanism of action:** The peripheral actions of *amphetamine* are mediated primarily through the cellular release of stored catecholamines (Figure 10.6). The alteration of behavior by *amphetamine* is probably due mainly to a release of *dopamine* rather than release of *norepinephrine*. In addition, *amphetamine* is a weak inhibitor of monoamine oxidase (MAO) (p.123).

2. **Actions:**

a. **Central nervous system:** *Amphetamine* stimulates the entire cerebrospinal axis, cortex, brain stem, and medulla. This results in increased alertness, decreased fatigue, depressed appetite, and insomnia. In high doses, convulsions can ensue. Tolerance to the euphoric, anorectic, and lethal dose, as well as psychological dependence, occur with regular use. Little or no tolerance to CNS toxicity occurs.

b. **Sympathetic nervous system:** In addition to its marked action on the CNS, amphetamine acts on the adrenergic system, indirectly stimulating the receptors through norepinephrine release (p.67).

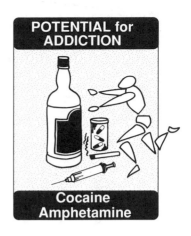

POTENTIAL for ADDICTION

Cocaine Amphetamine

A. No Amphetamine

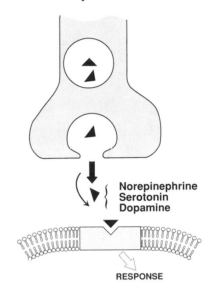

Norepinephrine
Serotonin
Dopamine

RESPONSE

B. With Amphetamine

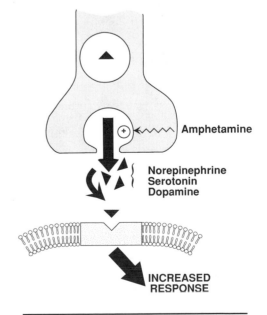

Amphetamine

Norepinephrine
Serotonin
Dopamine

INCREASED RESPONSE

Figure 10.6
Mechanism of action of amphetamine.

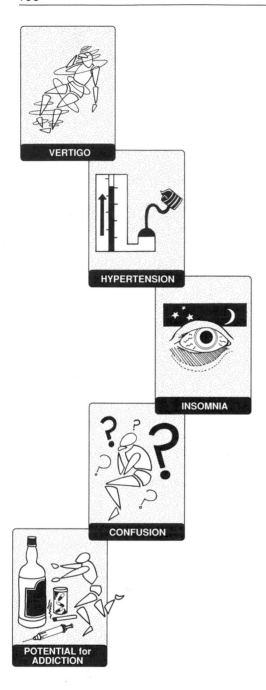

Figure 10.7
Adverse effects of amphetamines.

3. **Therapeutic uses:**

   a. **Attention deficit syndrome:** Some young children are hyperkinetic and lack the ability to be involved in any one activity for longer than a few minutes. *Amphetamine* and more recently the amphetamine derivative *methylphenidate* [meth ill FEN i date] alleviates many of the behavioral problems associated with this syndrome and reduces the hyperkinesia that the children demonstrate. Their attention is thus prolonged, allowing them to function better in a school atmosphere.

   b. **Narcolepsy:** *Methylphenidate* is used to treat narcolepsy, a disorder marked by an uncontrollable desire for sleep.

   c. **Appetite control:** *Amphetamines* diminish the appetite (anorexigenic action) by blocking the appetite centers in the lateral hypothalamus. Tolerance develops rapidly and within 1-2 weeks appetite suppression disappears, despite the continued use of the drug. Its use for this purpose is controversial.

4. **Pharmacology:** *Amphetamines* are completely absorbed from the gastrointestinal tract, metabolized by the liver, and excreted in the urine. The euphoria caused by *amphetamine* lasts 4-6 hours, or four to eight times longer than the effects of *cocaine*. Both drugs produce dependence, tolerance, and addiction.

5. **Adverse effects:**

   a. **Central effects:** Insomnia, irritability, weakness, dizziness, tremor, and hyperactive reflexes may occur (Figure 10.7). Confusion, delirium, panic states, and suicidal tendencies occur, especially in mentally ill patients. Chronic use produces a state of "*amphetamine* psychosis" that resembles an acute schizophrenic attack. Psychic and physical dependence on the drug occurs, but tolerance to *amphetamines* may occur within a few weeks. Overdosages are treated with *chlorpromazine* (p.129), which relieves the CNS symptoms and the hypertension, because of its α-blocking effects.

   b. **Cardiovascular effects:** These include palpitations, anginal pain, cardiac arrhythmias, hypertension, and eventual circulatory collapse. Headache, chills, and excessive sweating may occur. *Amphetamines* should not be given to patients with cardiovascular disease, because the drug stimulates the heart.

   c. **Gastrointestinal system effects:** Anorexia, nausea, vomiting, abdominal cramps, and diarrhea may occur.

   d. **Contraindications:** *Amphetamines* should not be used in patients with cardiovascular disease and in those receiving MAO inhibitors (p.123) or *guanethidine* (p.79).

III. CONVULSANTS AND RESPIRATORY STIMULANTS

A. Nikethamide and doxapram

Nikethamide [NIK eth a mide] and *doxapram* [DOX a pram] are respiratory stimulants used in treating acute ventilatory failure that often results from an overdose of CNS depressants, such as barbiturates. They may also be used to relieve postanesthetic respiratory depression. *Doxapram* stimulates both carotid chemoreceptors and the respiratory center, whereas *nikethamide* primarily stimulates the respiratory center. Both stimulate respiration in subconvulsive doses and increase tidal volume. In higher doses, convulsions occur that can be blocked by *diazepam* (p.94).

IV. HALLUCINOGENS

A few drugs have as their primary action the ability to induce altered perceptual states reminiscent of dreams. Many of these altered states are accompanied by bright, colorful changes in the environment and by a plasticity of constantly changing shapes and color. The individual under the influence of these drugs is incapable of normal decision making, since the drug interferes with rational thought. These compounds are known as hallucinogens or psychotomimetic drugs.

A. Lysergic acid diethylamide (LSD)

Multiple sites in the CNS are affected by *LSD*. The drug shows serotonin (5-HT) agonist activity at presynaptic receptors in the midbrain. It binds to both 5-HT_1 and 5-HT_2 receptors. Activation of the sympathetic nervous system occurs, which causes pupillary dilation, increased blood pressure, piloerection, and increased body temperature. Taken orally, low doses of *LSD* can induce hallucinations with brilliant colors. Alteration in mood occurs. Tolerance and physical dependence have occurred, but true dependence is rare. Adverse effects include hyperreflexia, nausea, and muscular weakness. Sometimes high doses produce long-lasting psychotic changes in susceptible individuals. *Haloperidol* (p.127) and other neuroleptics can block the hallucinatory action of *LSD* and quickly abort the syndrome.

B. Tetrahydrocannabinol

The main alkaloid contained in marijuana is $\Delta\text{-}^9$-tetrahydrocannabinol [tet ra hi dro can NAB i nol] (THC), which produces euphoria that is followed by drowsiness and relaxation, depending on the social situation. The THC impairs short-term memory and mental activity. It decreases muscle strength and impairs highly skilled motor activity, such as that required to drive a car. It increases appetite, causes xerostomia, visual hallucinations, delusions, and enhancement of sensory activity. The mechanism of action of THC is unknown. The THC shows effects immediately after smoking, but maximal effects take about 20 minutes. By 3 hours, the effects largely disappear.

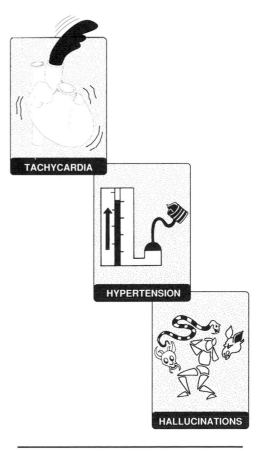

Figure 10.8
Adverse effects of tetrahydro-cannabinol.

Adverse effects include an increase in heart rate, blood pressure, and a reddening of the conjunctiva (Figure 10.8). At high doses, a toxic psychosis develops. Tolerance and mild physical dependence occur with continued frequent use of the drug. The THC is sometimes given for the severe emesis caused by some of the cancer chemotherapeutic agents (p.341).

C. Phencyclidine (PCP)

Phencyclidine [fen SI kli deen] ("angel dust") inhibits the re-uptake of *dopamine*, 5-HT, and *norepinephrine*. It also has anticholinergic activity, but strangely produces hypersalivation. *Phencyclidine*, an analog of *ketamine* (p.115), causes dissociative anesthesia (insensitivity to pain, without loss of consciousness) and analgesia. In this state, it produces numbness of extremities, staggered gait, slurred speech, and muscular rigidity. Sometimes hostile and bizarre behavior occurs. In increased dosage, anesthesia, stupor, or coma result, but strangely the eyes may remain open. Increased sensitivity to external stimuli exists, and the CNS actions may persist for a week. Tolerance often develops with continued use.

Study Questions   (see p.413 for answers).

Choose the ONE best answer.

10.1 Which of the following is NOT characteristic of cocaine overdosage?

    A. Dilation of the pupil.
    B. Euphoria.
    C. Tachycardia.
    D. Peripheral vasodilation.
    E. Hallucinations.

10.2 Which of the following statements about amphetamine is INCORRECT?

    A. Overdosage of amphetamine can be managed with chlorpromazine.
    B. Ampthetamine s used as an adjunct with MAO inhibitors.
    C. Amphetamine has a longer duration of action than cocaine.
    D. Amphetamine depresses the hunger center in the hypothalamus.
    E. Amphetamine acts on α- and β-adrenergic presynaptic terminals.

10.3 Which of the following statements concerning tetrahydrocannabinol (THC) is correct?

    A. THC decreases heart rate.
    B. THC increases muscle strength.
    C. THC decreases appetite.
    D. THC causes hypotension.
    E. THC antiemetic action.

Answer A if 1,2 and 3 are correct.
    B if 1 and 3 are correct.
    C if 2 and 4 are correct.
    D if only 4 is correct.
    E if 1,2,3 and 4 are all correct.

10.4 Phencyclidine
    1. produces dissociative anesthesia.
    2. is an analog of ketamine.
    3. can cause hostile and bizarre behavior.
    4. is nonaddicting.

10.5 Which of the follow drugs is/are correctly paired with their toxic effects?

    1. Amphetamine: Paranoid psychosis.
    2. Cocaine: Anxiety and depression.
    3. LSD: Hallucinations.
    4. Nicotine (low doses): Decreased heart rate and blood pressure.

Anesthetics

11

I. OVERVIEW

General anesthetics produce a state of unconsciousness with the absence of pain sensation over the entire body. These drugs are usually gases or volatile liquids inspired in combination with oxygen. These inhalation anesthetics are absorbed from the alveoli into the blood and then carried to the brain, where they diffuse rapidly across the lipid membranes and enter the brain tissue. Certain highly lipid-soluble barbiturates, such as *thiopental*, are also used as anesthetics, but are given by the intravenous route. They are called "fixed" anesthetics, since the injected dose produces a given state of anesthesia and is incapable of minute-to-minute control, as with the gaseous anesthetics. In contrast to general anesthetics, which are administered systemically and affect the central nervous system (CNS), local anesthetics are applied locally and block nerve conduction, abolishing sensation in a limited area of the body without producing unconsciousness. The anesthetic agents are summarized in Figure 11.1.

II. DEPTH OF ANESTHESIA

The depth of anesthesia can be divided into a series of four sequential stages; each is characterized by increased CNS depression that is caused by accumulation of the anesthetic drug in the brain. With ether, which produces a slow onset of anesthesia, all the stages are discernible. However, with halothane and many other commonly used anesthetics, the stages are difficult to clearly characterize because of the rapidity of onset of anesthesia.

A. Stage I: analgesia

Loss of pain sensation results from interference with sensory transmission in the spinothalamic tract. The patient is conscious and conversational. A reduced awareness of pain occurs as Stage II is approached.

B. Stage II: excitement

The patient experiences delirium and violent combative behavior. There is a rise and irregularity in blood pressure. The respiratory rate↑

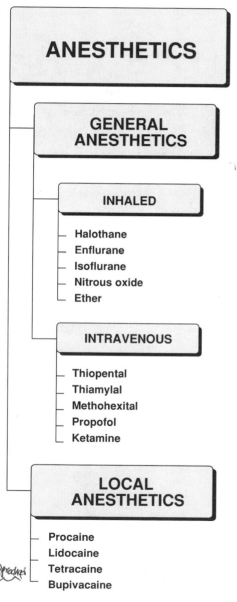

ANESTHETICS

GENERAL ANESTHETICS

INHALED
- Halothane
- Enflurane
- Isoflurane
- Nitrous oxide
- Ether

INTRAVENOUS
- Thiopental
- Thiamylal
- Methohexital
- Propofol
- Ketamine

LOCAL ANESTHETICS
- Procaine
- Lidocaine
- Tetracaine
- Bupivacaine

Figure 11.1
Summary of anesthetics.

rate may be increased. To avoid this stage of anesthesia, a short-acting barbiturate, such as *sodium pentothal*, is given intravenously before inhalation anesthesia is administered.

C. Stage III: surgical anesthesia

Regular respiration and relaxation of the skeletal muscles occur in this stage. Eye reflexes decrease progressively, until the eye movements cease and the pupil is fixed. Surgery may proceed during this stage.

D. Stage IV: medullary paralysis

Severe depression of the respiratory center and vasomotor center occur during this stage. Death can rapidly ensue.

III. KINETICS OF ANESTHESIA

Anesthesia can be divided into three stages: induction, maintenance, and recovery. Recovery is essentially the reverse of induction, and the two processes are considered together in this discussion.

A. Induction and recovery from anesthesia

Induction is defined as the period of time from onset of administration of the anesthetic to the development of effective surgical anesthesia in the patient. Recovery is the time from discontinuation of administration of anesthesia until consciousness is regained. Induction of anesthesia depends on how fast effective concentrations of the anesthetic drug reach the brain; recovery is the reverse of induction and depends on how fast the anesthetic drug is removed from the brain. For drugs administered by inhalation, the rates of onset and recovery are influenced by the following four factors:

1. **Solubility of anesthetic:** The solubility of an anesthetic gas is expressed as the blood/gas partition coefficient, which is the ratio of the concentration of gas in the blood relative to the gas equilibrium phase (Figure 11.2). Drugs with low or high solubility in blood differ in their speed of induction of anesthesia.

   a. **Low solubility:** When an anesthetic gas with low blood solubility, such as nitrous oxide (N_2O), diffuses from the alveoli into the circulation, little of the anesthetic dissolves in the blood. Therefore, the equilibrium between the inhaled anesthetic and arterial blood is rapidly achieved, and relatively few additional molecules of anesthetic are required to raise arterial tension. This results in rapid induction of anesthesia, prompt changes in the depth of anesthesia in response to changes in concentration of the inhaled drug, and short recovery times after discontinuing of the anesthetic (Figure 11.3).

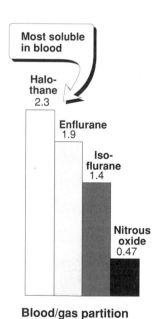

Most soluble in blood

Halo-thane
2.3

Enflurane
1.9

Iso-flurane
1.4

Nitrous oxide
0.47

Blood/gas partition coefficient

Figure 11.2
Blood/gas partition coefficients for the inhalational anesthetics.

b. **High solubility:** Anesthetics with greater solubility, such as halothane, dissolve more completely in the blood, and greater amounts of the anesthetic and longer periods of time are required to raise arterial tension. This results in increased times of induction and recovery, and slower changes in the depth of anesthesia in response to changes in the concentration of the inhaled drug (Figure 11.3).

2. **Rate of ventilation:** An increased rate of delivery of anesthetic gas to the lungs results in more anesthetic being delivered to the alveoli. This increases the rate at which the arterial blood approaches equilibrium. The effect of increased ventilation is most pronounced for anesthetics with high solubility in blood.

3. **Partial pressure of gas:** The rate at which an anesthetic enters the blood is directly proportional to the concentration of the anesthetic gas in the inspired gas mixture. Rapid induction with agents showing high solubility in blood requires "overpressure", that is, administration of a concentration that is higher than that required for maintenance of anesthesia. For example, 2.0% *halothane* may be administered during the first few minutes of induction. As soon as the desired state of anesthesia is reached, the *halothane* concentration is reduced to a maintenance level of 0.5%. This corresponds to the concept of a loading dose for nonvolatile drugs (p.17).

4. **Increased alveolar blood flow:** High blood flow causes more of the anesthetic agent to be removed from the alveoli, hastening anesthesia.

B. Maintenance of anesthesia

Maintenance is the time during which the patient is surgically anesthetized. Anesthesia is usually maintained by the administration of gases or volatile anesthetics, since these agents offer good minute-to-minute control over the depth of anesthesia.

IV. MOLECULAR MECHANISM OF ANESTHESIA

General anesthetics have the common property of increasing the threshold of action potentials and inhibiting the rapid increase in membrane permeability to sodium ion. The mechanism of these effects is not known but appears to result from changes in the physical state of the membrane, which interferes with normal function, for example the ability of the sodium channel to open rapidly. The anesthetics are unique in depressing CNS function by physicochemical disturbances in the neuron. No receptors have been found to interact with the anesthetics, and neurotransmitters do not appear to be involved in their action. This mode of action contrasts with other CNS agents (for example, opiates, neuroleptics, hypnotics), which affect the release or receptor binding of neurotransmitters in the CNS.

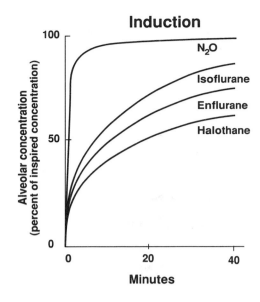

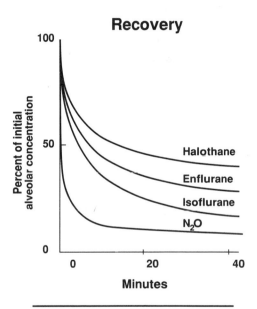

Figure 11.3
Changes in the alveolar blood concentration of the inhalation anesthetics with time.

V. GENERAL ANESTHETICS: INHALED

Inhaled gases are the mainstay of anesthesia and are primarily used for the maintenance of anesthesia after administration of an intravenous agent. Inhalation anesthetics have a benefit that is not available with intravenous agents, since the depth of anesthesia can be rapidly altered by changing the concentration of the inhaled anesthetic. Because most of these agents are rapidly eliminated from the body, they do not cause postoperative respiratory depression.

A. Potency

1. **Minimal alveolar concentration:** The potency of inhaled anesthetics is defined quantitatively as the minimum alveolar concentration (MAC), which is the concentration of anesthetic gas needed to eliminate movement among 50% of patients challenged by a standardized skin incision. The MAC is usually expressed as the percentage of gas in the mixture required to achieve the effect. Numerically, MAC is small for potent anesthetics, such as *halothane*, and large for less potent agents, such as N_2O. Therefore, the inverse of MAC is an index of potency of the anesthetic. By definition, 1 MAC of one gas produces equal anesthesia to 1 MAC of another gas. The MAC values are useful in comparing pharmacologic effects of different anesthetics (Figure 11.4). The more lipid-soluble an anesthetic, the lower the concentration of anesthetic needed to produce anesthesia. [Note: MAC is measured in patients with no premedication, because the concentration of the inhaled anesthetic required to produce surgical anesthesia may be reduced by the presence of another sedating drug, and MAC would thus be falsely estimated.]

2. **Additive effects:** When an anesthetic with a MAC of 0.5 is added to another anesthetic with a MAC of 0.5, the mixture does not always have a MAC of 1. Often the action of one anesthetic is synergistic with the effect of a second agent, but it may be different for each pair of drugs. For example, the dose of *halothane* required for anesthesia can be cut substantially by the simultaneous use of N_2O in sub-MAC doses; however, the MACs are not additive.

B. Halogenated gases

Each of the halogenated gases have characteristics beneficial for selected clinical applications. No one anesthetic is superior to another under all circumstances.

1. **Halothane:** The gas is a potent anesthetic, since its minimal anesthetic concentration is 0.74 vol %, and an overdose is easily given. *Halothane* [hal loe thane] lacks significant analgesic potency and is often used with other agents. *Halothane* is more extensively metabolized than *enflurane* or *isoflurane*, and in rare individuals, it may result in the formation of hepatotoxic intermediates. The resultant "halothane hepatitis" is a rare, unpredictable, but often lethal complication. *Enflurane* and *isoflurane* have a lower potential for hepatoxicity. [Note: *Halothane* is not

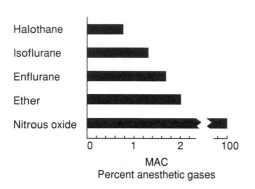

Figure 11.4
Minimal alveolar concentrations (MAC) for anesthetic gases.

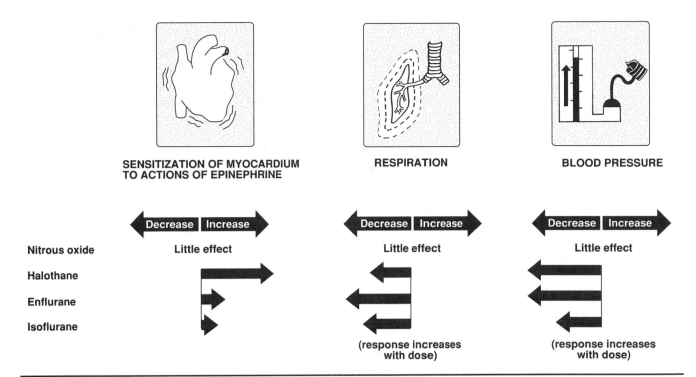

Figure 11.5
Cardiovascular and respiratory effects of inhalational anesthetics.

[handwritten margin notes:]
halothane
- potent anesth & OD is easily given
- but lacks signif. analgesia
∴ often used with other agents.
s/eff - hepatotoxic (hepatitis)
Enflurane & isoflurane less
hepatotoxic

not hepatotoxic in pediatric patients and that, combined with its pleasant odor, make it the agent of choice in pediatric patients.] In certain individuals *halothane* may cause malignant hyperthermia because of an increased metabolic state in skeletal muscle. The cardiovascular and respiratory actions of *halothane* and the other halogenated anesthetic gases are summarized in Figure 11.5.

2. **Enflurane:** This gas is less potent than *halothane*, but it produces rapid induction and recovery. About 2% of the agent is metabolized to fluoride ion, which is excreted by the kidney. *Enflurane* [EN floo rane] is contraindicated in patients with kidney failure.

3. **Isoflurane:** This is a new halogenated anesthetic that has low biotransformation and low organ toxicity. Unlike the other halogenated anesthetic gases, *isoflurane* [ey soe FLURE ane] does not induce cardiac arrhythmias and does not sensitize the heart to the action of catecholamines.

C. Nitrous oxide *[handwritten:]* SAFEST OF ALL ANESTHETIC provided 20% O₂ is always given with it

[handwritten:] 30% conc. of N₂O + O₂ in dental anesthesia

Nitrous oxide [nye truss OX ide] (N₂O or "laughing gas") is commonly employed in conjunction with other more potent anesthetics, since by itself, it does not produce surgical anesthesia. *Nitrous oxide* must never be given in concentrations greater than 80% for fear of hypoxia. This gas has the lowest solubility in blood of any of the anesthetic agents; therefore, it produces the fastest

[handwritten margin notes:]
disadv → does not produce muscle relaxation
adv → ① does not depress respiration
④ least effect of ↑ cerebral bld flow of all anesth.
⑤ least hepatotoxic
⑥ least effect on CVS
induction & recovery
① 30-40% conc it has strong analgesic actn

induction and recovery. In concentrations of 30-40%, it has a strong analgesic action. Often, it is used in conjunction with *thiopental* to maintain anesthesia. It does not depress respiration and has the least effect in increasing cerebral blood flow of all anesthetics. It is the least hepatotoxic of the anesthetics. It also has the least effect on the cardiovascular system and does not produce muscle relaxation. It probably is the safest of the anesthetics, provided that at least 20% oxygen is always given with it. It is often employed in concentrations of 30% in combination with oxygen for analgesia, particularly in dental surgery.

D. Ether

Ether is difficult to use in hot climates because of its low boiling point. One great disadvantage is that it is explosive when mixed with oxygen. In addition, it is an irritant to the respiratory tract and increases salivary and respiratory secretions. *Ether* is only of historical interest in Western societies because of the danger of explosion.

VI. GENERAL ANESTHETICS: INTRAVENOUS

Intravenous anesthetics are often used for the rapid induction of anesthesia, which is then maintained with an appropriate inhalation agent.

A. Barbiturates

Thiopental (p.96) is the most widely used intravenous general anesthetic. It is an ultra–short-acting barbiturate and has a high lipid solubility. When agents, such as *thiopental*, *thiamylal* [thye AM i tal], *methohexital* [meth oh HEX i tal], or the newest drug, *propofol* [pro POF ol], are administered intravenously, they quickly enter the CNS and depress function, often in less than 1 minute. However, diffusion out of the brain can occur very rapidly as well, because of redistribution of the drug to other body tissues, including skeletal muscle and ultimately adipose tissue (Figure 11.6). This latter site serves as a reservoir of drug from which the agent slowly leaks out and is metabolized and excreted. The short duration of anesthetic action is due to the decrease of its concentration in the brain below that necessary to produce anesthesia. The drugs may remain in the body for relatively long periods of time after their administration, since only about 15% of the dose of barbiturate entering the circulation is metabolized per hour in the liver. Thus, metabolism of *thiopental* is much slower than tissue redistribution. The barbiturates are not analgesic and require some type of supplementary analgesic administration during anesthesia, otherwise objectionable changes in blood pressure and autonomic function may ensue.

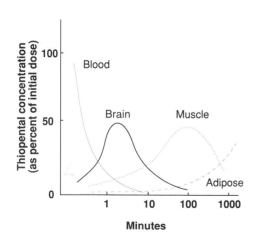

Figure 11.6
Redistribution of thiopental from brain to muscle and adipose tissue.

1. **Cardiovascular effects:** *Thiopental* depresses the arterial blood pressure. This effect is due to a decrease in cardiac output caused by myocardial depression, and it is dose dependent. There is no change in peripheral resistance. The drug impairs venous return to the heart and can cause venous pooling.

2. **Respiratory effects:** *Thiopental* depresses the respiratory center in a dose-dependent manner and decreases its sensitivity to carbon dioxide. It depresses oxygen consumption by brain tissue and decreases cerebral blood flow. The drug may also decrease hepatic blood flow and kidney blood flow. The drug may induce laryngospasm.

B. Ketamine

1. **Dissociative anesthesia:** *Ketamine* [KET a meen], a short-acting nonbarbiturate anesthetic, induces a dissociated state in which the patient appears awake but is unconscious and does not feel pain. Anesthesia produced by this drug is called "dissociative" and consists of amnesia, analgesia, and often rigidity or catatonia. Disorientation, hallucinations, and changes in perception often accompany its use. The drug is lipophilic and enters the brain circulation very quickly, but like the barbiturates, it can redistribute to other organs and tissues. It is metabolized in the liver, but small amounts can be excreted unchanged. *Ketamine* is used mainly in children and young adults for short procedures. *Ketamine* is not widely used because it increases cerebral blood flow and induces postoperative hallucinations.

2. **Actions:** *Ketamine* stimulates the central sympathetic outflow, which in turn, causes stimulation of the heart and increased blood pressure and cardiac output. It increases plasma catecholamine levels and increases blood flow.

VII. COMBINATION ANESTHETICS

General anesthesia ideally produces loss of consciousness, analgesia, inhibition of sensory and autonomic reflexes, and skeletal muscle relaxation. To achieve this state with a single agent may require a very deep stage of anesthesia that may not be desirable in all patients. Therefore, the anesthesiologist often employs a lighter stage of anesthesia, in combination with additional drugs, to produce sufficient relaxation and analgesia, for example, for surgical anesthesia. This approach uses the best properties of each anesthetic and minimizes dangerous adverse effects.

A. Balanced anesthesia

Full loss of both consciousness and pain-induced reflexes, along with muscle relaxation, is obtained with a combination of agents. The use of an ultra–short-acting barbiturate, an opioid analgesic, a muscle relaxant, and *nitrous oxide* to produce general anesthesia is termed "balanced anesthesia" (Figure 11.7). *Meperidine, morphine, fentanyl,* or *sufentanil* are widely used as opioid analgesic agents, in combination with the barbiturate, *thiopental. Tubocurarine* or another muscle relaxant is often used.

B. Neuroleptanesthesia

Neuroleptanesthesia is induced by the combined actions of a narcotic analgesic, and a neuroleptic agent, together with the inhala-

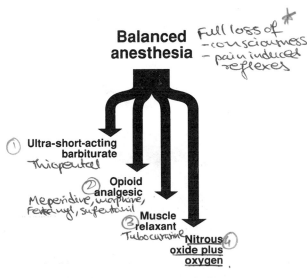

Balanced anesthesia

① **Ultra-short-acting barbiturate**

② **Opioid analgesic**

③ **Muscle relaxant**

④ **Nitrous oxide plus oxygen**

Figure 11.7
Components of balanced anesthesia.

Handwritten top margin: sideeff/- resp depression most common & serious complicat

Neurolept-anesthesia

Handwritten left margin: Consciousness is not lost ∴ useful in procedures where pt co-op reqd

Handwritten: effective analgesia Fentanyl

Handwritten: tranquility of motor activity droperidol

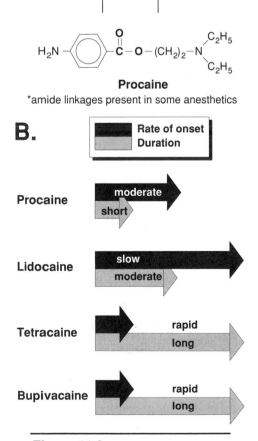

Narcotic analgesic

Neuroleptic agent

Nitrous oxide plus oxygen

Figure 11.8
Components of neuroleptanesthesia.

A.

| Lipophilic portion | Ester linkage* | Hydrophilic portion |

$$H_2N - \bigcirc - \overset{\overset{O}{\|}}{C} - O - (CH_2)_2 - N \overset{C_2H_5}{\underset{C_2H_5}{}}$$

Procaine

*amide linkages present in some anesthetics

B.

| Rate of onset / Duration |

Procaine — moderate / short

Lidocaine — slow / moderate

Tetracaine — rapid / long

Bupivacaine — rapid / long

Figure 11.9

A. Structural formula of procaine.
B. Pharmocokinetic properties of local anesthetics.

tion of *nitrous oxide* and oxygen (Figure 11.8). The most frequently used neuroleptic agents are *droperidol* combined with *fentanyl* (p.139). The neuroleptic properties of *droperidol* (see p.129) cause tranquility and reduced motor activity, whereas *fentanyl* produces effective analgesia. Consciousness is not lost during neurolept-analgesia; Therefore this drug combination is useful in certain diagnostic procedures that require cooperation of the patient. Respiratory depression is the most common and serious complication, and mechanical ventilation may be required.

VIII. LOCAL ANESTHETICS

These drugs are applied locally and block nerve conduction of sensory impulses from the periphery to the CNS. These agents abolish sensation (and in higher concentrations, motor activity) in a limited area of the body without producing unconsciousness. These drugs inhibit sodium channels of the nerve membrane. The small, unmyelinated nerve fibers, which conduct impulses for pain, temperature, and autonomic activity, are most sensitive to actions of local anesthetics.

All of the local anesthetics consist of a hydrophilic amino group linked through a connecting group of variable length to a lipophilic aromatic residue (Figure 11.9). Both potency and toxicity of the local anesthetics increase as the connecting group becomes longer. Adverse effects result from systemic absorption of toxic amounts of the locally applied anesthetic. Seizures are the most significant of these systemic effects. By adding the vasoconstrictor *epinephrine* to the local anesthetic, the rate of absorption is decreased (p.62). This both minimizes systemic toxicity and increases the duration of action.

Handwritten: Tetracaine & Bupivacaine most rapid onset & longest durat of action

IX. PREANESTHETIC MEDICATIONS

Often drugs are administered prior to anesthesia to allay anxiety, reduce pain, decrease excess salivation, and to combat nausea.

A. Anxiolytic drugs

Benzodiazepine derivatives, such as *diazepam* (p.91), provide preoperative sedation and attenuate CNS stimulation caused by local anesthetics.

B. Narcotic analgesics

Opioids such as *morphine* (p.134) or *fentanyl* (p.139) are often combined with general anesthetics of low potency, such as *N₂O*, to provide analgesia. Neuroleptic drugs, such as *promethazine* (p.129), and the antihistamine, *hydroxyzine* (p.390), are often administered concomitantly with opioids, because these agents potentiate the analgesic actions of the opioids without increasing the side effects.

C. Anticholinergic drugs

Atropine (p.45) and *scopolamine* (p.48) are used routinely for reduction of bronchial and salivary secretion to prevent fluid accumulation in the respiratory tract.

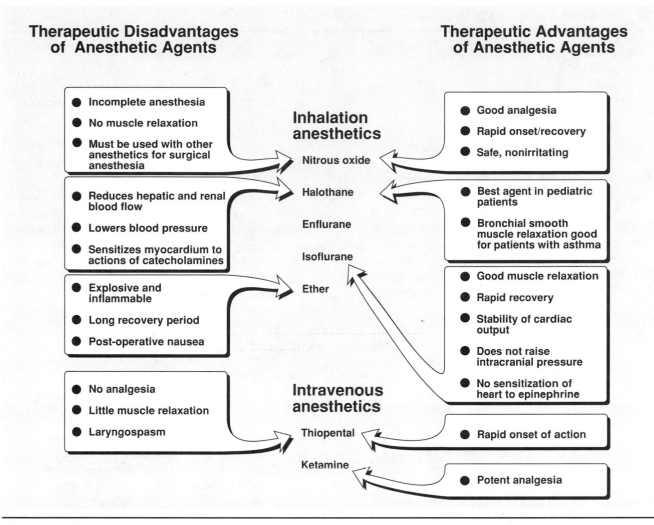

Figure 11.10
Therapeutic disadvantages and advantages of anesthetic agents.

D. Barbiturates

Secobarbital and *pentobarbital* (p.96) are used as preoperative sedatives. These drugs produce less postoperative nausea and vomiting than opioids.

E. Neuroleptics

Promethazine, *trimeprazine* or *chlorpromazine* are increasingly used as oral premedications, since these agents both sedate and have useful antiemetic properties.

X. MUSCLE RELAXANTS

Muscle relaxants cause reversible muscle paralysis. These agents are described in detail on p.49. They are used particularly for tracheal intubation, to facilitate assisted ventilation, to prevent laryngospasm during operations, and to produce sufficient muscle paralysis during surgery. Figure 11.10 summarizes the factors that influence the therapeutic applications of the anesthetic drugs.

Study Questions   (see p.414 for answers).

Answer A if 1,2 and 3 are correct.
   B if 1 and 3 are correct.
   C if 2 and 4 are correct.
   D if only 4 is correct.
   E if 1,2,3 and 4 are all correct.

11.1 Which of the following statements is/are correct?

  1. The more soluble the anesthetic gas, the slower it achieves equilibrium and the longer the induction time.
  2. Recovery is rapid from poorly soluble anesthetic gases and prolonged with agents having high blood solubility.
  3. Termination of anesthetic action of thiopental is primarily caused by redistribution of the drug from the brain to other tissues, particularly muscle.
  4. The more lipid soluble an anesthetic, the lower the concentration of anesthetic needed to produce anesthesia.

11.2 Which of the following statements is/are correct?

potency inversely related to MAC

  1. The potency of an anesthetic is proportional to the minimal anesthetic concentrations (MAC).
  2. Induction and recovery are rapid with nitrous oxide.
  3. Nitrous oxide is often used as a single agent in anesthesia.
  4. Halothane with a MAC of 0.76% is more potent than nitrous oxide with a MAC of 100%.

11.3 Which of the following statements concerning ketamine is/are correct?

  1. Ketamine is used mainly for children and young adults for short diagnostic procedures.
  2. Ketamine produces analgesia without unconsciousness. *pt is awake → dissociative state*
  3. Ketamine produces a high incidence of postanesthetic hallucinations.
  4. Ketamine inhibits the central sympathetic outflow. *stimulates, +ve ♡ & B.P & cardiac output*

Choose the ONE best answer.

11.4 Which of the following anesthetics is most likely to require administration of a muscle relaxant?

  A. Ethyl ether.
  B. Halothane.
  C. Methoxyflurane.
  D. Benzodiazepines.
  E. Nitrous oxide. *(No muscle relaxant prop)*

11.5 Which of the following anesthetics exhibits the shortest induction time when each agent is administered at a concentration that ultimately produces surgical anesthesia?

  A. Ethyl ether.
  B. Halothane.
  C. Methoxyflurane.
  D. Nitrous oxide. *coz of its low solubility, it rapidly saturates arterial bld reaching brain*
  E. Benzodiazepine.

11.6 Which of the following statements is true?

  A. Halothane produces anesthesia within 1-2 minutes of administration. *slow onset of actn coz of ↑ solubility in bld*
  B. Thiopental is commonly used as single agent for anesthesia.
  C. Halothane as well as thiopental produce depression of cardiovascular and respiratory system.
  D. Halothane is often hepatotoxic in pediatric patients.
  E. Halothane has less potential for hepatotoxicity than isoflurane.

Antidepressant Drugs

12

I. OVERVIEW

Depression is an affective disorder characterized by changes in mood (depression or mania). It is different from schizophrenia, which produces disturbances in thought. The symptoms of depression are intense feelings of sadness, hopelessness, despair, and the inability to experience pleasure in usual activities. Mania is characterized by the opposite behavior, that is, enthusiasm, rapid thought and speech patterns, and extreme self-confidence and impaired judgment.

All clinically useful antidepressant drugs (also called thymoleptics) potentiate, either directly or indirectly, the actions of *norepinephrine*, *dopamine*, and/or *serotonin* in the brain. (See Figure 12.1 for a summary of the antidepressant agents.) This, along with other evidence, lead to the biogenic amine theory, which proposes that depression is due to a deficiency of monoamines such as *norepinephrine* and *serotonin* at certain key sites in the brain. Conversely, mania is envisioned as caused by an overproduction of these neurotransmitters.

The amine theory of depression is probably overly simplistic, since it is now known that the antidepressant drugs, particularly the tricyclic antidepressants, affect many biological systems in addition to neurotransmitter uptake. It is not known which of these neurochemical systems is most responsible for the antidepressant activity.

II. TRICYCLIC/POLYCYCLIC ANTIDEPRESSANTS

The tricyclic and polycyclic antidepressants block *norepinephrine, dopamine*, and *serotonin* uptake into the neuron. Prolonged therapy probably leads to alterations in selected CNS receptors. The important drugs in this group are *imipramine* ([im IP ra meen], the prototype), *amitriptyline* [a mee TRIP ti leen], *desipramine* ([dess IP ra meen], a demethylated derivative of *imipramine*), *nortriptyline* [nor TRIP ti leen], *protriptyline* [proe TRIP te leen], and *doxepin* [DOX e pin]. *Amoxapine* [a MOX a peen] and *maprotiline* [ma PROE ti leen] are termed "second generation" to distinguish them from the older tricyclic antidepressants. [Note: These second generation drugs have actions similar to *imipramine*, although they exhibit slightly different pharmacokinetics.] All the tricyclic antidepressants (TCAs) have similar therapeutic efficacy, and the choice of drug depends on tolerance of side effects and duration of action. Patients that do not respond to one TCA may benefit from a different drug in this group.

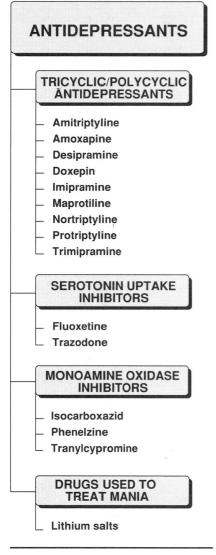

Figure 12.1
Summary of antidepressants.

119

A. Normal monoamine transmission

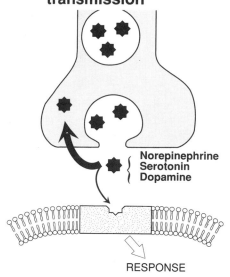

RESPONSE

B. Effect of tricyclic antidepressants

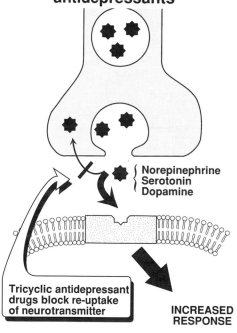

Tricyclic antidepressant drugs block re-uptake of neurotransmitter

INCREASED RESPONSE

Figure 12.2
Mechanisms of action of tricyclic and polycyclic antidepressant drugs.

A. Mode of action

1. **Inhibition of neurotransmitter uptake:** TCAs inhibit the neuronal re-uptake of *norepinephrine*, *dopamine*, and *serotonin* into presynaptic nerve terminals (Figure 12.2). By blocking the major route of neurotransmitter removal, the TCAs lead to increased concentrations of monoamines in the synaptic cleft, resulting in antidepressant effects. This theory has been discounted by some because of several observations. For example, the potency of the TCA in blocking neurotransmitter uptake often does not correlate with clinically observed antidepressant effects. Further, blockade of re-uptake of neurotransmitter occurs immediately after administration of the drug, but the antidepressant effect of the TCA requires several weeks of continued treatment. This suggests that decreased uptake of neurotransmitter is only an initial event which may not be related to the antidepressant effects. [Note: It has recently been suggested that monoamine receptor densities in the brain may change over a 2-4 week period with drug use and may be important in the onset of activity.]

2. **Blocking of receptors:** The TCAs also block serotoninergic, α-adrenergic, histamine, and muscarinic receptors. It is not known which, if any, of these account for therapeutic benefit.

B. Actions

1. **Mood elevation:** These drugs elevate mood, improve mental alertness, increase physical activity, and reduce morbid preoccupation in 50-70% of individuals with major depression. The onset of the mood-elevation is slow, requiring 2 weeks or longer. These drugs do not produce CNS stimulation or mood elevation in normal individuals, and drug abuse is seldom a problem.

2. **Tolerance:** Tolerance to the cholinergic properties of the TCAs develops within a short time. Some psychological dependence is possible, with slight withdrawal symptoms. The drugs can be used for prolonged treatment of depression without tolerance, which suggests that antimuscarinic activity is unrelated to its antidepressant action.

C. Therapeutic uses

1. **Severe endogenous depression:** The tricyclic antidepressants are the drugs most widely used to treat major depression.

2. **Phobias:** Some episodic phobias respond to TCA.

3. **Enuresis:** *Imipramine* has been used to control bed-wetting in children (older than 6 years) by causing contraction of the internal sphincter of the bladder. At present it is used cautiously, because of the inducement of cardiac arrhythmias and other serious cardiovascular problems.

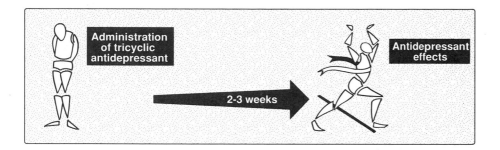

D. Pharmacology

1. **Absorption and distribution:** The TCAs are well absorbed on oral administration, and because of their lipophilic nature, are widely distributed and readily penetrate into the CNS. This lipid solubility also causes these drugs to have long half-lives, for example, 4-17 hours for *imipramine*. As a result of their variable first pass metabolism in the liver, these drugs have low and inconsistent bioavailability. Therefore the patient's response is used to adjust dosage. The initial treatment period is typically 4-8 weeks. The dosage can be gradually reduced unless relapse occurs.

2. **Fate:** These drugs are metabolized by the hepatic microsomal system (p.12) and conjugated with glucuronic acid. Ultimately, the TCAs are excreted as inactive metabolites via the kidney.

E. Adverse effects

1. **Antimuscarinic effects:** Blockade of acetylcholine receptors leads to blurred vision, xerostomia, urinary retention, constipation, and aggravation of glaucoma.

2. **Cardiovascular:** Increased catecholamine activity results in cardiac overstimulation, which can be life-threatening if an overdose of one of the drugs is taken. The slowing of atrioventricular conduction among depressed elderly patients is of particular concern.

3. **Orthostatic hypotension:** These drugs block α-adrenergic receptors, causing orthostatic hypotension and reflex tachycardia.

4. **Sedation:** Sedation may be prominent, especially during the first several weeks of treatment.

5. **Drug interactions:** See Figure 12.3.

6. **Precautions:** The tricyclic antidepressants should be used with caution in manic-depressive patients, since they may unmask manic behavior. The TCAs may aggravate epilepsy and glaucoma.

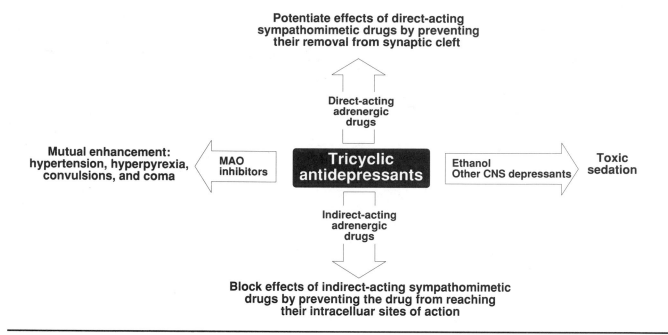

Figure 12.3
Drugs interacting with tricyclic antidepressants.

III. SEROTONIN-UPTAKE INHIBITORS

This new group of chemically unique antidepressant drugs specifically inhibits serotonin uptake (Figure 12.4). This contrasts with the tricyclic antidepressants, which nonselectively inhibit the uptake of *norepinephrine,* serotonin, and *dopamine.* Compared with tricyclic antidepressants, these drugs may cause fewer anticholinergic effects and lower cardiotoxicity. However, the serotonin re-uptake inhibitors should be used cautiously until their long-term effects have been evaluated.

A. Fluoxetine

Fluoxetine [floo OX e teen] is a new antidepressant that selectively inhibits serotonin re-uptake. *Fluoxetine* is as effective in the treatment of major depression as tricyclic antidepressants. The drug is free of most of the troubling side effects of tricyclic antidepressants, including anticholinergic effects, orthostatic hypotension, and weight gain. *Fluoxetine* has a long half-life—1-3 days for the parent compound and 7-15 days for the active metabolite, desmethylfluoxetine. Nausea, nervousness, insomnia, and headache are the most common side effects.

B. Trazodone

Trazodone [TRAY zoe done], like *fluoxetine,* inhibits serotonin re-uptake and has little effect on other neurotransmitter systems. *Trazodone* has shown efficacy comparable with tricyclic antidepressants, but the drug's side effect profile is superior to the older drugs. Few anticholinergic or cardiovascular side effects are observed with this drug. Adverse reactions include drowsiness, dizziness, headache, nausea, and rarely, priapism (persistent abnormal erection of the penis). *Trazodone* is useful in the treatment of patients with depression that is accompanied by marked agitation, anxiety, and insomnia, as well as those unable to tolerate anticholinergic side effects.

IV. MONOAMINE OXIDASE INHIBITORS

Monoamine oxidase (MAO) is a mitochondrial enzyme found in neural and other tissues, such as the gut and liver. In the neuron, MAO functions as a "safety valve" to oxidatively deaminate and inactivate any excess neurotransmitter molecules (*norepinephrine*, *dopamine*, and serotonin) that may leak out of synaptic vesicles when the neuron is at rest. The MAO inhibitors may irreversibly or reversibly inactivate the enzyme, permitting neurotransmitter molecules to escape degradation and therefore to both accumulate within the presynaptic neuron and to leak into the synaptic space. This causes activation of norepinephrine and serotonin receptors and may be responsible for the antidepressant action of these drugs.

Three MAO inhibitors are currently available: *phenelzine* [FEN el zeen], *isocarboxazid* [eye soe kar BOX a zid], and *tranylcypromine* [tran ill SIP roe meen]; no one drug is a prototype. Use of MAO inhibitors is now limited because the tricyclic antidepressants are more efficacious and less toxic.

A. Mode of action

1. **Inhibition of MAO:** Some MAO inhibitors, such as *isocarboxazid*, form stable complexes with the enzyme, causing irreversible inactivation. This results in increased stores of *norepinephrine*, serotonin and *dopamine* within the neuron and subsequent diffusion of excess neurotransmitter into the synaptic space (Figure 12.5).

2. **Inhibition of other oxidizing enzymes:** These drugs inhibit not only MAO in brain, but oxidases that catalyze oxidative deamination of drugs and potentially toxic substances, such as tyramine, which is found in certain foods. The MAO inhibitors therefore show a high incidence of drug-drug and drug-food interactions (see "Adverse effects", later).

B. Actions

1. **Mood elevation:** Although MAO is fully inhibited after several days of treatment, the antidepressant action of the MAO inhibitors, like that of the TCAs (p.119), is delayed several weeks.

2. **CNS stimulation:** *Phenelzine* and *tranylcypromine* have a mild amphetamine-like stimulant effect.

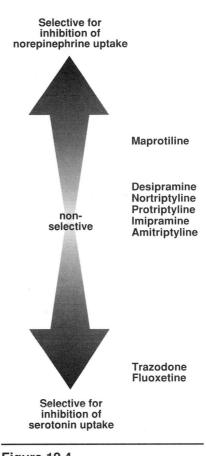

Selective for
inhibition of
norepinephrine uptake

Maprotiline

Desipramine
Nortriptyline
Protriptyline
Imipramine
Amitriptyline

non-
selective

Trazodone
Fluoxetine

Selective for
inhibition of
serotonin uptake

Figure 12.4
Relative selectivity of antidepressant drugs on the uptake of catecholamines.

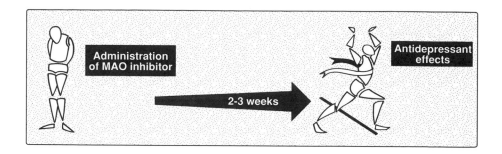

C. Therapeutic uses

1. **Moderate to severe depression:** Indicated for depressed patients who are unresponsive or allergic to tricyclic antidepressants or who experience strong anxiety.

2. **Treatment of hypersomnia:** Patients with low psychomotor activity may benefit from the stimulant properties of MAO inhibitors.

3. **Treatment of phobic states:** MAO inhibitors are useful in the treatment of phobic states.

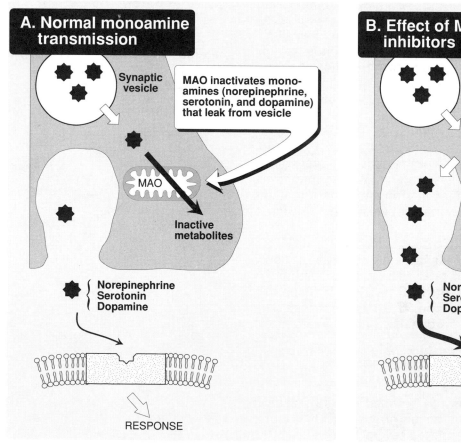

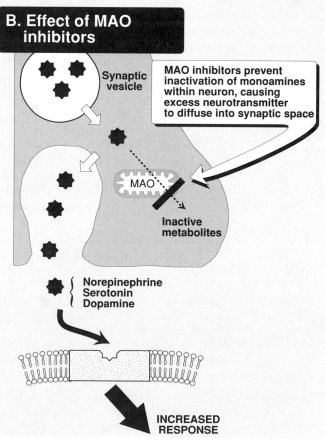

Figure 12.5
Mechanism of action of MAO inhibitors.

D. Pharmacology

1. **Absorption and distribution:** These drugs are well absorbed on oral administration, but antidepressant effects require 2-4 weeks of treatment. Enzyme regeneration, when irreversibly inactivated, varies but usually occurs several weeks after termination of the drug. Thus, when switching antidepressant agents, a minimum of 2 weeks delay must be allowed after termination of MAO-inhibitor therapy.

2. **Fate:** MAO inhibitors are metabolized and excreted rapidly in the urine.

E. Adverse effects

Severe and often unpredictable side effects limit the widespread use of MAO inhibitors.

1. **Hypertensive crises:** Tyramine, contained in certain foods, such as aged cheeses, chicken liver, beer, and red wines, is normally inactivated by MAO in the gut. Individuals receiving an MAO inhibitor are unable to degrade tyramine obtained from the diet. Tyramine causes the release of large amounts of stored catecholamines from nerve terminals. This results in headache, tachycardia, nausea, hypertension, cardiac arrhythmias, and stroke. Patients must be educated to avoid tyramine-containing foods. Treatment with MAO inhibitors can be dangerous in severely depressed patients with suicidal tendencies. *Phentolamine* (p.73) or *prazosin* (p.73) are helpful in the management of tyramine-induced hypertension. [Note: Treatment with MAO inhibitors may be dangerous in severely depressed patients with suicidal tendencies. Purposeful consumption of tyramine-containing foods is a possibility.]

2. Other adverse effects include drowsiness, orthostatic hypotension, blurred vision, dryness of the mouth, dysuria, and constipation.

V. LITHIUM SALTS

Lithium salts are used prophylactically in treating manic-depressive patients and in the treatment of manic episodes, they are also effective in treating 60-80% of patients exhibiting mania and hypomania. Although many cellular processes are altered by treatment with *lithium salts*, the mode of action is unknown. [Note: It is currently proposed that *lithium* acts by altering the cellular concentration of the second messenger, inositol triphosphate (IP$_3$, p.33).] *Lithium* is given orally. The ion is excreted by the kidney. *Lithium salts* are very toxic. Their safety factor and therapeutic index are extremely low and comparable to *digitalis*. Adverse effects include ataxia, tremors, confusion, and convulsions. *Lithium* causes no noticeable effect on normal individuals. It is not a sedative, euphoriant or depressant.

Figure 12.6 summarizes the therapeutic disadvantages and advantages of the antidepressant drugs.

Therapeutic Disadvantages of Antidepressant Agents   **Therapeutic Advantages of Antidepressant Agents**

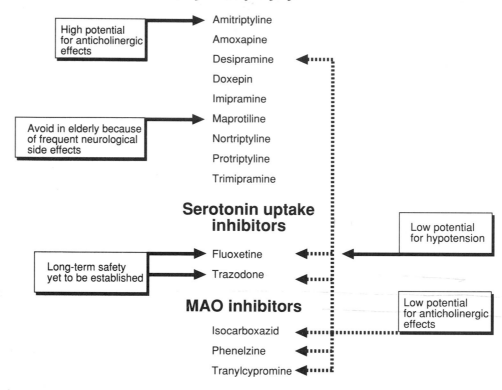

Tricyclics/polycyclics

High potential for anticholinergic effects → Amitriptyline

Amoxapine

Desipramine

Doxepin

Imipramine

Avoid in elderly because of frequent neurological side effects → Maprotiline

Nortriptyline

Protriptyline

Trimipramine

Serotonin uptake inhibitors

Low potential for hypotension

Long-term safety yet to be established → Fluoxetine

Trazodone

MAO inhibitors

Low potential for anticholinergic effects

Isocarboxazid

Phenelzine

Tranylcypromine

Figure 12.6
Therapeutic disadvantages and advantages of drugs used to treat depression.

Study Questions   (see p.415 for answers).

Choose the ONE best answer.

12.1 Which one of the following is an appropriate therapeutic use for imipramine?

    A. Insomnia.
    B. Epilepsy.
    C. Bed-wetting in children.
    D. Glaucoma.
    E. Mania.

12.2 MAO inhibitors are contraindicated with all of the following EXCEPT:

    A. Indirect adrenergic agents, such as ephedrine.
    B. Tricyclic antidepressants.
    C. Beer and cheese.
    D. Aspirin.
    E. Dopamine.

12.3 Which of the following statements concerning tricyclic antidepressants is correct?

    A. All the tricyclic antidepressants show similar therapeutic efficacy.
    B. Hypertension is a common adverse effect.
    C. The tricyclic antidepressants selectively inhibit uptake of norepinephrine into the neuron.
    D. These drugs show an immediate therapeutic effect.
    E. These drugs must be administered intramuscularly.

Neuroleptic Drugs

13

I. OVERVIEW

Neuroleptic drugs (also called antischizophrenic drugs, antipsychotic drugs, or major tranquilizers) are used primarily to treat schizophrenia but are also effective in other excited psychotic states, such as manic states and delirium. The neuroleptic drugs are competitive inhibitors at a variety of receptors, but their antipsychotic effects reflect competitive blocking of dopamine receptors. The neuroleptic drugs vary in their potency, but no one drug is clinically more effective than others. However, the trend is toward the use of high potency drugs, such as *thiothixene* [thye oh THIX een], *haloperidol* [ha loe PER i dole], and *fluphenazine* [floo FEN a zeen]. *Chlorpromazine* [klor PROE ma zeen], the prototype of the neuroleptic agents, is used infrequently because of its high incidence of serious side effects. Neuroleptic drugs are not curative and do not eliminate the fundamental thinking disorder, but often do permit the psychotic patient to function in a supportive environment.

II. SCHIZOPHRENIA

Schizophrenia is a particular type of psychosis, that is, a mental disorder caused by some inherent dysfunction of the brain. It is characterized by delusions, hallucinations (often in the form of voices), and thinking or speech disturbances. This mental disorder is a common affliction, occurring among about 1% of the population, or at about the same incidence as diabetes mellitus. The illness often initially affects people during adolescence and is a chronic and disabling disorder. Schizophrenia has a strong genetic component and probably reflects some fundamental biochemical abnormality, possibly an overactivity of the mesolimbic dopaminergic neurons.

III. NEUROLEPTIC DRUGS

The neuroleptic drugs can be divided into four major classifications based on the structure of the drug (Figure 13.1). This classification is of modest importance, because within each chemical group, different side chains have profound effects on the potencies of the drugs. The management of psychotic disorders can typically be achieved by familiarity with the effects of one or two drugs in each class.

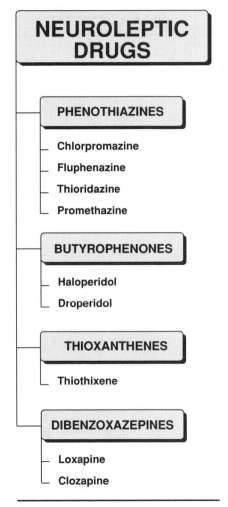

Figure 13.1
Summary of neuroleptic agents.

127

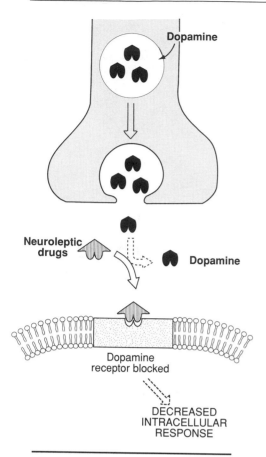

A. Mode of action

1. **Dopamine receptor-blocking activity in brain:** All the neuroleptic drugs block dopamine receptors in the brain and in the periphery (Figure 13.2). At least two types of dopamine receptors can be distinguished: D_1 receptors, which activate adenylate cyclase, and D_2 receptors, which inhibit adenylate cyclase. The neuroleptic drugs bind to both types of dopamine receptors. However, the clinical efficacy of the neuroleptic drugs correlates closely with their relative ability to block D_2 receptors in the mesolimbic system of the brain. The D_1 dopaminergic receptors are blocked only by high concentration of neuroleptics. The actions of the neuroleptic drugs are overturned by agents that raise dopamine concentration, for example, the drugs *L-dopa* (p.86) and *amphetamines* (p.105).

B. Actions

The antipsychotic actions of neuroleptic drugs reflect blockade at dopamine receptors. However, many of these agents also block cholinergic, adrenergic, and histamine receptors, causing a variety of side effects unrelated to antidopaminergic activity (Figure 13.3). Thus, the side effects of these drugs reflect the lack of absolute specificity for dopamine receptors.

1. **Antipsychotic actions:** The neuroleptic drugs reduce the hallucinations and agitation associated with schizophrenia by blocking dopamine receptors in the mesolimbic system of the brain. These drugs also have a calming effect and reduce spontaneous physical movement. In contrast to the CNS depressants, such as barbiturates, the neuroleptics do not depress intellectual function of the patient and motor incoordination is minimal. The antipsychotic effects usually take several weeks to occur, suggesting

Figure 13.2
Dopamine-blocking actions
of neuroleptic drugs.

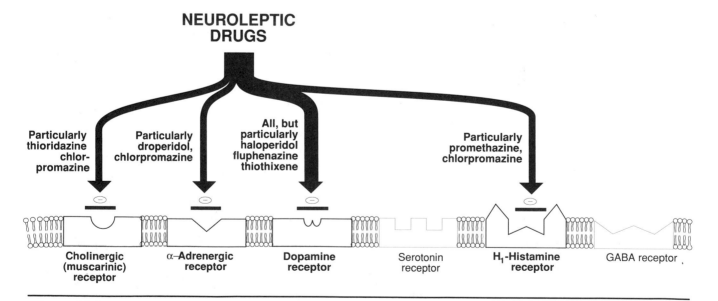

Figure 13.3
Neuroleptic drugs block at dopaminergic receptors as well as at adrenergic, cholinergic, and histamine-binding receptors. GABA = γ–aminobutyric acid.

that the therapeutic effects are related to secondary changes in the corticostriatal pathways.

2. **Extrapyramidal effects:** Parkinsonian symptoms, akathisia (motor restlessness), tardive dyskinesia (inappropriate postures of the neck, trunk, and limbs) occur with chronic treatment. Blocking of dopamine receptors in the nigrostriatal pathway probably causes these unwanted parkinsonian symptoms.

3. **Antiemetic effect:** With the exception of *thioridazine* [thye oh RID a zeen], most of the neuroleptic drugs have antiemetic effects that are mediated by blocking D_2 dopaminergic receptors of the chemoreceptor trigger zone of the medulla. Figure 13.4 summarizes the antiemetic uses of neuroleptic agents, along with the therapeutic applications of other drugs that combat nausea.

4. **Antimuscarinic effects:** All the neuroleptics, particularly *thioridazine* and *chlorpromazine*, have anticholinergic effects, including blurred vision, dry mouth, sedation, confusion, and inhibition of gastrointestinal and urinary smooth muscle, leading to constipation and urinary retention.

5. **Blockade of a-adrenergic receptors:** Blockade of these receptors causes orthostatic hypotension and lightheadedness.

6. **Hypothermia:** The neuroleptics alter temperature-regulating mechanisms and can produce poikilothermia.

7. **Endocrine effects:** In the pituitary, neuroleptics block D_2 receptors, leading to an increase in prolactin release.

C. Therapeutic uses

1. **Treatment of schizophrenia:** The neuroleptics are the only efficacious treatment of schizophrenia. Not all patients respond, and complete normalization of behavior is seldom achieved. However, patients typically have fewer hallucinations and delusions.

2. **Prevention of severe nausea and vomiting:** The neuroleptics, with the exception of *thioridazine*, are useful in the treatment of drug-induced nausea. Nausea arising from emotion and pregnancy should be treated with sedatives and antihistamines, rather than with these powerful drugs. *Scopolamine* (p.48) is the drug of choice for treatment of motion sickness.

3. **Agitated depression:** The neuroleptic drugs may be used as tranquilizers to manage agitated and disruptive behavior.

4. **Other:** Neuroleptics are used in combination with narcotic analgesics for treatment of chronic pain with severe anxiety. *Chlorpromazine* is used to treat intractable hiccups. *Droperidol* [droe PER i dole] is a component of neuroleptanesthesia (p.115). *Promethazine* [proe METH a zeen] is not a good antipsychotic drug, but the agent is used in treating pruritus because of its antihistamine properties (p.390).

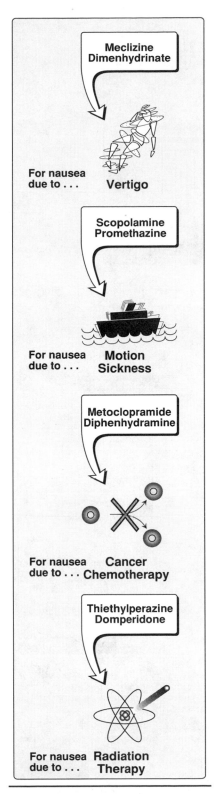

Figure 13.4
Therapeutic application of antiemetic agents.

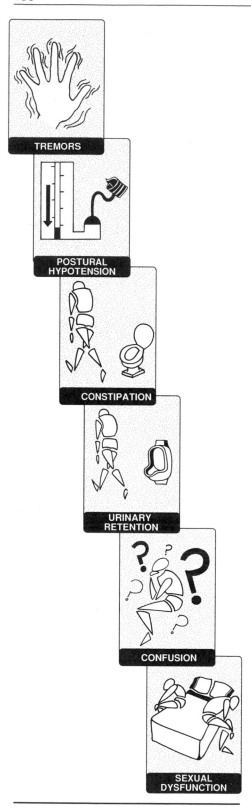

Figure 13.5
Adverse effects commonly observed in individuals treated with neuroleptic drugs.

D. Absorption and metabolism

1. **Absorption, distribution, and fate:** The neuroleptics show variable absorption after oral administration. These agents readily pass into the brain, have a large volume of distribution, bind well to plasma proteins, and are metabolized to many different substances by the P-450 system in the liver. *Fluphenazine enanthate* and *flupentixol decanoate* are long-acting (up to to 3 weeks) neuroleptics, administered by injection. These drugs are increasingly used in treating outpatients and individuals who are noncompliant. However, about 30% of these patients develop extrapyramidal symptoms.

2. **Tolerance:** The neuroleptic drugs produce some tolerance but little physical dependence.

E. Adverse effects

Adverse effects of the neuroleptic drugs occur in practically all patients and are significant in about 80% (Figure 13.5).

1. **Parkinsonian effects:**

   a. The inhibitory effects of dopaminergic neurons are normally balanced by the excitatory actions of cholinergic neurons. Blocking dopamine receptors alters this balance, causing a relative excess of cholinergic influence and resulting in extrapyramidal motor effects. However, if cholinergic activity is also blocked, a new, more nearly normal balance is restored, and extrapyramidal effects are minimized. This can be achieved by administration of an anticholinergic drug, such as *benztropine*. The therapeutic tradeoff is fewer extrapyramidal effects in exchange for the side effects of parasympathetic blockade (p.47). [Note: Often, the parkinsonian actions persist, despite the anticholinergic drugs.]

   b. Those drugs that exhibit strong anticholinergic activity, such as *thioridazine*, show few extrapyramidal disturbances, since the cholinergic activity is strongly dampened. This contrasts with *haloperidol* and *fluphenazine*, which have low anticholinergic activity and produce extrapyramidal effects because of the preferential blocking of dopaminergic transmission without the blocking of cholinergic activity.

   c. *Clozapine* [KLOE za peen] has a low potential for causing extrapyramidal symptoms and lower risk of tardive dyskinesia. The drug appears to be superior to *haloperidol* and *chlorpromazine* in treating the symptoms of schizophrenia. *Clozapine* can produce bone marrow suppression and cardiovascular side effects. *Clozapine* may be useful in patients who are refractory to traditional therapy. Figure 13.6 summarizes the pharmacological properties of *clozapine*, *chlorpromazine*, and *haloperidol*.

2. **Tardive dyskinesia:**

   a. Long-term treatment with neuroleptics can cause this motor disorder. Patients display involuntary movements, including lateral jaw movements and "fly-catching" motions of the tongue. A prolonged holiday from neuroleptics may cause the symptoms to diminish or disappear within 3 months. However, in many individuals, dyskinesia is irreversible and persists after discontinuation of therapy.

b. Tardive dyskinesia is postulated to result from an increased number of dopamine receptors that are synthesized in response to long-term dopamine receptor blockage. This makes the neuron supersensitive to the actions of dopamine and allows the dopaminergic input to this structure to overpower the cholinergic input, causing excess movement in the patient.

3. **CNS depression:** Drowsiness occurs, usually during the first 2 weeks of treatment. Confusion is sometimes encountered.

4. **Antimuscarinic effects:** The neuroleptics often produce dry mouth, urinary retention, constipation, and loss of accomodation.

5. **Orthostatic hypotension:** The neuroleptics block α-adrenergic receptors, resulting in lowered blood pressure and orthostatic hypotension.

6. **Endocrine alteration:** The neuroleptics depress the hypothalamus, causing amenorrhea, galactorrhea, infertility, and impotence.

7. **Cautions and contraindications:**

a. Acute agitation accompanying withdrawal from alcohol or other drugs may be aggravated by the neuroleptics. Stabilization with a simple sedative, such as a benzodiazepine (p.91), is the preferred treatment.

b. *Chlorpromazine* is contraindicated in patients with cardiovascular disease, since this drug can lead to arrhythmias.

c. The neuroleptics can aggravate epilepsy.

Figure 13.7 summarizes the therapeutic uses of the neuroleptic drugs.

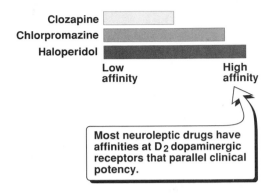

Relative affinities at D_2 receptors

Most neuroleptic drugs have affinities at D_2 dopaminergic receptors that parallel clinical potency.

Clozapine differs from typical neuroleptic drugs in having a similar affinity for both D_1 and D_2 dopaminergic receptors.

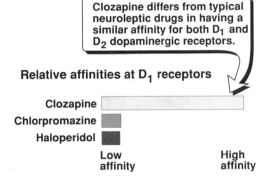

Relative affinities at D_1 receptors

Figure 13.6
Relative affinity of clozapine, chlorpromazine and haloperidol at D_1 and D_2 dopaminergic receptors

Study Questions   (see p.415 for answers)

Choose the ONE best answer.

13.1 The neuroleptic drugs.

A. show a wide range of efficacy in treating schizophrenia.
B. all show the potential for causing tardive dyskinesia.
C. bind selectively to D_2-dopaminergic receptors.
D. are useful in the treatment of epilepsy.
E. show antipsychotic effects immediately on administration.

13.2 The neuroleptic drugs

A. cause altered mental acuity.
B. all cause similar extrapyramidal effects.
C. are highly addictive.
D. can produce orthostatic hypotension.
E. are excreted unchanged.

Drug	Therapeutic notes
Fluphenazine	Available as slow release depot form
Droperidol	Used in neuroleptanalgesia; not used in schizophrenia
Haloperidol	Little adrenergic or muscarinic activity
Thiothixene	
Loxapine	Pronounced extrapyramidal effects
Thioridazine	Strong muscarinic antagonist
Chlorpromazine	Used infrequently because of adverse effects

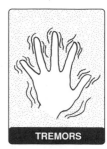

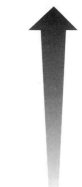

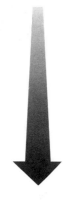

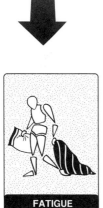

FATIGUE

TREMORS

Sedation and cardiovascular effects commonly seen with agents in the lower portion of table

Parkinsonian effects commonly seen with agents in the upper portion of table

Figure 13.7
Summary of neuroleptic agents.

13.3 All of the following are observed in patients taking neuroleptic agents EXCEPT:

A. Drowsiness.
B. Hypotension.
C. Altered endocrine function.
D. Diarrhea.
E. Urinary retention.

13.4 Which of the following is a therapeutic application of the neuroleptic agents?

A. Acute mania.
B. Motion sickness.
C. Glaucoma.
D. Insomnia.
E. Hypertension.

Opioid Analgesics and Antagonists

14

I. OVERVIEW

Opioids are natural or synthetic compounds that produce morphine-like effects (see Figure 14.1 for a summary of the opioid drugs). The term opiates is reserved for drugs obtained from opium, such as *morphine* and *codeine*. These drugs act by binding to specific opioid receptors in the central nervous system (CNS) to produce effects that mimic the action of endogenous peptide neurotransmitters, for example, the endorphins. *Morphine* and *codeine*, isolated from the poppy, relieve severe pain and are essential in current treatment of major diseases, trauma, and surgery. However, their widespread availability has led to drug abuse.

II. OPIOID RECEPTORS

Opioids interact with specific protein receptors on the membranes of certain cells in the CNS and the gastrointestinal tract. The major effects of the opioids are mediated by three families of receptors, designated by the Greek letters, μ, κ and σ, each of which exhibits a different specificity for the drug(s) it binds (Figure 14.2). Additional receptors for the opioids are known; for example, the δ receptor is a specific target for enkephalin peptides, and is involved with behavior and euphoria.

A. Distribution of receptors

Opioid receptors are present at the highest density in five general areas of the brain known to be involved in integrating information about pain.

1. **Brainstem:** Opioid receptors mediate respiration, cough, nausea and vomiting, maintenance of blood pressure, pupillary diameter, and control of stomach secretions.

2. **Medial thalamus:** This area mediates deep pain that is poorly localized and emotionally influenced.

3. **Spinal cord:** Receptors in the substantia gelatinosa are involved with the receipt and integration of incoming sensory information, leading to the attenuation of painful afferent stimuli.

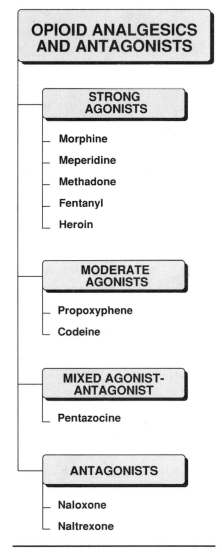

Figure 14.1
Summary of opioid analgesics and antagonists.

133

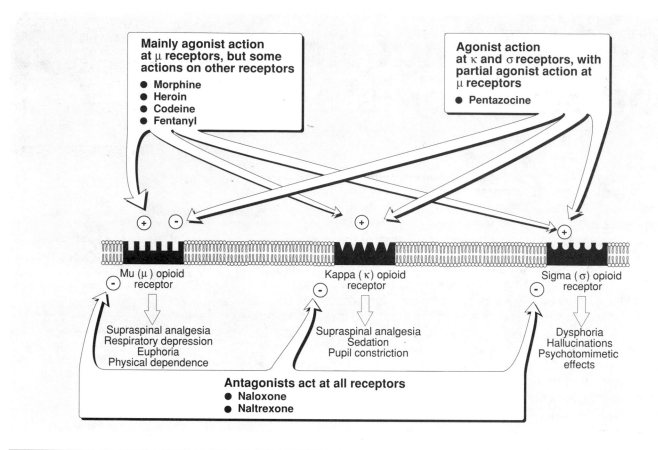

Figure 14.2
Actions of agonists and antagonists at opioid receptors.

4. **Hypothalamus:** Receptors here affect neuroendocrine secretion.

5. **Limbic system:** The greatest concentration of opiate receptors in the limbic system is located in the amygdala. These receptors probably do not exert analgesic action, but they may influence emotional behavior.

III. STRONG AGONISTS

Morphine [MOR feen] is the major analgesic drug contained in crude opium and is the prototype agonist. *Codeine* [KOE deen] is present in lower concentrations and is inherently less potent. The opioid agonists all have similar actions; these drugs show a high affinity for μ receptors, varying affinities for δ and κ receptors, and low affinity for σ receptors.

A. Morphine

1. **Mechanism of action:** Opioids exert their major effects by interacting with opioid receptors in the CNS and the gastrointestinal tract. Opioids cause hyperpolarization of nerve cells, inhibition

of nerve firing, and presynaptic inhibition of transmitter release. *Morphine* acts at μ receptors in lamina I and II of the substantia gelatinosa of the spinal cord and decreases the release of substance P, which modulates pain perception in the spinal cord. *Morphine* also appears to inhibit the release of many excitatory transmitters from nerve terminals carrying nociceptive (painful) stimuli.

2. **Actions:**

a. **Analgesia:** *Morphine* causes analgesia (relief of pain without the loss of consciousness). Opioids relieve pain both by enhancing the pain threshold at the spinal cord level, and more importantly, by altering the brain's interpretation of pain. Patients treated with *morphine* are still aware of the presence of pain, but the sensation is not unpleasant. The maximum analgesic efficacy and the potential for addiction for representative agonists is shown in Figure 14.3.

b. **Euphoria:** *Morphine* produces a powerful sense of contentment and well-being. Euphoria may be caused by stimulation of the ventral tegmentum.

c. **Respiration:** *Morphine* causes respiratory depression by reduction of the sensitivity of respiratory center neurons to carbon dioxide. This occurs with ordinary doses of *morphine* and is accentuated as the dose increases until, ultimately, respiration ceases. Respiratory depression is the most common cause of death in acute opioid overdose.

d. **Depression of cough reflex:** *Morphine* and *codeine* have antitussive properties. In general, cough suppression does not correlate closely with analgesic and respiratory depressant properties of opioid drugs. The receptors involved in the antitussive action appear to be different than those involved in analgesia.

e. **Miosis:** The pinpoint pupil, characteristic of *morphine* use, results from stimulation of μ and κ receptors. *Morphine* excites the Edinger-Westphal nucleus of the oculomotor nerve, which causes enhanced parasympathetic stimulation to the eye. There is little tolerance to the effect, and all addicts demonstrate pin-point pupils. This is important diagnostically, because most other causes of coma and respiratory depression produce dilation of the pupil.

f. **Emesis:** *Morphine* directly stimulates the chemoreceptor trigger zone in the area postrema, which causes vomiting. However, the emesis does not produce unpleasant sensations.

g. **Gastrointestinal tract:** *Morphine* relieves diarrhea and dysentery. It decreases motility of smooth muscle and increases tone. It increases pressure in the biliary tract. *Morphine* also increases the tone of the anal sphincter. Overall, *morphine* produces constipation, with little tolerance developing.

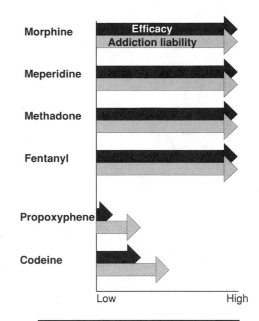

Figure 14.3
A comparison of the maximum efficacy and addiction/abuse liability of commonly used narcotic analgesics.

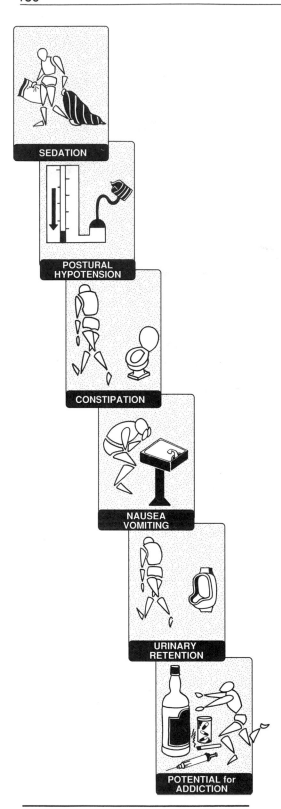

Figure 14.4
Adverse effects commonly observed in individuals treated with opioids.

h. **Cardiovascular:** *Morphine* has no major effects on the blood pressure or heart rate. Because of respiratory depression and carbon dioxide retention, cerebral vessels dilate and increase the cerebrospinal fluid (CSF) pressure. Therefore, *morphine* is usually contraindicated in individuals with severe brain injury.

i. **Histamine release:** *Morphine* releases histamine from mast cells, causing urticaria, sweating, and vasodilation.

j. **Hormonal actions:** *Morphine* inhibits release of gonadotropin-releasing hormone and corticotropin-releasing hormone and decreases the concentration of luteinizing hormone, follicle-stimulating hormone, adrenocorticotropic hormone, and β-endorphin. Testosterone and cortisol levels decrease. *Morphine* increases prolactin and growth hormone release by diminishing dopaminergic inhibition.

3. **Therapeutic uses:**

a. **Analgesia:** Despite intensive research, few other drugs have been developed that are as effective in the treatment of pain. Opioids induce sleep, and in clinical situations when pain is present and sleep is necessary, opiates may be used to supplement the sleep-inducing properties of barbiturates. [Note: The sedative-hypnotic drugs are not usually analgesic, and may have diminished sedative effect in the presence of pain (p.92).]

b. **Treatment of diarrhea:** *Morphine* decreases the motility of smooth muscle and increases tone (see earlier).

c. **Relief of cough:** *Morphine* suppresses the cough reflex; however, *codeine* or *dextromethorphan* are more widely used.

4. **Pharmacology**

a. **Administration:** The absorption of *morphine* from the gastrointestinal tract is slow and erratic, and the drug is usually not given orally. *Codeine*, by contrast, is well absorbed when given by mouth. Significant first-pass metabolism of *morphine* occurs in the liver; therefore, parenteral injections produce a greater response. The opiates have been commonly administered for nonmedical purposes by inhalation of the smoke from burning crude opium, which provides a rapid onset of drug action.

b. **Distribution:** *Morphine* rapidly enters all body tissues, including the fetus of pregnant women. Infants born of addicted mothers show physical dependence on opiates and exhibit withdrawal symptoms if opioids are not administered. Only a small percentage of *morphine* crosses the blood-brain barrier, since *morphine* is the least lipophilic of the common opioids. This contrasts with the more fat-soluble opioids, such as *fentanyl* and *heroin*, which readily penetrate into the brain and rapidly produce an intense "rush" of euphoria.

c. **Metabolism:** *Morphine* is metabolized in the liver to the glucuronide and is excreted primarily in the urine, with small quantities of the conjugate appearing in the bile. The duration of action of *morphine* is 4-5 hours

5. **Adverse effects:** Severe respiratory depression occurs. Other effects include vomiting, dysphoria, allergy-enhanced hypotensive effects, and low blood volume (Figure 14.4). The elevation of intracranial pressure, particularly in head injury, can be serious. It enhances cerebral and spinal ischemia. In prostatic hypertrophy, *morphine* may cause acute urinary retention. A serious action is stoppage of respiratory exchange in emphysema or cor pulmonale patients. If employed in such individuals, respiration must be carefully watched.

6. **Tolerance and physical dependence:** Repeated use produces tolerance to the respiratory depressant, analgesic, euphoric, and sedative effects of *morphine*. However, tolerance usually does not develop to the pupil-constricting and constipating effects of the drug. Physical dependence readily occurs with *morphine* and with some of the other agonists to be described (see Figure 14.3). Withdrawal produces a series of autonomic, motor and psychological responses that incapacitates the individual and causes serious, almost unbearable symptoms. However, it is very rare that the effects are so profound as to cause death.

7. **Drug interactions:** The depressant actions of *morphine* are enhanced by phenothiazines (p.127), monoamine oxidase inhibitors (p.123), and tricyclic antidepressants (p.119 and Figure 14.5). Low doses of *amphetamine* (p.105) strangely enhance analgesia. *Hydroxyzine* (p.390) also enhances analgesia.

B. Meperidine

Meperidine [me PER i deen] is a synthetic opioid that can be given orally. However, it is less effective orally than when given parenterally.

1. **Mechanism of action:** *Meperidine* binds to opioid receptors, particularly κ receptors.

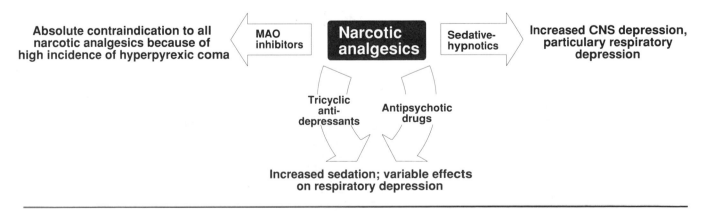

Figure 14.5
Drugs interacting with narcotic analgesics.

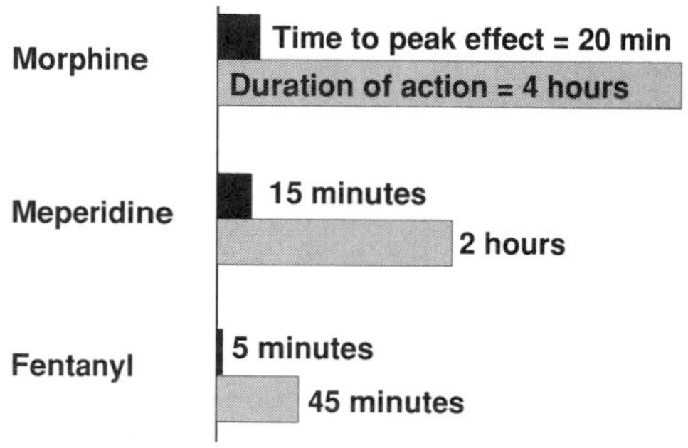

2. **Actions:**

   a. **Respiration:** Depression of respiration is similar to that of *morphine*.

   b. **Cardiovascular:** There is no significant cardiovascular action when given orally. On intravenous (IV) administration, the drug produces a decrease in peripheral resistance and an increase in peripheral blood flow. On IV use, it may cause an increase in cardiac rate. As with *morphine*, *meperidine* dilates cerebral vessels and increases cerebrospinal fluid pressure.

   c. **Smooth muscle:** Like *morphine*, *meperidine* contracts smooth muscle but to a lesser extent. In the gastrointestinal tract, it impedes motility, and constipation results on chronic use.

   d. **Eye:** *Meperidine* does not cause pinpoint pupils, but rather causes the pupils to dilate because of an atropine-like activity.

3. **Therapeutic uses:** *Meperidine* provides analgesia for any type of severe pain. Unlike *morphine*, *meperidine* is not clinically useful in the treatment of diarrhea or cough. *Meperidine* produces less of an increase in urinary retention than does *morphine*.

4. **Pharmacology:** Unlike *morphine*, *meperidine* is well absorbed from the gastrointestinal tract and is useful when an orally administered, potent analgesic is needed. However, *meperidine* is most often administered intramuscularly. The drug has a duration of action of 2-4 hours, which is shorter than that of *morphine* (4-6 hours, see Figure 14.6). *Meperidine* is metabolized in the liver and excreted in the urine.

5. **Adverse effects:** Large doses of *meperidine* cause tremors, muscle twitches, and rarely convulsions. The drug differs from opioids in that in large doses it dilates the pupil and causes hyperactive reflexes. When used with major neuroleptics, depression is greatly enhanced. *Meperidine* is addictive and can substitute for *morphine* or *heroin* in use by addicts.

Figure 14.6
Time to peak effect and duration of action of several opioids administered intravenously.

C. Methadone

Methadone [METH a done] is a synthetic, orally effective opioid that is approximately equal in potency to *morphine*, but it induces less euphoria and has a longer duration of action.

1. **Mechanism of action:** *Methadone* has its greatest action on μ receptors.

2. **Actions:** The analgesic activity of *methadone* is equivalent to *morphine*. *Methadone* shows strong analgesic action when administered orally, which contrasts with *morphine*, which is only partially absorbed from the gastrointestinal tract. The miotic and respiratory depressant actions of *methadone* have average half-lives of 24 hours. *Methadone* increases biliary pressure like *morphine* and is also constipating.

3. **Therapeutic uses:** *Methadone* is well absorbed orally. The drug has been used in the controlled withdrawal of addicts from *heroin* and *morphine*. Orally administered, *methadone* is substituted for the injected opioid. The patient is then slowly removed from *methadone*. *Methadone* causes a milder withdrawal syndrome, which also develops more slowly than that seen during withdrawal from *morphine*.

4. **Pharmacology:** *Methadone* has a longer duration of action than does *morphine*. It has the ability to accumulate in the tissues and remains there for long periods by binding to protein. The drug is biotransformed in the liver and excreted in the urine mainly as inactive metabolites.

5. **Adverse effects:** *Methadone* can produce addiction like *morphine*. The withdrawal syndrome is much milder but is more protracted (days to weeks) than with opiates.

D. Fentanyl

Fentanyl [FEN ta nil] has 80 times the analgesic potency of *morphine*. This highly potent opioid has a rapid onset and short duration of action (15-30 minutes). When combined with *droperidol* (p.116) it produces a dissociative anesthesia.

E. Heroin

Heroin [HAIR o in] does not occur naturally but is produced by acetylation modification of *morphine*, which leads to a three-fold increase in potency. *Heroin* is more lipid soluble and crosses the blood-brain barrier more rapidly than *morphine*, causing a more exaggerated euphoria when the drug is taken by injection. It has no accepted medical use in the United States.

IV. MODERATE AGONISTS

A. Propoxyphene

Propoxyphene [proe POX i feen] is a derivative of *methadone*. The dextro isomer is used as an analgesic to relieve mild to moderate pain. The levo isomer is not analgesic but has antitussive action. Given parenterally, *propoxyphene* produces analgesia that is equivalent to less than half that of *codeine*. When given orally, it is only about one third as active as *codeine*. *Propoxyphene* is often used in combination with *aspirin* for a greater degree of analgesia than with either alone. It is well absorbed orally, with peak plasma levels occurring in 1 hour, and it is metabolized in the liver. *Propoxyphene* can produce nausea, anorexia, and constipation. In toxic doses, it can cause respiratory depression, convulsions, hallucinations and confusion. When toxic doses are used, a very serious problem can arise in some individuals with resultant cardiotoxicity and pulmonary edema. [Note: When used with alcohol and sedatives, a severe CNS depression is produced and death by respiratory depression and cardiotoxicity can result. This respiratory depression and sedation can be antagonized by *naloxone* (p.141), but the cardiotoxicity cannot.]

B. Codeine

Codeine [KOE deen] is a much less potent analgesic than *morphine*, but it has a higher oral efficacy. *Codeine* shows good antitussive activity at doses that do not cause analgesia. The drug has a lower abuse potential than *morphine* and rarely produces addiction. The analgesic action is quite weak and equivalent to aspirin. *Codeine* produces less euphoria than *morphine*. [Note: In most nonprescription cough preparations *codeine* has been replaced by newer drugs, such as *dextromethorphan* (p.210), a synthetic cough depressant that has no analgesic action and a low potential for abuse.]

V. MIXED AGONIST-ANTAGONISTS

Drugs that stimulate one receptor but block another are termed mixed agonists-antagonists. The effects of these drugs depend on previous exposure to opioids. In individuals who have not recently received opioids, mixed agonist-antagonists show agonist activity and are used to relieve pain. In the patient with opioid dependence, the agonist-antagonists drugs may show primarily blocking effects, that is, produce withdrawal symptoms. Most of the drugs in this group cause dysphoria, rather than euphoria, mediated by activation of σ receptors

A. Pentazocine

Pentazocine [pen TAZ oh seen] acts as an agonist on κ receptors and a lesser agonist on the μ receptors. *Pentazocine* also shows weak antagonist activity at μ and δ receptors. *Pentazocine* promotes analgesia caused by action on the spinal cord, and it is used to relieve moderate pain. It may be administered either orally or parenterally. *Pentazocine* produces less euphoria than *morphine*. In higher doses, the drug causes respiratory depression and decreases the activity of the gastrointestinal tract. High doses increase blood pressure and can cause hallucinations, nightmares, tachycardia, and dizziness. In angina, *pentazocine* increases the mean aortic pressure and pulmonary artery pressure and thus increases the work of the heart. The drug decreases renal plasma flow. Despite its antagonist action, *pentazocine* does not antagonize the respiratory depression of *morphine*, but it can precipitate a withdrawal syndrome in a *morphine* abuser. *Pentazocine* should also not be used with agonists such as *morphine*, since the antagonist action of *pentazocine* may block the analgesic effects of *morphine*. Tolerance develops to repeated use and addiction.

VI. ANTAGONISTS

The opioid antagonists bind with high affinity to opioid receptors but fail to activate the receptor-mediated response. Administration of opioid antagonists produces no profound effects in normal individuals. However, in patients addicted to opioids, antagonists rapidly reverse the effect of agonists, such as *heroin*, and precipitate the symptoms of opiate withdrawal.

A. Naloxone

Naloxone [nal OX one] is used to reverse the coma and respiratory depression of opioid overdose. It rapidly displaces all receptor-bound opioid molecules and therefore is able to reverse the effect of a heroin overdose (Figure 14.7). Within 30 seconds of intravenous injection of *naloxone*, the respiratory depression and coma characteristic of high doses of *heroin* are reversed, causing the patient to be revived and alert. *Naloxone* has a half-life of 60-100 minutes. *Naloxone* is a competitive antagonist at μ, κ and σ, receptors. *Naloxone* has 10-fold higher affinity for μ receptors than for κ receptors. This may explain why *naloxone* readily reverses respiratory depression with only minimal reversal of analgesia that results from agonist stimulation of κ receptors in the spinal cord. *Naloxone* produces no pharmacological effects in normal individuals, but it can precipitate withdrawal symptoms in *morphine* or *heroin* abusers.

B. Naltrexone

Naltrexone [nal TREX one] has actions similar to *naloxone*. This drug has a longer duration of action than *naloxone*, and a single oral dose of *naltrexone* blocks the effect of injected *heroin* for up to 48 hours. *Naltrexone* is used in opiate-dependence maintenance programs.

VII. OPIOID PEPTIDES (OPIOPEPTINS)

A. Enkephalins

Enkephalins are naturally occurring opioid agonists. They function as neurotransmitters of specific neuronal systems in the brain that mediate the integration of sensory inputs associated with pain and emotional behavior. These endogenous neurotransmitters are pentapeptides that bind to the opioid receptors and exhibit actions similar to *morphine*; these transmitters are blocked by *naloxone*. The opioid drugs act by mimicking the action of these endogenous neurotransmitters. Increased levels of enkephalins may be responsible for acupuncture-induced analgesia. The two best characterized examples of this group are met-enkephalin and leu-enkephalin.

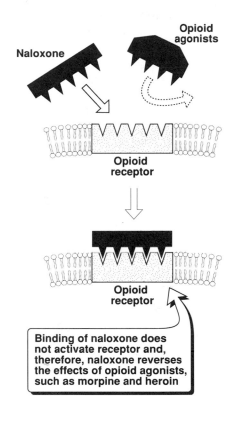

Figure 14.7
Competition of naloxone with opioid agonists.

Study Questions (see p.416 for answers).

Answer A if 1,2 and 3 are correct.
    B if 1 and 3 are correct.
    C if 2 and 4 are correct.
    D if only 4 is correct.
    E if 1,2,3 and 4 are all correct.

14.1 Which of the following actions of morphine do not develop tolerance?

    1. Respiratory depression.
    2. Pinpoint pupils.
    3. Euphoria.
    4. Constipation.

14.2 Codeine

1. is more effective than morphine in suppressing
   the cough reflex.
2. is equivalent to morphine in producing
   euphoria.
3. is a much less potent analgesic than morphine.
4. is a synthetic opioid.

14.3 Naloxone

1. produces respiratory depression in individuals
   who have not previously taken opioids.(Levallorphan)
2. antagonizes the actions of morphine.
3. has a short (10-15 minutes) duration of action.
4. can prompt the appearance of withdrawal
   symptoms in the heroin addict.

Choose the ONE best answer.

14.4 All of the following statements concerning
methadone are correct EXCEPT:

A. It has less potent analgesic activity than that of
   morphine. *[similar]*
B. It has a longer duration of action than that of
   morphine.
C. It is effective by oral administration.
D. Methadone causes a milder withdrawal
   syndrome than morphine.
E. It has its greatest action on μ receptors.

14.5 Which of the following statements about
pentazocine is INCORRECT?

A. It is a mixed agonist-antagonist.
B. It may be administered orally or parenterally.
C. It produces less euphoria than morphine.
D. It is often combined with morphine for
   maximal analgesic effects.
E. High doses of pentazocine increase blood
   pressure.

14.6 Which of the following statements about
morphine is INCORRECT?

A. It is used therapeutically to relieve pain caused
   by severe head injury.
B. Its withdrawal symptoms can be relieved by
   methadone.
C. It causes constipation.
D. It is most effective by parenteral
   administration.
E. It rapidly enters all body tissues, including the
   fetus of a pregnant woman.

Drugs Used to Treat Epilepsy

15

I. OVERVIEW OF EPILEPSY

Epilepsy is widespread among the general population with an incidence of 0.6%, representing 1.5 million affected individuals in the United States. Epilepsy is not a single entity; it is a family of different recurrent seizure disorders that have in common the sudden, excessive and disorderly discharge of cerebral neurons. This results in abnormal movements or perceptions that are of short duration but that tend to recur. The site of the electrical discharge determines the symptoms that are produced. For example, epileptic seizures may cause convulsions if the motor cortex is involved. The seizures may also include visual, auditory, or olfactory hallucinations if the parietal or occipital cortex plays a role. Drug therapy is the most widely effective mode of treatment for epilepsy (see Figure 15.1 for a summary of the antiepileptic drugs). Seizures can be controlled completely in approximately 50% of epileptic patients, and meaningful improvement is achieved in at least one half of the remaining patients.

A. Etiology

The neuronal discharge in epilepsy results from the firing of a small group of neurons that are localized in a specific area of the brain called the primary focus. Anatomically, this focal area may appear perfectly normal. Usually there is no identifiable cause for epilepsy, although the focal areas that are functionally abnormal may be triggered into activity by changes in any of a variety of environmental factors, including alteration in blood gasses, pH, electrolytes, or glucose availability.

1. **Primary epilepsy:** When no specific anatomical cause for the seizure, such as trauma or neoplasm, is evident the syndrome is called idiopathic or primary epilepsy. These seizures may be produced by an inherited abnormality in the central nervous system (CNS). Patients are treated chronically with antiepileptic drugs, often for life.

2. **Secondary epilepsy:** A number of reversible disturbances, such as tumors, head injury, hypoglycemia, meningeal infection, or rapid withdrawal of alcohol from an alcoholic, can precipitate seizures. Antiepileptic drugs are given until the primary cause of the seizures can be corrected. Seizures secondary to stroke or trauma may cause irreversible CNS damage.

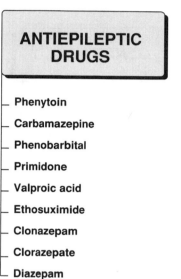

ANTIEPILEPTIC DRUGS

- Phenytoin
- Carbamazepine
- Phenobarbital
- Primidone
- Valproic acid
- Ethosuximide
- Clonazepam
- Clorazepate
- Diazepam

Figure 15.1
Summary of agents used in the treatment of epilepsy.

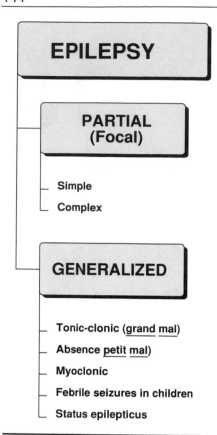

Figure 15.2
Classification of epilepsy.

B. Classification of epilepsy

Seizures have been classified into two broad groups, partial (or focal), and generalized (Figure 15.2). Choice of drug treatment is based on the classification of the epilepsy being treated.

1. **Partial:** The symptoms of each seizure type depend on the site of neuronal discharge and on the extent to which the electrical activity spreads to other neurons in the brain. Partial seizures may progress, becoming generalized tonic-clonic seizures.

   a. **Simple partial:** These seizures are caused by a group of hyperactive neurons exhibiting abnormal electrical activity and are confined to a single focus in the brain; the electrical disorder does not spread. The patient does not lose consciousness and often exhibits abnormal activity of a single limb or muscle group that is controlled by the region of the brain experiencing the disturbance. The patient may also show sensory distortions. Simple partial seizures may occur at any age.

   b. **Complex partial:** These seizures exhibit complex sensory hallucinations, mental distortion, and loss of consciousness. Motor dysfunction may involve chewing movements, diarrhea, urination. Most (80%) of individuals with complex partial epilepsy experience their initial seizures before age 20 years.

2. **Generalized:** These seizures begin locally, but they rapidly spread to produce abnormal electrical discharge throughout both hemispheres of the brain. Generalized seizures may be convulsive or nonconvulsive; the patient usually has an immediate loss of consciousness.

   a. **Tonic-clonic (grand mal):** This is the most commonly encountered and the most dramatic form of epilepsy. Seizures result in loss of consciousness, followed by tonic then clonic phases. The seizure is followed by a period of confusion and exhaustion.

   b. **Absence (petit mal):** These seizures involve a brief, abrupt, and self-limiting loss of consciousness. The onset occurs in patients at ages 3-5 years and lasts until puberty. The patient stares and exhibits rapid eye-blinking, which lasts for 3-5 seconds.

   c. **Myoclonic:** These seizures consist of short episodes of muscle contractions that may reoccur for several minutes. Myoclonic seizures are rare, occur at any age, and are often a result of permanent neurologic damage acquired as a result of hypoxia, uremia, encephalitis, or drug poisoning.

   d. **Febrile seizures:** Young children (3 months to 5 years of age) frequently develop seizures with illness accompanied by high fever. The febrile seizures consist of generalized tonic-clonic convulsions of short duration.

   e. **Status epilepticus:** Seizures are rapidly recurrent.

C. Mechanism of action of antiepileptic drugs

Drugs that are effective in seizure reduction can either block the initiation of the electrical discharge from the focal area, or more commonly, prevent the spread of the abnormal electrical discharge to adjacent brain areas.

II. ANTIEPILEPTIC DRUGS

Initial drug treatment to suppress or reduce the incidence of seizures is based on the specific type of seizure (Figure 15.3). Thus, the tonic-clonic (grand mal) seizures are treated differently than absence seizures (petit mal). Several drugs may be equally effective, and the toxicity of the agent is often a major consideration in drug selection. Monotherapy is instituted with a single agent until seizures are controlled or toxic signs occur. When therapy with a single drug is ineffective, a second drug may be added to the therapeutic regimen. Antiepileptic therapy for tonic-clonic seizures should never be terminated abruptly, otherwise seizures will result.

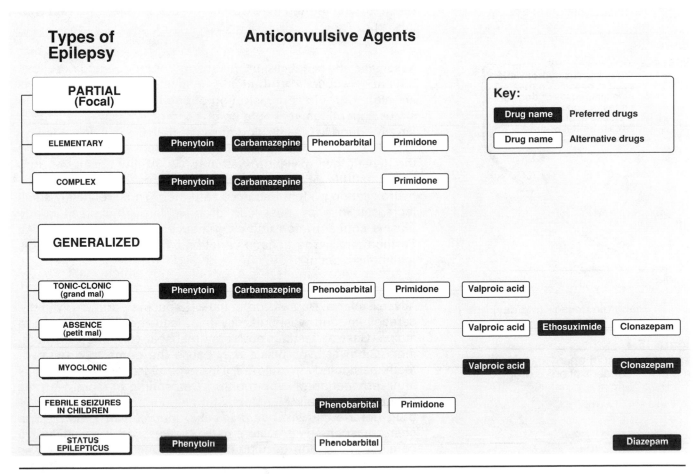

Figure 15.3
Therapeutic indications for anticonvulsant agents.

A. Phenytoin

Phenytoin [FEN i toy in] (formerly called *diphenylhydantoin*) is effective in suppressing tonic-clonic and partial seizures and was frequently the drug chosen for initial therapy, particularly in treating adults. More recently, its use is diminishing.

1. **Mechanism of action:** *Phenytoin* stabilizes neuronal membranes to depolarization by decreasing the flux of sodium ions in neurons in the resting state or during depolarization. It also reduces the influx of calcium ions during depolarization as well as suppressing repetitive firing of neurons.

2. **Actions:** *Phenytoin* is not a generalized CNS depressant like the barbiturates, but it does produce some degree of drowsiness and lethargy without progression to hypnosis. *Phenytoin* reduces the propagation of abnormal impulses in the brain.

3. **Therapeutic uses:** *Phenytoin* is highly effective for all partial seizures (elementary and complex), for tonic-clonic seizures, and in the treatment of status epilepticus caused by recurrent tonic-clonic seizures (Figure 15.3). The drug is not indicated for children under 5 years of age. *Phenytoin* is not effective for absence seizures, which often may worsen in such a patient treated with this drug.

4. **Absorption and Metabolism:** Oral absorption of *phenytoin* is slow, but once it occurs, distribution is rapid and brain concentrations are high. Chronic administration of *phenytoin* is always oral; in status epilepticus, it should be given intravenously. The drug is largely bound to plasma albumin. Less than 5% of a given dose is excreted unchanged in the urine. *Phenytoin* is metabolized by the hepatic hydroxylation system (p.12). At low doses the drug has a half-life of 24 hours, but as the dosage increases, the hydroxylation system becomes saturated. Thus, relatively small increases in each dose can produce large increases in the plasma concentration and drug-induced toxicity (Figure 15.4). Furthermore, large genetic variations in the rate of the drug's metabolism occur.

5. **Adverse effects:** Depression of the CNS occurs particularly in the cerebellum and vestibular system, causing nystagmus and ataxia. Gastrointestinal problems (nausea, vomiting) are common. Gingival hyperplasia may cause the gums to grow over teeth, particularly in children. This hyperplasia slowly regresses after termination of drug therapy. Coarsening of facial features occurs in children. Megaloblastic anemia occurs because the drug interferes with vitamin B_{12} metabolism[1]. Behavioral changes, such as confusion, hallucination, and drowsiness are common. Inhibition of antidiuretic hormone release occurs as well as hyperglycemia and glycosuria caused by inhibition of insulin secretion. *Phenytoin* is also an anti-arrhythmic drug. Treatment with *phenytoin* should not be stopped abruptly.

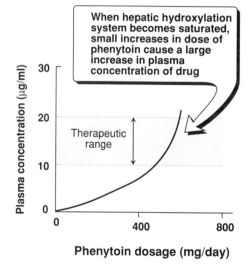

Figure 15.4
Nonlinear effect of phenytoin dosage on plasma concentration of drug.

6. **Teratogenic effects:**

   a. *Phenytoin* causes teratogenic effects in offspring of mothers given the drug during pregnancy. "Fetal hydantoin syndrome" includes cleft lip, cleft palate, congenital heart disease, as well as slowed growth and mental deficiency.

   b. Almost half of untreated epileptic women have an increased seizure frequency during pregnancy. This can lead to anoxic episodes, which yield a higher incidence of congenital birth defects if the epilepsy is untreated. Antiepileptic drugs are given at the lowest possible dose to control seizures.

7. **Drug interactions:**

   a. Inhibition of microsomal metabolism of *phenytoin* in the liver is caused by *chloramphenicol, dicumarol, cimetidine, sulfonamides,* and *isoniazid.* When used chronically, these drugs increase the concentration of *phenytoin* in plasma by preventing its metabolism. A decrease in plasma concentration of *phenytoin* is caused by *carbamazepine*, which enhances *phenytoin* metabolism (Figure 15.5).

   b. *Phenytoin* induces the P-450 system (p.12) which leads to an increase in the metabolism of other antiepileptics, anticoagulants, oral contraceptives, *quinidine* and *doxycycline, cyclosporine, mexiletine, methadone,* and *levodopa.*

B. Carbamazepine

1. **Actions:** *Carbamazepine* [kar ba MAZ a peen] reduces the propagation of abnormal impulses in the brain by blocking sodium channels, thereby inhibiting the generation of repetitive action potentials in the epileptic focus.

2. **Therapeutic uses:** *Carbamazepine* is highly effective for all partial seizures (elementary and complex) and is often the drug of first choice. In addition the drug is highly effective for tonic-clonic seizures and is used to treat trigeminal neuralgia. It has occasionally been used in manic-depressive patients to ameliorate the symptoms.

3. **Absorption and metabolism:** *Carbamazepine* is absorbed slowly and is erratically distributed on oral administration. It enters the brain rapidly because of its high lipid solubility. *Carbamazepine* induces the drug metabolizing enzymes in the liver, and its half-life therefore decreases with chronic administration. The enhanced hepatic P-450 system activity also increases the metabolism of other antiepileptic drugs.

4. **Adverse effects:** Chronic administration of *carbamazepine* can cause stupor, coma, and respiratory depression, along with drowsiness, vertigo, ataxia, and blurred vision. The drug is irritating to the stomach, and nausea and vomiting may occur. Aplastic anemia, agranulocytosis, and thrombocytopenia have occurred

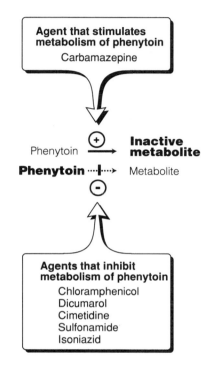

Figure 15.5
Drugs affecting the metabolism of phenytoin.

in some patients. This drug has the potential for inducing serious liver toxicity. Therefore, anyone being treated with *carbamazepine* should have frequent liver function tests.

5. **Drug interactions:** The hepatic metabolism of *carbamazepine* is inhibited by several drugs (Figure 15.6). Toxic symptoms may arise if the dose is not adjusted.

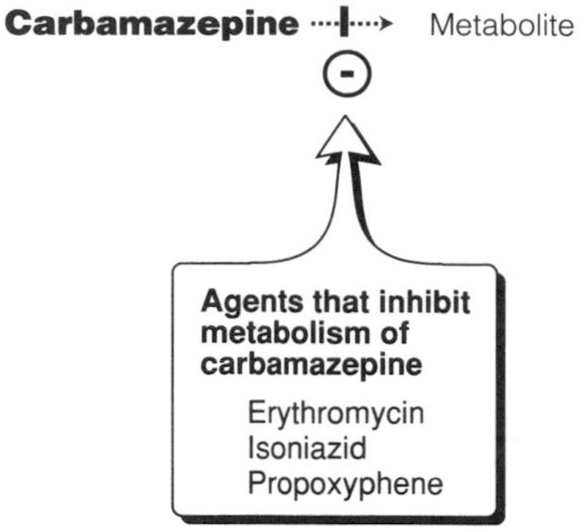

Carbamazepine ·····┃····▸ Metabolite

Figure 15.6
Drugs affecting the metabolism of carbamazepine.

C. Phenobarbital

1. **Actions:** *Phenobarbital* (p.96) has antiepileptic activity, limiting the spread of seizure discharges in the brain and elevating the seizure threshold. Its mechanism of action is unknown but may involve potentiation of the inhibitory effects of γ-aminobutyric acid-mediated neurons (see p.96). Doses required for antiepileptic action are lower than those that cause pronounced CNS depression.

2. **Therapeutic uses:** *Phenobarbital* provides a 50% favorable response rate for elementary partial seizures, but it is not very effective for complex partial seizures. The drug has been regarded as the first choice in treating seizures in children, including febrile seizures. However, *phenobarbital* can depresses cognitive performance in children treated for febrile seizures, and the drug should be used cautiously. *Phenobarbital* is also used to treat recurrent tonic-clonic seizures, especially in patients that do not respond to *diazepam* plus *phenytoin*. *Phenobarbital* is also used as a mild sedative to relieve anxiety, nervous tension and insomnia (see p.96), although benzodiazepines (p.91) are superior.

3. **Absorption and metabolism:** *Phenobarbital* is well absorbed orally. The drug freely penetrates the brain. Approximately 75% of the drug is inactivated by the hepatic microsomal system, the remaining drug is excreted unchanged by the kidney. *Phenobarbital* is a potent inducer of P-450 system, and when given chronically, it enhances the metabolism of other agents (see p.98).

4. **Adverse effects:** Sedation, ataxia, nystagmus, vertigo, and acute psychotic reactions may occur with chronic use. Nausea and vomiting are seen as well as a morbilliform rash in sensitive individuals. Agitation and confusion occur at high doses. Rebound seizures can occur on discontinuance of *phenobarbital*.

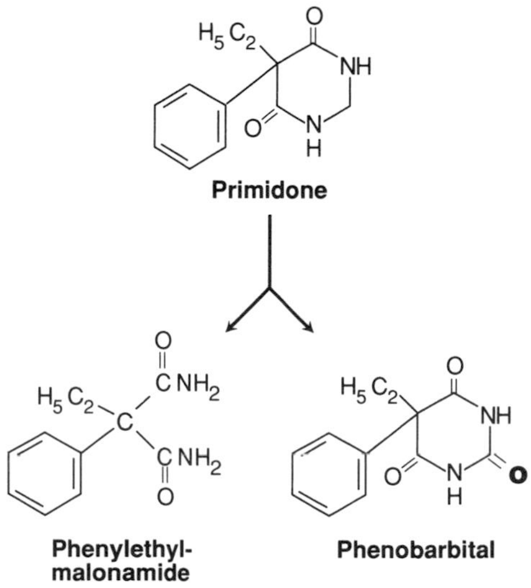

Figure 15.7
Metabolism of primidone.

D. Primidone

Primidone [PRI mi done] is a derivative of *phenobarbital*, and resembles *phenobarbital* in anticonvulsant activity.

1. **Therapeutic uses:** *Primidone* is an alternate choice in partial seizures and tonic-clonic seizures. Much of *primidone*'s efficacy comes from its metabolites *phenobarbital* and phenylethylmalonamide (Figure 15.7). *Phenobarbital* is effective against tonic-clonic and elementary partial seizures, and phenylethylmalonamide is effective against complex partial seizures. *Primidone* is often used with *carbamazepine* and *phenytoin*, allowing

smaller doses of these agents to be used. It is ineffective in absence seizures.

2. **Absorption and metabolism:** *Primidone* is well absorbed orally. It exhibits poor protein binding. It is converted to phenylethylmalonamide and to *phenobarbital* which have longer half-lives than the parent drug.

3. **Adverse effects:** This drug has the same adverse effects as those seen with *phenobarbital*.

E. Valproic acid

1. **Actions:** *Valproic* [val PROE ic] acid reduces the propagation of abnormal electrical discharge in the brain. It may enhance γ-aminobutyric acid action at inhibitory synapses.

2. **Therapeutic uses:** *Valproic acid* is the most effective agent available for treatment of myoclonic seizures. The drug diminishes absence seizures but is a second choice because of its hepatotoxic potential. *Valproic acid* also reduces the incidence and severity of tonic-clonic seizures.

3. **Absorption and metabolism:** The drug is effective orally and is rapidly absorbed. About 90% is bound to plasma proteins. Only 3% is excreted unchanged; the rest is metabolized by the liver. The metabolites are active. The glucuronide metabolites are excreted in the urine. *Valproic acid* is metabolized by the P-450 system, but it does not induce enzyme synthesis.

4. **Adverse effects:** *Valproic acid* can cause nausea and vomiting. Sedation, ataxia, and tremor are common (Figure 15.8). Hepatic toxicity may cause a rise in hepatic enzymes in plasma, which should be monitored frequently. In some individuals, a rash and alopecia may occur. Bleeding times may increase because of both thrombocytopenia and an inhibition of platelet aggregation. *Valproic acid* inhibits *phenobarbital* metabolism and increases circulating levels of the barbiturate.

F. Ethosuximide

1. **Actions:** *Ethosuximide* [eth oh SUX i mide] reduces propagation of abnormal electrical activity in the brain

2. **Therapeutic uses:** *Ethosuximide* is the first choice in absence seizures.

3. **Absorption and metabolism:** *Ethosuximide* is well absorbed orally. It is not bound to plasma proteins. About 25% of the drug is excreted unchanged in the urine, and 75% is metabolized to inactive metabolites in the liver by the microsomal P-450 system. *Ethosuximide* does not induce P-450 enzyme synthesis.

4. **Adverse effects:** The drug is irritating to the stomach, and nausea and vomiting may occur on chronic administration. Drowsiness, lethargy, dizziness, restlessness, agitation, anxiety, and the inability to concentrate are often observed. In sensitive individuals, a Stevens-Johnson syndrome or urticaria may occur, as well as leukopenia, aplastic anemia, and thrombocytopenia.

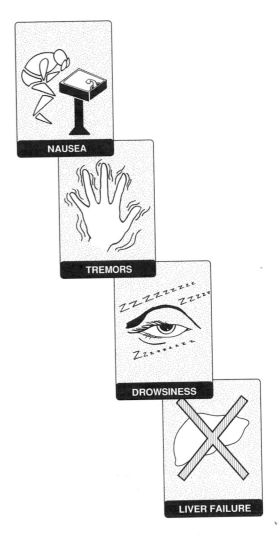

NAUSEA

TREMORS

DROWSINESS

LIVER FAILURE

Figure 15.8
Some adverse effects of valproic acid.

G. Benzodiazepines

Several of the benzodiazepines show antiepileptic activity. *Clonazepam* [kloe NA zi pam] and *clorazepate* are used for chronic treatment, whereas *diazepam* is the drug of choice in the acute treatment of status epilepticus. *Clonazepam* suppresses seizure spread from the epileptogenic focus, and it is effective in all types of seizures other than tonic-clonic.

1. **Actions:** This drug reduces propagation of abnormal electrical activity in the brain.

2. **Therapeutic uses:** *Diazepam* is the drug of choice for status epilepticus and is given intravenously. *Clonazepam* is effective in absence and myoclonic seizures, but tolerance develops. *Clorazepate* is effective in partial seizures when used in conjunction with other drugs.

3. **Adverse effects:** Of all the antiepileptics, the benzodiazepines are the safest and most free from severe side effects. All benzodiazepines have sedative properties; thus, drowsiness, somnolence, and fatigue can occur with higher dosage as well as ataxia, dizziness and behavior changes. Respiratory depression and cardiac depression may occur when given intravenously in acute situations.

Study Questions   (see p.417 for answers).

Answer A if 1,2 and 3 are correct.
    B if 1 and 3 are correct.
    C if 2 and 4 are correct.
    D if only 4 is correct.
    E if 1,2,3 and 4 are all correct.

15.1 Which of the following correctly pairs an antiepileptic drug with its therapeutic indication?

1. Ethosuximide: Absence seizures.
2. Phenobarbital: Febrile seizures in children.
3. Diazepam: Status epilepticus.
4. Phenytoin: Absence seizures.

15.2 Which of the following statements concerning phenytoin is/are correct?

1. Phenytoin causes less sedation than phenobarbital.
2. Phenytoin is not indicated for children under 5 years of age.
3. Phenytoin is not effective for absence seizure.
4. The plasma half-life increases as the dose is increased.

15.3 Which of the following drugs are useful in treating complex partial seizures?

1. Phenytoin.
2. Phenobarbital.
3. Carbamazepine.
4. Valproic acid.

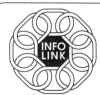

[1]See *cobalamin* n **Biochemistry** for the role of vitamin B_{12} in metabolism and cell growth (see index).

Treatment of Congestive Heart Failure

16

I. OVERVIEW OF CONGESTIVE HEART FAILURE

Congestive heart failure (CHF) is a condition in which the heart is unable to pump sufficient blood to meet the needs of the body. CHF can be caused by an impaired ability of the cardiac muscle to contract or by an increased workload imposed on the heart. This condition is accompanied by abnormal increases in blood volume and interstitial fluid, and the heart, veins, and capillaries are therefore generally dilated with blood. Hence the term "congestive" heart failure, since the symptoms include pulmonary congestion with left heart failure and peripheral edema with right heart failure. Common causes of chronic failure are coronary artery disease or hypertension, whereas acute failure can result from myocardial infarction.

The therapeutic goal for CHF is to increase cardiac output. Therefore, CHF is treated with drugs that increase the strength of the cardiac muscle (positive inotropic action, see Figure 16.1) and diuretic agents that decrease extracellular fluid volume (p.211). Often drug-induced vasodilation reduces the load on the myocardium and thus provides relief. Antiarrhythmic agents occasionally are required to normalize cardiac rate and rhythm. [Note: The agents summarized in Figure 16.1 relieve the symptoms of cardiac insufficiency but do not reverse the underlying pathologic condition.] Knowledge of the physiology of cardiac muscle contraction is clearly essential to an understanding of the compensatory responses evoked by the failing heart, as well as the actions of drugs used to treat CHF.

II. PHYSIOLOGY OF MUSCLE CONTRACTION

The myocardium, like smooth and skeletal muscle, responds to stimulation by depolarization of the membrane; this is followed by shortening of the contractile proteins and ends with relaxation and return to the resting state (Figure 16.2). However, unlike skeletal muscle, which shows graded contractions depending on the number of muscle cells stimulated, the cardiac muscle cells are interconnected in groups that respond to stimuli as a unit, contracting together whenever a single cell is stimulated.

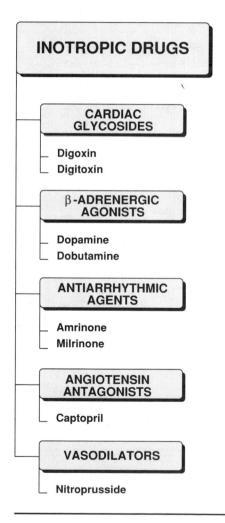

Figure 16.1
Summary of Inotropic drugs.

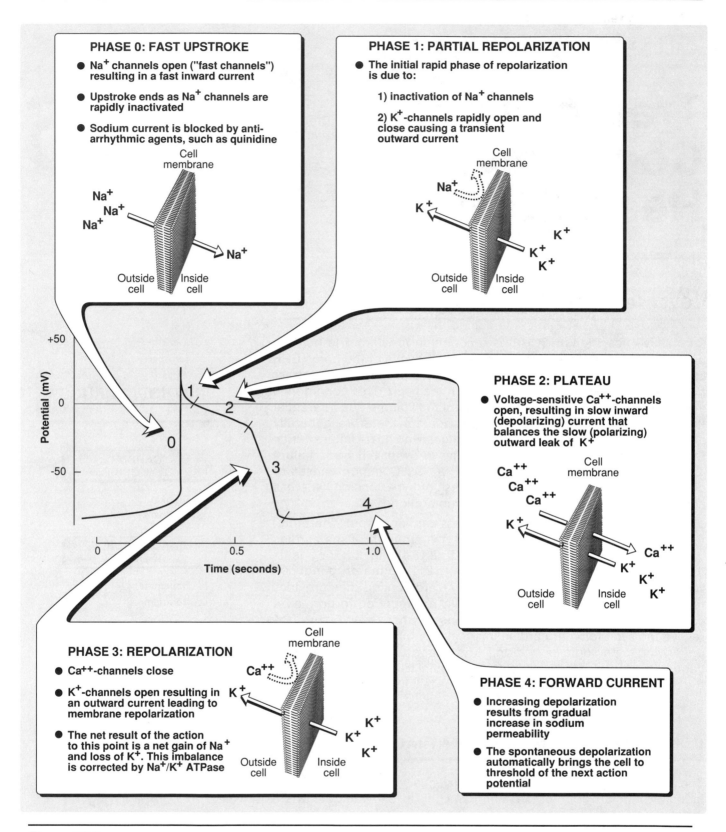

PHASE 0: FAST UPSTROKE

- Na^+ channels open ("fast channels") resulting in a fast inward current
- Upstroke ends as Na^+ channels are rapidly inactivated
- Sodium current is blocked by anti-arrhythmic agents, such as quinidine

Cell membrane
Na^+
Na^+
Na^+
Na^+
Outside cell   Inside cell

PHASE 1: PARTIAL REPOLARIZATION

- The initial rapid phase of repolarization is due to:

  1) inactivation of Na^+ channels

  2) K^+-channels rapidly open and close causing a transient outward current

Cell membrane
Na^+
K^+
K^+
K^+
K^+
Outside cell   Inside cell

PHASE 2: PLATEAU

- Voltage-sensitive Ca^{++}-channels open, resulting in slow inward (depolarizing) current that balances the slow (polarizing) outward leak of K^+

Cell membrane
Ca^{++}
Ca^{++}
Ca^{++}
K^+
Ca^{++}
K^+
K^+
K^+
Outside cell   Inside cell

PHASE 3: REPOLARIZATION

- Ca^{++}-channels close
- K^+-channels open resulting in an outward current leading to membrane repolarization
- The net result of the action to this point is a net gain of Na^+ and loss of K^+. This imbalance is corrected by Na^+/K^+ ATPase

Cell membrane
Ca^{++}
K^+
K^+
K^+
Outside cell   Inside cell

PHASE 4: FORWARD CURRENT

- Increasing depolarization results from gradual increase in sodium permeability
- The spontaneous depolarization automatically brings the cell to threshold of the next action potential

Potential (mV)
+50
0
-50

0   0.5   1.0
Time (seconds)

1
2
0
3
4

Figure 16.2
Action potential of a Purkinje fiber.

A. Action potential

Cardiac muscle cells are electrically excitable. However, unlike the cells of other muscles and nerves, the cells of cardiac muscle show a spontaneous, intrinsic rhythm generated by specialized "pacemaker" cells located in the sinoatrial (SA) and atrioventricular (AV) nodes. The cardiac cells also have an unusually long action potential, which can be divided into five phases (0 to 4). Figure 16.2 illustrates the major ions contributing to depolarization and polarization of cardiac cells. These ions pass through channels in the sarcolemmal membrane and thus create a current. The channels open and close at different times during the action potential; some respond primarily to changes in ion concentration, whereas others are either ATP- or voltage-sensitive.

B. Cardiac contraction

The contractile machinery of the myocardial cell is essentially the same as in striated muscle. The force of contraction of the cardiac muscle is directly related to the concentration of free (unbound) cytosolic calcium. Therefore agents that increase these calcium levels (or increase the sensitivity of the contractile machinery to calcium) result in an increase in the force of contraction (inotropic effect). [Note: The inotropic agents increase the contractility of the heart by altering the mechanisms that control the concentration of intracellular calcium.]

1. **Sources of free intracellular calcium:** Calcium comes from two sources. The first is from outside the cell, where opening of voltage-sensitive calcium channels causes an immediate rise in free cytosolic calcium. The second source is the release of calcium from the sarcoplasmic reticulum and mitochondria, which further increases the cytosolic level of calcium (Figure 16.3).

2. **Removal of free cytosolic calcium:** If free cytosolic calcium levels were to remain high, the cardiac muscle would be in a constant state of contraction, rather than showing a periodic contraction. Mechanisms of removal include two alternatives.

   a. **Sodium-calcium exchange:** Calcium is removed by a sodium-calcium exchange reaction that reversibly exchanges calcium ions for sodium ions across the cell membrane (Figure 16.3). This interaction between the movement of calcium and sodium ions is significant, since changes in intracellular sodium can affect cellular levels of calcium.

   b. **Uptake of calcium by the sarcoplasmic reticulum and mitochondria:** Calcium is also recaptured by the sarcoplasmic reticulum and the mitochondria. More than 99% of the intracellular calcium is located in these organelles, and even a modest shift between these stores and free calcium can lead to large changes in the concentration of free cytosolic calcium.

C. Compensatory physiological responses of heart muscle in CHF

The failing heart evokes three major compensatory mechanisms to enhance cardiac output (Figure 16.4).

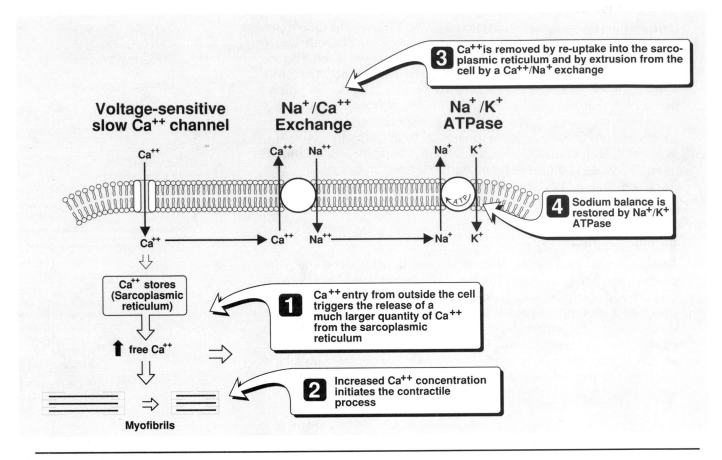

Figure 16.3
Ion movements during the contraction of cardiac muscle.

1. **Increased sympathetic activity:** Activation of β-adrenergic receptors in the heart results in an increase in heart rate and a greater force of contraction of the heart muscle (Figure 16.4). In addition, vasoconstriction enhances venous return and increases cardiac output. These compensatory responses increase the work of the heart and, therefore, can contribute to the further decline in cardiac function.

2. **Fluid retention:** A fall in cardiac output decreases blood flow to the kidney, prompting the release of renin, with a resulting increase in the synthesis of angiotensin II and aldosterone (p.380). This results in increased peripheral resistance and retention of sodium and water. Blood volume increases, and more blood is returned to the heart. If the heart is unable to pump this extra volume, venous pressure increases and edema of the peripheral tissues and lungs occurs (Figure 16.4). These compensatory responses increase the work of the heart and, therefore, can contribute to the further decline in cardiac function.

3. **Myocardial hypertrophy:** The heart increases in size, and the chambers dilate. Initially, stretching of the heart muscle leads to a stronger contraction of the heart. However, excessive elongation of the fibers results in weaker contractions.

D. Decompensated heart failure

If the mechanisms listed above adequately restore cardiac output, then the heart failure is said to be compensated. If the adaptive mechanisms fail to maintain cardiac output, the heart failure is termed decompensated.

III. CARDIAC GLYCOSIDES

The cardiac glycosides are often called digitalis or digitalis glycosides because most of the drugs come from the digitalis (foxglove) plant. They are a group of chemically similar compounds that can increase the contractility of the heart muscle and are therefore widely used in treating heart failure. Like the antiarrhythmic drugs described in Chapter 17, the cardiac glycosides influence the sodium and/or calcium ion flows in the cardiac muscle, thereby increasing contraction of the atrial and ventricular myocardium (positive inotropic action). The digitalis glycosides show only a small difference between a therapeutically effective dose and doses that are toxic or even fatal. Therefore, the drugs have a low therapeutic index (p.20). The digitalis glycosides include *digitoxin* [di ji TOX in], and the most widely used agent, *digoxin* [di JOX in].

A. Mode of action:

1. **Regulation of cytosolic calcium concentration:** Cardiac glycosides combine reversibly with the sodium-potassium ATPase of the cardiac cell membrane (Figure 16.5), resulting in an inhibition of pump activity. This causes an increase in the intracellular sodium concentration, which favors the transport of calcium into the cell and decreases calcium exodus from the cell, via the sodium-calcium exchange mechanism (Figure 16.5). The elevated intracellular calcium levels result in an increase in the systolic force of contraction.

2. **Increased contractility of the cardiac muscle:** Administration of digitalis glycosides increases the force of cardiac contractility causing the cardiac output to more closely resemble that of the normal heart (Figure 16.6). An increased myocardial contraction leads to a decrease in diastolic volume, thus increasing the efficiency of contraction. The resulting improved circulation leads to reduced sympathetic activity, which then reduces peripheral resistance. Together, these effects cause a reduction in heart rate. [Note: In the normal heart, the positive inotropic effect of digitalis is counteracted by compensatory autonomic reflexes.]

B. Therapeutic uses:

Digitalis is therapeutically most effective in the treatment of congestive heart failure caused by ischemic or congenital heart disease. It is also effective in hypertensive heart disease that is not controlled by antihypertensive therapy.

C. Pharmacology

All digitalis glycosides possess the same pharmacological actions, but they vary in potency and pharmacokinetics (Figure 16.7). These

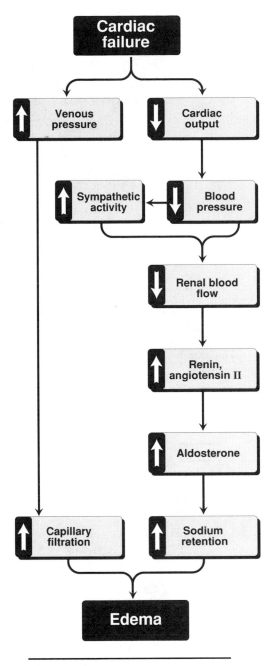

Figure 16.4
Cardiovascular consequences of heart failure.

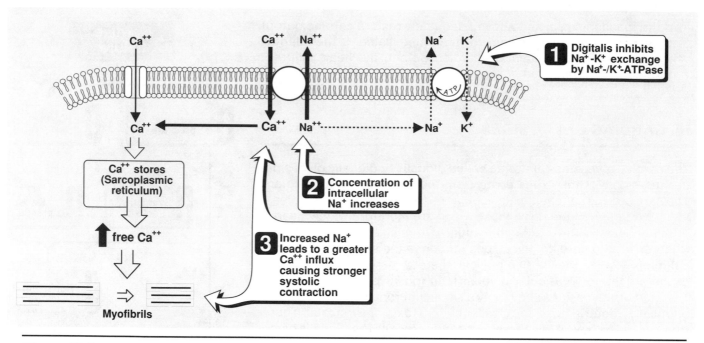

Figure 16.5
Mechanism of action of cardiac glycosides, or digitalis.

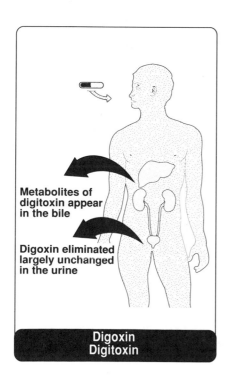

drugs are absorbed after oral administration. Note that *digitoxin* binds strongly to proteins in the extravascular space, resulting in a large volume of distribution. *Digoxin* has the advantage of a relatively short half-life, which allows better treatment of toxic reactions. *Digoxin* also has a more rapid onset of action, making it useful in emergency situations. *Digoxin* is eliminated largely unchanged in the urine. *Digitoxin* is extensively metabolized by the liver before excretion in the feces, and hepatic disease may require decreased doses.

D. Adverse effects

Digitalis toxicity is one of the most commonly encountered adverse drug reactions. Side effects can often be managed by discontinuing cardiac glycoside therapy, determining serum potassium levels, and if indicated, by giving potassium supplements. Severe toxicity resulting in ventricular tachycardia requires administration of antiarrhythmic drugs if serum potassium is not elevated (p.158), and the use of antibodies (FAB fragments) to *digoxin*. Types of side effects include:

1. **Cardiac effects:** The major effect is progressively more severe dysrhythmia, moving from decreased or blocked atrioventricular conduction, paroxysmal atrial tachycardia, to the conversion of atrial flutter to atrial fibrillation, premature ventricular depolarization, ventricular fibrillation, and finally, to complete heart

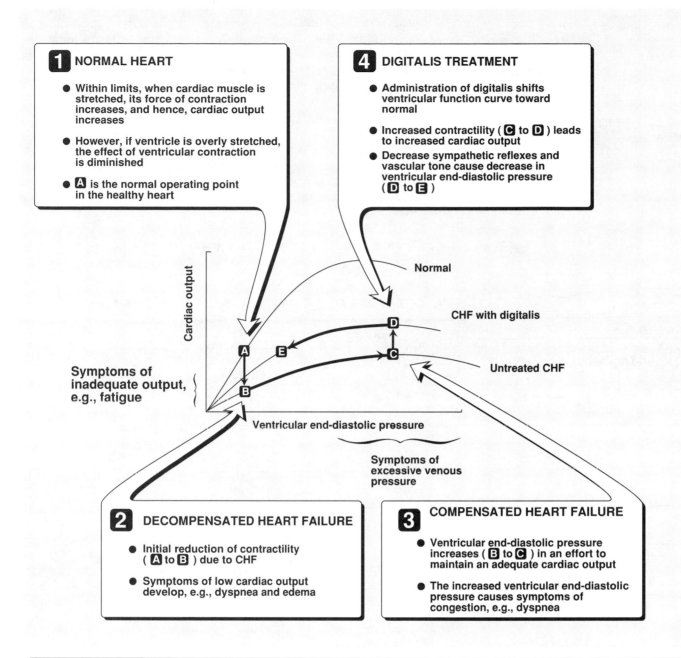

1 NORMAL HEART

● Within limits, when cardiac muscle is stretched, its force of contraction increases, and hence, cardiac output increases

● However, if ventricle is overly stretched, the effect of ventricular contraction is diminished

● **A** is the normal operating point in the healthy heart

4 DIGITALIS TREATMENT

● Administration of digitalis shifts ventricular function curve toward normal

● Increased contractility (**C** to **D**) leads to increased cardiac output

● Decrease sympathetic reflexes and vascular tone cause decrease in ventricular end-diastolic pressure (**D** to **E**)

Cardiac output

Normal

CHF with digitalis

Untreated CHF

Symptoms of inadequate output, e.g., fatigue

Ventricular end-diastolic pressure

Symptoms of excessive venous pressure

2 DECOMPENSATED HEART FAILURE

● Initial reduction of contractility (**A** to **B**) due to CHF

● Symptoms of low cardiac output develop, e.g., dyspnea and edema

3 COMPENSATED HEART FAILURE

● Ventricular end-diastolic pressure increases (**B** to **C**) in an effort to maintain an adequate cardiac output

● The increased ventricular end-diastolic pressure causes symptoms of congestion, e.g., dyspnea

Figure 16.6
Ventricular function curves in the normal heart, in congestive heart failure (CHF), and in CHF treated with digitalis.

block. A decrease in intracellular potassium is the primary predisposing factor in these effects.

2. **Gastrointestinal effects:** Anorexia, nausea, and vomiting are commonly encountered adverse effect.

3. **CNS effects:** Headache, fatigue, confusion, blurred vision, alteration of color perception, and haloes on dark objects are CNS effects.

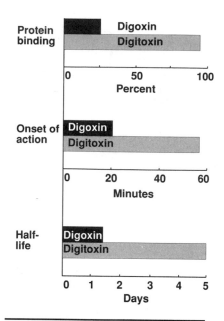

Figure 16.7
A comparison of the properties of
digoxin and digitoxin.

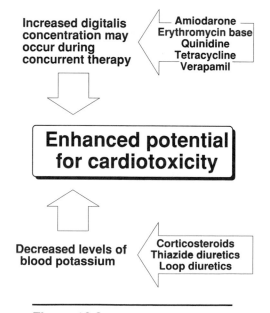

Figure 16.8
Drugs interacting with digoxin and
other digitalis glycosides.

E. Factors predisposing to digitalis toxicity:

1. **Electrolytic disturbances:** Hypokalemia can precipitate serious arrhythmias. Reduction of serum potassium levels is most frequently observed in patients receiving *thiazide* or loop diuretics and can usually be prevented by use of a potassium-sparing diuretic or supplementation with potassium chloride. Hypercalcemia, hypernatremia, hypermagnesemia, and alkalosis also predispose to digitalis toxicity.

2. **Drugs:** *Quinidine* reduces the renal clearance of *digoxin* and alters the volume of distribution. This increases the toxicity of *digoxin*. Potassium-depleting diuretics, corticosteroids, and a variety of other drugs can also increase digitalis toxicity (Figure 16.8).

3. **Disease states:** Hypothyroidism, hypoxia, renal failure, and myocarditis are predisposing factors to digitalis toxicity.

IV. ALTERNATIVE THERAPIES IN HEART FAILURE

Chronic heart failure is typically managed by reduction in physical activity, low intake of sodium, and treatment with cardiac glycosides and diuretics. [Note: The major beneficial action of diuretics is to decrease preload by decreasing blood volume and venous return.] However, the low therapeutic index of the cardiac glycosides has prompted the search for alternate therapies.

A. β-Adrenergic agonists

β-Adrenergic stimulation improves cardiac performance by their positive inotropic effects and vasodilation. *Dopamine* (p.64) and *dobutamine* (p.66) are the two most commonly used inotropic agents other than digitalis. Each of these agonists leads to an increase in intracellular cAMP, which results in the activation of protein kinase (p.33). Slow calcium channels are one important site of phosphorylation by protein kinase. When phosphorylated, the entry of calcium ion into the myocardial cells increases, thus enhancing contraction (Figure 16.9). [Note: *Dopamine* and *dobutamine* produce less tachycardia and fewer peripheral vascular effects than do drugs such as *epinephrine* (p.61) and *isoproterenol* (p.64).]

B. Antiarrhythmic agents

Amrinone [AM ri none] and *milrinone* [MIL ri none] are phosphodiesterase inhibitors that increase the intracellular concentration of cAMP (Figure 16.9). This results in an increase in intracellular calcium, and therefore cardiac contractility, as discussed above for the β-adrenergic agonists. [Note: *Amrinone* is available in the United States, but *milrinone* is not approved.]

Since *amrinone* is given only by the intravenous route, it is mainly for short-term management of congestive heart failure. *Amrinone* is associated with reversible thrombocytopenia, whereas *milrinone* does not affect platelets.

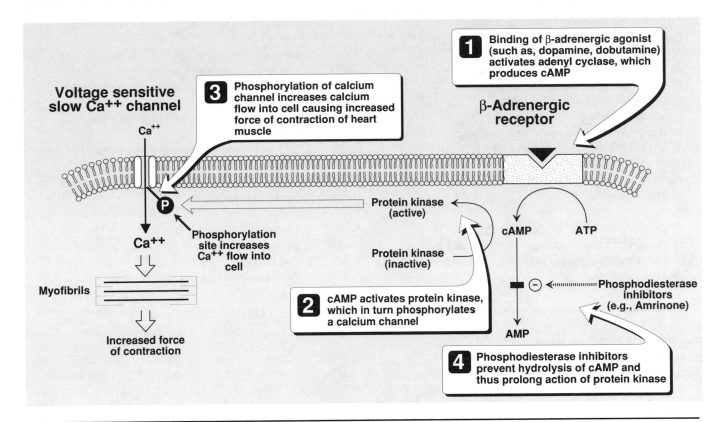

Figure 16.9
Sites of action of β-adrenergic agonists on heart muscle.

C. Vasodilators

Vasodilators provide an important advance in the treatment of congestive heart failure beyond the benefits obtained with *digitalis* and diuretics (p.211). Dilation of venous blood vessels leads to a decrease in cardiac preload by increasing venous capacitance; arterial dilators reduce systemic arteriolar resistance and decrease afterload. *Captopril* (p.383) is the vasodilator of choice for patients with congestive heart failure. Other vasodilators, such as *nitroprusside* [nye troe PRUSS ide], are also useful since many of these drugs dilate both venous and arterial beds (p. 183). This reduces the work of the heart. [Note: *Prazosin* (p. 182) is the vasodilator used as the outpatient equivalent of *nitroprusside*.]

Study Questions   (see p.418 for answers).

Choose the ONE best answer.

16.1 Which of the following most directly describes the mechanism of action of digitalis?

A. Inhibits sodium-potassium ATPase.
B. Decreases intracellular sodium concentration.
C. Increases the intracellular level of ATP.
D. Stimulates production of cAMP.
E. Decreases release of calcium from the sarcoplasmic reticulum.

16.2 All of the following are therapeutically useful in the treatment of congestive heart failure EXCEPT:

A. a vasodilator such as hydralazine.
B. a cardiac glycoside such as digoxin.
C. a β-adrenergic agonist such as norepinephrine.
D. a diuretic such as hydrochlorothiazide.
E. a β blocker such as propranolol.

16.3 All of the following are useful in the treatment of digitalis overdose EXCEPT:

A. Digoxin immune FAB fragments.
B. Dietary potassium supplements for patients being treated concomitantly with diuretics.
C. Lidocaine.
D. Phenytoin.
E. Quinidine.

Answer A if 1,2 and 3 are correct.
       B if 1 and 3 are correct.
       C if 2 and 4 are correct.
       D if only 4 is correct.
       E if 1,2,3 and 4 are all correct.

16.4 Which of the following statements is/are correct?

1. Digoxin is more widely used than digitoxin because it has a shorter half-life.
2. Serum levels of digoxin can be increased by quinidine.
3. Digitoxin is used in patients with renal insufficiency.
4. Digoxin is eliminated primarily in the bile.

16.5 Which of the following aggravates a digitalis-induced arrhythmia?

1. Decreased serum calcium.
2. Increasing heart rate with epinephrine.
3. Decreased serum sodium.
4. Decreased serum potassium.

Antiarrhythmic Drugs

I. OVERVIEW

In contrast to skeletal muscle, which contracts only when it receives a stimulus, the heart contains specialized cells that exhibit automaticity, that is, they can intrinsically generate rhythmic action potentials in the absence of external stimuli. These "pacemaker" cells differ from other myocardial cells in showing a slow, spontaneous depolarization during diastole (Phase 4) caused by an inward positive current carried by sodium (p.152). This depolarization is fastest in the sinoatrial (SA) node (the normal initiation site of the action potential) and decreases throughout the normal conduction pathway through the atrioventricular (AV) node to the bundle of His and the Purkinje system. Dysfunction of impulse generation or conduction at any of a number of sites in the heart can cause an abnormality in cardiac rhythm. Management of cardiac arrhythmias is concerned with reducing or abolishing the frequency of beats arising from sources other than the SA node (ectopic beats) and with restoring or approximating normal sinus rhythm. Figure 17.1 summarizes the drugs used to treat cardiac arrhythmias.

II. CAUSES OF ARRHYTHMIAS

Most arrhythmias arise either from alteration in impulse generation, leading to enhanced or abnormal automaticity, or from an abnormality in impulse conduction, which can result in the reentry phenomenon.

A. Abnormalities in impulse generation

1. **Enhanced normal automaticity:** The SA node shows the fastest rate of Phase 4 depolarization and therefore, exhibits a higher rate of discharge than that occurring in other pacemaker cells exhibiting automaticity. The SA node thus normally sets the pace of contraction for the myocardium, and latent pacemakers are depolarized by impulses coming from the SA node. However, if cardiac sites other than the SA node show enhanced automaticity, they may generate competing stimuli, and arrhythmias may arise.

2. **Abnormal automaticity:** Myocardial cells damaged, for example, by hypoxia or potassium imbalance, may remain partially depolarized during diastole. These cells may therefore reach the firing

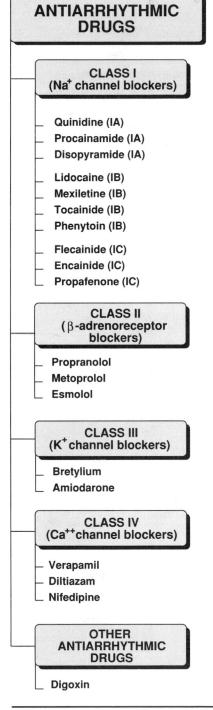

ANTIARRHYTHMIC DRUGS

CLASS I
(Na⁺ channel blockers)

- Quinidine (IA)
- Procainamide (IA)
- Disopyramide (IA)

- Lidocaine (IB)
- Mexiletine (IB)
- Tocainide (IB)
- Phenytoin (IB)

- Flecainide (IC)
- Encainide (IC)
- Propafenone (IC)

CLASS II
(β-adrenoreceptor blockers)

- Propranolol
- Metoprolol
- Esmolol

CLASS III
(K⁺ channel blockers)

- Bretylium
- Amiodarone

CLASS IV
(Ca⁺⁺ channel blockers)

- Verapamil
- Diltiazem
- Nifedipine

OTHER ANTIARRHYTHMIC DRUGS

- Digoxin

Figure 17.1
Summary of antiarrhythmic drugs.

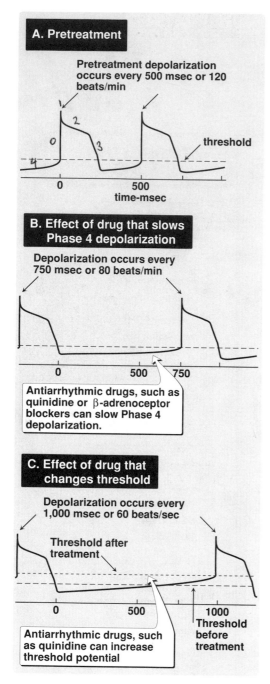

Figure 17.2
Actions of antiarrhythmic drugs on action potential of Purkinje fiber cell.

threshold earlier than normal cells and may induce abnormal automatic discharges.

3. **Effect of drugs on automaticity:** Most of the antiarrhythmic agents suppress automaticity (1) by decreasing the slope of Phase 4 (diastolic) depolarization and/or (2) by raising the threshold of discharge to a less negative voltage (Figure 17.2). Such drugs cause the frequency of discharge to decrease, an effect that is more pronounced in cells with ectopic pacemaker activity than in normal cells.

B. Abnormalities in impulse conduction

1. **Reentry:** Impulses from higher pacemaker centers are normally conducted down pathways that bifurcate to activate the entire ventricular surface (Figure 17.3). A phenomenon called reentry can occur if a unidirectional block caused by myocardial injury or a prolonged refractory period results in an abnormal conduction pathway. Consider a single Purkinje fiber with two conduction pathways to ventricular muscle. An impulse normally travels down both limbs of the conduction path. However, if myocardial injury results in a unidirectional block, the impulse may only be conducted down pathway #1 (see Figure 17.3). If the block in pathway #2 is in the forward direction only, the impulse may travel in a retrograde fashion through pathway #2 and reenter the point of bifurcation. This short-circuit pathway results in reexcitation of the ventricular muscle, causing premature contraction or sustained ventricular arrhythmia.

2. **Effects of drugs on conduction abnormalities:** Antiarrhythmic agents prevent reentry either by improving conduction in the abnormal pathway (reconverting a unidirectional block to normal, forward conduction) or by slowing conduction and/or increasing the refractory period to convert a unidirectional block into a bidirectional block. Reentry is the most common cause of arrhythmias and can occur at any level of the cardiac conduction system.

III. CLASS I ANTIARRHYTHMIC DRUGS

The antiarrhythmic drugs can be classified according to their predominant effects on the action potential (Figure 17.4). Although this classification is convenient, it is not entirely clear-cut, because many of the drugs have actions relating to more than one class or may have active metabolites with a different class of action. Class I antiarrhythmic drugs act by blocking voltage-sensitive sodium channels by the same mechanism as local anesthetics (p.116). The decreased rate of entry of sodium slows the rate of rise of Phase 0 of the action potential. [Note: At therapeutic doses, these drugs have little effect on the resting, fully polarized membrane.] Class I antiarrhythmic drugs therefore generally cause a decrease in excitability and conduction velocity.

A. Use-dependence

Class I drugs bind most rapidly to sodium channels that are open; therefore, these drugs show a greater degree of blockade when the channels are opened frequently. This property is called use-dependence (or state-dependence) and enables these drugs to block cells that are discharging at an abnormally high frequency without interfering with the normal low-frequency beating of the heart. The Class I drugs have been subdivided into three groups according to their effect on the duration of the action potential. Class IA agents slow the rate of rise of the action potential and prolong the ventricular effective refractory period, thus slowing conduction. They have an intermediate speed of association with activated/inactivated sodium channels, and an intermediate rate of dissociation from resting channels (Figure 17.4). Class IB drugs have little effect on the rate of depolarization, but rather they decrease the duration of the action potential by shortening repolarization. They rapidly interact with sodium channels. Class IC agents markedly depress the rate of rise of the membrane action potential, and therefore they cause marked conduction slowing but have little effect on the duration of the membrane action potential or the ventricular effective refractory period. They bind slowly to sodium channels.

B. Quinidine

Quinidine [KWIN i deen] is the prototype Class IA drug. At high doses, it can actually precipitate dysrhythmias, which can lead to fatal ventricular fibrillation. Because of quinidine's toxic potential, calcium antagonists, such as *verapamil*, are increasingly replacing this drug in clinical use.

1. **Mechanism of action:** *Quinidine* binds to open and inactivated sodium channels and prevents sodium influx, thus slowing the

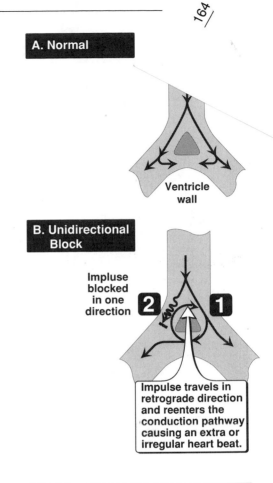

A. Normal

Ventricle wall

B. Unidirectional Block

Impulse blocked in one direction **2** **1**

Impulse travels in retrograde direction and reenters the conduction pathway causing an extra or irregular heart beat.

Figure 17.3
Schematic representation of reentry.

Classification of Drug	Mechanism of Action	Comment
IA	Na⁺ channel blocker	Slows Phase zero depolarization
IB	Na⁺ channel blocker	Shortens Phase 3 repolarization
IC	Na⁺ channel blocker	Markedly slows Phase zero depolarization
II	β Adrenoreceptor blocker	Suppresses Phase 4 depolarization
III	K⁺ channel blocker	Prolongs Phase 3 repolarization
IV	Ca⁺⁺ channel blocker	Shortens action potential

Figure 17.4
Actions of antiarrhythmic drugs.

rapid upstroke during Phase 0 (p.152). It also decreases the slope of Phase 4 spontaneous depolarization. The combined effects work together to efficiently block sodium channels, that is, *quinidine* actually enhances its own binding to the sodium channel by increasing the duration of the action potential, thus causing the channels to be open longer, allowing more drug to bind.

2. **Actions:** *Quinidine* inhibits ectopic arrhythmias and ventricular arrhythmias caused by increased normal automaticity. *Quinidine* also prevents reentry arrhythmias by producing bidirectional block through decreasing membrane responsiveness and prolonging the effective refractory period. The drug has little effect on normal automaticity. [Note: *Quinidine* can induce a tachycardia in normal individuals because of its atropine-like effect.]

3. **Therapeutic uses:** *Quinidine* is used in the treatment of a wide variety of arrhythmias, including atrial, AV junctional, and ventricular tachyarrhythmias. *Quinidine* is used to maintain sinus rhythm after direct current cardioconversion of atrial flutter or fibrillation and to prevent frequent ventricular tachycardia.

4. **Pharmacology:** *Quinidine sulfate* is rapidly and almost completely absorbed after oral administration.

5. **Adverse effects:** A potential adverse effect of *quinidine* (or any antiarrhythmic drug) is exacerbation of the arrhythmia. *Quinidine* may cause SA and AV block or asystole. At toxic levels, the drug may induce ventricular tachycardia. Cardiotoxic effects are exacerbated by hyperkalemia. *Quinidine* can increase the steady state concentration of *digoxin* by displacement of *digoxin* from tissue binding sites. Nausea, vomiting, and diarrhea are commonly observed. Large doses may induce the symptoms of cinchonism, for example, blurred vision, tinnitus, headache, disorientation, and psychosis. The drug has a mild α-adrenergic blocking action as well as an atropine-like effect. Drugs interacting with *quinidine* are shown in Figure 17.5

C. Procainamide

1. **Actions:** This Class IA drug, a derivative of the local anesthetic *procaine* (p.116), shows actions similar to those of *quinidine*.

2. **Pharmacology:** *Procainamide* [pro kane A mide] is absorbed following oral administration. [Note: The intravenous route is rarely used because hypotension occurs if the drug is too rapidly infused.] *Procainamide* has a relatively short half-life of 2-3 hours. A portion of the drug is acetylated in the liver to N-acetylprocainamide (NAPA), which has little effect on the maximum polarization of Purkinje fibers but prolongs the duration of the action potential. Thus, NAPA has properties of a Class III drug. NAPA is eliminated via the kidney, and dosages of *procainamide* may need to be adjusted in patients with renal failure.

3. **Adverse effects:** With chronic use, *procainamide* causes a high incidence of side effects, including a reversible lupus ery-

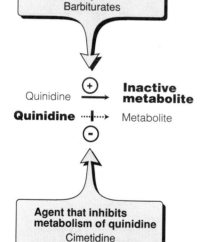

Figure 17.5
Drugs affecting the metabolism of quinidine.

thematosus-like syndrome that develops in 25 - 30% of patients. Toxic concentrations of *procainamide* may cause asystole or induction of ventricular arrhythmias. CNS side effects include depression, hallucination and psychosis. With this drug, gastrointestinal intolerance is less frequent than with *quinidine*.

D. Disopyramide

1. **Actions:** This Class IA drug shows actions similar to those of *quinidine*. *Disopyramide* [di so PEER a mide] produces a negative inotropic effect that is greater than the weak effect exerted by *quinidine* and *procainamide*, and unlike the latter drugs, *disopyramide* causes peripheral vasoconstriction. The drug may produce a clinically important decrease in myocardial contractility in patients with preexisting impairment of left ventricular function. *Disopyramide* is used for treatment of ventricular arrhythmia as an alternative to *procainamide* or *quinidine*.

2. **Pharmacology:** Approximately one half of the orally ingested drug is excreted unchanged by the kidneys. About 30% of the drug is converted by the liver to the less active mono-N-dealkylated metabolite.

3. **Adverse effects:** *Disopyramide* shows effects of anticholinergic activity, for example, dry mouth, urinary retention, blurred vision, and constipation.

E. Lidocaine

Lidocaine [LYE doe kane] is a Class IB drug. The IB agents rapidly associate with and dissociate from sodium channels. Thus the actions of Class IB agents are manifested when the cardiac cell is depolarized or firing rapidly. [Note: Class IB drugs are particularly useful in treating ventricular arrhythmias.]

1. **Actions:** *Lidocaine*, an anesthetic, causes a reduction in the Phase 0 of the action potential. It therefore shortens the duration of the action potential. Unlike *quinidine*, *lidocaine* suppresses abnormal automaticity. *Lidocaine*, like *quinidine*, abolishes ventricular reentry.

2. **Therapeutic uses:** *Lidocaine* is useful in treating ventricular arrhythmias arising during myocardial ischemia, such as that experienced during a myocardial infarction. The drug does not slow conduction and thus has little effect on atrial or AV junction arrhythmias.

3. **Pharmacology:** *Lidocaine* is given intravenously because of extensive first-pass transformation by the liver, which precludes oral administration. The drug is dealkylated and eliminated almost entirely by the liver, consequently dosage adjustment may be necessary in patients with liver dysfunction.

4. **Adverse effects:** *Lidocaine* has a fairly wide toxic-to-therapeutic ratio, shows little impairment of left ventricular function, and has

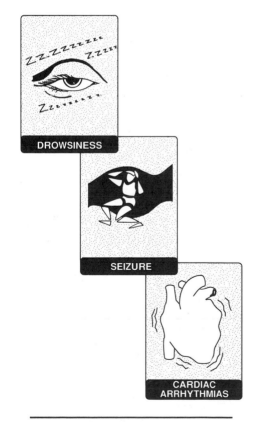

Figure 17.6
Adverse effects commonly observed with lidocaine.

no negative inotropic effect. The CNS effects include drowsiness, slurred speech, paresthesias, agitation, confusion, and convulsions; cardiac arrhythmias may also occur (Figure 17.6).

F. Mexiletine and tocainide

These are Class IB drugs with actions similar to those of lidocaine. These agents can be administered orally. *Mexiletine* [mex IL e teen] is used for chronic treatment of ventricular arrhythmias associated with previous myocardial infarction. *Tocainide* [toe KAY nide] is used for treatment of ventricular tachyarrhythmias. *Tocainide* has pulmonary toxicity, which may lead to pulmonary fibrosis.

G. Phenytoin

This antiepileptic drug (p.146) has antiarrhythmic properties similar to those of *lidocaine*. *Phenytoin* [FEN i toy in] is useful in *digitalis*-induced arrhythmias and is sometimes used in children with ventricular arrhythmias.

H. Flecainide

Flecainide [fle KAY nide] is a Class IC drug. These drugs slowly dissociate from resting sodium channels and show prominent effects, even at normal heart rates. These drugs are approved only for refractory ventricular arrhythmias. However recent data have cast doubts on the safety of the classic drugs.

1. **Actions:** *Flecainide* suppresses Phase 0 upstroke in Purkinje and myocardial fibers. This causes marked slowing of conduction in all cardiac tissue, with a minor effect on the duration of the action potential and refractoriness. Automaticity is reduced by an increase in the threshold potential rather than a decrease in the slope of Phase 4 depolarization.

2. **Therapeutic uses:** *Flecainide* is useful in treating refractory ventricular arrhythmias. It is particularly useful in suppressing premature ventricular contraction. *Flecainide* has a negative inotropic effect and can aggravate congestive heart failure.

3. **Pharmacology:** *Flecainide* is absorbed orally, undergoes minimal biotransformation, and has a half-life of 16-20 hours.

4. **Adverse effects:** *Flecainide* can cause dizziness, blurred vision, headache, and nausea. Like other Class IC drugs, *flecainide* can aggravate preexisting arrhythmias or induce life-threatening ventricular tachycardia that is resistant to treatment.

I. Encainide and propafenone

These Class IC drugs show actions similar to those of *flecainide*. *Propafenone* [proe POF en one] and *encainide* [en KAY nide], like *flecainide*, slow conduction in all cardiac tissues and are considered broad spectrum antiarrhythmic agents. Figure 17.7 summarizes some of the actions of Class I antiarrhythmic drugs.

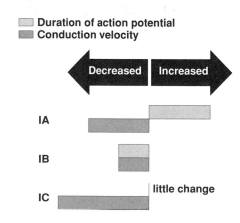

Figure 17.7
Effect of Na+ channel blockers (Class IA, IB, IC) on the cardiac action potential.

IV. CLASS II ANTIARRHYTHMIC DRUGS

The Class II agents include the β-adrenergic antagonists. These drugs diminish Phase 4 depolarization, thus depressing automaticity, prolonging AV conduction, and decreasing heart rate and contractility. These agents are useful in treating tachyarrhythmia caused by increased sympathetic activity. They are also used for atrial flutter and fibrillation, and for AV nodal reentrant tachycardia.

A. Propranolol

Propranolol reduces the incidence of sudden arrhythmic death after myocardial infarction (the most common cause of death in this group of patients). The mortality rate in the first year after a heart attack is significantly reduced by *propranolol*, partly because of its ability to prevent ventricular arrhythmias. *Propranolol* is described in detail on p.77.

B. Metoprolol and pindolol

Propranolol is the β-adrenergic antagonist most widely used in the treatment of cardiac arrhythmias. However, β_1-specific drugs, such as *metoprolol* (p.77) reduce the risk of bronchospasm, and drugs with partial agonist activity, such as *pindolol* (p.78), may decrease the frequency of cardiac failure.

C. Esmolol

Esmolol [ESS moe lol] is a very short-acting β blocker for intravenous administration in acute surgical arrhythmias.

V. CLASS III ANTIARRHYTHMIC DRUGS

Class III agents block potassium channels and thus diminish the outward potassium current, which leads to repolarization of the cardiac cells. These agents prolong the duration of the action potential without altering Phase 0 of depolarization or the resting membrane potential (Figure 17.8). Instead, they prolong the effective refractory period.

A. Bretylium

1. **Actions:** *Bretylium* [bre TIL ee um] differs from Class I antiarrhythmic drugs in that it does not slow the rise of Phase 0 of the cardiac action potential and does not reduce the slope of Phase 4 spontaneous depolarization. *Bretylium* has a number of direct and indirect electrophysiological actions, the most prominent of which are prolongation of the refractory period and raising of the intensity of the electrical current necessary to induce ventricular fibrillation in the His-Purkinje system.

2. **Therapeutic uses:** *Bretylium* is reserved for life-threatening ventricular arrhythmias, especially recurrent ventricular fibrillation or tachycardia.

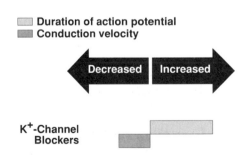

Figure 17.8
Effect of K$^+$ channel blockers (Class II) on the cardiac action potential.

3. **Pharmacology:** *Bretylium* is poorly absorbed from the gastrointestinal tract and therefore is usually administered parenterally. The drug is excreted unchanged in the urine, and dosage may have to be adjusted in patients with kidney dysfunctions.

4. **Adverse effects:** *Bretylium* can cause severe postural hypotension.

B. Amiodarone

1. **Actions:** *Amiodarone* [a MEE oh da rone] contains iodine and is related structurally to thyroxine. It has complex effects showing Class I, II, III and IV actions. Its dominant effect is prolongation of the action potential duration and the refractory period. *Amiodarone* has anti-anginal as well as antiarrhythmic activity.

2. **Therapeutic uses:** *Amiodarone* is effective in the treatment of severe refractory supraventricular and ventricular tachyarrhythmia. Its clinical usefulness is limited by its toxicity.

3. **Pharmacology:** *Amiodarone* is incompletely absorbed after oral administration. The drug is unusual in having a prolonged half-life of several weeks. Full clinical effects may not be achieved until 6 weeks after initiation of treatment.

4. **Adverse effects:** *Amiodarone* shows a variety of toxic effects. After long-term use, more than one half of the patients receiving the drug show side effects sufficiently severe to prompt its discontinuation. Some of the more common effects include interstitial pulmonary fibrosis, gastrointestinal tract intolerance, tremor, ataxia, dizziness, hyper- or hypothyroidism, liver toxicity, photosensitivity, neuropathy, muscle weakness, and blue skin discoloration caused by iodine accumulation in the skin.

VI. CLASS IV ANTIARRHYTHMIC DRUGS

The Class IV drugs are calcium channel blockers. They decrease the inward current carried by calcium, resulting in a decrease in the rate of Phase 4 spontaneous depolarization and slowed conduction in tissues dependent on calcium currents, such as the AV node. Although voltage-sensitive calcium channels occur in many different tissues, the major effect of calcium-channel blockers are on vascular smooth muscle and the heart. *Verapamil* shows greater action on the heart than on vascular smooth muscle, whereas *nifedipine*, a calcium channel-blocker used to treat hypertension (p.181) exerts a stronger effect on vascular smooth muscle than on the heart. *Diltiazem* is intermediate in its actions.

A. Verapamil and diltiazem

1. **Actions:** Calcium enters cells by voltage-sensitive channels and by receptor-operated channels that are controlled by the binding of agonists, such as catecholamines, to membrane receptors (Figure 17.9). Calcium channel blockers, such as *verapamil* [ver

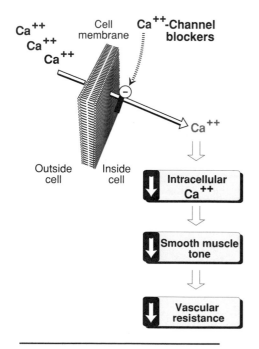

Figure 17.9
Action of calcium channel blockers.

AP a mill] and *diltiazem* [dil TYE a zem], are more effective against voltage-sensitive channels, which causes a decrease in the slow inward current that triggers cardiac contraction (p.152). *Verapamil* and *diltiazem* bind only to open, depolarized channels, thus preventing repolarization until the drug dissociates from the channel. These drugs are therefore use-dependent (p.163), that is, they block most effectively when the heart is beating rapidly, since in a normally paced heart, the calcium channels have time to repolarize, and the bound drug dissociates from the channel before the next conduction pulse. By decreasing the inward current carried by calcium, *verapamil* and *diltiazem* slow conduction and prolong the effective refractory period in tissues dependent on calcium currents, such as the AV node. These drugs are therefore effective in treating arrhythmias that must traverse calcium-dependent cardiac tissues.

2. **Therapeutic uses:** *Verapamil* and *diltiazem* are more effective against atrial than ventricular dysrhythmias. They are useful in

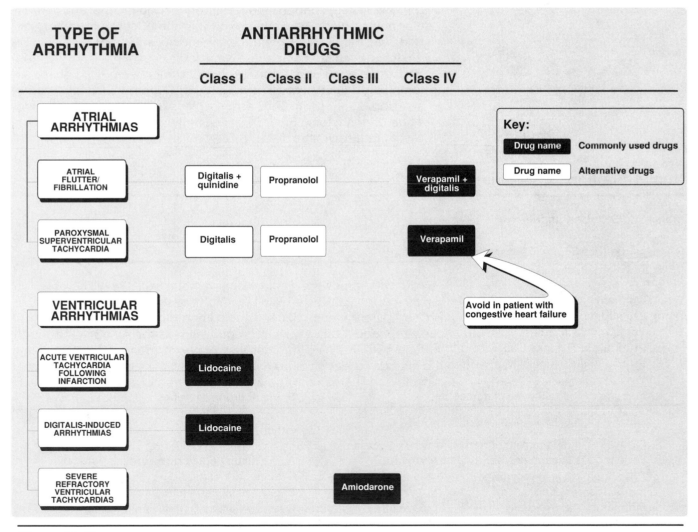

Figure 17.10
Therapeutic indications for antiarrhythmic agents.

treating reentrant supraventricular tachycardia and reducing ventricular rate in atrial flutter and fibrillation. In addition these drugs are used to treat hypertension (p.181) and angina (p.172).

3. **Pharmacology:** *Verapamil* and *diltiazem* are absorbed after oral administration. *Verapamil* is extensively metabolized by the liver; thus, care should be taken in administration of this drug to patients with hepatic dysfunction.

4. **Adverse effects:** *Verapamil* and *diltiazem* have negative inotropic properties and therefore may be contraindicated in patients with preexisting depressed cardiac function. Both drugs can also cause a decrease in blood pressure caused by peripheral vasodilation.

VII. OTHER ANTIARRHYTHMIC DRUGS

A. Digoxin

Digoxin (p.155) shortens the refractory period in atrial and ventricular myocardial cells while prolonging the effective refractory period and diminishing conduction velocity in Purkinje fibers. *Digoxin* is used to control the ventricular response rate in atrial fibrillation and flutter. At toxic concentrations, *digoxin* causes ectopic ventricular beats that may result in ventricular tachycardia and fibrillation. [Note: This arrhythmia is usually treated with *lidocaine* or *phenytoin*.] Figure 17.10 summarizes the therapeutic uses of the antiarrhythmic drugs.

Study Questions   (see p.419 for answers).

Choose the ONE best answer.

17.1 All of the following pairs correctly match a drug with its action EXCEPT?

    A. Quinidine: Blocks Na^+ channels.
    B. Bretylium: Blocks K^+ channels.
    C. Verapamil: Blocks Ca^{++} channels.
    D. Propranolol: Blocks β adrenoceptors.
    E. Procainamide: Blocks K^+ channels.

17.2 Which one of the following statements is INCORRECT?

    A. Lidocaine must be given parenterally.
    B. Lidocaine is used mainly for atrial arrhythmias.
    C. Procainamide is associated with a reversible lupus phenomenon.
    D. Quinidine is active orally.
    E. All antiarrhythmic drugs can suppress cardiac contractions.

17.3 Which one of the following statements is INCORRECT?

    A. Quinidine prolongs repolarization and the effective refractory period.
    B. Mexiletine shortens repolarization and decreases the effective refractory period.
    C. Propranolol increases Phase 4 depolarization.
    D. Verapamil shortens the duration of the action potential.
    E. Amiodarone prolongs repolarization.

17.4 Antiarrhythmic drugs

    A. may act by converting unidirectional block to a bidirectional block.
    B. often cause an increase in cardiac output.
    C. as a group have mild side effects.
    D. all affect Na^+ channels in the cell membrane.
    E. are equally useful in atrial and ventricular arrhythmias.

Antianginal Drugs

18

I. OVERVIEW

Angina pectoris is a characteristic chest pain caused by coronary blood flow that is insufficient to meet the oxygen demands of the myocardium. The imbalance between oxygen delivery and utilization may result from a spasm of the vascular smooth muscle or from obstruction of blood vessels caused by atherosclerotic lesions. Angina is characterized by a sudden, severe pressing substernal pain radiating to the left arm. It is treated with (1) drugs that increase perfusion of the myocardium by relaxing coronary arteries (for example, organic nitrates that decrease coronary vasoconstriction or spasm, and the vasodilating calcium channel-blockers) and/or (2) β blockers that decrease the oxygen demands of the heart. Variant angina is due to spontaneous coronary spasm, either at work or at rest, rather than by increases in myocardial oxygen requirements. It is controlled by organic nitrates or calcium channel blockers, but β blockers are contraindicated. (See Figure 18.1 for a summary of these antianginal agents.)

II. ORGANIC NITRATES

Organic nitrates (and nitrites) are simple nitric and nitrous acid esters of alcohols. They differ in their volatility; for example, *isosorbide dinitrate* is solid at room temperature, *nitroglycerin* is only moderately volatile, whereas *amyl nitrate* is extremely volatile. These compounds cause a rapid reduction in myocardial oxygen demand followed by rapid relief of the angina.

A. Nitroglycerin

1. **Actions:**

   a. The organic nitrates, such as *nitroglycerin* [nye troe GLI ser in], are thought to relax vascular smooth muscle by their intracellular conversion to nitrite ions and then to nitric oxide (NO), which in turn activates guanylate cyclase and increases the cells' cGMP content. Elevated cGMP ultimately leads to dephosphorylation of the myosin light chain, resulting in smooth muscle relaxation (Figure 18.2).

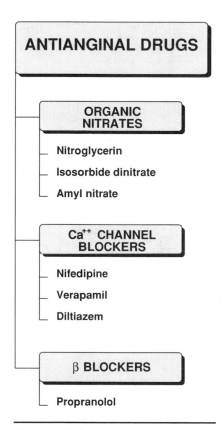

ANTIANGINAL DRUGS

ORGANIC NITRATES
- Nitroglycerin
- Isosorbide dinitrate
- Amyl nitrate

Ca++ CHANNEL BLOCKERS
- Nifedipine
- Verapamil
- Diltiazem

β BLOCKERS
- Propranolol

Figure 18.1
Summary of antianginal drugs.

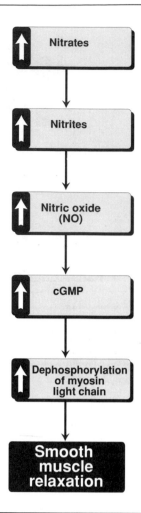

Figure 18.2
Effects of nitrates and nitrites on smooth muscle.

b. At low doses, dilation of the large veins occurs, causing pooling of blood in the veins and diminished preload (venous return to the heart). This results in a reduction in the central venous pressure and reduction of diastolic filling and cardiac output. Little effect on the arterioles exists, and the decreased stroke output is compensated by reflex tachycardia. Therefore, the arterial pressure does not change significantly. *Nitroglycerin* causes a decrease in myocardial oxygen consumption because of decreased cardiac output.

c. At higher doses, *nitroglycerin* dilates arterioles, causing a decrease in peripheral resistance and a drop in blood pressure. [Note: Baroreceptors can then cause a reflex sympathetic discharge leading to stimulation of the heart rate, which may aggravate the angina.]

2. **Therapeutic uses:** In addition to the treatment of angina, organic nitrites are useful in the treatment of cyanide poisoning. It is imperative to institute therapy as quickly as possible because cyanide binds tightly to the ferric ion (Fe^{+++}) of cytochrome oxidase, which effectively inhibits all ATP production by the electron transport chain. Since cyanide interacts with ferric iron, a solution of *sodium nitrite* that converts a portion of the patient's hemoglobin (Fe^{++}) to methemoglobin (Fe^{+++}) is slowly injected. The methemoglobin competes for the cyanide, forming cyanmethemoglobin and regenerating the cytochrome oxidase (Figure 18.3). Alternatively, the patient may inhale *amyl nitrite*, which also promotes the formation of methemoglobin. Next a solution of *sodium thiosulfate* is slowly administered intravenously. The reaction of *thiosulfate* with cyanide forms the relatively innocuous thiocyanate ion.

3. **Pharmacology:** Significant first-pass metabolism of *nitroglycerin* occurs in the liver. Therefore, it is common to give the drug either sublingually or via a transdermal patch. *Amyl nitrate* is administered through inhalation.

4. **Adverse effects:** High doses of organic nitrates can cause postural hypotension (as described above) that results in dizziness, headache, facial flushing, and tachycardia.

B. Isosorbide dinitrate

Isosorbide dinitrate [eye soe SOR bide] is an orally active nitrate. The drug is not readily metabolized by the liver or smooth muscle and has a lower potency than *nitroglycerin* in relaxing smooth muscle.

III. CALCIUM CHANNEL BLOCKERS

The calcium-channel blockers inhibit the entrance of calcium into cardiac and smooth muscle cells of the coronary and systemic arterial beds. All calcium channel blockers are therefore vasodilators that cause a decrease in smooth muscle tone and vascular resistance. (See p.168 for a description of the mechanism of action of this group of

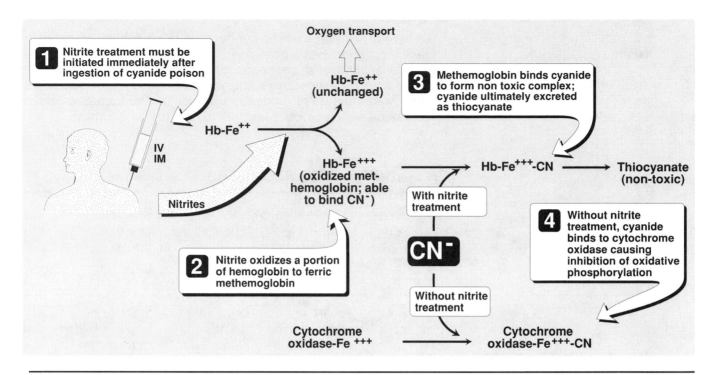

Figure 18.3
Treatment of cyanide poisoning with nitrites.

drugs.) At clinical doses, these agents affect primarily the resistance of vascular smooth muscle and the myocardium. [Note: *Verapamil* mainly affects the myocardium, whereas *nifedipine* exerts a greater effect on smooth muscle in the peripheral vasculature. *Diltiazem* is intermediate in its actions.]

A. Nifedipine

Nifedipine [nye FED i peen] functions mainly as an arteriolar vasodilator. This drug has no effect on cardiac conduction or heart rate. *Nifedipine* is administered orally and has a short half-life (about 4 hours) requiring multiple dosing. The vasodilation effect of *nifedipine* is useful in treatment of variant angina caused by spontaneous coronary spasm. *Nifedipine* can cause flushing, headache, hypotension, and peripheral edema as side effects of its vasodilation activity.

B. Verapamil

Verapamil slows cardiac conduction directly and thus decreases heart rate. However, this cardiac suppression is largely balanced by reflex activation, with the net balance being modest cardiac suppression. *Verapamil* causes greater cardiac suppression than *nifedipine*, but it is a weaker vasodilator. *Verapamil* is contraindicated in patients with preexisting depressed cardiac function or AV conduction abnormalities. It also causes constipation. *Verapamil* should be used with caution in digitalized patients, since it may increase *digoxin* levels.

C. Diltiazem

Diltiazem has cardiovascular effects that are similar to those of *verapamil*. It reduces the heart rate, although to a lesser extent than *verapamil*, and also decreases blood pressure. In addition, *diltiazem* can relieve coronary artery spasm and is therefore particularly useful in patients with variant angina. The incidence of adverse side effects is low.

IV. β-ADRENERGIC BLOCKERS

The β-adrenergic blocking agents suppress the activation of the heart by blocking β_1 receptors (p.74). They also reduce the work of the heart by decreasing cardiac output and causing a slight decrease in blood pressure. *Propranolol* [proe PRAN oh lole] is the prototype of this class of compounds. The β blockers reduce the frequency and severity of angina attacks. These agents are particularly useful in the treatment of patients with myocardial infarction. The β blockers can be used with nitrates to increase exercise duration and tolerance. They are, however, contraindicated in patients with bronchospasm, asthma, diabetes, or peripheral vascular disease. [Note: Calcium channel blockers are useful for patients with these complaints.] See p.74 for a discussion of the mechanism of action, pharmacology, and adverse effects associated with β-blockers.

Study Questions   (see p.420 for answers).

Choose the ONE best answer.

18.1 The β-adrenergic blockers, such as propranolol, are contraindicated as a treatment of angina in patients with all of the following conditions EXCEPT:

A. Congestive heart failure.
B. Asthma.
C. Hypertension.
D. Insulin-dependent diabetes.
E. Peripheral vascular disease.

18.2 All of the following statements concerning nitroglycerin are correct EXCEPT?

A. It causes an elevation of intracellular cGMP.
B. It undergoes significant first-pass metabolism in the liver.
C. It may cause significant reflex tachycardia.
D. It significantly decreases AV conduction.
E. It can cause postural hypotension.

18.3 Which one of the following is most effective in treating the ischemic pain of variant angina?

A. Propranolol.
B. Sodium nitroprusside.
C. Atropine.
D. Isosorbide dinitrate.
E. Nifedipine.

18.4 Which one of the following adverse effects is associated with nitroglycerin?

A. Hypertension.
B. Throbbing headache.
C. Bradycardia.
D. Sexual dysfunction.
E. Anemia.

Antihypertensive Drugs

19

I. OVERVIEW

Hypertension is defined as a sustained diastolic blood pressure greater than 90 mm Hg accompanied by an elevated systolic blood pressure (>140 mm Hg). Hypertension results from increased peripheral vascular smooth muscle tone, which leads to increased arteriolar resistance and reduced capacitance of the venules. Elevated blood pressure is an extremely common disorder affecting approximately 15% of the population of the United States (60 million people). Although many of these individuals have no symptoms, chronic hypertension can lead to congestive heart failure, myocardial infarction, renal damage, and cerebrovascular accidents. These complications correlate best with the diastolic pressure. The incidence of morbidity and mortality significantly decreases when hypertension is diagnosed early and is properly treated.

II. ETIOLOGY OF HYPERTENSION

Although hypertension may occur secondary to other disease processes, more than 90% of patients have essential hypertension, a disorder of unknown origin affecting the blood pressure-regulating mechanism. A family history of hypertension increases the likelihood that an individual will develop hypertensive disease. Essential hypertension occurs four times more frequently among blacks than among whites, and it occurs more often among middle-aged males than among middle-aged females. Environmental factors such as a stressful lifestyle, high dietary intake of sodium, obesity, and smoking all further predispose an individual to the occurence of hypertension. Figure 19.1 summarizes the drugs used to treat hypertension.

III. MECHANISMS FOR CONTROLLING BLOOD PRESSURE

Arterial blood pressure is regulated within a narrow range to provide adequate perfusion of the tissues without causing damage to the vascular system, particularly the arterial intima. Arterial blood pressure is directly proportional to the product of the cardiac output and the peripheral vascular resistance (Figure 19.2). In both normal and hypertensive individuals, cardiac output and peripheral resistance are controlled mainly by two overlapping control mechanisms: the bar-

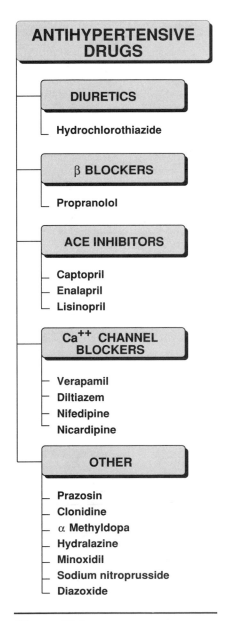

ANTIHYPERTENSIVE DRUGS

DIURETICS
- Hydrochlorothiazide

β BLOCKERS
- Propranolol

ACE INHIBITORS
- Captopril
- Enalapril
- Lisinopril

Ca⁺⁺ CHANNEL BLOCKERS
- Verapamil
- Diltiazem
- Nifedipine
- Nicardipine

OTHER
- Prazosin
- Clonidine
- α Methyldopa
- Hydralazine
- Minoxidil
- Sodium nitroprusside
- Diazoxide

Figure 19.1
Summary of antihypertensive drugs.

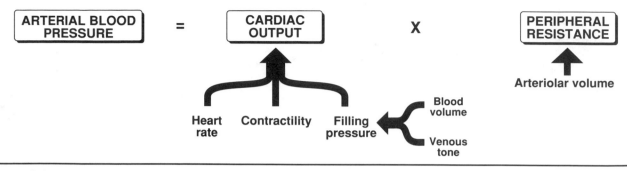

Figure 19.2
Major factors influencing blood pressure.

oreflexes mediated by the sympathetic nervous system and the renin-angiotensin-aldosterone system (Figure 19.3). Most antihypertensive drugs lower blood pressure by reducing cardiac output and/or decreasing peripheral resistance.

A. Baroreceptors and the sympathetic nervous system

Baroreflexes involving the sympathetic nervous system are responsible for the rapid moment-to-moment regulation of blood pressure. A fall in blood pressure causes pressure-sensitive neurons (baroreceptors in the aortic arch and carotid sinuses) to send fewer impulses to cardiovascular centers in the spinal cord. This prompts a reflex response of increased sympathetic and decreased parasympathetic output to the heart and vasculature, resulting in vasoconstriction and increased cardiac output. These changes result in a compensatory rise in blood pressure (Figure 19.3 and p.29).

B. Renin-angiotensin-aldosterone system

The kidney provides for the long-term control of blood pressure by altering the blood volume. Baroreceptors in the kidney respond to reduced arterial pressure (and to sympathetic stimulation of β adrenoceptors) by releasing the enzyme renin (Figure 19.3). This peptidase converts angiotensinogen to angiotensin I, which is in turn converted to angiotensin II in the presence of angiotensin converting enzyme (ACE, see p.380). Angiotensin II is the body's most potent circulating vasoconstrictor causing an increase in blood pressure. Furthermore, angiotensin II stimulates aldosterone secretion, leading to increased renal sodium absorption and an increase in blood volume, which contribute to a further increase in blood pressure (see p.380 for a more complete discussion of angiotensin).

IV. TREATMENT STRATEGIES

Mild hypertension can often be controlled with a single drug. More severe hypertension may require treatment with several drugs that are selected to minimize adverse effects of the combined regimen. Treatment is initiated with any of four drugs depending on the individual

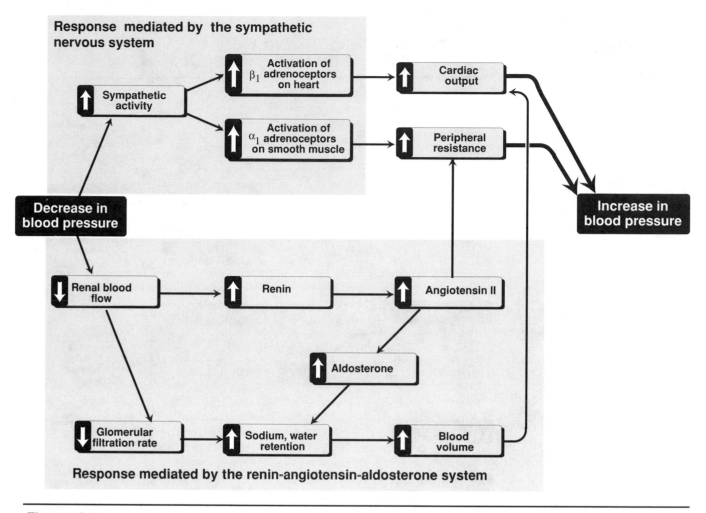

Figure 19.3
Response of the autonomic nervous system and the renin-angiotensin-aldosterone system to a decrease in blood pressure.

patient: a diuretic, a β blocker, an ACE inhibitor, or a calcium channel blocker. If blood pressure is inadequately controlled, a second drug is added. A β blocker is usually added if the initial drug was a diuretic, or a diuretic is added if the first drug was a β blocker. A vasodilator can be added as a third step for those patients who fail to respond.

A. Individualized care

Certain subsets of the hypertensive population respond better to one class of drug than another. Furthermore, hypertension may coexist with other diseases that may be aggravated by some of the antihypertensive drugs. For example, Figure 19.4 shows the preferred therapy in hypertensive patients with various concomitant diseases. In such cases, it is important to match antihypertensive drugs to the particular patient. Figure 19.5 shows the frequency of concomitant disease in the hypertensive patient population.

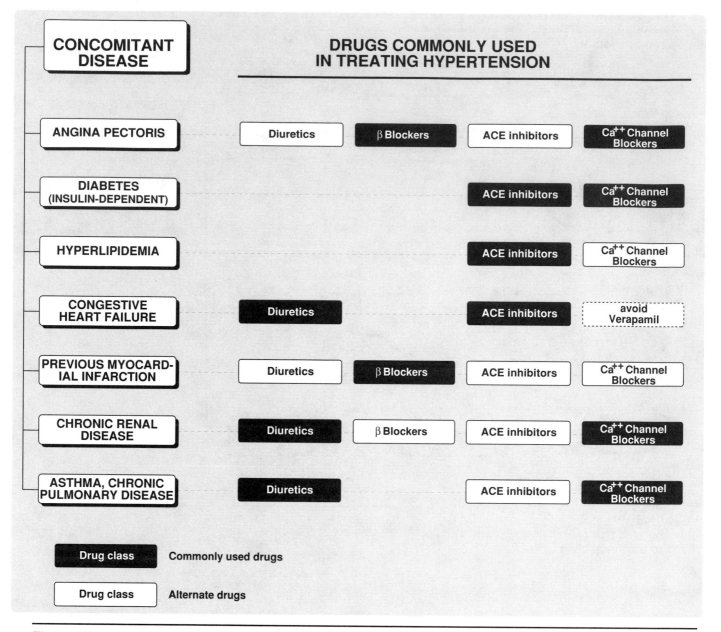

Figure 19.4
Treatment of hypertension in patients with concomitant diseases.

B. Patient compliance in antihypertensive therapy

Lack of patient compliance is the most common reason for failure of antihypertensive therapy. The hypertensive patient is usually asymptomatic and is diagnosed by routine screening before the occurence of overt organ damage. Thus, therapy is directed at preventing disease that may occur in the future, rather than in relieving present discomfort of the patient. The adverse effects associated with the hypertensive therapy may influence the patient more than future benefits. Thus, it is important to enhance compliance by carefully selecting a drug regimen that minimizes adverse effects.

V. ANTIHYPERTENSIVE DRUGS

All antihypertensive agents act by interfering with the mechanisms that control cardiac output or peripheral resistance.

A. Thiazide diuretics

All oral diuretic drugs are effective in the treatment of hypertension, but the *thiazides* have found the most widespread use.

1. **Actions:** *Thiazide* diuretics, such as *hydrochlorothiazide* [hye droe klor oh THYE a zide], lower blood pressure, initially by increasing sodium and water excretion. This causes a decrease in extracellular volume, resulting in a decrease in cardiac output and renal blood flow (Figure 19.6). With long-term treatment, plasma volume approaches a normal value, but peripheral resistance decreases. *Spironolactone* [speer on oh LAK tone], a potassium-sparing diuretic, is often used with *thiazides*. A complete discussion of diuretics is found on p.211.

2. **Therapeutic uses:** *Thiazide* diuretics decrease blood pressure in both the supine and standing positions; postural hypotension is rarely observed, except in elderly, volume-depleted patients. These agents counteract the sodium and water retention observed with other agents used in the treatment of hypertension (for example, *hydralazine*). *Thiazides* are therefore useful in combination therapy with a variety of other antihypertensive agents including β blockers and ACE inhibitors. *Thiazide* diuretics are particularly useful in the treatment of black or elderly patients and in those with chronic renal disease.

3. **Pharmacology:** *Thiazide* diuretics can be administered orally. They induce considerable disturbances in electrolyte balance. For example, blood levels of K^+ and Mg^{++} are reduced, and Ca^{++} is retained by the body (p.217).

4. **Adverse effects:** *Thiazide* diuretics induce hypokalemia and hyperuricemia in 70% of patients, and hyperglycemia in 10% of patients. Serum potassium levels should be monitored closely in patients who are predisposed to cardiac arrhythmias (particularly individuals with left ventricular hypertrophy, ischemic heart disease, or chronic congestive heart failure) and who are concurrently being treated with both *thiazide* diuretics and *digitalis* glycosides (Figure 16.8). Diuretics should be avoided in the treatment of hypertensive diabetics or patients with hyperlipidemia.

B. β-Adrenoceptor blocking agents

1. **Actions:** The β blockers reduce blood pressure primarily by decreasing cardiac output (Figure 19.7). They may also decrease sympathetic outflow from the CNS and inhibit the release of renin from the kidneys, thus decreasing the formation of angiotensin II and secretion of aldosterone. The prototype β blocker is *propranolol* which acts at both $β_1$ and $β_2$ receptors. All of the β blockers have actions similar to *propranolol*, regardless

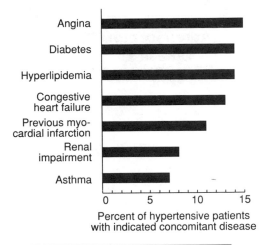

Figure 19.5
Frequency of occurrence of concomitant disease among the hypertensive patient population.

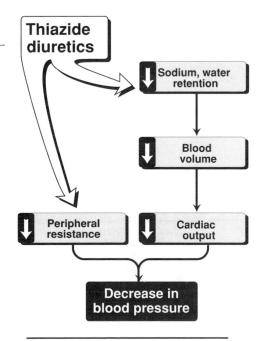

Figure 19.6
Actions of thiazide diuretics.

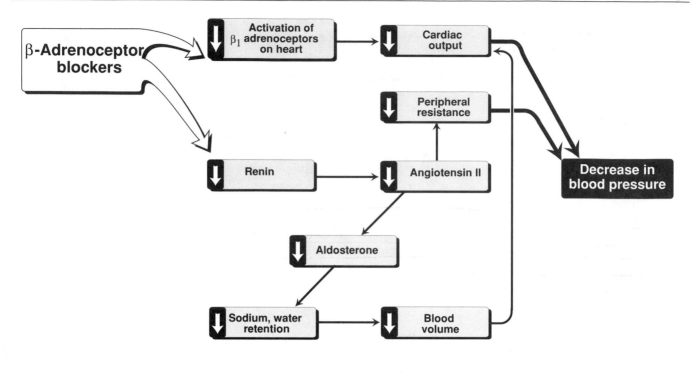

Figure 19.7
Actions of β adrenoceptor blocking agents.

of their special features. If *propranolol* is contraindicated, then other β blockers should not be used. (See p.74 for a complete discussion of β blockers.)

2. **Therapeutic uses:**

   a. The β blockers are useful in treating conditions that may coexist with hypertension, such as supraventricular tachyarrhythmia, previous myocardial infarction, angina pectoris, glaucoma, and migraine headache.

   b. The β blockers are more effective for treating hypertension in white than in black patients, and in young patients compared to the elderly. [Note: Conditions that discourage the use of β blockers (e.g. severe chronic obstructive lung disease, chronic congestive heart failure, severe symptomatic occlusive peripheral vascular disease) are more commonly found in the elderly and in diabetics.]

3. **Pharmacology:** The β blockers may take several weeks to develop their full effects.

4. **Adverse effects:**

   a. The β blockers should be avoided in treating patients with asthma, angina, and peripheral vascular disease.

b. The β blockers may cause CNS side effects such as depression, fatigue, lethargy, insomnia, and hallucinations.

c. The β blockers may disturb lipid metabolism, decreasing high-density-lipoproteins (HDL) and increasing plasma triacylglycerol.

C. ACE inhibitors

1. Actions:

a. The angiotensin-converting enzyme (ACE) inhibitors lower blood pressure by reducing peripheral vascular resistance without reflexively increasing cardiac output, rate, or contractility. The currently available ACE inhibitors are *captopril* [KAP toe pril], *enalapril* [e NAL a pril], and *lisinopril* [lye SIN oh pril]. These drugs block the enzyme that cleaves angiotensin I to form the potent vasoconstrictor, angiotensin II (Figure 19.8). These agents also diminish the rate of bradykinin inactivation (see Figure 39.5, p.383). Vasodilation occurs as a result of the combined effects of lower vasoconstriction caused by diminished levels of angiotensin II and the potent vasodilation effect of increased bradykinin.

b. By reducing circulating angiotensin II levels, ACE inhibitors also decrease the secretion of aldosterone, resulting in decreased sodium and water retention.

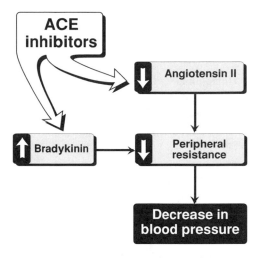

Figure 19.8
Actions of ACE inhibitors.

2. Therapeutic uses:

a. Like β blockers, ACE inhibitors are most effective in hypertensive patients who are white and young. However, when used in combination with a diuretic, the effectiveness of ACE inhibitors is similar in white and black hypertensive patients.

b. Unlike β blockers, ACE inhibitors are effective in the management of patients with chronic congestive heart failure.

3. Adverse effects: Side effects are rare, but include hypercalcemia in patients with impaired renal function, rashes, fever, hypotension, neutropenia, and loss of taste. Although ACE inhibitors are generally well tolerated, they can cause reversible acute renal failure in patients with severe bilateral renal artery stenosis.

D. Calcium channel blockers

1. Actions: The currently approved agents, *verapamil, diltiazem, nifedipine*, and *nicardipine* reduce arterial pressure by inhibiting calcium ion influx into the vascular smooth muscle cells, which results in a decrease in smooth muscle tone and vascular resistance (Figure 19.9). [Note: These agents specifically inhibit calcium-selective channels carrying a slow inward current during depolarization.] All calcium channel blockers are therefore vasodilators. See p.169 for a discussion of the calcium channel blockers.

Dilation of coronary vessels

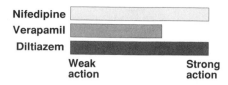

AV Conduction

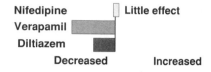

Frequency of adverse effects

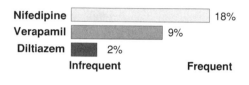

Figure 19.9
Actions of calcium channel blockers.

2. **Therapeutic uses:** Calcium channel blockers have an intrinsic natriuretic effect; therefore, they do not usually require the addition of a diuretic. These agents are useful in the treatment of hypertensive patients who also have asthma, diabetes, angina, and peripheral vascular disease.

3. **Pharmacology:** These agents have short half-lives ($t_{1/2}$=3-4 hours) following an oral dose. Treatment is required three times a day to maintain good control of hypertension. However, *verapamil* is now available in a sustained-release form, which requires only one daily dose.

4. **Adverse effects:** Although infrequent, side effects include constipation in 10% of patients, dizziness, headache, and a feeling of fatigue caused by a decrease in blood pressure. *Verapamil* should be avoided in treating patients with congestive heart failure.

E. α-Adrenergic blocking agents

Prazosin (p.73) produces a competitive block of α_1 adrenoceptors. It decreases peripheral vascular resistance and lowers arterial blood pressure by causing the relaxation of both arterial and venous smooth muscle. The drug causes only minimal changes in cardiac output, renal blood flow, and glomerular filtration rate. Therefore, tachycardia and increased renin release do not occur. Postural hypotension may occur in some individuals. *Prazosin* is used to treat mild to moderate hypertension and is prescribed in combination with *propranolol* or a diuretic for additive effects.

F. Centrally acting adrenergic drugs

1. **Clonidine:** This α_2 agonist diminishes central adrenergic outflow. Clonidine [KLOE ni deen] is used primarily for the treatment of mild to moderate hypertension that has not responded adequately to treatment with diuretics alone. *Clonidine* does not decrease renal blood flow or glomerular filtration and therefore is useful in the treatment of hypertension complicated by renal disease. *Clonidine* is absorbed well after oral administration and is excreted by the kidney. Because it causes sodium and water retention, *clonidine* is usually administered in combination with a diuretic. Adverse effects are generally mild, but the drug can produce sedation and drying of nasal mucosa.

2. **α-Methyldopa:** The α-adrenergic agonist diminishes the adrenergic outflow from the CNS, leading to reduced total peripheral resistance and a decreased blood pressure. Cardiac output is not decreased and blood flow to vital organs is not diminished. Because blood flow to the kidney is not diminished by its use, *α-methyldopa* [meth ill DOE pa] is especially valuable in treating hypertensive patients with renal insufficiency. The most common side effects of *α-methyldopa* are sedation and drowsiness.

G. Vasodilators

The direct-acting smooth muscle relaxants, such as *hydralazine* and *minoxidil*, have traditionally not been used as primary drugs to treat hypertension (p.177). Vasodilators act by producing relaxation of vascular smooth muscle, which increases vasodilation and therefore decreases blood pressure. These agents produce reflex stimulation of the heart, resulting in the competing symptoms of increased myocardial contractility, heart rate, and oxygen consumption. These actions may prompt angina pectoris, myocardial infarction, or cardiac failure in predisposed individuals. Vasodilators also increase plasma renin concentration, resulting in sodium and water retention. These undesirable side effects can be blocked by concomitant use of a diuretic and a β blocker.

1. **Hydralazine:** This drug causes direct vasodilation, acting primarily on arteries and arterioles. This results in a decreased peripheral resistance, which in turn, prompts a reflex elevation in heart rate and cardiac output. *Hydralazine* [hye DRAL a zeen] is used to treat moderately severe hypertension. It is almost always administered in combination with a β blocker such as *propranolol* (to balance the reflex tachycardia) and a diuretic (to decrease sodium retention). Together, the three drugs decrease cardiac output, plasma volume, and peripheral vascular resistance. Adverse effects include headache, nausea, sweating, arrhythmia, and precipitation of angina. A lupus-like syndrome can occur with high dosage, but it is reversible on discontinuation of the drug.

2. **Minoxidil:** This drug causes dilation of resistance vessels (arterioles) but not of capacitance vessels (venules). *Minoxidil* [mi NOX i dill] is administered orally for treatment of severe to malignant hypertension that is refractory to other drugs. Reflex tachycardia may be severe and require the concomitant use of a diuretic and a β blocker. *Minoxidil* causes serious sodium and water retention, leading to volume overload, edema, and congestive heart failure. [Note: *Minoxidil* treatment also causes hypertrichosis (the growth of body hair). This drug is now used topically to treat alopecia (hair loss).]

VI. HYPERTENSIVE EMERGENCY

Hypertensive emergency is a rare, but life-threatening situation in which the diastolic blood pressure is either over 150 mm Hg in an otherwise healthy person, or 130 mm Hg in an individual with preexisting complications, such as encephalopathy, cerebral hemorrhage, left ventricular failure, or aortic stenosis. The therapeutic goal is to rapidly reduce blood pressure.

A. Sodium nitroprusside

Nitroprusside administered intravenously, causes prompt vasodilation, with reflex tachycardia. It is capable of reducing blood pressure in all patients, regardless of the cause of hypertension. The drug has little effect outside the vascular system, acting equally on arterial and venous smooth muscle. [Note: Because *nitroprusside* also acts on the veins, it can reduce cardiac preload.] *Nitroprusside* is metabolized rapidly ($t_{1/2}$ of minutes) and requires continuous infusion to maintain hypotensive action. *Sodium nitroprusside*

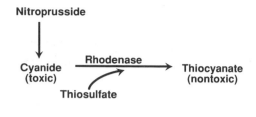

Figure 19.10
Detoxification of cyanide with
thiosulfate and rhodenase

exerts few adverse effects except for those of hypotension caused by overdose. Cyanide ion production may occur from *nitroprusside* although cyanide toxicity is rare. This can be effectively treated with an infusion of *rhodanase,* a normal mitochondrial enzyme, that combines cyanide with thiosulfate to produce thiocyanate, which is less toxic and is eliminated by the kidneys (Figure 19.10). [Note: *Nitroprusside* is poisonous if given orally because of its hydrolysis to cyanide.]

B. Diazoxide

Diazoxide [dye az OX ide] is a direct-acting arteriolar vasodilator. It has vascular effects like those of *hydralazine*. For patients with coronary insufficiency, *diazoxide* is administered intravenously with a β blocker which diminishes reflex activation of the heart. *Diazoxide* is useful in the treatment of hypertensive emergencies, particularly malignant hypertension, hypertensive encephalopathy, and eclampsia. Excessive hypotension is the most serious toxicity.

Study Questions   (see p.420 for answers).

Answer A if 1,2 and 3 are correct.
   B if 1 and 3 are correct.
   C if 2 and 4 are correct.
   D if only 4 is correct.
   E if 1,2,3 and 4 are all correct.

19.1 Which of the following statements is/are correct?

1. Cerebral hemorrhage is a common complication of severe hypertension.
2. Hypertension results from increased vascular smooth muscle tone which leads to increased arteriolar resistance and reduced capacitance of the venules.
3. Prazosin is likely to produce postural hypotension.
4. Antihypertensive therapy is designed to relieve the symptoms of high blood pressure.

19.2 Administration of ACE inhibitors leads to

1. Decreased blood pressure.
2. Decreased aldosterone levels.
3. Increased bradykinin.
4. Increased cardiac performance.

Choose the ONE best answer.

19.3 Which of the following patients is most suited for primary therapy with hydrochlorothiazide?

   A. Patients with gout.
   B. Patients with hyperlipidemia.
   C. Young hypertensive patients with rapid resting heart rates.
   D. Black patients and elderly patients.
   E. Patients with impaired renal function.

19.4 All of the following produce a significant decrease in peripheral resistance except:

   A. Chronic administration of diuretics.
   B. Hydralazine.
   C. β-blocker.
   D. ACE inhibitors.
   E. Clonidine.

19.5 Which one of the following acts at central presynaptic α_2 receptors?

   A. Minoxidil.
   B. Verapamil.
   C. Clonidine.
   D. Enalapril.
   E. Hydrochlorothiazide.

Drugs Affecting Blood

20

I. OVERVIEW

This chapter describes drugs useful in treating three important dysfunctions of blood: thrombosis, bleeding, and anemia. Thrombosis—the formation of an unwanted clot within the blood vessels or heart—is the most common abnormality of hemostasis. Bleeding disorders involving failure of hemostasis are less common than thromboembolic diseases and include hemophilia and vitamin K deficiency. Anemias caused by nutritional deficiencies can be treated with dietary supplementation. See Figure 20.1 for a summary of drugs affecting blood.

II. NORMAL RESPONSE TO VASCULAR TRAUMA

Physical trauma to the vascular system, such as a puncture or cut, initiates a complex series of interactions between platelets, endothelial cells, and the coagulation cascade. This results in the formation of a platelet-fibrin plug. The creation of an unwanted thrombus involves many of the same steps, except that the triggering stimulus is a pathological condition in the vascular system rather than physical trauma.

A. Formation of a clot

1. **Role of platelets and fibrin:** Platelets respond to vascular trauma by an "activation" process, which involves three steps: adhesion to the site of injury, release of intracellular granules, and aggregation of the platelets (Figure 20.2). Platelets first adhere to exposed collagen in the subendothelial layers of injured blood vessels, triggering the release of platelet granules containing chemical mediators, which promote platelet aggregation and the formation of a plug composed of the viscous contents of lysed platelets. This rapidly arrests bleeding. Local stimulation of the coagulation cascade by factors released from the injured tissue and platelets results in the formation of thrombin. Thrombin, in turn, catalyzes the conversion of fibrinogen to fibrin, which is incorporated into the plug. Subsequent cross-linking of the fibrin strands stabilizes the clot and forms a hemostatic plug.

2. **Thrombus** versus **embolus:** A clot that adheres to a vessel wall is called a thrombus, whereas an intravascular clot that floats within the blood is termed an embolus. Thus, a detached throm-

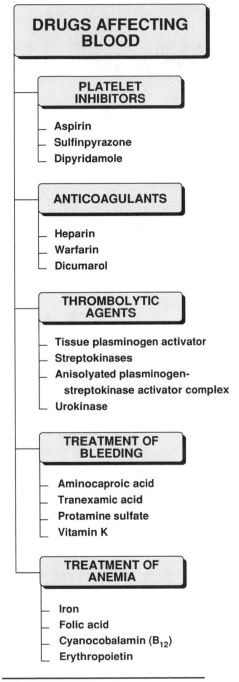

DRUGS AFFECTING BLOOD

PLATELET INHIBITORS
- Aspirin
- Sulfinpyrazone
- Dipyridamole

ANTICOAGULANTS
- Heparin
- Warfarin
- Dicumarol

THROMBOLYTIC AGENTS
- Tissue plasminogen activator
- Streptokinases
- Anisolyated plasminogen-streptokinase activator complex
- Urokinase

TREATMENT OF BLEEDING
- Aminocaproic acid
- Tranexamic acid
- Protamine sulfate
- Vitamin K

TREATMENT OF ANEMIA
- Iron
- Folic acid
- Cyanocobalamin (B_{12})
- Erythropoietin

Figure 20.1
Summary of drugs used in treating dysfunctions of blood.

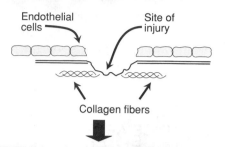

1 Damage to vessel exposes collagen of subendothelium

2 Platelet adhesion and release of granules

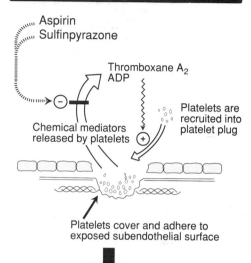

Platelets cover and adhere to exposed subendothelial surface

3 Platelet aggregation and formation of fibrin plug

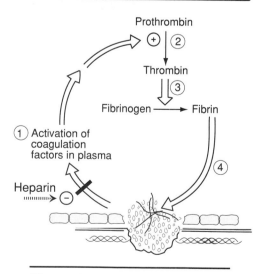

Figure 20.2
Formation of a hemostatic plug.

bus becomes an embolus. Both thrombi and emboli are dangerous, since they may occlude blood vessels and deprive tissues of oxygen and nutrients. Arterial thrombosis most often involves medium-sized vessels rendered thrombogenic by surface lesions of endothelial cells caused by atherosclerosis. In contrast, venous thrombosis is triggered by blood stasis or inappropriate activation of the coagulation cascade, often as a result of a defect in the normal defense hemostatic mechanisms.

B. Fibrinolysis

During platelet plug formation, the fibrinolytic pathway is locally activated. Plasminogen is enzymatically processed to plasmin (fibrinolysin) by plasminogen activators present in the tissue. Plasmin interferes in clot propagation and dissolves the fibrin network as wounds heal. At present, a number of fibrinolytic enzymes are available for treatment of myocardial infarctions or pulmonary emboli (p.192).

III. PLATELET ACTIVATION

The outer membrane of platelets contains a variety of receptors that function as sensors capable of responding to physiological signals present in the plasma (Figure 20.3). These chemical stimuli are classified as platelet-activating if they promote platelet aggregation and the subsequent release of granules stored in the platelet. Conversely, other chemical signals are classified as platelet-inhibiting, if they inhibit platelet activation and the release of platelet granules. Whether platelets remain in a quiescent state or become activated is determined by the balance of activating and inhibiting chemical signals.

A. Chemical signals that oppose platelet activation

1. **Elevated prostacyclin levels:** In a normal, undamaged vessel, platelets circulate freely, since the balance of chemical signals indicate that the vascular system is not damaged. For example, prostacyclin (p.362), synthesized by the intact endothelial cells and released into plasma, binds to a specific set of platelet membrane receptors that are coupled to the synthesis of cAMP as an intracellular message (p.33). Elevated levels of intracellular cAMP inhibit platelet activation, and the subsequent release of platelet aggregation agents (Figure 20.3).

2. **Decreased plasma levels of thrombin and thromboxanes:** The platelet membrane also contains receptors that can bind thrombin (the protease that converts fibrinogen to fibrin), thromboxanes, and exposed collagen. When occupied, each of these receptor types triggers a series of reactions leading to the release into the circulation of intracellular granules and ultimately to platelet aggregation. However, in the intact, normal vessel, circulating levels of thrombin and thromboxanes are low and the intact endothelium covers the collagen present in the subendothelial layers. The corresponding platelet receptors are thus unoc-

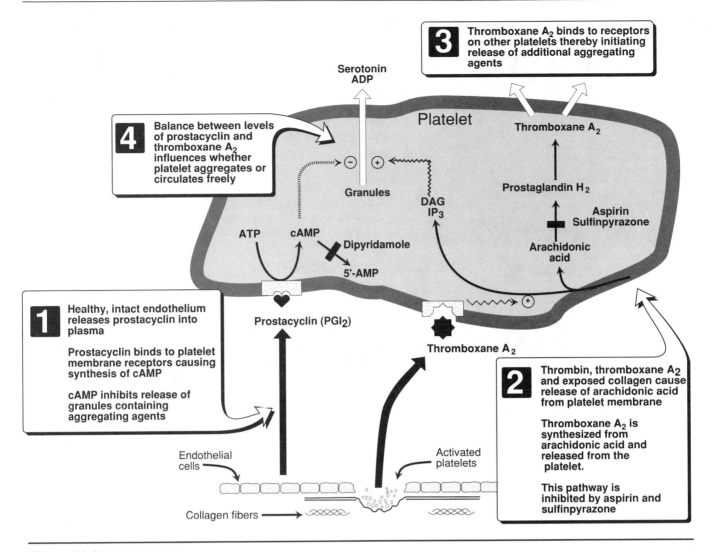

Figure 20.3
Chemical mediators influencing platelet activation and aggregation
(relative size of platelets and endothelial cells are not to scale).

cupied and therefore remain inactive. Platelet activation and aggregation are not initiated.

B. Chemical signals that promote platelet aggregation

1. **Decreased prostacyclin levels:** Damaged endothelial cells synthesize less prostacyclin, resulting in a localized decrease in prostacyclin levels. The binding of prostacyclin to platelet receptors is decreased, and thus lower levels of intracellular cAMP permit platelet aggregation.

2. **Exposed collagen:** Within seconds of vascular injury, platelets adhere to and virtually cover the exposed collagen of the subendothelium. Receptors on the surface of the platelet are activated by the collagen of this underlying connective tissue, which triggers the release of platelet granules containing ADP and seroto-

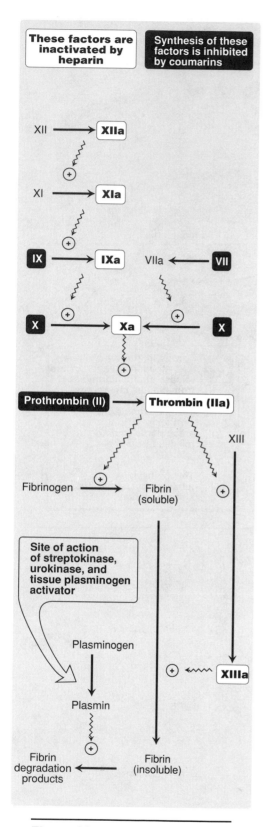

Figure 20.4
Formation of fibrin clot and its ultimate dissolution.

nin. This process is sometimes referred to as the "platelet release reaction," and the platelet is then said to be activated.

3. **Increased synthesis of thromboxanes:** Stimulation of platelets by thrombin, collagen, and ADP results in activation of platelet membrane phospholipases, which liberate arachidonic acid from membrane phospholipid. Arachidonic acid is first converted to prostaglandin H_2 by cyclooxygenase, an enzyme that is irreversibly inactivated by *aspirin* (p.363). Prostaglandin H_2 is metabolized to thromboxane A_2, which is released into the plasma. Thromboxane A_2 produced by the aggregating platelets further promotes the clumping process that is essential to the rapid formation of a hemostatic plug (Figure 20.3).

IV. BLOOD COAGULATION

The coagulation process that generates thrombin consists of two interrelated pathways—the extrinsic and the intrinsic systems. The extrinsic system is initiated by the activation of clotting Factor VII, and the release of tissue thromboplastin—a phospholipid and protein mixture. The intrinsic system is triggered by the activation of clotting Factor XII, following its contact with exposed collagen fibers in the subendothelium of damaged blood vessels. Both systems involve a cascade of enzymatic reactions that sequentially transform various plasma factors (proenzymes) to their active (enzymatic) forms, ultimately producing thrombin (Figure 20.4). Thrombin, a serine protease that plays a key role in coagulation, catalyzes the conversion of fibrinogen to fibrin, a glycoprotein that forms the mesh-like matrix of the blood clot. Thrombin also activates clotting Factor XIII (necessary for stabilizing and crosslinking the fibrin molecules into an insoluble clot) as well as activating other blood clotting factors. If thrombin is not formed, or its function is impeded, for example, with antithrombin III, coagulation is inhibited.

V. PLATELET AGGREGATION INHIBITORS

Platelet aggregation inhibitors decrease the formation or the action of chemical signals that promote platelet aggregation.

A. Aspirin

Aspirin [AS pir in] blocks thromboxane A_2 synthesis from arachidonic acid in platelets by irreversibly acetylating and thus inhibiting cyclo-oxygenase, a key enzyme in prostaglandin synthesis (see p.363 for a discussion of the actions of aspirin on platelets). The *aspirin*-induced inhibition of thromboxane A_2 synthetase and the resulting suppression of platelet aggregation last for the life of the platelet—approximately 7-10 days. *Aspirin* is currently employed in the prophylactic treatment of transient cerebral ischemia, to reduce the incidence of recurrent myocardial infarction and to decrease mortality in postmyocardial infarction patients.

B. Sulfinpyrazone

Sulfinpyrazone [sul fin PEER a zone] is therapeutically employed as a uricosuric agent (p.377). However, it can also inhibit platelet functions, including release of platelet factors and adherence to subendothelial cells (see Figure 20.2). Unlike *aspirin*, *sulfinpyrazone* can also prolong the survival of platelets in patients with various disorders.

C. Dipyridamole

Dipyridamole [dye peer ID a mole], a coronary vasodilator, is employed to prophylactically treat angina pectoris. It is usually given in combination with *aspirin*. *Dipyridamole* increases intracellular levels of cyclic AMP by inhibiting cyclic nucleotide phosphodiesterase. This may potentiate the effect of prostacyclin (PGI$_2$) to antagonize platelet stickiness and therefore decrease platelet adhesion to thrombogenic surfaces (see Figure 20.2). The meager data available suggest that *dipyridamole* makes only a marginal contribution to the antithrombotic action of *aspirin*. In combination with *warfarin*, however, *dipyridamole* is effective in inhibiting embolization from prosthetic heart valves.

VI. ANTICOAGULANTS

Two types of drugs are employed in preventing blood coagulation, *heparin* and the *vitamin K* antagonists. Their mechanisms of action differ, as do their clinical uses.

A. Heparin

Heparin [HEP a rin] is an injectable, rapidly-acting anticoagulant that is often used acutely to interfere with the formation of thrombi. *Heparin* occurs normally complexed to histamine as a macromolecule in mast cells where its physiological role is unknown. It is obtained for commercial use from porcine intestine or bovine lung tissue. *Heparin* is a straight-chain anionic glycosaminoglycan[1]. It is strongly acidic because of the presence of sulfate and carboxylic acid groups.

1. **Mechanism of Action:** Although *heparin* acts indirectly by binding to antithrombin III, its anticoagulant effect is immediate and maximal anticoagulation occurs within minutes after direct intravenous *heparin* injection (unlike oral anticoagulants, such as *warfarin*, whose maximum activity may require 8-12 hours). Antithrombin III, sometimes referred to as heparin cofactor, is an α-globulin that inhibits serine proteases, including several of the clotting factors, e.g., thrombin (Figure 20.5). However, in the absence of *heparin*, antithrombin III only slowly interacts with thrombin. The binding of *heparin* to antithrombin III to form a complex rapidly enhances the proteolytic activity of antithrombin III by accelerating the binding of this complex to its substrate. However, chronic or intermittent administration of *heparin* can lead to a reduction in antithrombin III activity and increase the risk of thrombosis. To minimize this risk low dose heparin therapy is usually employed.

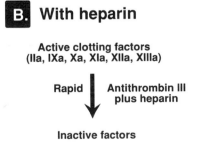

Figure 20.5
Heparin binds to antithrombin III and enhances its proteolytic activity.

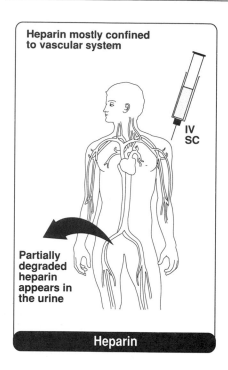

Heparin mostly confined to vascular system

IV
SC

Partially degraded heparin appears in the urine

Heparin

2. **Therapeutic uses:**

Heparin abolishes fibrin formation and thus limits the expansion of thrombi. *Heparin* is the major antithrombotic drug for the treatment of deep vein thrombosis and pulmonary embolism. It prevents additional complications and decreases the incidence of recurrent thromboembolic episodes. Clinically, *heparin* is used prophylactically to prevent postoperative venous thrombosis in patients undergoing elective surgery, and in the acute phase of myocardial infarction. *Heparin* also has the advantage of an immediate onset of action, which is rapidly terminated on suspension of therapy.

3. **Pharmacology:**

   a. **Absorption:** *Heparin* must be given parenterally either in a deep subcutaneous site or intravenously, because the drug does not readily cross membranes. *Heparin* is often administered intravenously in a bolus to achieve rapid anticoagulation. Continuous infusion is then maintained for 7-10 days, titering the dose of *heparin* so that the partial thromboplastin time is 1.5-2.5 times the normal control.

   b. **Fate:** Although generally restricted to the circulation, *heparin* is taken up by the reticuloendothelial system and undergoes hepatic degradation to inactive products. *Heparin* therefore has a longer half-life in patients with hepatic cirrhosis. The inactive metabolites as well as some of the parent *heparin* are excreted into the urine, therefore renal insufficiency also prolongs the half-life. [Note: *Heparin* does not cross the placental barrier.]

4. **Adverse effects:**

   a. **Bleeding complications:** The chief complication of *heparin* therapy is hemorrhage. Careful monitoring of bleeding time is required to minimize this problem. *Protamine sulfate* is administered to counter excessive bleeding caused by *heparin*. It inactivates *heparin* by combining ionically with it to form a stable complex. The incidence of hemorrhage complication is also reduced with continuous infusion, rather than intermittent administration.

   b. **Hypersensitivity reactions:** Reactions such as chills, fever, urticaria, or anaphylactic shock are possible, especially since the *heparin* preparation is obtained from animal sources and may therefore be antigenic.

   c. **Thrombocytopenia:** A decrease in the number of circulating platelets may occur after about 8 days of therapy. In some patients, *heparin*-induced platelet aggregation is followed by the formation of antiplatelet antibodies. Discontinuance of the drug then becomes necessary. Should *heparin*-induced thromboembolism occur, therapy with a drug that inhibits platelet aggregation or an oral anticoagulant is instituted in place of the *heparin*.

d. **Contraindications:** *Heparin* is contraindicated for patients who are hypersensitive to it or have bleeding disorders, for alcoholics, and for patients who have had surgery of the brain, eye, or spinal cord. *Heparin* was previously considered to be non-teratogenic, but recent data show a higher than expected rate of stillbirths associated with its use.

B. Warfarin

The coumarin anticoagulants, which include *warfarin* [WAR far in] and *dicumarol* [dye KOO ma role] (formerly *bishydroxycoumarin*) owe their action to their ability to antagonize the cofactor functions of *vitamin K*. Initially used as a rodenticide, *warfarin* is now widely employed clinically as an oral anticoagulant. However, conflicting opinions exist concerning the usefulness of these agents in clinical situations such as myocardial infarction and hip arthroplasty.

1. **Mechanism of action:**

   Several of the protein factors that are involved in the coagulation reactions depend on *vitamin K* as a cofactor in their activation, (including Factors II, VII, IX, and X; see Figure 20.4). This activation involves the factors undergoing vitamin K-dependent post-translational modification, whereby a number of their glutamic acid residues are carboxylated to form γ-carboxyglutamic acid residues (Figure 20.6). The γ-carboxyglutamyl residues serve an essential role in the activity of these clotting factors during hemostasis. *Warfarin* or *dicumarol* treatment results in the production of inactive clotting factors, since they lack the γ-carboxyglutamyl side chains necessary for calcium binding and subsequent activity. Unlike *heparin*, the anticoagulant effects of *warfarin* are not observed until 8-12 hours after drug administration. The anticoagulant effects of *warfarin* can be overcome by the administration of *vitamin K*. However, reversal by *vitamin K* takes approximately 24 hours.

2. **Pharmacology:**

   a. **Absorption:** The sodium salt of *warfarin* is rapidly and completely absorbed after oral administration. Though food may delay absorption, it does not affect the extent of absorption. The drug is 99% bound to plasma albumin, which prevents its diffusion into the CSF, urine, and breast milk. However, drugs having a greater affinity for the binding site, such as sulfonamides, can displace the anticoagulant and lead to a transient elevated activity (p.10).

   b. **Fate:** The products of *warfarin* metabolism are inactive and, after conjugation to glucuronic acid, are excreted in the urine and stool.

3. **Adverse effects:**

   a. **Bleeding disorders:** The principal untoward reaction is hemorrhage. Therefore, it is important to monitor the anticoagulant effect. Minor bleeding may be treated by withdrawal of the

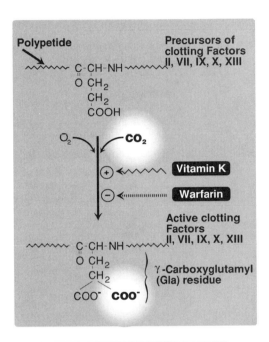

Figure 20.6
Mechanism of action of warfarin.

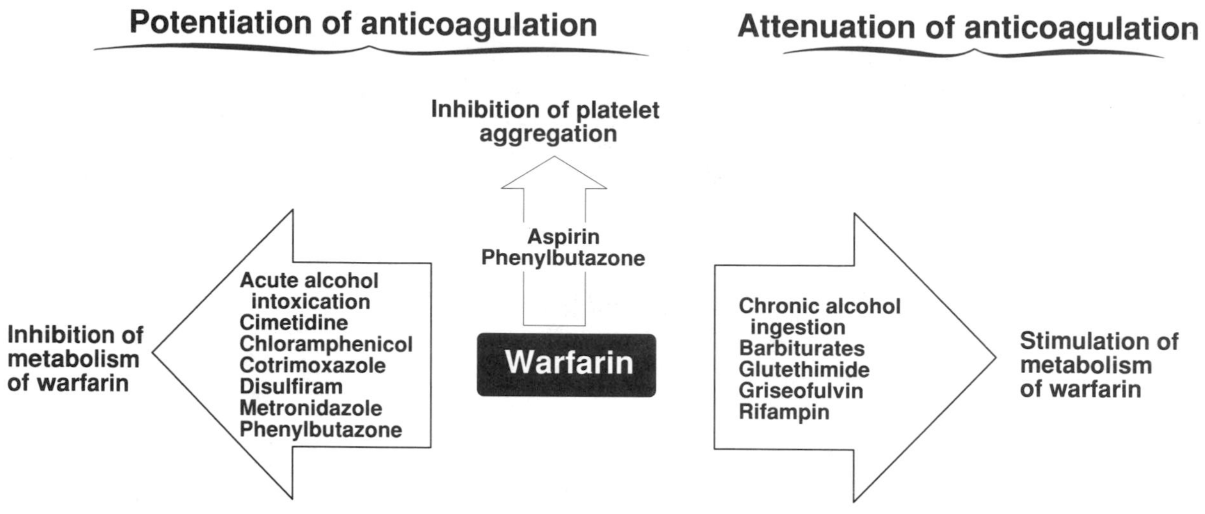

Potentiation of anticoagulation   ## Attenuation of anticoagulation

Inhibition of platelet aggregation

Aspirin
Phenylbutazone

Inhibition of metabolism of warfarin

Acute alcohol intoxication
Cimetidine
Chloramphenicol
Cotrimoxazole
Disulfiram
Metronidazole
Phenylbutazone

Warfarin

Chronic alcohol ingestion
Barbiturates
Glutethimide
Griseofulvin
Rifampin

Stimulation of metabolism of warfarin

Figure 20.7
Drugs affecting the anticoagulant effect of warfarin.

drug and administration of oral *vitamin K₁*; severe bleeding requires greater doses of the vitamin given intravenously. Whole blood, frozen plasma, or plasma concentrates of the blood factors may also be employed to arrest hemorrhaging.

b. **Drug interactions:** A number of drug interactions that potentiate the anticoagulant effects of these agents have been identified. A summary of the most important of these interactions is shown in Figure 20.7.

c. Disease states can also influence the hypoprothrombinemic state of the patient and influence the response to the anticoagulants. For example, a *vitamin K* deficiency, hepatic disease, which impairs synthesis of the clotting factors, and hypermetabolic states, which increase catabolism of the vitamin K-dependent clotting factors, can all augment the response to the oral anticoagulants.

VII. THROMBOLYTIC DRUGS

Acute thromboembolic disease may be treated by the administration of agents that activate the conversion of plasminogen to plasmin, a serine protease that hydrolyzes fibrin and thus dissolves clots (Figure 20.8). The first such agents to be approved, *streptokinase* and *urokinase*, cause a systemic fibrinolytic state which can lead to bleeding problems. *Tissue-type plasminogen activator (tPA)* acts more locally on the thrombotic fibrin to produce fibrinolysis and is a potentially important agent in treating thromboembolic disease. (See Figure 20.9 for a comparison of the commonly used thrombolytic agents.) Clinical experience has shown about equal efficacy between streptokinase and tPA.

A. Common characteristics of thrombolytic agents

1. **Actions:** The thrombolytic agents share some common features. All act either directly or indirectly to convert plasminogen to plasmin which in turn cleaves fibrin (Figure 20.8). All of these agents are effective in dissolving thrombi. In each case, clot dissolution and reperfusion occurs with a higher frequency when therapy is initiated early after clot formation, since clots become more resistant to lysis as they age.

2. **Administration:** Intracoronary delivery of the drugs is the most reliable in terms of achieving recanalization. However, cardiac catheterization may not be possible in the 2-6 hour "therapeutic window," beyond which significant myocardial salvage become less likely. Thus thrombolytic agents are usually administered intravenously, since this route is rapid, inexpensive, and does not have the risks of catheterization.

3. **Therapeutic uses:** Originally used for the treatment of deep-vein thrombosis and serious pulmonary embolism, thrombolytic drugs are now being used with increasing frequency to treat acute peripheral arterial thrombosis and emboli, and for unclotting catheters and shunts. A major use of thrombolytic drugs is in the management of acute myocardial infarction because the agents are now administered intravenously, rather than by the cumbersome intracoronary injection used previously.

4. **Adverse effects:** The thrombolytic agents do not distinguish between the fibrin of an unwanted thrombus and the fibrin of a beneficial hemostatic plug. Thus, the thrombolytic agents have hemorrhage as a major side effect. For example, a previously unsuspected lesion, such as a peptic ulcer, may hemorrhage following injection of a thrombolytic agent (Figure 20.10). They are contraindicated in patients with a healing wound, pregnancy, or a recent cerebrovascular accident. Continued presence of thrombogenic stimuli may precipitate the formation of a second thrombus after lysis of the initial clot. Consequently, *heparin* is simultaneously administered to protect against rethrombosis in the case of *tissue-type plasminogen activator* (*tPA*) and *urokinase*.

B. Tissue-type plasminogen activator

Tissue-type plasminogen activator is a serine protease originally derived from cultured human melanoma cells, but it is now obtained in therapeutic quantities as a product of recombinant DNA technology.

1. **Mechanism of action:** *tPA* has a low affinity for free plasminogen, but it rapidly activates plasminogen bound to fibrin in a thrombus or a hemostatic plug. Thus, *tPA* is said to be "fibrin selective" and has the advantage of lysing only fibrin, without unwanted degradation of other proteins, notably fibrinogen. This contrasts with *urokinase* and *streptokinase*, which act on free plasminogen and induce a thrombolytic state. This advantage seems to be realized at low doses of *tPA*, but at high doses, a thrombolytic state is induced with the risk of hemorrhage.

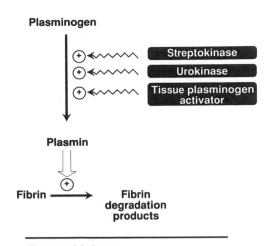

Figure 20.8
Activation of plasminogen by fibrinolytic agents.

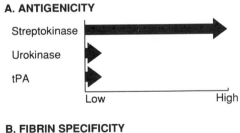

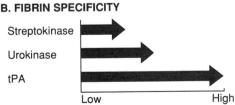

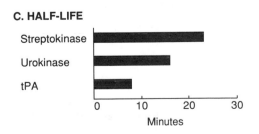

Figure 20.9
A comparison of commonly used thrombolytic agents. tPA= tissue-type plasminogen activator.

A. Untreated patient

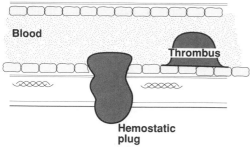

Blood

Thrombus

Hemostatic plug

B. Patient treated with plasminogen activator

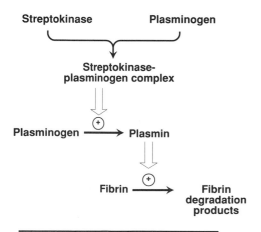

Blood

Bleeding

Figure 20.10
Degradation of an unwanted thrombus and a beneficial hemostatic plug by plasminogen activators.

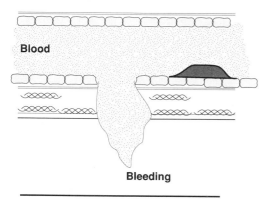

Streptokinase   Plasminogen

Streptokinase-plasminogen complex

Plasminogen $\xrightarrow{(+)}$ Plasmin

Fibrin $\xrightarrow{(+)}$ Fibrin degradation products

Figure 20.11
Mechanism of action of streptokinase.

2. **Therapeutic uses:** Currently *tPA* is only approved for the treatment of myocardial infarction. *Tissue-type plasminogen activator* seems to be superior to *streptokinase* and *urokinase* in dissolving older clots; *tPA* may ultimately be approved for other applications.

3. **Adverse effects:** Bleeding complications, including cerebral hemorrhages, may occur. Therefore *heparin* is administered simultaneously with *tPA* to enhance reperfusion and decrease the rate at which second thrombi form.

C. Streptokinase

Streptokinase [strep toe KYE nase] is an extracellular protein derived from purified culture broth of Group C β-hemolytic streptococci.

1. **Mechanism of action:** *Streptokinase* has no enzymic activity; instead it forms an active complex with plasminogen, which then converts uncomplexed plasminogen to the active enzyme plasmin (Figure 20.11). In addition to the hydrolysis of fibrin plugs, the complex also catalyzes the degradation of fibrinogen as well as clotting Factors V and VII.

2. **Therapeutic uses:** *Streptokinase* is approved for use in acute pulmonary embolism, deep venous thrombosis, acute myocardial infarction, arterial thrombosis, and occluded access shunts.

3. **Pharmacology:** *Streptokinase* therapy is instituted within 4 hours of a myocardial infarction and continued for 1 to 3 days. Thromboplastin time is monitored and maintained at two to five times control value. On discontinuation of treatment, either *heparin* or oral anticoagulants are administered.

4. **Adverse effects**

   a. **Bleeding disorders:** Activation of circulating plasminogen leads to elevated levels of plasmin, which may precipitate bleeding by dissolving hemostatic plugs (Figure 20.12). In the rare instance of life-threatening hemorrhage, *aminocaproic acid* (see p.195) may be administered.

   b. **Hypersensitivity:** *Streptokinase* is a foreign protein and is antigenic. Rashes, fever, and rarely, anaphylaxis occur. Since most individuals have had a streptococcal infection sometime in their lives, circulating antibodies against *streptokinase* are likely to be present in most patients. These antibodies can combine with *streptokinase* and neutralize its fibrinolytic properties. Therefore, sufficient quantities of *streptokinase* must be administered to overwhelm the antibodies and provide a therapeutic concentration of plasmin. Fever, allergic reactions, and therapeutic failure may be associated with the presence of antistreptococcal antibodies in the patient. The incidence of allergic reactions is approximately 3%.

   [Note: *Anistreplase* [Ani strep lase] (*anisolyated plasminogen streptokinase activator complex*) was synthesized to improve the kinetics of *streptokinase-plasminogen*. The lysine at the active site of plasminogen is acylated so that fibrinolysis does not occur during injection. However, the ability to bind to fibrin is retained. The complex is semiselective for hydrolysis at the clot site. The plasma half-life is long (2 hours) compared to *streptokinase*. It is well tolerated on rapid injection, and reperfusion results compare favorably with *streptokinase*. Like other thrombolytic agents, bleeding is a complication, as well as arrhythmias and hypotension.]

D. Urokinase

1. **Mechanism of action:** *Urokinase* [yoor oh KIN ase] is an enzyme capable of directly degrading both fibrin and fibrinogen (Figure 20.12). *Urokinase* was originally isolated from human urine, but it is now obtained from cultures of human fetal renal cells. *Urokinase* is more expensive than *streptokinase* and is usually employed in patients who are sensitive to *streptokinase*. It is not a foreign protein and is therefore nonantigenic.

2. **Therapeutic uses:** *Urokinase, like streptokinase,* is effective in treating severe pulmonary emboli and deep vein thrombosis. Although some practitioners feel that thrombolytic therapy is the treatment of choice in all cases of pulmonary emboli, most still feel it should be reserved for patients with massive pulmonary emboli and hypertension.

3. **Adverse effects:** Bleeding complications are the most important side effects.

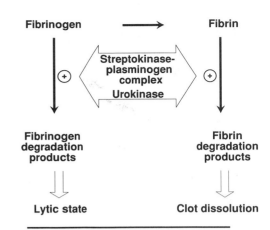

Figure 20.12
Streptokinase and urokinase degrade both fibrin and fibrinogen.

VIII. DRUGS USED TO TREAT BLEEDING

Bleeding problems may have their origin in naturally occurring pathological conditions, for example, hemophilia, or as a result of fibrinolytic states that may arise after gastrointestinal surgery or prostatectomy. The use of anticoagulants may also give rise to hemorrhaging. Certain natural proteins and *vitamin K* as well as synthetic antagonists are effective in controlling this condition. Hemophilia is a consequence of a deficiency in plasma coagulation factors, most frequently Factors VIII and IX. Concentrated preparations of these factors are available from human donors. However, they hold the risk of transferring viral infections.

A. Aminocaproic acid and tranexamic acid

Fibrinolytic states can be controlled by the administration of *aminocaproic acid* [a mee noe ka PROE ic] or *tranexamic acid* [tran ex AM ic]. Both agents are synthetic and inhibit plasminogen activation.

B. Protamine sulfate

Protamine sulfate [PROE ta meen] antagonizes the anticoagulant effects of *heparin*. This protein is derived from fish sperm or testes and is high in arginine content, which explains its basicity. The positively charged protein interacts with the negatively charged *heparin* to form a stable complex without anticoagulant activity. *Protamine sulfate* itself can interfere in coagulation when it is given in the absence of *heparin*, since the basic protein interacts with platelets and fibrinogen. Adverse effects include hypersensitivity, as well as dyspnea, flushing, bradycardia, and hypotension when rapidly injected.

C. Vitamin K

That *vitamin K* administration can stem bleeding problems due to the oral anticoagulants is not surprising, since those substances act by interfering in the action of the vitamin (Figure 20.6). *Vitamin K* is one of the fat-soluble vitamins found in green leafy vegetables and produced by intestinal flora.[2] The absorption of *vitamin K* from the intestinal tract requires bile salts. Intravenous administration should be slow to avoid dyspnea, chest pain, and possibly death. The response to *vitamin K* is slow, requiring about 24 hours.

IX. AGENTS USED TO TREAT ANEMIA

Anemia is defined as a below-normal plasma hemoglobin concentration resulting from a decreased number of circulating red blood cells or an abnormally low total hemoglobin content per unit of blood volume. Anemia can be caused by chronic blood loss, bone marrow abnormalities, increased hemolysis, infections, malignancy, endocrine deficiencies, and a number of other disease states. A large number of drugs cause toxic effects on blood cells, hemoglobin production, or erythropoietic organs, which in turn causes anemia. In addition, nutritional anemias are caused by dietary deficiencies of substances necessary for normal erythropoiesis. These substances include iron, folic acid, and, to a lesser extent, vitamin B_{12} (cyanocobalamin).

A. Iron

Iron is stored in intestinal mucosal cells (in an iron/protein complex called ferritin) until needed by the body. Iron deficiency results from acute or chronic blood loss, from insufficient intake during periods of accelerated growth in children, or in heavily menstruating or pregnant women. Iron deficiency anemia is therefore essentially the result of negative iron balance that begins with a depletion of iron stores and results in the development of hypochromic microcytic anemia. Dietary iron supplementation is required to correct the deficiency. Iron salts such as ferrous sulfate are the standard form of iron supplements. Gastrointestinal disturbances caused by local irritation are the most common adverse effects caused by iron supplements.

B. Folic acid

The primary use of *folic acid* is in treating deficiency states that arise from inadequate levels of *folate* caused by increased demand (e.g., pregnancy and lactation) or by poor absorption caused by

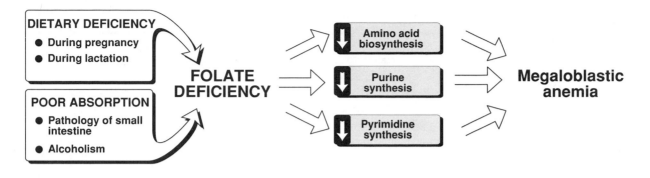

Figure 20.13
Causes and consequences of folic acid depletion.

disorders of the small intestine, alcoholism, or treatment with drugs, which are dihydrofolate reductase inhibitors (for example, *methotrexate, trimethoprim*, p.268). A primary result of folic acid deficiency is megaloblastic anemia, caused by diminished synthesis of purines and pyrimidines, leading to an inability of erythropoietic tissue to make DNA and divide (Figure 20.13).[3] [Note: It is important to evaluate the cause of the megaloblastic anemia prior to instituting therapy, since vitamin B_{12} deficiency indirectly causes symptoms of this disorder (see following paragraph).] *Folic acid* is well absorbed in the jejunum unless pathology is present. If excess amounts of the vitamin are ingested, they are excreted in the urine and feces. *Folic acid* administered orally has no known toxicity.

C. Cyanocobalamin (B12)

Deficiencies of *vitamin B_{12}* can result from either low dietary levels or, more commonly, from poor absorption due to the failure of gastric parietal cells to produce intrinsic factor (as in pernicious anemia) or to a loss of activity of the receptor needed for intestinal uptake of the vitamin.[4] Less specific malabsorption syndromes or gastric resection can also cause vitamin deficiency. Depending on the type of deficiency, the vitamin may be administered orally (for dietary deficiencies), intramuscularly, or deep subcutaneously (for pernicious anemia). [Note: *Folic acid* administration alone reverses the hematologic abnormality and thus masks the B_{12} deficiency which can then proceed to severe neurological dysfunction and disease; therefore megaloblastic anemia should not be treated with *folic acid* alone, but rather with a combination of *folate* and *vitamin B_{12}*.] Therapy must be continued for the lives of patients suffering from pernicious anemia. There are no known adverse effects of this vitamin.

D. Erythropoietin

Erythropoietin is a glycoprotein, normally produced by the kidney, that regulates red cell proliferation and differentiation in bone marrow. Human *erythropoietin*, produced by recombinant DNA technology, is effective in the treatment of anemia caused by end-stage renal disease.

Study Questions   (see p.421 for answers).

Choose the ONE best answer.

20.1 The anticoagulant activity of warfarin can be potentiated by all of the following EXCEPT:

   A. Rifampin.
   B. Aspirin.
   C. Phenylbutazone.
   D. Cimetidine.
   E. Disulfiram.

Answer A if 1,2 and 3 are correct.
   B if 1 and 3 are correct.
   C if 2 and 4 are correct.
   D if only 4 is correct.
   E if 1,2,3 and 4 are all correct.

20.2 Which of the following statements is/are correct?

   1. Aspirin does not affect prostacyclin synthesis in endothelial cells.
   2. Aspirin has been shown to decrease the probability of a second myocardial infarct.
   3. The anticoagulatory effect of heparin requires 12-24 hours to develop.
   4. Heparin is a major antithrombotic drug for the treatment of deep vein thrombosis and pulmonary embolism.

20.3 Which of the following statements concerning warfarin is/are correct?

   1. Warfarin treatment results in the production of inactive clotting factors that lack γ-carboxy-glutamyl side chains necessary for calcium binding and subsequent activation.
   2. Warfarin must be given intravenously.
   3. The anticoagulant effects of warfarin can be overcome by the administration of vitamin K.
   4. Warfarin can be used to prevent the clotting of blood drawn for chemical analysis.

20.4 Which of the following statements concerning thrombolytic agents is/are correct?

   1. Hemorrhage is a major side effect.
   2. Streptokinase is a proteolytic enzyme specific for fibrin-bound plasminogen.
   3. Clot dissolution occurs with a higher frequency when therapy is initiated rapidly after clots begin to form.
   4. Streptokinase, urokinase, and tissue plasminogen activator (tPA) are equally specific for cleavage of plasminogen bound to fibrin.

20.5 Which of the following compounds promotes platelet aggregation?

   1. Thromboxane A_2.
   2. ADP.
   3. Collagen.
   4. Prostacyclin.

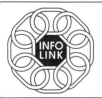

[1]See *heparin* in **Biochemistry** for structure and function of glycosaminoglycans (see index).

[2]See *vitamin K* in **Biochemistry** for structure and function of this vitamin).

[3]See *folic acid* in **Biochemistry** for role of folic acid in metabolism, nucleic acid synthesis and cell growth.

[4]See *cobalamin* in **Biochemistry** for the role of vitamin B_{12} in metabolism and cell growth.

Antihyperlipidemic Drugs

21

I. OVERVIEW

Coronary heart disease (CHD) is the cause of about half of all deaths in the United States. CHD has been shown to be correlated with the levels of plasma cholesterol- and/or triacylglycerol-containing lipoprotein particles. These particles, which are initially synthesized by the intestinal mucosa and the liver and undergo extensive metabolism in the plasma, play an essential role in the transport of lipids between tissues. [Note: Because lipids are insoluble in aqueous solutions, they must be transported in the plasma from tissue to tissue bound to proteins, hence the name, lipoprotein.] Their levels can be elevated by environmental causes, such as diet, or by inherited genetic defects in the appropriate synthesis or degradation of these compounds. Drugs used in the treatment of elevated serum lipids (hyperlipidemias) generally are targeted to (1) decrease production of a lipoprotein by the tissues, (2) increase catabolism of a lipoprotein in the plasma, or (3) increase removal of cholesterol from the body (Figure 21.1).

II. HYPERLIPIDEMIAS

The hyperlipidemias are a complex group of diseases that can be designated either primary or secondary depending on their causes.

A. Primary hyperlipidemias

Primary hyperlipidemias can be divided into two groups: (1) those resulting from a single inherited gene defect, or more commonly, (2) those caused by a combination of genetic and environmental factors. Figure 21.2 illustrates the normal metabolism of serum lipoproteins, and the characteristics of the major genetic hyperlipidemias.

B. Secondary hyperlipidemias

Secondary hyperlipidemias are the result of a more generalized metabolic problem, such as diabetes mellitus, excessive alcohol intake, hypothyroidism, or primary biliary cirrhosis. Therapeutic strategies for treating hyperlipidemia caused by one of these disorders include dietary intervention plus a regimen of drugs used to treat the primary cause of the hyperlipidemia.

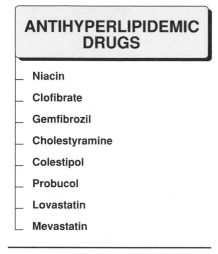

ANTIHYPERLIPIDEMIC DRUGS

- Niacin
- Clofibrate
- Gemfibrozil
- Cholestyramine
- Colestipol
- Probucol
- Lovastatin
- Mevastatin

Figure 21.1
Summary of antihyperlipidemic drugs.

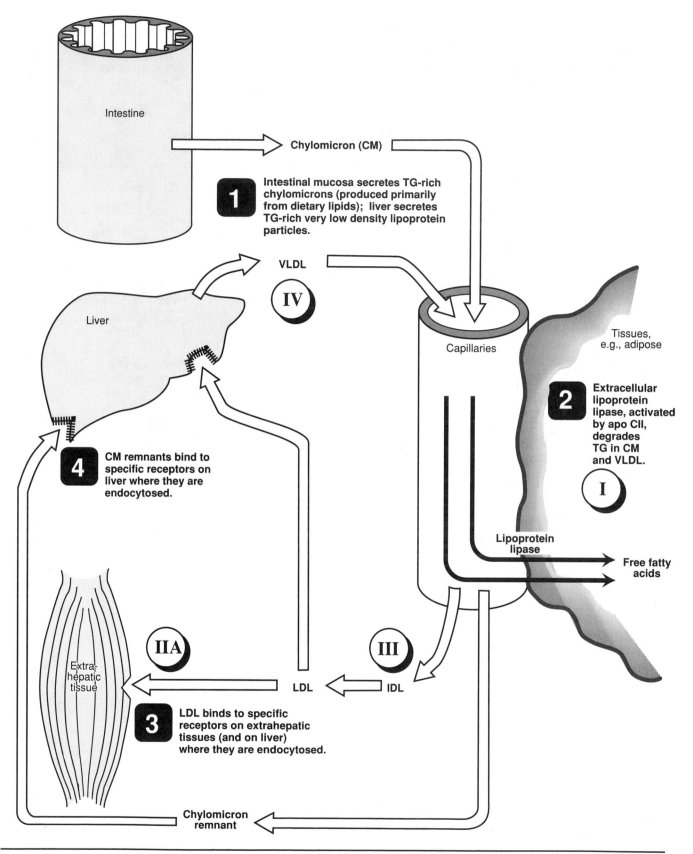

Figure 21.2

Metabolism of plasma lipoproteins and related genetic diseases. CM=chylomicron, TG=triacylglycerol, VLDL=very low density lipoprotein, LDL=low density lipoprotein, IDL=intermediate density lipoprotein, apo CII= apoprotein CII found in chylomicrons and VLDL. The Roman numerals in the white circles refer to specific genetic types of hyperlipidemias summarized on the facing page.

Type I [FAMILIAL HYPERCHYLOMICRONEMIA]

- Massive fasting hyperchylomicronemia even following normal dietary fat intake, resulting in greatly elevated serum triacylglycerol.
- Deficiency of lipoprotein lipase or deficiency of normal apoprotein CII (rare).
- Type I is not associated with an increase in coronary heart disease.
- Treatment: Low fat diet. No drug therapy is effective for Type I hyperlipidemia.

Type IIA [FAMILIAL HYPERBETALIPOPROTEINEMIA]

- Elevated LDL with normal VLDL levels due to block in LDL degradation, therefore increased serum cholesterol but normal triacylglycerol.
- Caused by decreased numbers of normal LDL receptors.
- Ischemic heart disease is greatly accelerated.
- Treatment: Low cholesterol and low saturated fat in the diet. Heterozygotes: Cholestyramine or colestipol, and/or lovastatin or mevastatin. Homozygotes: As above, plus niacin.

Type IIB [FAMILIAL COMBINED (MIXED) HYPERLIPIDEMIA]

- Similar to IIA except VLDL are also increased, resulting in elevated serum triacylglycerol as well as cholesterol.
- Relatively common.
- Treatment: Dietary restriction of cholesterol and saturated fat and alcohol. Drug therapy similar to IIA except heterozygotes also receive niacin.

Type III [FAMILIAL DYSBETALIPOPROTEINEMIA]

- Serum concentrations of IDL are increased resulting in increased triacylglycerol and cholesterol levels.
- Cause is either overproduction or underutilization of IDL, prehaps due to a mutant apoprotein.
- Xanthomas and accelerated coronary and peripheral vascular disease develop in patients by middle age.
- Treatment: Weight reduction (if necessary). Dietary restriction of cholesterol and alcohol. Drug therapy includes niacin and clofibrate (or gemfibrozil), or lovastatin (or mevastatin).

Type IV [FAMILIAL HYPERTRIGLYCERIDEMIA]

- VLDL levels are increased, while LDL levels are normal or decreased, resulting in normal to elevated cholesterol, and greatly elevated circulating triacylglycerol levels.
- Cause is either overproduction or decreased removal of VLDL in serum.
- This is a relatively common disease. It has few clinical manifestations other than accelerated ischemic heart disease.
- Treatment: Weight reduction (if necessary) is of primary importance. Dietary restriction of controlled carbohydrate, modified fat, low alcohol consumption. If necessary, drug therapy includes niacin and/or gemfibrozil (or clofibrate), or lovastatin (or mevastatin).

Type V [FAMILIAL MIXED HYPERTRIGLYCERIDEMIA]

- Serum VLDL and chylomicrons are elevated. LDL is normal or decreased. This results in elevated cholesterol and greatly elevated triacylglycerol levels.
- Cause is either increased production or decreased clearance of VLDL and chylomicrons.
- Treatment: Weight reduction (if necessary) is important. Diet should include protein, low fat and controlled carbohydrate, and no alcohol. If necessary, drug therapy includes niacin, clofibrate and/or gemfibrozil, or lovastatin (or mevastatin).

Figure 21.2 (continued).

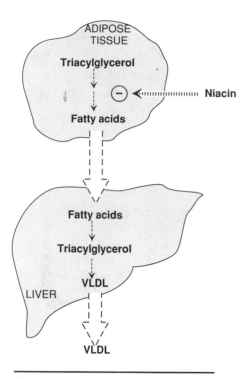

Figure 21.3
Niacin inhibits lipolysis in adipose tissue, resulting in decreased hepatic VLDL synthesis.

III. DRUGS THAT LOWER SERUM LIPOPROTEIN CONCENTRATION

A. Niacin

1. **Mechanism of action**: *Niacin* [NYE a sin] strongly inhibits lipolysis in adipose tissue—the primary producer of circulating free fatty acids. The liver normally utilizes these circulating fatty acids as a major precursor for triacylglycerol synthesis. Thus, *niacin* causes a decrease in liver triacylglycerol synthesis, which is required for very low density lipoprotein (VLDL) production (Figure 21.3). Low density lipoprotein (LDL, the cholesterol-rich lipoprotein) is derived from VLDL in the plasma. Therefore a reduction in the VLDL concentration also results in a decreased plasma LDL concentration. Thus, both plasma triacylglycerol (in VLDL) and cholesterol (in VLDL and LDL) are lowered (Figure 21.4).

2. **Therapeutic uses**: *Niacin* lowers plasma levels of both cholesterol and triacylglycerol. Therefore, it is particularly useful in the treatment of Type IIb hyperlipoproteinemia, where both VLDL and LDL are elevated. *Niacin* is also used to treat other severe hypercholesterolemias, often in combination with other antihyperlipidemic agents (p. 204).

3. **Pharmacology**: *Niacin* (*nicotinic acid*) is administered orally. It is converted in the body to nicotinamide, which is incorporated into the cofactor nicotinamide adenine dinucleotide (NAD$^+$). *Niacin* and its nicotinamide derivative are excreted in the urine.[1] [Note: Nicotinamide does *not* decrease plasma lipid levels.]

4. **Adverse effects**: The most common side effects of *niacin* therapy are an intense cutaneous flush (accompanied by an uncomfortable feeling of warmth) and pruritus. Administration of *aspirin* prior to taking *niacin* decreases the flush, which is prostaglandin-mediated. Some patients also experience nausea and abdominal pain.

B. Clofibrate

1. **Mechanism of action**: *Clofibrate* [kloe FYE brate] causes a decrease in plasma triacylglycerol levels by increasing the activity of lipoprotein lipase, thereby increasing the removal of VLDL from the plasma (Figure 21.5). *Clofibrate* can also cause a lowering of plasma cholesterol by inhibiting cholesterol synthesis in the liver (the mechanism is not yet known) and by causing an increase in cholesterol excretion via the bile to the feces.

2. **Therapeutic uses**: *Clofibrate* is used in the treatment of hypertriglyceridemias, causing a significant decrease in plasma triacylglycerol levels. It is particularly useful in treating Type III hyperlipidemia, where intermediate density lipoproteins (IDL) particles accumulate. Patients with Type IV (elevated VLDL) or Type V (elevated VLDL plus chylomicron) disease may also benefit from *clofibrate* treatment.

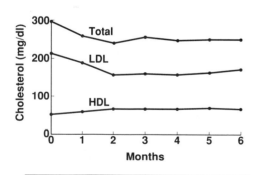

Figure 21.4
Plasma levels of cholesterol in hyperlipidemic patients during treatment with niacin.

3. **Pharmacology**: *Clofibrate* is completely absorbed after an oral dose. It is totally converted to the active *clofibric acid,* which distributes widely in body tissues bound to albumin. *Clofibric acid* and its glucuronide conjugate are excreted in the urine.

4. **Adverse effects**:

   a. The most common adverse effects of *clofibrate* therapy are nausea and gastrointestinal disturbances. These lessen as the therapy progresses.

   b. Because *clofibrate* causes an increase in cholesterol excretion via the bile, drug treatment may result in the formation of gallstones.

   c. *Clofibrate* competes with the coumarin anticoagulants for binding sites on plasma proteins, thus potentiating anticoagulant activity. Prothrombin levels should therefore be monitored when a patient is taking both these drugs. Similarly, the drug may elevate the levels of sulfonyl ureas.

C. Gemfibrozil

1. **Mechanism of action**: *Gemfibrozil* [gem FI broe zil] decreases the rate of incorporation of long-chain fatty acids into triacylglycerol. This results in a decreased production of VLDL in the liver. Like *clofibrate, gemfibrozil* also increases lipoprotein lipase activity (see Figure 21.5). Therefore, *gemfibrozil* causes a lowering in plasma triacylglycerol concentrations both by decreasing VLDL synthesis in the liver and by increasing VLDL removal from the plasma. *Gemfibrozil* also has the effect of increasing liver production of HDL.

2. **Therapeutic uses**: Like *clofibrate, gemfibrozil* is particularly useful in treating patients with hypertriglyceridemias resulting from elevated serum VLDLs or IDLs, namely those with Types III, IV, and V hyperlipidemias.

3. **Pharmacology**: *Gemfibrozil* is almost totally absorbed after oral administration. Most of the dose is excreted unchanged in the urine.

4. **Adverse effects**: Gastrointestinal disturbance and rash are the most common adverse effects of *gemfibrozil* treatment. Like *clofibrate, gemfibrozil* also potentiates the activity of coumarin anticoagulants.

D. Cholestyramine and colestipol (bile acid binding resins)

1. **Mechanism of action**: *Cholestyramine* [koe less TEAR a meen] and *colestipol* [koe LES ti pole] are taken orally and are anion exchange resins that bind negatively charged bile acids in the small intestine (Figure 21.6). The resin/bile acid complex is excreted in the feces, thus preventing the bile acids from returning to the liver by the enterohepatic circulation.

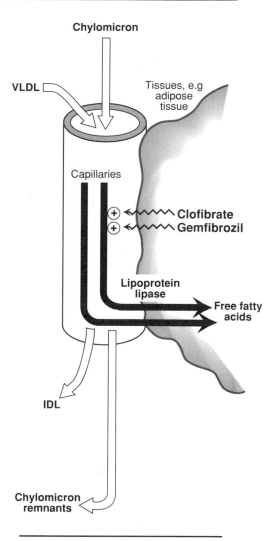

Figure 21.5
Activation of lipoprotein lipase by clofibrate and gemfibrozil.

A. Untreated hyperlipidemic patient

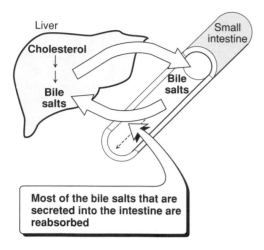

Most of the bile salts that are secreted into the intestine are reabsorbed

B. Hyperlipidemic patient treated with bile acid binding resins

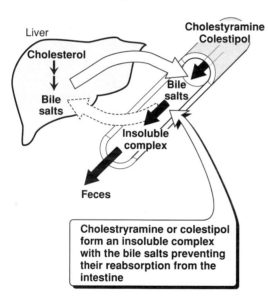

Cholestryramine or colestipol form an insoluble complex with the bile salts preventing their reabsorption from the intestine

Figure 21.6
Mechanism of bile acid binding resins.

a. Lowering the bile acid concentration in the hepatocytes causes an increased conversion of cholesterol to bile acids resulting in a replenished supply of these compounds, which are essential components of the bile.

b. This causes a decrease in the intracellular cholesterol concentration, which activates an increased uptake of LDL particles. [Note: This increased uptake is mediated by an increase in the number of cell-surface LDL receptors.] In some patients, an increase in plasma HDL levels is observed.

c. The final outcome of this sequence of events is a decreased plasma cholesterol concentration (Figure 21.6).

2. **Therapeutic uses** : The bile acid binding resins are the drugs of choice (often in combination with *niacin,* p. 202) in treating Type IIa and IIb hyperlipidemias. [Note: In those rare individuals who are homozygous for Type IIa, i.e., where functional LDL receptors are totally lacking, these drugs have little effect on plasma LDL levels.]

3. **Pharmacology**: *Cholestyramine* and *colestipol* are taken orally. Because they are insoluble in water and are very large (having molecular weights of greater than 10^6), they are neither absorbed nor metabolically altered by the intestine. They are totally excreted in the feces.

4. **Adverse effects**:

   a. The most common side effects are gastrointestinal disturbances, such as constipation and nausea.

   b. Absorption of fat-soluble vitamins, such as A, D, E, and K, can be impaired if high doses of the resin are present.

   c. *Cholestyramine* and *colestipol* interfere with the intestinal absorption of many drugs, for example, *tetracycline, phenobarbital, digitoxin,* and *warfarin.* Therefore, other drugs should be taken at least 1-2 hours before, or 6 hours after, the bile acid binding resins.

E. Probucol

1. **Mechanism of action**: *Probucol* [PROE byoo kole] lowers serum cholesterol by causing an increased uptake of LDL particles from the plasma. This uptake does not use the primary LDL receptors but rather activates a normally low-affinity uptake mechanism. Unfortunately, HDL^2 levels are also lowered by *probucol.* [Note: *Probucol* does not affect plasma triacylglycerol levels.]

2. **Therapeutic uses**: *Probucol* is useful in treating Type IIA hypercholesterolemia, although less so than the bile acid binding resins. Because a low HDL level is at least as great a risk for atherosclerosis as an elevated LDL level, the usefulness of this drug is limited to instances where other antihyperlipidemic agents are ineffective.

3. **Pharmacology**: *Probucol* is so lipid-soluble as to be poorly absorbed after an oral dose (the normal method of administration; see p.5 for discussion of drug solubility and extent of absorption). It accumulates in fatty tissues and is excreted via the bile into the feces.

4. **Adverse effects**: Mild gastrointestinal disturbance is the only common adverse effect. This generally disappears with continued treatment.

F. Lovastatin and Mevastatin

1. **Mechanism of action**:

   a. *Lovastatin* [loe vah STAT in] (formerly called *mevinolin*) and *mevastatin* [me vah STAT in] (formerly called *compactin*) contain chemical groups that are structural analogs of 3-hydroxy-3-methylglutarate (HMG), a precursor of cholesterol. These drugs are inhibitors of HMG-CoA reductase, the rate-limiting step in cholesterol synthesis[3]. By inhibiting de novo cholesterol synthesis, they deplete the intracellular supply of cholesterol (Figure 21.7).

   b. Depletion of intracellular cholesterol causes the cell to increase the number of specific cell-surface LDL receptors that can bind and internalize circulating LDLs—a significant source of cholesterol. Thus, the plasma cholesterol level is decreased both by lowered cholesterol synthesis and by increased catabolism of LDL.

   c. *Lovastatin* and *mevastatin,* like *cholestyramine,* cause an increase in plasma HDL levels in some patients, resulting in an additional lowering of risk for coronary heart disease.

2. **Therapeutic uses**: *Lovastatin* and *mevastatin* are effective in lowering plasma cholesterol levels in patients who are heterozygous for familial hypercholesterolemia. However, patients who are homozygous for this disease lack LDL receptors entirely and therefore benefit much less from treatment with these drugs. Patients with Type III, IV, or V hyperlipidemias can also receive benefit from treatment with *lovastatin* or *mevastatin*. [Note: These drugs are often given in combination with treatment by other antihyperlipidemic drugs, see later.]

3. **Pharmacology**: Because of their strong lipophilic nature, only about 30% of an oral dose of these drugs is absorbed by the body. *Lovastatin* and *mevastatin* are almost entirely removed from the portal circulation by the liver, and little appears in the systemic circulation. They are removed from the body via the bile to the feces.

4. **Adverse effects**: *Lovastatin* and *mevastatin* have shown few short-term adverse effects. Long-term studies using these drugs have not yet been completed, but a rise in serum liver enzymes in some individuals requires immediate withdrawal from the drug. These drugs are contraindicated in pregnancy and should not be used in children or teen-agers.

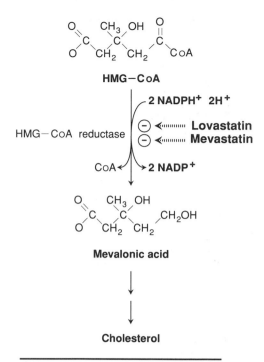

Figure 21.7
Inhibition of HMG-CoA reductase by lovastatin and mevastatin.

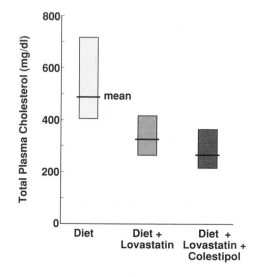

Figure 21.8
Response of total plasma cholesterol in patients with heterozygous familial hypercholesterolemia to diet (low cholesterol, low saturated fat) and hyperlipidemic drugs.

G. Combination Drug Therapy

It is sometimes necessary to employ two antihyperlipidemia drugs in order to achieve a significant decrease in plasma lipid levels. For example, in Type II hyperlipidemias, patients are commonly treated with a combination of *niacin* plus a bile acid binding agent, such as *cholestyramine.* [Note: Remember that *cholestyramine* causes an increase in LDL receptors that clears the plasma of circulating LDL, whereas *niacin* decreases synthesis of VLDL and therefore also the synthesis of LDL.] The combination of an HMG-CoA reductase inhibitor with a bile acid binding agent has also been shown to be useful in lowering LDL cholesterol (Figure 21.8).

Study Questions   (see p.421 for answers).

Choose the ONE best answer.

21.1 Which one of the following is the most common side effect of antihyperlipidemic drug therapy?

   A. Elevated blood pressure.
   B. Gastrointestinal disturbance.
   C. Neurological problems.
   D. Heart palpitations.
   E. Migraine headaches.

21.2 Which ONE of the following hyperlipidemias is characterized by elevated plasma levels of chylomicrons and has no drug therapy available to lower the plasma lipoprotein levels?

   A. Type I.
   B. Type II.
   C. Type III.
   D. Type IV.
   E. Type V.

21.3 Which ONE of the following drugs decreases *de novo* cholesterol synthesis by inhibiting the enzyme 3-hydroxy-3-methylglutaryl CoA reductase?

   A. Clofibrate.
   B. Niacin.
   C. Cholestyramine.
   D. Lovastatin.
   E. Pyridoxine.

QUESTIONS 21.4–21.7

DIRECTIONS: The group of questions below consists of five drugs (A-E) followed by a list of numbered statements. For each numbered statement, select the ONE drug from the list (A-E) that is most closely associated with it. Each drug may be selected once, more than once, or not at all.

Match each drug with the statement that best describes its mode of action:

   A. Niacin.
   B. Clofibrate.
   C. Cholestyramine.
   D. Probucol.
   E. Mevastatin.

21.4 Binds bile acids in the intestine, thus preventing their return to the liver via the enterohepatic circulation.

21.5 Causes a decrease in plasma triacylglycerol levels by increasing the activity of lipoprotein lipase.

21.6 Causes a decrease in liver triacylglycerol synthesis by limiting available free fatty acids needed as building blocks for this pathway.

21.7 Inhibits 3-hydroxy-3-methylglutaryl CoA reductase, the rate-limiting step in cholesterol synthesis.

[1]See *niacin* in **Biochemistry** for structure and function of the vitamin (see index).

[3]See *cholesterol, synthesis* in **Biochemistry** for the reactions and regulation of cholesterol biosynthesis.

[2]See *HDL* in **Biochemistry** for a discussion of the beneficial effect of elevated serum levels of HDL lipoproteins.

Drugs Affecting the Respiratory System

22

I. OVERVIEW

Drugs affecting the respiratory system either act directly on the bronchial airways or affect CNS mechanisms controlling respiration. Those drugs acting on the respiratory tree most often relax bronchial smooth muscle or modify bronchial mucous secretion. Drugs used to treat asthma, rhinitis, and cough are summarized in Figure 22.1.

II. DRUGS USED TO TREAT ASTHMA

Airflow obstruction in asthma is due to the inflammation of the bronchial wall, contraction of the bronchiolar smooth muscle, and increased mucous secretion, causing shortness of breath, coughing, and wheezing respiration. An asthmatic attack may be precipitated by inhalation of allergens (such as dust, pollen, or animal dander), which interact with mast cells coated with IgE, generated in response to a previous exposure to the allergen (Figure 22.2). The mast cells release mediators, such as histamine, leukotrienes, and chemotactic factors, which promote bronchiolar spasm and mucosal thickening from edema and cellular infiltration. However, many asthmatic attacks are not related to recent exposure to an allergen, but rather reflect bronchial hyperactivity of unknown origin that is somehow related to inflammation of the airway mucosa. The symptoms of asthma may be effectively treated by several drugs, but none of the agents provide a cure for this obstructive lung disease.

A. Adrenergic agonists

The adrenergic agonists with β activity are the drugs of choice for mild, intermittent asthma. These potent bronchodilators relax airway smooth muscle and inhibit the release of substances from mast cells that cause bronchoconstriction. The agents most commonly used are *epinephrine, ephedrine,* and *isoproterenol*. β_2-Selective agents, such as *metaproterenol, terbutaline,* and *albuterol* offer the advantage of providing maximally attainable bronchodilation without the undesired effect of α or β_1 stimulation (see p.59 for the receptor-specific actions of adrenergic agonists). Toxic side effects are minimized when the drugs are delivered by inhalation rather than by systemic routes.

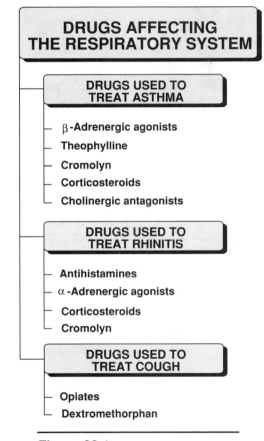

DRUGS AFFECTING THE RESPIRATORY SYSTEM

DRUGS USED TO TREAT ASTHMA

- β-Adrenergic agonists
- Theophylline
- Cromolyn
- Corticosteroids
- Cholinergic antagonists

DRUGS USED TO TREAT RHINITIS

- Antihistamines
- α-Adrenergic agonists
- Corticosteroids
- Cromolyn

DRUGS USED TO TREAT COUGH

- Opiates
- Dextromethorphan

Figure 22.1
Summary of drugs affecting the respiratory system.

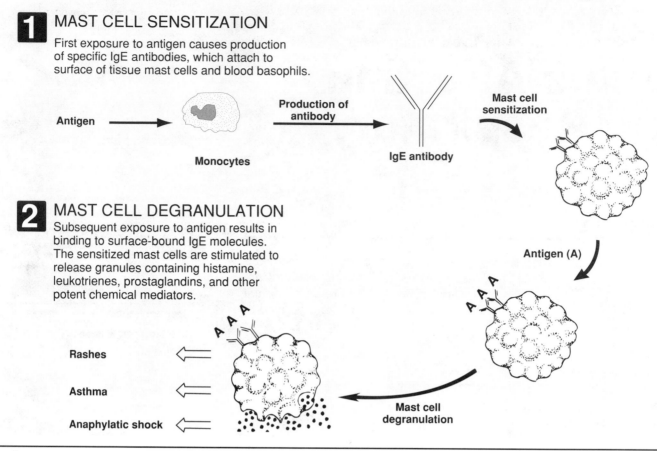

1 MAST CELL SENSITIZATION

First exposure to antigen causes production of specific IgE antibodies, which attach to surface of tissue mast cells and blood basophils.

Antigen → Monocytes

Production of antibody → IgE antibody

Mast cell sensitization

2 MAST CELL DEGRANULATION

Subsequent exposure to antigen results in binding to surface-bound IgE molecules. The sensitized mast cells are stimulated to release granules containing histamine, leukotrienes, prostaglandins, and other potent chemical mediators.

Antigen (A)

Rashes

Asthma

Anaphylatic shock

Mast cell degranulation

Figure 22.2
Hypersensitivity reactions mediated by IgE molecules.

B. Theophylline

When the asthmatic symptoms cannot be controlled with adrenergic agents, addition of the methylxanthine derivative, *theophylline* (p.102), may be appropriate. *Theophylline* is a bronchodilator that relieves airflow obstruction in acute asthma and decreases the symptoms of the chronic disease. The drug is well absorbed by the gastrointestinal tract, and several sustained-release preparations are available. Overdoses of the drug may cause seizures or arrhythmias. Figure 22.3 shows drugs that interact with *theophylline.*

C. Cromolyn

Cromolyn [KROE moe lin] is an effective prophylactic agent that stabilizes the membrane of mast cells and prevents mediator release, probably by blocking calcium gates. The drug is not useful in managing an acute asthmatic attack. For use in asthma, *cromolyn* is administered by inhalation of a microfine powder, or as an aerosolized solution. Because it is poorly absorbed, only minor adverse effects are associated with it. Pretreatment with *cromolyn* blocks allergen-induced and exercise-induced bronchoconstriction. *Cromolyn* is also useful in reducing the symptoms of allergic rhinitis. Not all patients respond to *cromolyn* therapy, but those who do respond to treatment show improvement that is roughly equal to the improvement obtained from maintenance *theophylline* therapy.

D. Corticosteroids

Corticosteroid aerosols, such as *beclomethasone* (p.256), *flunisolide*, and *triamcinolone* [trye am SIN oh lone] are useful in the treatment of chronic asthma. Anti-inflammatory steroids reduce inflammation by reversing mucosal edema, decreasing the permeability of capillaries, and inhibiting the release of leukotrienes. Bronchial reactivity is greatly reduced. Patients with severe exacerbation of asthma (status asthmaticus) may require intravenous administration of *methylprednisolone* (p.255). Once the patient has improved, the dose of drug is gradually reduced, leading to discontinuance in 1 to 4 weeks. Steroids are not indicated for the treatment of acute asthma.

E. Cholinergic antagonists

Anticholinergic agents are less effective than β-adrenergic agonists. However, inhaled *ipratropium,* a quaternary derivative of *atropine* (p.45), is useful in patients unable to take adrenergic agonists.

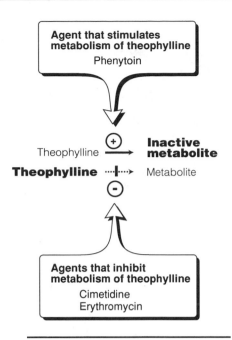

Figure 22.3
Drugs affecting the metabolism of theophylline.

III. DRUGS USED TO TREAT RHINITIS

Rhinitis is an inflammation of the mucous membranes of the nose. It is most commonly caused by viruses or by hypersensitivity responses to airborne allergens.

A. Antihistamines

H_1-Histamine receptor blockers, such as *diphenhydramine, chlorpheniramine, cyproheptadine,* and *promethazine* (p.390), are useful in treating the symptoms of allergic rhinitis caused by histamine release.

B. α-Adrenergic agonists

α-Adrenergic agonists ("nasal decongestants") constrict dilated arterioles in the nasal mucosa and reduce airway resistance. When administered as an aerosol, these drugs have a rapid onset of action and show few systemic effects. These agents should be used no longer than several days; rebound nasal congestion often occurs upon discontinuance of these drugs. Oral administration results in longer duration of action but increased systemic effects. Rebound nasal congestion is a common adverse effect after long term use of α-adrenergic agents.

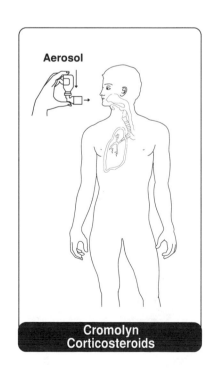

C. Corticosteroids

Corticosteroids, such as *beclomethasone* and *flunisolide,* are effective when administered as nasal sprays to reduce systemic side effects. Treatment of chronic rhinitis does not show improvement until 1-2 weeks after starting therapy.

D. Cromolyn

Intranasal *cromolyn* may be useful, particularly when administered before contact with an allergen.

IV. DRUGS USED TO TREAT COUGH

A. Antitussive agents

1. **Opiates:** *Codeine, hydrocodone,* and *hydromorphone* decrease the sensitivity of CNS cough center to peripheral stimuli and decrease mucosal secretion. These actions occur at doses lower than required for analgesia (see p.140 for a more complete discussion of the opiates).

2. **Dextromethorphan:** This synthetic derivative of *morphine* suppresses the response of the cough center, but it has no analgesic or addictive potential. *Dextromethorphan* [dex troe meth OR fan] is less constipating than *codeine.*

Study Questions   (see p.422 for answers).

Choose the ONE best answer.

22.1 All of the following statements regarding the treatment of asthma are true EXCEPT:

A. β_2-Specific adrenergic agonists are most effective in treating asthma.
B. Corticosteroid aerosols are useful in the treatment of chronic asthma.
C. Ipratropium is useful in patients unable to take adrenergic agonists.
D. Cromolyn is used in treating an acute asthmatic attack.
E. Cromolyn prevents the release of inflammatory mediators from mast cell.

22.2 All of the following statements are true EXCEPT:

A. Propranolol is contraindicated in asthma.
B. Metaproterenol produces less tachycardia than isoproterenol when both drugs are given at doses producing equal bronchodilation.
C. H_1 histamine receptor blockers, such as diphenhydramine, are useful in treating the symptoms of allergic rhinitis.
D. Dextromethorphan, being a derivative of morphine, has strong analgesic properties.
E. Rebound nasal congestion is a common adverse effect of prolonged use of α-adrenergic agonists.

Diuretic Drugs

23

I. OVERVIEW

Drugs inducing a state of increased urine flow are called diuretics. These agents are ion transport inhibitors that decrease the reabsorption of Na^+ at different sites in the nephron. As a result, Na^+ and other ions such as Cl^- enter the urine in greater amounts than normal, along with water, which is carried passively to maintain osmotic equilibrium. Diuretics thus increase the volume of the urine and often change the pH as well as the ionic composition of the urine and blood. The efficacy of the different classes of diuretics vary considerably, with the increase in secretion of Na^+ varying from less then 2% for the weak, potassium-sparing diuretics, to over 20% for the potent loop diuretics. Their major clinical uses are in managing disorders involving abnormal fluid retention (edema) or in treating hypertension where their diuretic action causes a decreased blood volume, which leads to a reduction in blood pressure. In this chapter, the diuretic drugs (Figure 23.1) are discussed in the order of their site of action along the nephron (Figure 23.2).

II. REGULATION OF FLUID AND ELECTROLYTES BY THE KIDNEYS

A. Normal kidney function

Approximately 16 - 20% of the blood plasma entering the kidneys is filtered from the glomerular capillaries into Bowman's capsule. The filtrate, although normally free of proteins and blood cells, does contain most low molecular weight plasma components in approximately the same concentrations as are found in the plasma. These include glucose, sodium bicarbonate, amino acids, and other organic solutes, plus electrolytes, such as Na^+, K^+, and Cl^-. The kidney regulates the ionic composition and volume of urine by the reabsorption or secretion of ions and/or water at five functional zones along the nephron, namely the proximal convoluted tubule, the descending loop of Henle, the ascending loop of Henle, the distal convoluted tubule, and the collecting duct (Figure 23.2).

1. **Proximal convoluted tubule**: In the extensively convoluted proximal tubule located in the cortex of the kidney, almost all of the glucose, bicarbonate, amino acids, and other metabolites are

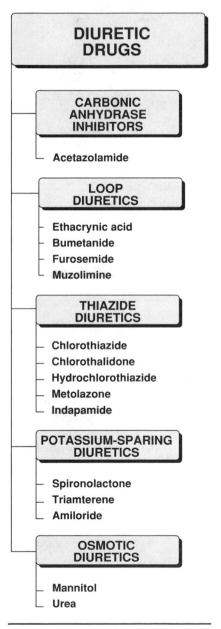

DIURETIC DRUGS

CARBONIC ANHYDRASE INHIBITORS
- Acetazolamide

LOOP DIURETICS
- Ethacrynic acid
- Bumetanide
- Furosemide
- Muzolimine

THIAZIDE DIURETICS
- Chlorothiazide
- Chlorothalidone
- Hydrochlorothiazide
- Metolazone
- Indapamide

POTASSIUM-SPARING DIURETICS
- Spironolactone
- Triamterene
- Amiloride

OSMOTIC DIURETICS
- Mannitol
- Urea

Figure 23.1
Summary of diuretic drugs.

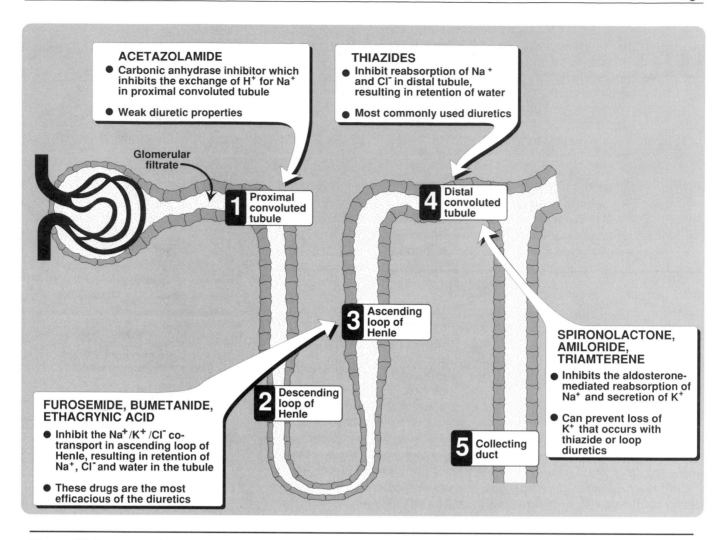

Figure 23.2
Major locations of ion and water exchange in the nephron, showing sites of action of the diuretic drugs.

reabsorbed. Approximately two thirds of the Na^+ is also reabsorbed in the proximal tubule; chloride and water follow passively to maintain electrical and osmolar equality. If it were not for the extensive reabsorption of solutes and water in the proximal tubule, the mammalian organism would rapidly become dehydrated and lose its normal osmolarity.

a. **Acid secretory system:** The proximal tubule is the site of organic acid and base secretory systems (Figure 23.3). The organic acid secretory system secretes a variety of organic acids (such as uric acid, some antibiotics, diuretics) from the bloodstream into the proximal tubule's lumen. Most diuretic drugs are delivered to the tubular fluid via this system. The organic acid secretory system is saturable, and diuretic drugs in the blood stream compete for transfer with endogenous organic acids, such as uric acid. This explains the hyperuricemia seen with certain of the diuretic drugs, such as *furosemide* or *chlorothiazide.*

2. **Descending loop of Henle:** The remaining filtrate, which is isotonic, next enters the descending limb of the loop of Henle and passes into the medulla of the kidney. The osmolarity increases along the descending portion of the loop of Henle because of the countercurrent mechanism. This results in a tubular fluid with a three-fold increase in salt concentration.

3. **Ascending loop of Henle:** The cells of the ascending tubular epithelium are unique in the body in being impermeable to water. In addition, these cells actively reabsorb Cl⁻ while Na⁺ follows passively to maintain electrical neutrality. The ascending loop is thus a diluting section of the nephron. This continuous reabsorption of Cl⁻ and Na⁺ from the ascending limb insures that about 25% of tubular fluid sodium chloride returns to the interstitial fluid, helping to maintain the high osmolarity of the interstitial fluid. Since the loop of Henle is a major site for reabsorption of salt, drugs affecting this site, such as loop diuretics, appear to be the most efficacious of all the classes of diuretics.

4. **Distal convoluted tubule:** Sodium is actively reabsorbed by the cells of the distal convoluted tubule, and Cl⁻ and water follow passively. At the terminal end of the distal tubule is the Na^+–K^+ exchange site, which fine tunes the K^+ content of the urine (see Figure 23.3). The reabsorption of Na^+ and the secretion of K^+ are stimulated by aldosterone, which is released from the adrenal cortex in response to elevated levels of circulating angiotensin II (p.380).

5. **Collecting duct:** The collecting duct is the site of action of vasopressin (antidiuretic hormone [ADH], see Figure 23.3). ADH enhances the reabsorption of water from the epithelial cells of the collecting duct, an action mediated by increased levels of cAMP.

B. Kidney function in disease

In many diseases the amount of sodium chloride reabsorbed by the kidney tubules is abnormally high. This leads to the retention of water, an increase in blood volume, and expansion of the extravascular fluid compartment, resulting in edema of the tissues. Several commonly encountered causes of edema include:

1. **Congestive heart failure:** The decreased ability of the failing heart to sustain adequate cardiac output causes the kidney to respond as if there were a decrease in blood volume. The kidney, as part of the normal compensatory mechanism, retains more salt and water as a means of raising blood volume and increasing the amount of blood that is returned to the heart. However, the diseased heart cannot increase its output, and the increased vascular volume results in edema (see p.154 for causes and treatment of congestive heart failure).

2. **Hepatic ascites:** Ascites, the accumulation of fluid in the abdominal cavity, is a common complication of cirrhosis of the liver.

   a. Blood flow in the portal system is often obstructed in cirrhosis, resulting in an increased blood pressure. Further, colloidal

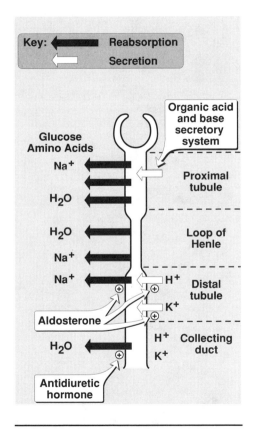

Figure 23.3
Sites of transport of solutes and water along the nephron.

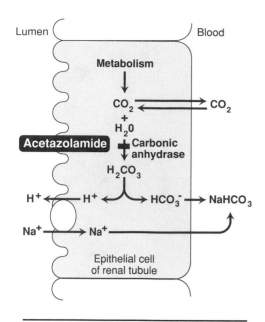

Figure 23.4
Role of carbonic anhydrase in sodium retention by epithelial cells of renal tubule.

osmotic pressure of the blood is decreased as a result of impaired synthesis of plasma proteins by the diseased liver. High blood pressure and low osmolarity of the blood cause fluid to escape from the portal vascular system and collect in the abdomen.

b. Fluid retention is also promoted by elevated levels of circulating aldosterone. This secondary hyperaldosteronism results from the decreased ability of the liver to inactivate the steroid hormone and leads to increased Na^+ and water reabsorption, increased vascular volume, and exacerbation of fluid accumulation.

3. **Nephrotic syndrome:** When damaged by disease, the glomerular membranes allow plasma proteins to enter the glomerular ultra-filtrate. The loss of protein from the plasma reduces the colloidal osmotic pressure resulting in edema. The low plasma volume stimulates aldosterone secretion through the renin-angiotensin-aldosterone system (p.380). This leads to retention of Na^+ and fluid, further aggravating the edema.

4. **Premenstrual edema:** Edema associated with menstruation is the result of imbalances in hormones such as estrogen excess, which facilitates the loss of fluid into the extracellular space. Diuretics can reduce the edema, but they are without effect on the emotional tension of the premenstrual syndrome.

III. CARBONIC ANHYDRASE INHIBITORS

Acetazolamide [a set a ZOLE a mide] is a sulfonamide without antibacterial activity. Its main action is to inhibit the enzyme carbonic anhydrase in the proximal tubular epithelial cells. However, carbonic anhydrase inhibitors are more often used for their other pharmacological actions rather than for their diuretic effect, because these agents are much less efficacious than the thiazides or loop diuretics.

A. Acetazolamide

1. **Mechanism of action:** Acetazolamide inhibits carbonic anhydrase, a normal component of plasma. [Note: Carbonic anhydrase catalyzes the reaction of CO_2 and H_2O leading to H^+ and HCO_3^- (bicarbonate).] Hydrogen ions (H^+) are normally excreted in exchange for Na^+, which is then retained in the proximal and distal convoluted tubules (Figure 23.4). The carbonic anhydrase inhibitors have only a weak effect on Na^+ retention, since the loop of Henle, which is downstream from the proximal tubule (the drug's major site of action), is able to reabsorb a large fraction of the excess NaCl in the fluid leaving from the proximal tubule. [Note: changes in the composition of urinary electrolytes induced by *acetazolamide* are summarized in Figure 23.5.]

2. **Therapeutic uses:**

a. **Treatment of glaucoma:** The most common use of *acetazolamide* is to reduce the elevated intraocular pressure of glau-

Decreased urinary secretion ⟵ ⟶ **Increased urinary secretion**

| Na^+ |
| K^+ |
| Ca^{++} |
| Volume of urine |

Figure 23.5
Relative changes in the composition of urine induced by acetazolamide.

coma. *Acetazolamide* decreases the production of aqueous humor, probably by blocking carbonic anhydrase in the ciliary body of the eye. It is useful in the chronic treatment of glaucoma but should not be used for an acute attack; *pilocarpine* (p.40) is preferred for acute attack because of its immediate action. Often, *acetazolamide* is used to enhance the actions of *pilocarpine* or the β-adrenergic blockers (p.76) in the treatment of severe, chronic glaucoma.

b. **Epilepsy:** *Acetazolamide* is sometimes used in the treatment of epilepsy—both grand mal and petit mal. It reduces the severity and magnitude of the seizures. Often *acetazolamide* is used chronically in conjunction with antiepileptic medication to enhance the action of these other drugs.

c. **Mountain sickness:** Less commonly *acetazolamide* can be used in the prophylaxis of acute mountain sickness among healthy, physically active individuals who rapidly ascend above 10,000 feet. *Acetazolamide* given nightly for 5 days before the ascent prevents the weakness, breathlessness, dizziness, nausea, and cerebral and pulmonary edema characteristic of the syndrome.

3. **Pharmacology**: As a diuretic, *acetazolamide* is given orally once a day. For glaucoma, it is given topically two to four times daily.

4. **Adverse effects:** Metabolic acidosis (mild), potassium depletion, drowsiness, and paresthesia may occur.

IV. LOOP OR HIGH-CEILING DIURETICS

Furosemide [fur OH se mide], *bumetanide* [byoo MET a nide] and *ethacrynic acid* [eth a KRIN ik] are three diuretics that have their major action on the ascending limb of the loop of Henle (Figure 23.2). Compared to all other classes of diuretics, these drugs have the highest efficacy in mobilizing Na$^+$ and Cl$^-$ from the body. *Ethacrynic acid* has a steeper dose-response curve (p.19) than *furosemide*; it shows greater side effects than those seen with the other loop diuretics and is not as widely used. *Bumetanide* is much more potent than *furosemide*, and its use is increasing.

A. Bumetanide, furosemide, ethacrynic acid

1. **Mechanism of action:** Loop diuretics inhibit the Na$^+$/K$^+$/Cl$^-$ co-transport of the luminal membrane in the ascending limb of the loop of Henle. Therefore reabsorption of Na$^+$, K$^+$, and Cl$^-$ is decreased (Figure 23.5). The loop diuretics are the most efficacious of the diuretic drugs, because the ascending limb accounts for the reabsorption of 30-40% of filtered NaCl and downstream sites are not able to compensate for this increased Na$^+$ excretion.

2. **Actions:** The loop diuretics act promptly, even among patients who have poor renal function or who have not responded to thiazides or other diuretics. Changes in the composition of the

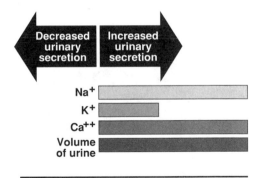

Figure 23.6
Relative changes in the composition of urine induced by loop diuretics.

urine induced by loop diuretics are shown in Figure 23.6. [Note: Loop diuretics increase the Ca^{++} content of urine, while thiazide diuretics (p.217) decrease the Ca^{++} concentration of the urine.] The loop diuretics cause decreased renal vascular resistance and increased renal blood flow.

3. **Therapeutic uses:**

   a. **Edematous state:** The loop diuretics are the drugs of choice for reducing the acute pulmonary edema of congestive heart failure. Because of their rapid onset of action, the drugs are useful in emergency situations, such as acute pulmonary edema, which calls for a rapid, intense diuresis.

   b. **Hypercalcemia:** Loop diuretics stimulate tubular Ca^{++} secretion and are therefore useful in treating hypercalcemia.

   c. **Elevated intracranial pressure:** A decrease in elevated intracranial pressure can be effected by these agents.

4. **Pharmacology:** Loop diuretics are administered orally or parenterally; their duration of action is relatively brief, 1-4 hours.

5. **Adverse effects:**

   a. **Ototoxicity:** Hearing can be affected adversely by the loop diuretics, particularly when used in conjunction with the aminoglycoside antibiotics (p.288). Permanent damage may result with continued treatment. Vestibular function is less likely to be disturbed, but it too may be affected by combined treatment.

   b. **Hyperuricemia:** *Furosemide* and *ethacrynic acid* compete with uric acid for the renal and biliary secretory systems, thus blocking its secretion and thereby causing or exacerbating gouty attacks.

   c. **Acute hypovolemia:** Loop diuretics can cause a severe and rapid reduction in blood volume, with the possibility of hypotension, shock, and cardiac arrhythmias.

   d. **Potassium depletion:** The heavy load of Na^+ presented to the distal tubule results in increased exchange of tubular Na^+ for K^+, with the possibility of inducing hypokalemia. The loss of K^+ from cells in exchange for H^+ leads to hypokalemic alkalosis. Potassium depletion can be averted by use of potassium-sparing diuretics or dietary supplementation with K^+. The adverse effects of the loop diuretic are summarized in Figure 23.7.

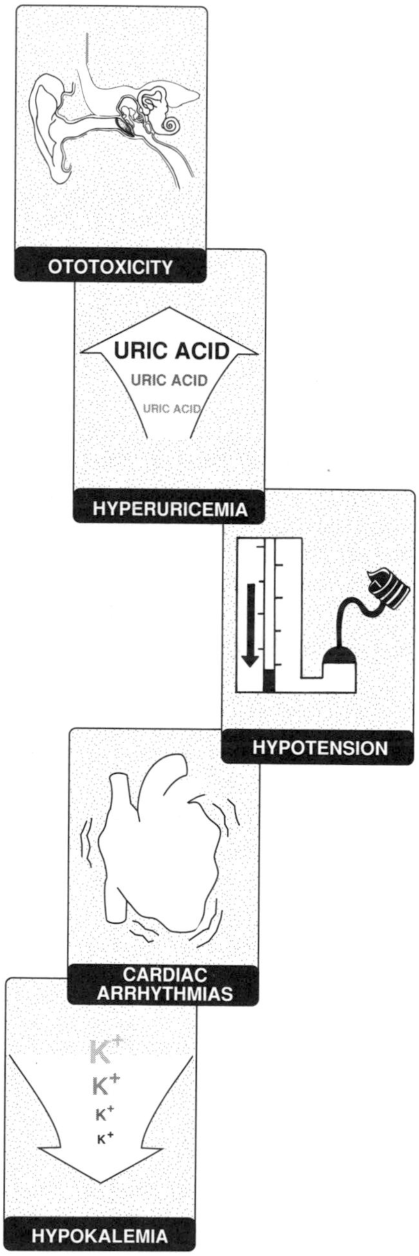

B. Muzolimine

Muzolimine is a new loop diuretic that has a high pK (9.2) and is very lipophilic. It undergoes hepatic metabolism, and the bile is the major route of excretion. Its half-life is prolonged over that of the older loop diuretics, lasting 10-20 hours. *Muzolimine* is effective in treating advanced renal failure.

Figure 23.7
Summary of adverse effects commonly observed with loop diuretics.

V. THIAZIDES AND RELATED AGENTS

The thiazides are the most widely used of the diuretic drugs. They are sulfonamide derivatives and are related in structure to the carbonic anhydrase inhibitors. The thiazides have significantly greater diuretic activity than *acetazolamide,* and they act on the kidney by different mechanisms. All thiazides affect the distal tubule, and all have equal maximum diuretic effect, differing only in potency, expressed on a per-milligram basis.

A. Chlorothiazide

Chlorothiazide [klor oh THYE a zide], the prototype drug, was the first modern diuretic that was active orally and was capable of affecting the severe edema of cirrhosis and congestive heart failure with a minimum of side effects. Its properties are representative of the thiazide group, although newer derivatives such as *hydrochlorothiazide* or *chlorthalidone* are now used more commonly.

1. **Mechanism of action:** The thiazide derivatives act mainly in the distal tubule to decrease the reabsorption of Na^+ by inhibition of a Na^+/Cl^- cotransporter on the luminal membrane. They have a lesser effect in the proximal tubule (Figure 23.2). As a result, these drugs increase the concentration of Na^+ and Cl^- in the tubular fluid. The acid-base balance is not usually affected.

2. **Actions:**

   a. **Increased excretion of Na+ and Cl-:** *Chlorothiazide* causes diuresis with increased Na^+ and Cl^- excretion, which can result in the excretion of a very hyperosmolar urine. This latter effect is unique among the other diuretic classes, which are unlikely to produce a hyperosmolar urine. The diuretic action is not affected by the acid-base status of the body, nor does *chlorothiazide* use by an individual change the acid-base status of the blood. The ionic composition of the urine during therapy is given in Figure 23.8.

   b. **Loss of K+:** Because thiazides increase the Na^+ in the filtrate arriving at the distal tubule, more K^+ is also exchanged for Na^+. Thus, prolonged use of these drugs results in continual loss of K^+ from the body. Therefore, it is imperative to measure serum K^+ once per month to assure that hypokalemia does not develop. Often, K^+ can be supplemented by diet alone, such as increasing the intake of citrus fruits, bananas, and prunes. In some cases, K^+ salt supplementation may be necessary.

   c. **Decreased urinary calcium excretion:** Thiazide diuretics decrease the Ca^{++} content of urine, that is they promote the reabsorption of Ca^{++}. This contrasts with the loop diuretics (p.215), which increase the Ca^{++} concentration of the urine.

   d. **Reduced peripheral vascular resistance:** An initial reduction in blood pressure results from a decrease in blood volume and therefore a decrease in cardiac output (p.179). With continued therapy, volume recovery occurs, but continued hypotensive effects result from reduced peripheral vascular resistance caused by relaxation of arteriolar smooth muscle.

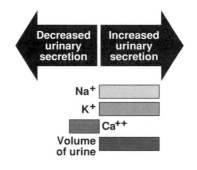

Figure 23.8
Relative changes in the composition of urine induced by thiazide diuretics.

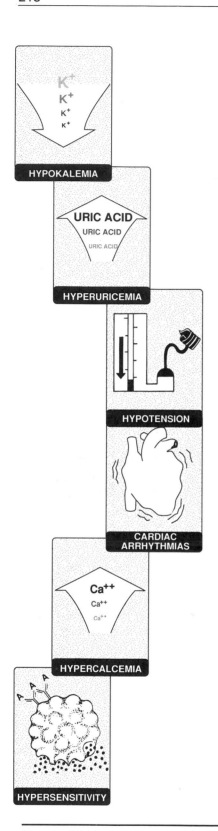

Figure 23.9
Summary of adverse effects commonly observed with thiazide diuretics.

3. **Therapeutic uses:**

  a. **Hypertension:** Clinically, the thiazides have long been the mainstay of antihypertensive medication, since they are inexpensive, convenient to administer, and well tolerated. They are effective in reducing systolic and diastolic blood pressure for extended periods in the majority of patients with mild to moderate essential hypertension (see p.175 for details on treatment of hypertension). After 3-7 days of treatment, the blood pressure stabilizes at a lower level and can be maintained indefinitely by a daily dosage level of the drug, which causes lower peripheral resistance without having a major diuretic effect. Many patients can be continued for years on the thiazides alone, although a small percentage of patients require additional medication, such as β-adrenergic blockers (p.179).

  b. **Congestive heart failure:** Thiazides can be the diuretic of choice in reducing extracellular volume in mild to moderate congestive heart failure (p.151). If the thiazide fails, loop diuretics may be useful.

  c. **Nephrosis:** Patients with nephrotic syndrome accompanied by edema are initially treated with loop diuretics, and only if this treatment fails, are they given thiazides.

  d. **Hypercalciuria:** The thiazides can be useful in treating idiopathic hypercalciuria because they inhibit urinary Ca^{++} excretion. This is particularly beneficial to patients with calcium oxalate stones in the urinary tract.

  e. **Diabetes insipidus:** Thiazides have the unique ability to produce a hyperosmolar urine. Thiazides can substitute for the antidiuretic hormone in the treatment of diabetes insipidus. The urine volume of such individuals may drop from 11 L/day to about 3 L/day when treated with the drug.

4. **Pharmacology:** The drugs are effective orally. Most thiazides take 1-3 weeks to produce a stable reduction in blood pressure, and they exhibit a prolonged biological half-life (40 hours). All thiazides are secreted by the organic acid secretory system of the kidney (p.212).

5. **Adverse effects:**

  a. **Potassium depletion:** Hypokalemia is the most frequent problem encountered with the thiazide diuretics and can predispose patients on *digitalis* to ventricular arrhythmias (Figure 23.9). Activation of the renin-angiotensin-aldosterone system by the decrease in intravascular volume contributes significantly to urinary K^+ losses. The K^+ deficiency can be overcome by *spironolactone*, which interferes with aldosterone action, or by administering *triamterene*, which acts to retain K^+ (p.220). Low sodium diets blunt the potassium depletion caused by thiazide diuretics.

b. **Hyperuricemia:** Thiazides increase serum uric acid by decreasing the amount of acid excreted by the organic acid secretory system. Being insoluble, the uric acid deposits in the joints, and a full-blown attack of gout may result. It is important, therefore, to perform periodic blood tests for uric acid levels.

c. **Volume depletion:** This can cause orthostatic dizziness or light-headedness.

d. **Hypercalcemia:** The thiazides inhibit the secretion of Ca^{++}, sometimes leading to elevated levels of Ca^{++} in the blood.

e. **Hyperglycemia:** Patients with diabetes mellitus, who are taking thiazides for hypertension, may become hyperglycemic and have difficulty in maintaining appropriate blood sugar levels.

f. **Hypersensitivity:** Bone marrow suppression, dermatitis, necrotizing vasculitis, and interstitial nephritis are very rare.

B. Hydrochlorothiazide

Hydrochlorothiazide is a thiazide derivative that has proven to be more popular than the parent drug. This is because it has far less ability to inhibit carbonic anhydrase as compared to *chlorothiazide.* It is also more potent, so that the required dose is considerably less than that of *chlorothiazide.* On the other hand, the efficacy is exactly the same as that of the parent drug.

C. Chlorthalidone

Chlorthalidone [klor THAL i done] is a thiazide derivative that behaves like *hydrochlorothiazide.* It has a very long duration of action and therefore is often used to treat hypertension. It is given once per day for this therapy.

D. Thiazide analogs

1. *Metolazone* [me TOLE a zone] is more potent than the thiazides and, unlike the thiazides, causes Na^+ excretion in advanced renal failure.

2. *Indapamide* [in DAP a mide] is a lipid soluble, nonthiazide diuretic that has a long duration of action. At low doses, it shows significant antihypertensive action with minimal diuretic effects. *Indapamide* is metabolized and excreted by the gastrointestinal tract and the kidneys; it therefore is less likely to accumulate in patients with renal failure and may be useful in their treatment.

VI. POTASSIUM-SPARING DIURETICS

These agents act in the distal tubule to inhibit Na^+ reabsorption, K^+ secretion, and H^+ secretion. Potassium-sparing diuretics are used primarily when aldosterone is present in excess. The major use of potassium-sparing agents is in the treatment of hypertension, most often in combination with a thiazide.

A. Spironolactone

1. **Mechanism of action:** *Spironolactone* [speer on oh LAK tone] is a synthetic aldosterone antagonist that competes with aldosterone for intracellular cytoplasmic receptor sites. The *spironolactone*-receptor complex is inactive, that is, it prevents translocation of the receptor complex into the nucleus of the target cell, and thus does not bind to DNA. This results in a failure to produce proteins that are normally synthesized in response to aldosterone. These mediator proteins normally stimulate the Na^+–K^+ exchange sites of the distal tubule. Thus, a lack of mediator proteins prevents Na^+ reabsorption and therefore K^+ and H^+ secretion.

2. **Actions:** In most edematous states, blood levels of aldosterone are high, which is instrumental in retaining Na^+ (p.213). When *spironolactone* is given to a patient with elevated circulating levels of aldosterone, the drug antagonizes the activity of the hormone, resulting in retention of K^+ and excretion of Na^+ (Figure 23.10). Where there are no significant circulating levels of aldosterone, such as in Addison's Disease (primary adrenal insufficiency), no diuretic effect of the drug occurs.

3. **Therapeutic uses:**

   a. **Diuretic:** Although *spironolactone* has a low efficacy in mobilizing Na^+ from the body in comparison with the other drugs, the drug has the useful property of causing the retention of K^+ (Figure 23.10). Because of this latter action, *spironolactone* is often given in conjunction with a thiazide or loop diuretic to prevent K^+ excretion that would otherwise occur with these drugs.

   b. **Secondary hyperaldosteronism:** *Spironolactone* is the only potassium-sparing diuretic that is routinely used alone to induce net negative salt balance. It is particularly effective in clinical situations associated with secondary hyperaldosteronism.

4. **Pharmacology:** *Spironolactone* is completely absorbed orally and is strongly bound to proteins. It is rapidly converted to an active metabolite, *canrenone,* which is available commercially for intravenous injection. The action of *spironolactone* is largely due to the effect of *canrenone,* which has mineralocorticoid-blocking activity. *Spironolactone* induces hepatic cytochrome P-450.

5. **Adverse effects:**

   a. **Hormonal activity:** Because *spironolactone* chemically resembles some of the sex steroids, it does have minimal hormonal activity and may induce gynecomastia in males and menstrual irregularities in females. Because of this, the drug should not be given on a chronic basis. It is most effectively employed in mild edematous states where it is given for a few days at a time.

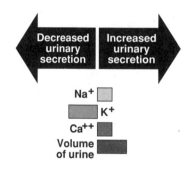

Figure 23.10
Relative changes in the composition of urine induced by potassium-sparing diuretics.

b. **Other:** Hyperkalemia, nausea, lethargy, and mental confusion can occur.

B. Amiloride and Triamterene

Amiloride [a MIL oh ride] and *triamterene* [trye AM ter een] block Na$^+$ transport channels resulting in a decrease in Na$^+$–K$^+$ exchange; they have K$^+$-sparing diuretic actions similar to that of *spironolactone*. However, the ability of these drugs to block the K$^+$–Na$^+$ exchange site in the distal tubule does not depend on the presence of aldosterone. Thus, they have diuretic activity even in individuals with Addison's Disease. They, like *spironolactone,* are not very efficacious diuretics. Both *triamterene* and *amiloride* are frequently used in combination with other diuretics, usually for their potassium-sparing properties. For example, much like *spironolactone,* they prevent K$^+$ loss that occurs with thiazides and *furosemide.* The side effects of *triamterene* are leg cramps and the possibility of increased blood urea nitrogen (BUN) as well as uric acid and K$^+$ retention. Figure 23.10 shows the changes in the composition of the urine following administration of potassium-sparing diuretic drugs.

VII. OSMOTIC DIURETICS

A number of simple, hydrophilic, chemical substances that are filtered through the glomerulus, such as *mannitol* [MAN i tole] and *urea* [yu REE ah], result in some degree of diuresis. This is due to their ability to carry water with them into the tubular fluid. If the substance that is filtered subsequently undergoes little or no reabsorption, then the filtered substance will cause an increase in urinary output. Only a small amount of additional salt may also be excreted. Because osmotic diuretics are used to effect increased water excretion rather than Na$^+$ excretion, they are not useful in treating conditions in which Na$^+$ retention occurs. They are used to maintain urine flow following acute toxic ingestion of substances capable of producing acute renal failure.

Figure 23.11 summarizes the relative changes in urinary composition induced by diuretic drugs.

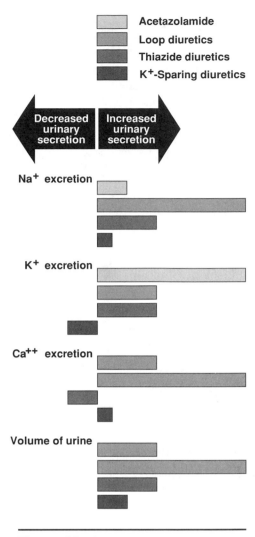

Figure 23.11
Summary of relative changes in urinary composition induced by diuretic drugs.

Study Questions   (see p.423 for answers).

Answer A if 1,2 and 3 are correct.
    B if 1 and 3 are correct.
    C if 2 and 4 are correct.
    D if only 4 is correct.
    E if 1,2,3 and 4 are all correct.

23.1 Which of the following diuretics can produce hypokalemia by continued use?

    1. Spironolactone.
    2. Acetazolamide.
    3. Amiloride.
    4. Hydrochlorothiazide.

23.2 Which of the following diuretics markedly increase(s) the excretion of calcium from the body?

    1. Acetazolamide.
    2. Chlorothiazide.
    3. Furosemide.
    4. Spironolactone.

23.3 Hydrochlorothiazide can produce which of the following actions?

1. Hyperkalemia.
2. Hyperuricemia.
3. Increase in blood pressure.
4. Hyperglycemia in diabetic patients.

23.4 In an addisonian patient, which of the following agents would have diuretic actions?

1. Amiloride.
2. Chlorothiazide.
3. Triamterene.
4. Spironolactone.

23.5 Hyperkalemia is observed with which of the following diuretics?

1. Chlorothiazide.
2. Furosemide.
3. Acetazolamide.
4. Spironolactone.

23.6 Which of the following correctly pairs the diuretic drug with one of its adverse effects?

1. Furosemide: Ototoxicity.
2. Chlorthalidone: Hyperuricemia.
3. Spironolactone: Gynecomastia (development of enlarged breasts) in males.
4. Acetazolamide: Metabolic acidosis.

23.7 Chlorothiazide increases the urinary excretion of

1. Sodium.
2. Calcium.
3. Potassium.
4. Uric acid.

23.8 Loop diuretics are useful in the treatment of which of the following conditions?

1. Congestive heart failure.
2. Acute pulmonary edema.
3. Ascites.
4. Hypocalcemia.

23.9 In which of the following patients would a loop diuretic be contraindicated, or used with caution?

1. Diabetics.
2. Gouty patients.
3. Patients with hypercalcemia.
4. Patients being treated with aminoglycoside antibiotics.

Gastrointestinal Drugs

24

I. OVERVIEW

A number of drugs described in other chapters are also useful in the treatment of gastrointestinal disorders. For example, the antimuscarinic agents *atropine* and *scopolamine* (p.45) diminish motility of the smooth muscle of the gut, whereas the morphine derivative *diphenoxylate* increases the tone of the gastrointestinal tract and decreases peristaltic activity. These drugs are thus useful in the treatment of severe diarrhea. Drugs that are used almost exclusively to treat gastrointestinal tract disorders include those employed to heal peptic ulcers and those used to treat constipation (Figure 24.1).

II. DRUGS USED TO TREAT PEPTIC ULCERS

Enhanced hydrochloric acid secretion is a primary factor in the pathologic nature and pain of peptic ulcer. Therefore the treatment of peptic ulcer can be accomplished in three ways: by decreasing the stimuli that cause acid secretion, by neutralizing the acid after it is released, or by providing agents that protect the gastric mucosa from damage.

A. Inhibitors of gastric acid production

Gastric acid secretion is controlled by activation of four types of receptors located in the cell membrane of the parietal cell (Figure 24.2). The receptor-mediated binding of acetylcholine, histamine, or gastrin results in the activation of an ATP-dependent proton pump that secretes hydrochloric acid (HCl) into the lumen of the stomach. In contrast, the binding of prostaglandin E_2 to its receptor diminishes gastric acid production. Histamine and prostaglandin E_2 have opposing actions on adenylate cyclase, whereas gastrin and acetylcholine induce an increase in intracellular calcium levels.

1. Histamine H2 receptor blockers

a. Histamine has a powerful effect on the secretory cells of the stomach, stimulating acid (and to a lesser extent pepsin) secretion. It does so by binding to H_2 receptor on the parietal cells of the stomach, thereby initiating a cyclic AMP-mediated cascade of activity (p.388).

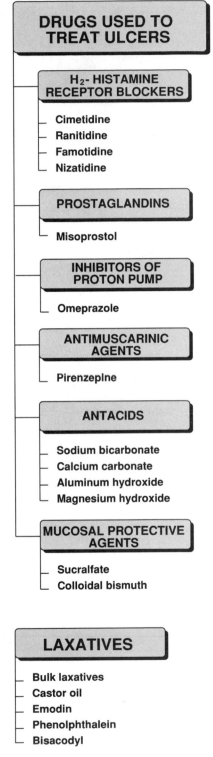

DRUGS USED TO TREAT ULCERS

H_2- HISTAMINE RECEPTOR BLOCKERS
- Cimetidine
- Ranitidine
- Famotidine
- Nizatidine

PROSTAGLANDINS
- Misoprostol

INHIBITORS OF PROTON PUMP
- Omeprazole

ANTIMUSCARINIC AGENTS
- Pirenzepine

ANTACIDS
- Sodium bicarbonate
- Calcium carbonate
- Aluminum hydroxide
- Magnesium hydroxide

MUCOSAL PROTECTIVE AGENTS
- Sucralfate
- Colloidal bismuth

LAXATIVES
- Bulk laxatives
- Castor oil
- Emodin
- Phenolphthalein
- Bisacodyl

Figure 24.1
Summary of gastrointestinal drugs.

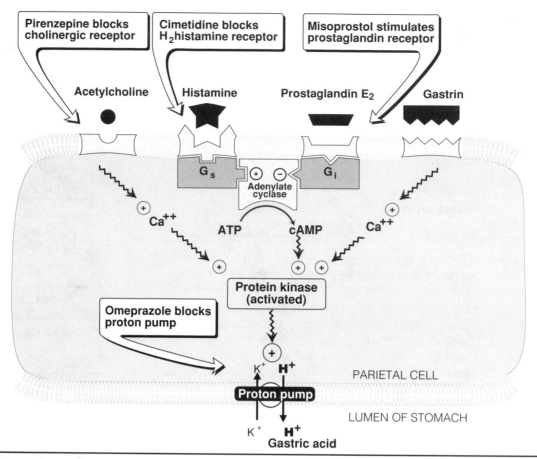

Figure 24.2
Effects of acetylcholine, histamine, prostaglandin E_2 and gastrin on gastric acid secretion by the parietal cell of stomach; G_s and G_i are membrane proteins that mediate the stimulatory or inhibitory effect of receptor binding to adenylate cyclase.

b. Drugs such as *cimetidine, ranitidine, famotidine,* and *nizatidine* competitively block the H_2 histamine receptor, thus decreasing acid secretion and promoting healing of the ulcer among 90% of patients within 3-4 weeks. These drugs are taken orally, distribute widely throughout the body (including in breast milk and across the placenta), and are excreted in the urine. Side effects are minimal.

c. The H_2 histamine receptor blockers are of great value in treating patients with Zollinger-Ellison syndrome where a gastrin-secreting tumor causes a continuous release of hydrochloric acid (see p.390 for a more complete discussion of histamine receptor blockers).

2. **Prostaglandins**

a. *Misoprostol* [miz o PROS ol], a methylester analog of prostaglandin E1, with antisecretory and cytoprotective properties has been approved for the prevention of anti-inflammatory agent-induced ulceration (see pp. 367, 380 for a discussion of gastrointestinal problems associated with nonsteroidal anti-inflammatory drugs [NSAIDs]). The drug represents the first synthetic, orally active prostaglandin evaluated for the treatment of peptic ulcer disease.

b. *Misoprostol* is superior to placebo and *cimetidine* in reducing mucosal damage resulting from the chronic administration of NSAIDs. Patients with peptic ulcer disease produce less gastroduodenal prostaglandins than patients without ulcers and thus may have a relative deficiency of mucosal prostaglandin synthesis.

c. *Misoprostol* causes ulcer healing and pain relief in both gastric and duodenal ulcer. These therapeutic effects are significantly superior to placebo therapy and comparable to those achieved with high or conventional doses of *cimetidine*. *Misoprostol* heals a significant proportion of duodenal ulcers that are refractory to treatment with H_2 histamine receptor antagonists.

3. Inhibitors of proton pump

a. *Omeprazole* [om PRAY zole] is the first H^+-K^+-adenosine triphosphatase antagonist available for clinical use. *Omeprazole* inhibits the gastric (H^+, K^+)-ATPase, a membrane-bound proton pump that is the final step in the secretion of gastric acid (see Figure 24.2). Pepsin and intrinsic factor secretion are unaffected. *Omeprazole* is effective in the management of gastric acid hypersecretion and symptom relief in patients with the Zollinger-Ellison syndrome and in the treatment of patients with ulcers resistant to histamine H_2-receptor antagonists. Most patients require only a once-daily dose.

b. *Omeprazole* has been found to be safe and is well tolerated. Side effects are few and do not differ from those observed during H_2-blocker treatment.

4. Antimuscarinic agents

a. Cholinergic antagonists such as *pirenzepine* (p.38) are used as adjuncts to the H_2 histamine receptors blockers, particularly in patients that do not respond to treatment with the histamine antagonists alone.

b. In contrast to the classic anticholinergics, *pirenzepine* shows a greater specificity against the secretory function of the stomach, with less effect against salivary glands and smooth muscle.

B. Antacids

Weak bases react with gastric acid to form water and a salt (Figure 24.3), thereby raising the pH of the stomach contents. Systemic antacids are highly soluble and are rapidly absorbed from the gut. This may cause systemic alkalosis. Nonsystemic antacids are less soluble and exert their antacid action locally in the gastrointestinal

A. Systemic antacids

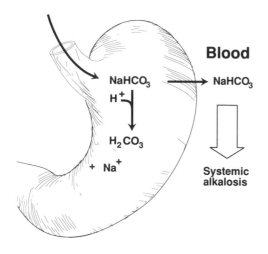

B. Nonsystemic antacids

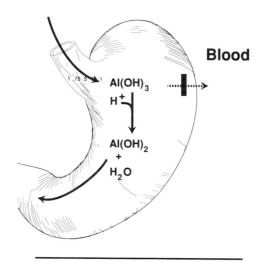

Figure 24.3

Comparison of systemic and nonsystemic antacids.

tract, producing no drastic changes in acid-base balance. The non-systemic antacids are preferred because of safety as well as their longer duration of action. In medical practice, the systemic type of antacid has been discontinued, although drugs of this type (such as *sodium bicarbonate* and *sodium citrate*) are still available in over-the-counter remedies. Use of antacids may alter the absorption of other drugs because of the change in gastric pH (p.4).

1. **Systemic antacids**: *Sodium bicarbonate* ($NaHCO_3$) is a very effective antacid. It can, however, increase gastric pH to an alkaline level, which is undesirable because it stimulates additional HCl secretion. Adverse side effects include its systemic absorption, which may cause transient metabolic alkalosis. In addition, the release of carbon dioxide in the stomach can cause belching, flatulence, and abdominal distension.

2. **Nonsystemic antacids**: Calcium, aluminum, and magnesium salts all have the ability to buffer the pH of the stomach contents to approximately 4. At that pH, little excess acid is secreted and pepsin activity is diminished.

   a. *Calcium carbonate* ($CaCO_3$) is widely available over the counter. It can reduce pain and aid healing of duodenal ulcer and esophagitis. Approximately 10% of the product of neutralization, calcium chloride, is absorbed causing potential hypercalcemia if the antacid is taken in large amounts.

   b. *Aluminum hydroxide* [$Al(OH)_3$] reacts with HCl to produce aluminum chloride, which is insoluble and may cause constipation. $Al(OH)_3$ binds to phosphate and a number of drugs (for example, *tetracycline*), preventing their absorption.

   c. *Magnesium hydroxide* [$Mg(OH)_2$, "milk of magnesia"] forms salts following reaction with acid. The magnesium salts are relatively insoluble, which slows their removal from the stomach. These salts act as good cathartics by attracting fluid into the gastrointestinal tract. [Note: Many antacid preparations combine both aluminum and magnesium hydroxides, the purpose being to prevent diarrhea caused by the magnesium salt or constipation caused by the aluminum salt.]

C. Mucosal protective agents

These compounds selectively protect the gastric mucosa either by forming a synthetic covering over the gastric surface or by stimulating the secretion of mucus.

1. *Sucralfate* [soo KRAL fate], aluminum sucrose sulfate, selectively binds to necrotic ulcer tissue. It acts as a barrier to HCl and pepsin and is particularly effective in healing duodenal ulcers. Because it requires an acidic pH for activation, *sucralfate* should not be administered with H_2 blockers or antacids. The drug is not absorbed systemically.

2. Colloidal bismuth preparations coat and bind to both gastric and duodenal ulcer tissue. They protect the ulcer from acid and pepsin.

III. LAXATIVES

Laxatives are commonly used to increase the movement of food down the gastrointestinal tract. These drugs can be classified on the basis of their mechanism of action, for example, as irritants or stimulants of the gut or as bulk agents.

A. Bulk laxatives

1. These agents include, for example, hydrophilic colloids and fibers from fruits and vegetables, agar, methyl cellulose, psyllium seeds, and bran. They distend the intestine, thus stimulating peristaltic movement.

2. Saline cathartics are salts of nonabsorbable ions, such as magnesium. They attract fluid into the gut by increasing the osmotic pressure. The resulting distension of the intestine increases peristaltic activity.

B. Irritants and stimulants

Castor oil is broken down in the small intestine to ricinoleic acid, which is very irritating to the gut and causes increased intestinal motility. Cascara, senna, and aloe contain *emodin,* which stimulates colonic activity. *Phenolphthalein* and *bisacodyl* are also stimulants of the colon.

Study Questions   (see p.424 for answers).

Choose the ONE best answer.

24.1 All of the following drugs are correctly matched to their actions EXCEPT

    A. Cimetidine: Blocks H_2 histamine receptors.
    B. Misoprostol: Inhibits adenylate cyclase.
    C. Omeprazole: Activates adenylate cyclase.
    D. Sucralfate: Protects ulcerated mucosa.
    E. Pirenzepine: Selectively blocks muscarinic receptors in stomach.

24.2 Which of the following is a bulk-forming laxative?

    A. Castor oil.
    B. Psyllium.
    C. Colloidal bismuth.
    D. Sucralfate.
    E. Phenolphthalein.

24.3 The use of an aluminum-containing antacid is most likely to cause?

    A. Constipation.
    B. Diarrhea.
    C. Hypertension.
    D. Headache.
    E. Nausea.

24.4 Which one of the following statements is correct?

    A. Histamine and prostaglandin E_2 have opposing actions on the secretion of gastric acid.
    B. Gastrin and acetylcholine induce a decrease in intracellular calcium levels.
    C. Omeprazole blocks muscarinic receptors of the parietal cell.
    D. Pirenzepine is similar to atropine in its actions.
    E. Famotidine blocks the action of gastrin on the parietal cell.

Hormones of the Pituitary and Thyroid

25

I. OVERVIEW

The nervous system and the endocrine system are the two mechanisms coordinating body functions and transmitting messages between individual cells and tissues. The nervous system communicates by electrical impulses directed through neurons to other neurons or to specific target cells, such as muscle or gland cells. Nerve impulses generally act within milliseconds. In contrast, the endocrine system releases hormones into the blood stream, which carries these chemical messengers to target cells throughout the body. Hormones have a much broader range of response times than do nerve impulses, requiring from seconds to days or longer to cause a response that may last for weeks or months. The two regulatory systems are closely interrelated. In several instances, the release of hormones is stimulated or inhibited by the nervous system, whereas some hormones can stimulate or inhibit nerve impulses. Chapters 25-27 in this text focus on drugs that affect the synthesis and/or secretion of specific hormones. In this chapter, the central role of the hypothalamic and pituitary hormones in regulating body functions is briefly presented. In addition, drugs affecting thyroid hormone synthesis and/or secretion are discussed (Figure 25.1).

II. HYPOTHALAMIC AND PITUITARY HORMONES

The hormones secreted by the hypothalamus and the anterior pituitary are all peptides or proteins that act by binding to specific hormone receptor sites on their target tissues (Figure 25.2). These hormones are administered either intramuscularly (IM) or subcutaneously (SC) but not orally, since they are destroyed by the proteolytic enzymes of the digestive tract. Each hypothalamic regulatory hormone controls the release of a specific hormone from the anterior pituitary. The hypothalamic hormones shown in Figure 25.2 are primarily used for diagnostic purposes (i.e., to determine pituitary insufficiency). The hypothalamus also synthesizes the hormones vasopressin and oxytocin, which are transported to the posterior pituitary where they are stored or released. Although a number of pituitary hormone preparations are currently used therapeutically for cases of specific hormonal deficiencies (examples of which are described below), most of these agents have limited therapeutic applications.

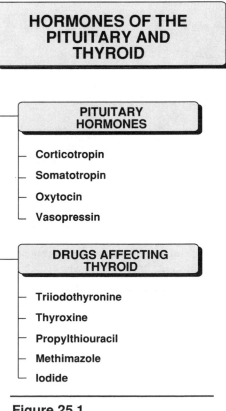

HORMONES OF THE PITUITARY AND THYROID

PITUITARY HORMONES

- Corticotropin
- Somatotropin
- Oxytocin
- Vasopressin

DRUGS AFFECTING THYROID

- Triiodothyronine
- Thyroxine
- Propylthiouracil
- Methimazole
- Iodide

Figure 25.1
Some of the hormones of the pituitary and thyroid.

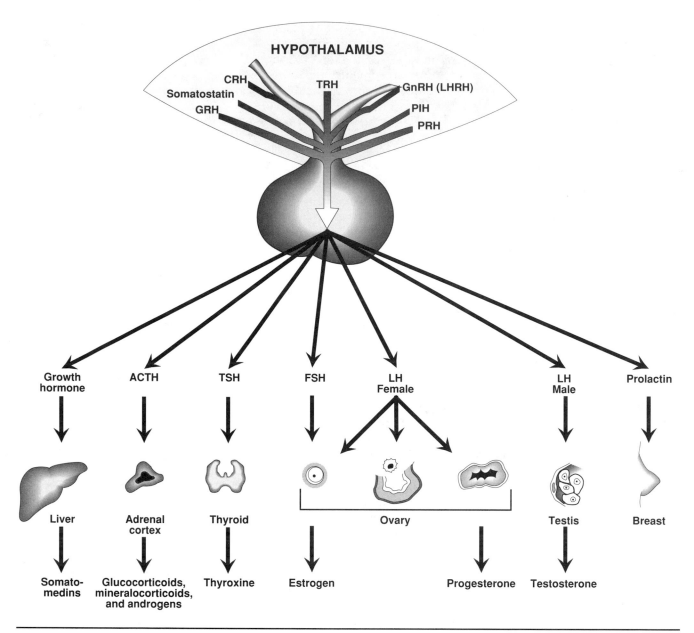

Figure 25.2
Hypothalamic-releasing hormones and actions of anterior pituitary hormones. GRH= growth hormone-releasing hormone; TRH= thyrotropin-releasing hormone; CRH= corticotropin-releasing hormone; GnRH (LHRH)= gonadotropin-releasing hormone (luteinizing hormone-releasing hormone); PIH= prolactin-inhibiting hormone (dopamine); and PRH= prolactin-releasing hormone; ACTH= adrenocorticotropic hormone; TSH= thyrotropin-stimulating hormone; FSH= follicle-stimulating hormone; LH= luteinizing hormone.

A. Adrenocorticotropic hormone (ACTH or corticotropin)

Corticotropin [kor ti koe TROE pin] is a peptide that is extracted from the anterior pituitary of domestic animals. Corticotropin binds to specific receptors on the adrenal cortex. The activated receptor, acting via cAMP, stimulates the rate-limiting step in the adrenocorticosteroid synthetic pathway, causing the synthesis and release of cortisol, the adrenal androgens, and mineralocorticoids[1]. The

availability of synthetic adrenocorticosteroids with specific properties has limited the use of corticotropin to serving principally as a
diagnostic tool for differentiating primary adrenal insufficiency
(Addison's disease, associated with adrenal atrophy) from secondary adrenal insufficiency (caused by inadequate secretion of ACTH
by the pituitary). *Cosyntropin,* a synthetic agent similar to corticotropin, is now used routinely for this diagnostic purpose.

B. Growth hormone (somatropin)

Somatropin [soe ma TROE pin] is a large polypeptide, now produced
synthetically by recombinant DNA technology. Somatotropin influences a wide variety of biochemical processes. The drug is used
in the treatment of growth-hormone deficiency in children. [Note: A
therapeutically equivalent drug, *samatrem,* contains an extra terminal methionyl group not found in somatropin.]

C. Oxytocin

Oxytocin [ox i TOE sin] is a nonapeptide extracted from animal
posterior pituitaries. It stimulates uterine contraction and is sometimes used to induce or reinforce labor.

D. Vasopressin

Vasopressin [vay soe PRESS in] (antidiuretic hormone, ADH), like
oxytocin, is a nonapeptide extracted from animal posterior pituitaries. Vasopressin increases water permeability in the collecting tubules of the kidney, leading to an antidiuretic effect. The major use
of vasopressin is to treat pituitary diabetes insipidus.

III. THYROID HORMONES

The thyroid gland facilitates normal growth and maturation by maintaining the level of metabolism in the tissues that is optimal for their
normal function. The two major thyroid hormones are T_3 (triiodothyronine, the most active form), and T_4 (thyroxine). Although the thyroid
gland is not essential for life, inadequate secretion of thyroid hormone
(hypothyroidism) results in bradycardia, poor resistance to cold, and
mental and physical slowing (in children this can cause mental retar-
dation and dwarfism). If, however, an excess of thyroid hormones is
secreted (hyperthyroidism), tachycardia and cardiac arrhythmias,
body wasting, nervousness, tremor, and excess heat production can
occur. In mammals, the thyroid gland also secretes the hormone
calcitonin, a serum calcium-lowering hormone.

A. Regulation of thyroid hormone synthesis and secretion

1. **Synthesis:** The thyroid gland is made up of multiple follicles that
   consist of a single layer of epithelial cells surrounding a lumen
   filled with colloid (thyroglobulin), the storage form of thyroid
   hormone. A diagram of the steps in thyroid hormone synthesis is
   shown in Figure 25.3.

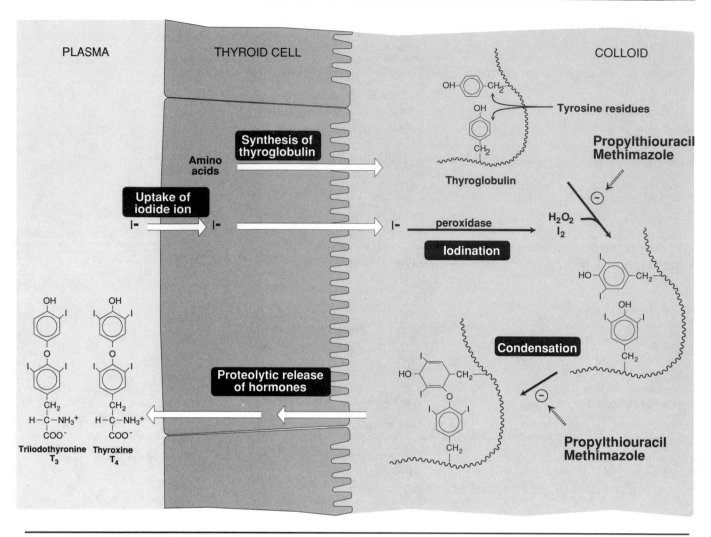

Figure 25.3
Biosynthesis of thyroid hormones.

2. **Secretion:** Thyroid function is controlled by the tropic hormone thyrotropin-stimulating hormone (TSH, thyrotropin), a glycoprotein synthesized by the anterior pituitary (Figure 25.2). Secretion of TSH by the anterior pituitary is stimulated by the hypothalamic thyrotropin-releasing hormone (TRH) and is inhibited by feedback of high circulating thyroid hormone levels.

B. Treatment of hyperthyroidism (thyrotoxicosis)

Excessive amounts of thyroid hormones in the circulation can be caused by a number of disease states, including Graves' disease, toxic adenoma, goiter, and thyroiditis, among others. The goal of therapy is to decrease synthesis and/or release of additional hormone. This can be accomplished by removing part or all of the thyroid gland, by inhibiting synthesis of the hormones, or by blocking release of the hormones from the follicle.

1. Removal of part or all of the thyroid

This can be accomplished either surgically or by destruction of the gland by radioactive iodine (^{131}I), which is selectively taken up by the thyroid follicular cells.

2. Inhibition of thyroid hormone synthesis

The thioamides, *propylthiouracil* [proe pill thye oh YOOR a sil] and *methimazole* [meth IM a zole], inhibit both the iodination of tyrosyl groups and the coupling of iodotyrosines to form T_3 and T_4 (see Figure 25.3). They have no effect on the thyroglobulin already stored in the gland; therefore observation of any clinical effect of these drugs may be delayed until thyroglobulin stores are depleted. The thioamides are well absorbed from the gastrointestinal tract, but they have short half-lives; thus, several doses are required per day. Relatively rare adverse effects include agranulocytosis, rash, and edema.

3. Blockage of hormone release

A pharmacological dose of *iodide* inhibits the iodination of tyrosines, thus decreasing the supply of stored thyroglobulin. *Iodide* also inhibits thyroid hormone release by mechanisms not yet understood. Today, *iodide* is rarely used as sole therapy. However, it is employed to treat potentially fatal thyrotoxic crisis (thyroid storm), or it is used prior to surgery, since it decreases the vascularity of the thyroid gland. *Iodide* is not useful for long-term therapy, since the thyroid ceases to respond to the drug after a few weeks. *Iodide* is administered orally. Adverse effects are relatively minor and include sore mouth and throat, rashes, ulcerations of mucous membranes, and a metallic taste in the mouth.

Study Questions   (see p.425 for answers).

Choose the ONE best answer.

25.1 Symptoms of hyperthyroidism include all of the following EXCEPT

A. tachycardia.
B. nervousness.
C. poor resistance to cold.
D. body wasting.
E. tremor.

25.2 Which of the following best describes the effect of propylthiouracil on thyroid hormone production?

A. It blocks the release of thyrotropin-releasing hormone.
B. It inhibits uptake of iodide by thyroid cells.
C. It prevents the release of thyroid hormone from thyroglobulin.
D. It blocks iodination and coupling of tyrosines in thyroglobulin to form thyroid hormones.
E. It blocks the release of hormones from the thyroid gland.

Answer A if 1,2 and 3 are correct.
      B if 1 and 3 are correct.
      C if 2 and 4 are correct.
      D if only 4 is correct.
      E if 1,2,3, and 4 are all correct.

25.3 Drugs used in the treatment of hyperthyroidism
     include:

    1. Propylthiouracil.
    2. Iodide.
    3. Methimazole.
    4. Triiodothyronine.

Chapter 25

[1]See *steroid hormones, synthesis* in **Biochemistry** for a
discussion of the actions of ACTH (see index).

Insulin and Oral Hypoglycemic Drugs

26

I. OVERVIEW

The pancreas is both an endocrine gland that produces the peptide hormones *insulin* and glucagon and an exocrine gland that produces digestive enzymes. *Insulin* and glucagon play an important role in regulating the metabolic activities of the body, and in doing so, help maintain the homeostasis of blood glucose levels. Hyperinsulinemia (due, for example, to a pancreatic tumor) can cause severe hypoglycemia. More commonly, a relative or absolute lack of *insulin* (such as in diabetes mellitus) can cause serious hyperglycemia. The latter state can be treated by administration of *insulin* preparations or with other hypoglycemic agents (Figure 26.1).

II. METABOLIC ROLES OF INSULIN AND GLUCAGON

High serum glucose stimulates an increase in *insulin* release from β cells of the pancreas. Increased serum *insulin* serves to lower blood glucose levels by driving the carbohydrate into cells unable to take up glucose in the absence of *insulin.* Low serum glucose causes a decrease in *insulin* release and stimulates an increase in the secretion of glucagon from the α cells of the pancreas. Elevated serum glucagon causes a mobilization of energy storage forms (for example glycogen, triacylglycerol, protein) whose building blocks (sugars, fats, amino acids) can be used to fuel gluconeogenesis in the liver, producing glucose.[1]

III. DIABETES MELLITUS

Diabetes is not a single disease; instead, it is a heterogeneous group of syndromes all characterized by an elevation of blood glucose caused by a relative or absolute deficiency of *insulin.* Frequently the inadequate release of *insulin* is aggravated by an excess of glucagon. Diabetics can be conveniently divided into two groups, based on their requirements for *insulin.*[2]

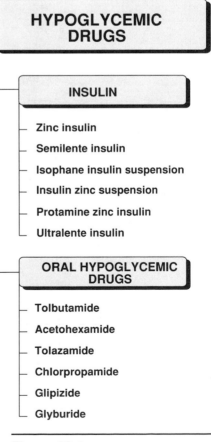

HYPOGLYCEMIC DRUGS

INSULIN

- Zinc insulin
- Semilente insulin
- Isophane insulin suspension
- Insulin zinc suspension
- Protamine zinc insulin
- Ultralente insulin

ORAL HYPOGLYCEMIC DRUGS

- Tolbutamide
- Acetohexamide
- Tolazamide
- Chlorpropamide
- Glipizide
- Glyburide

Figure 26.1
Summary of hypoglycemic agents.

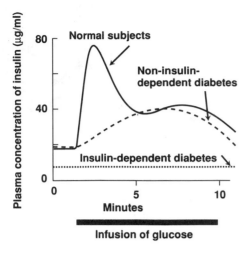

Figure 26.2
Release of insulin that occurs
in response to constant infusion
of glucose in normal subjects and
in diabetic patients.

A. Type I diabetes (insulin-dependent diabetes mellitus, IDDM)

1. **Cause of the disease:** Insulin-dependent diabetes is characterized by an absolute deficiency of *insulin* caused by massive β-cell lesions or necrosis. Loss of β-cell function may be due to invasion by viruses, the action of chemical toxins, or most commonly through the actions of autoimmune antibodies directed against the β cell. As a result of the destruction of β cells, the pancreas fails to respond to ingestion of glucose, and the Type I diabetic shows symptoms of *insulin* deficiency. Insulin-dependent diabetics require exogenous *insulin* to avoid ketoacidosis.

2. **Occurrence of the disease:** Insulin-dependent diabetics constitute 10-20% of the 6 million diabetics in the United States. The disease occurs most commonly among juveniles, but it can occur among adults.

3. **Treatment of Type I diabetes:** Normally, after ingestion of a meal, a burst of *insulin* secretion occurs in response to transient increases in the levels of circulating glucose and amino acids. In the postabsorptive period, β-cell secretion maintains low, basal levels of circulating *insulin.* However, the Type I diabetic has virtually no functional β cells and can neither respond to variations in circulating fuels nor maintain even a basal secretion of *insulin* (Figure 26.2). The diabetic must rely on exogenous (injected) *insulin* in order to control the hyperglycemia and ketoacidosis. The goal in administering *insulin* to Type I diabetics is to maintain blood glucose concentrations as close to normal as possible and to avoid wide swings in blood glucose levels that may contribute to the long-term complications of the disease.

B. Type II diabetes (non-insulin-dependent diabetes mellitus, NIDDM)

1. **Cause of the disease:** In non-insulin-dependent diabetes, the pancreas retains some β-cell capacity, resulting in *insulin* levels that vary from below normal to above normal, but in all cases, *insulin* levels are less than that required to maintain glucose homeostasis (Figure 26.2). Patients with Type II diabetes are often obese. Type II diabetes is frequently accompanied by target organ *insulin* resistance that results in a decreased responsiveness to both endogenous and exogenous *insulin.* In some cases, *insulin* resistance can be due to a decreased number of *insulin* receptors. Other patients show an as yet undefined defect in the events that occur after *insulin* binds to its receptor on the cell membrane.

2. **Occurence of the disease:** Patients with Type II disease constitute 80-90% of the diabetics in the United States. It is almost completely determined by genetic factors. No involvement of viruses or autoimmune antibodies is apparent. The metabolic alterations observed are milder than those described for the insulin-dependent form of the disease.

3. **Treatment of Type II diabetes:** The goal in treating Type II diabetes is to maintain blood glucose concentrations within normal limits and to prevent the development of long-term complications of diabetes mellitus. Weight reduction and dietary modification often correct the hyperglycemia of Type II diabetes. *Sulfonylurea* drugs (hypoglycemic agents) or *insulin* therapy may be required to achieve satisfactory serum glucose levels. [Note: See Figure 26.3 for a summary comparison of Type I and Type II diabetes mellitus.]

	Insulin-dependent diabetes *Type I*	Non-insulin-dependent diabetes *Type II*
Age of onset	Usually during childhood or puberty	Frequently over age 35
Nutritional status at time of onset of disease	Frequently undernourished	Obesity usually present
Prevalence	10-20% of diagnosed diabetics	80-90% of diagnosed diabetics
Genetic predisposition	Moderate	Very strong
Defect or deficiency	β cells destroyed eliminating production of insulin	Inability of β cells to produce appropriate quantities of insulin; insulin resistance; other unknown defects

Figure 26.3
Comparison of insulin-dependent diabetes and non-insulin-dependent diabetes.

IV. INSULIN

Insulin [IN suh lin] is a small protein made up of two polypeptide chains that are connected by disulfide bonds. It is synthesized and secreted by the β cells of the pancreas.[3]

A. Insulin structure and secretion

Insulin is highly negatively charged because of the presence of a large proportion of dicarboxylic amino acids. This enables the hormone to bind both to positively charged proteins in the circulation and to insulin receptors on receptive cell membranes. *Insulin* secretion is regulated not only by blood glucose levels but also by other hormones and autonomic mediators. [Note: Glucose given by injection has a lower effect on *insulin* secretion than does glucose taken orally, because orally taken glucose stimulates production of digestive hormones by the gut, which in turn stimulate *insulin* secretion by the pancreas.]

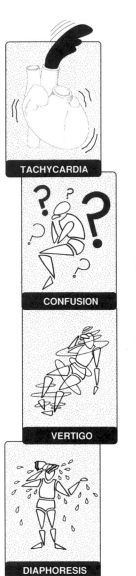

Symptoms caused
by hypoglycemia

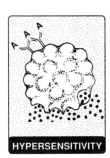

Figure 26.4
Adverse effects observed with insulin;
Note: lipodystrophy is a local atrophy
or hypertrophy of subcutaneous fatty
tissue at the site of injections.

B. Sources of insulin

Insulin can be isolated from animal sources (for example, beef and pork). Human *insulin* is also produced synthetically (i.e., through recombinant DNA technology or through substitution of a specific amino acid in pork *insulin,* which converts the structure into human *insulin*). Human *insulin* is absorbed more quickly from its site of injection than are the beef or pork hormones. Thus, the duration of action of human *insulin* is shorter and doses must be adjusted.

C. Insulin administration

Insulin is a protein. Therefore, if it were taken orally, it would be degraded in the gastrointestinal tract. *Insulin* must therefore be administered by injection. However, if *insulin* is injected intravenously, its plasma half-life is less than 9 minutes; thus *insulin* is normally administered subcutaneously. [Note: *Insulin* is degraded by the enzyme insulinase, found mainly in the liver and kidney.] *Insulin* preparations vary primarily in their times of onset of activity and duration of activity (Figure 26.5). This is due in large part to the size and composition of the *insulin* crystals in the preparations. [Note: As the *insulin* preparation becomes less soluble it becomes longer acting.]

D. Adverse reactions to insulin

The symptoms of hypoglycemia are the most serious and common adverse reactions to an overdose of *insulin* (Figure 26.4). Long-term diabetics often do not produce adequate amounts of the counterregulatory hormones (glucagon, epinephrine, cortisol, and growth hormone) that normally provide an effective defense against hypoglycemia. Other adverse reactions include lipodystrophy and allergic reactions.

V. INSULIN PREPARATIONS

A. Rapid action insulin preparations

1. *Crystalline zinc insulin* (*CZI*, "regular insulin") is purified *insulin* extracted from pork or beef pancreas or synthetically prepared human *insulin* that is crystallized as a zinc salt. [Note: The positively charged zinc binds to the negatively charged *insulin,* causing crystallization.] The *CZI* is usually given subcutaneously (or intravenously in emergencies) and lowers blood sugar within minutes (Figure 26.5).

2. *Semilente insulin* ("prompt *insulin* zinc suspension") is a suspension of amorphous *insulin* derived from beef or pork. It is used most commonly as a supplement for intermediate or prolonged action forms of *insulin. Semilente insulin* is only given subcutaneously.

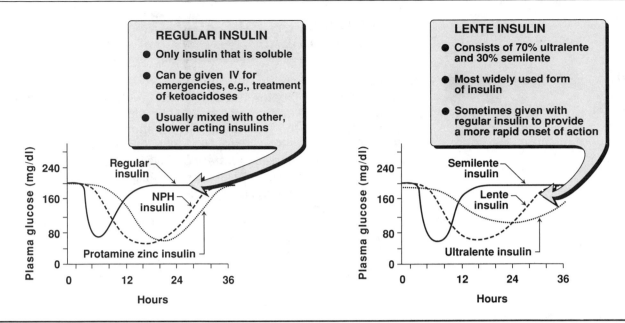

Figure 26.5
Extent and duration of action of various types of insulin (in a fasting diabetic). NPH= neutral protamine Hagedorn.

B. Intermediate action insulin preparations

1. *Isophane insulin suspension* ("neutral protamine Hagedorn", *NPH*) is a suspension of crystalline zinc *insulin* with the positively charged peptide mixture called protamine, at neutral pH. Its duration of action is intermediate between *CZI* and *protamine zinc insulin* (*PZI*), which is described below. This is due to delayed absorption of the *insulin* because of conjugation of the *insulin* with protamine to form a less soluble complex. The *NPH* should only be given subcutaneously (never intravenously) and is useful in treating all forms of diabetes except diabetic ketoacidosis or in emergency hyperglycemia.

2. *Insulin zinc suspension* ("Lente insulin") is a mixture of 30% *semilente insulin* ("prompt acting") and 70% *ultralente insulin* ("prolonged acting"). It is given only subcutaneously and is used for previously untreated diabetics who require *insulin*.

C. Prolonged action insulin preparations

1. *Protamine zinc insulin* (*PZI*) is prepared by treating *CZI* with protamine at neutral pH, resulting in a fine precipitate. Injected subcutaneously, *PZI* slowly reaches its maximum effect in about 24 hours.

2. *Extended insulin zinc suspension* ("ultralente insulin") is a crystalline zinc *insulin* that is poorly soluble. It therefore has a delayed onset and prolonged duration of action. *Ultralente insulin* is often combined with *semilente insulin* to produce *lente insulin*, a preparation that combines the solubility properties of both components.

VI. ORAL HYPOGLYCEMIC AGENTS: SULFONYLUREAS

These agents are useful in the treatment of patients who have non-insulin-dependent diabetes but cannot be managed by diet alone. Their mechanisms of actions include: (1) stimulation of *insulin* release from the β cells of the pancreas, (2) reduction of serum glucagon levels, and (3) increased binding of *insulin* to target tissues and receptors. Sulfonylureas, such as *tolbutamide* [tole BYOO ta mide], *chlorpropamide* [klor PROE pa mide], *tolazamide* [tole AZ a mide], *acetohexamide* [a seat oh HEX a mide], and the second generation derivatives, *glyburide* [GLYE byoor ide] and *glipizide* [GLIP i zide], are given orally, metabolized by the liver, and excreted by the liver or kidney. [Note: These drugs are contraindicated in patients with hepatic or renal insufficiency, since delayed excretion of the drug may cause hypoglycemia.] Figure 26.6 and 26.7 summarize the properties of the oral hypoglycemic agents.

Study Questions   *(see p.425 for answers).*

Choose the ONE best answer.

26.1 Which one of the following series of insulin preparations correctly ranks these agents according to their onsets of action from the most rapid to the slowest?

A. Ultralente insulin > isophane insulin > protamine insulin.

B. Protamine insulin > zinc insulin > ultralente insulin.

C. Isophane insulin > zinc insulin > protamine insulin.

D. Zinc insulin > ultralente insulin > protamine insulin.

E. Zinc insulin > Isophane insulin > ultralente insulin.

26.2 Which one of the following statements is correct?

A. Sulfonylureas decrease the secretion of insulin.

B. Tolbutamide is effective in Type I diabetics.

C. Sulfonylureas increase release of insulin and increase insulin-sensitivity of target tissue.

D. Glipizide increases glucagon secretion.

E. Chlorpropamide blocks insulin receptors.

26.3 Which one of the following statements is correct?

A. Insulin can be administered orally.

B. Insulin is always required therapy in Type II diabetics.

C. Protamine is added to insulin to decrease the rate of absorption of the hormone.

D. Sulfonylureas are useful in the treatment of ketoacidosis.

E. Insulin acts by binding to receptors in the nucleus of target tissue.

26.4 All of the following are correct EXCEPT:

A. One of the most common side effects of oral hypoglycemic agents is gastrointestinal disturbances.

B. The most serious consequence of insulin overdose is hypoglycemia.

C. Weight reduction is often of therapeutic help in obese Type II diabetics.

D. Sulfonylureas are contraindicated in patients with hepatic insufficiency.

E. Insulin and glucagon have similar effects on metabolism.

[1]See *glucagon, actions* in **Biochemistry** for a summary of the actions of glucagon on energy metabolism (see index).

[2]See *diabetes* in **Biochemistry** for a more detailed description of Type I and Type II diabetes.

[3]See *insulin* in **Biochemistry** for a description of the synthesis and actions of insulin.

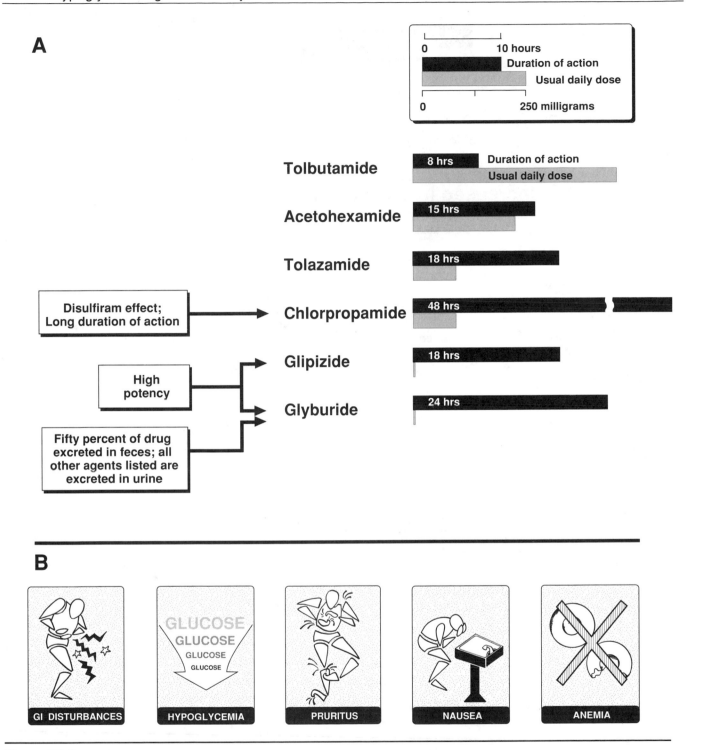

Figure 26.6
Summary of (A) the properties of and (B) the adverse effects observed with oral hypoglycemic agents.

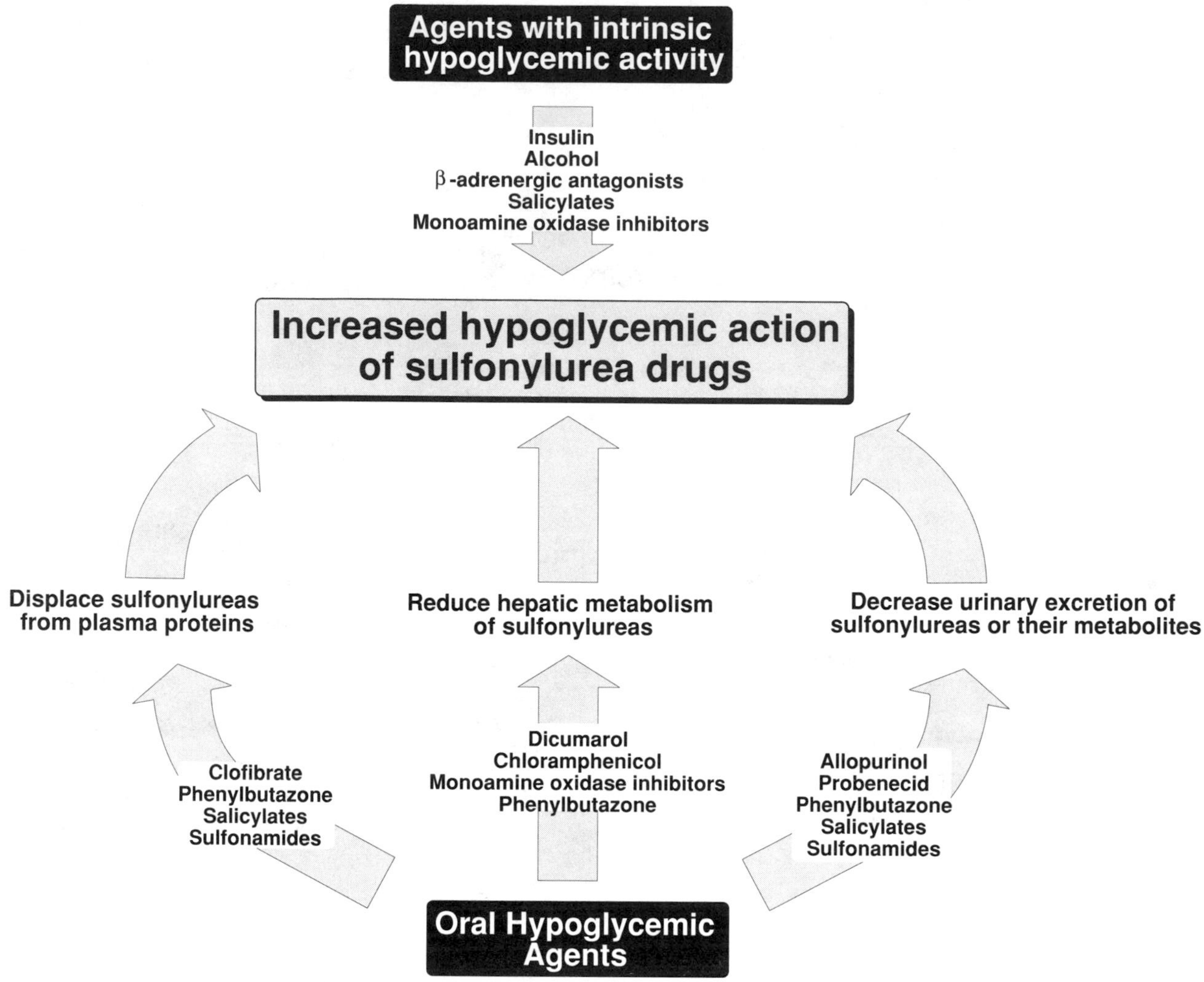

Agents with intrinsic hypoglycemic activity

Insulin
Alcohol
β-adrenergic antagonists
Salicylates
Monoamine oxidase inhibitors

Increased hypoglycemic action of sulfonylurea drugs

Displace sulfonylureas
from plasma proteins

Reduce hepatic metabolism
of sulfonylureas

Decrease urinary excretion of
sulfonylureas or their metabolites

Clofibrate
Phenylbutazone
Salicylates
Sulfonamides

Dicumarol
Chloramphenicol
Monoamine oxidase inhibitors
Phenylbutazone

Allopurinol
Probenecid
Phenylbutazone
Salicylates
Sulfonamides

Oral Hypoglycemic Agents

Figure 26.7
Drugs interacting with sulfonylurea drugs.

Steroid Hormones

27

I. OVERVIEW

Steroid sex hormones produced by the gonads and adrenals are necessary for conception, embryonic maturation, and development of primary and secondary sexual characteristics at puberty. The synthesis and release of the gonadal hormones are controlled by the gonadotropic hormones of the anterior pituitary, the luteinizing hormone (LH) and the follicle-stimulating hormone (FSH), which in turn are regulated by the gonadotropin-releasing hormone (GnRH) produced by the hypothalamus (p.229). The gonadal hormones are therapeutically used primarily in replacement therapy and in contraceptive preparations.

The adrenal cortex produces two major classes of steroid hormones: the adrenocorticosteroids (glucocorticoids and mineralocorticoids) and the adrenal androgens. Their synthesis is stimulated by adrenocorticotropic hormone (ACTH), which is a hormone that is synthesized in the anterior lobe of the pituitary gland and that acts primarily on the cortex of the adrenal gland (p.229). Analogs of the naturally occurring adrenocorticosteroids have been synthesized in an attempt to increase specificity and potency of the hormone activities. Inhibitors of adrenal cortical steroids are used to treat hormonal dysfunctions in which these compounds are produced in excess. Hormones of the adrenal cortex are also used in replacement therapy, in the management of rheumatoid arthritis and of other diseases requiring an anti-inflammatory agent, in the treatment of severe allergic reactions, and in the treatment of some cancers (p.353). Figure 27.1 summarizes the steroid hormones referred to in this chapter.

II. ESTROGENS

The major estrogens produced by women are estradiol, estrone, and estriol. The ovary is the primary source of estradiol, whereas the liver converts estradiol to estrone and estriol. In addition, the adrenal gland can synthesize estrogens, and other tissues (e.g., fat tissue, hair follicles, the liver, and skeletal muscle) can convert circulating androstenedione and testosterone (secreted by the testes) into estrogens. [Note: It is the adrenal gland by which estrogens are produced in men and postmenopausal women.] These naturally occurring steroids are subject to a large first-pass metabolism and are not administered orally. To circumvent this problem, esters of estradiol may be given intramuscularly. The synthetic estrogens exhibit less first-pass metabolism and thus increase the effectiveness of the hormone when administered orally. Nonsteroidal compounds with estrogenic activity,

STEROID HORMONES

ESTROGENS
- Estradiol
- Estrone
- Estriol
- Diethylstilbestrol
- Quinestrol
- Chlorotrianisene
- Ethinyl estradiol
- Mestranol

ANTIESTROGENS
- Clomiphene
- Tamoxifen

PROGESTINS
- Medroxyprogesterone
- Norethindrone
- Hydroxyprogesterone
- Norgestrel

ANTIPROGESTIN
- Mifepristone

ANDROGENS
- Testosterone cypionate
- Fluoxymesterone
- Danazol
- Testolactone

ANTIANDROGENS
- Cyproterone acetate
- Flutamide

Figure 27.1
Summary of steroid hormones.
(figure continues on next page)

STEROID HORMONES
(continued)

CORTICOSTEROIDS

— Hydrocortisone
— Cortisone
— Prednisone
— Prednisolone
— Methylprednisolone
— Triamcinolone
— Betamethasone
— Dexamethasone
— Paramethasone
— Fludrocortisone
— Desoxycorticosterone
— Beclomethasone

INHIBITORS OF ADRENOCORTICOID BIOSYNTHESIS

— Metyrapone
— Aminoglutethimide
— Ketoconazole

Figure 27.1 (continued)
Summary of steroid hormones.

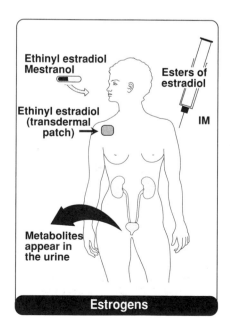

Estrogens

for example, *diethylstilbestrol* [dye eth il stil BESS trol] [*DES*], *quinestrol* [kwin ESS trole], and *chlorotrianisene* [klor oh trye AN i seen], have been synthesized and are used clinically.

A. Mechanism of action

Steroid hormones cross the cell membrane by diffusion and bind with high affinity to specific receptor proteins present in the cytoplasm (Figure 37.4). The activated steroid-receptor complex enters the nucleus and interacts with nuclear chromatin to stimulate hormone-specific RNA synthesis, resulting in the synthesis of specific proteins that mediate a number of physiologic functions. [Note: The steroid hormones may elicit the synthesis of different RNA species in different target tissues and are therefore both receptor- and tissue-specific.]

B. Therapeutic uses of estrogens

Estrogens have been used extensively for replacement therapy in patients deficient in this hormone. Such a deficiency can be due to lack of development of the ovaries, menopause, or castration. Estrogens are also frequently used, often in conjunction with other steroid hormones, for contraception.

1. **Postmenopausal hormone therapy:** Estrogen therapy is used in treating menopausal women experiencing "hot flashes", atrophic vaginitis, and in women who wish to reduce the risk of osteoporosis. For women who have not undergone a hysterectomy, a progestin is usually included with the estrogen therapy, since the combination therapy reduces the risk of endometrial carcinoma associated with estrogen treatment. For women whose uterus has been surgically removed, unopposed estrogen therapy is recommended, since progestins may unfavorably alter the high density/low density lipoprotein (HDL/LDL) ratio. [Note: The doses of estrogen used in replacement therapy are approximately 1/5 of the doses used effectively in oral contraception, described on p.248. Thus the adverse effects of estrogen replacement therapy tend to be less severe than side effects seen in women taking estrogen for contraceptive purposes.] For many patients, the multiple benefits of estrogen replacement therapy, summarized in Figure 27.2, exceed the risks.

2. **Primary hypogonadism:** Estrogen therapy, usually in combination with progestins, is instituted to stimulate development of secondary sex characteristics in young women (11 to 13 years of age) with hypogonadism.

3. **Treatment of metastatic breast cancer:** If estrogen receptors can be demonstrated in the neoplastic tissue, administration of large doses of estrogen may lead to arrest or regression of breast tumor growth. The mechanism of the effect is unknown. [Note: This is paradoxical, since estrogen at normal levels stimulates growth of breast tissue.]

4. **Contraception:** The most frequent use of synthetic estrogens is for contraception, often in combination with progestin. This topic is discussed on p.248.

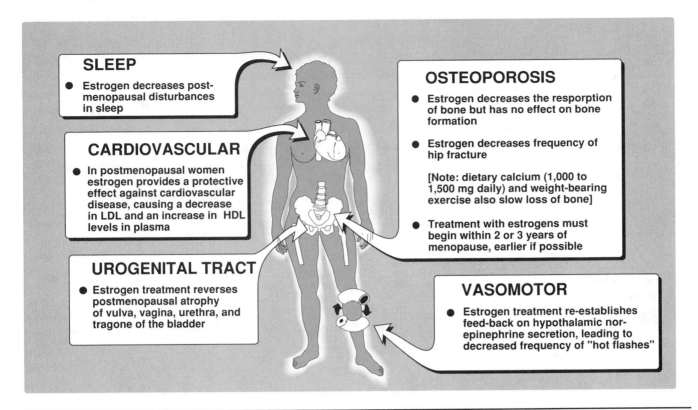

Figure 27.2
Benefits associated with postmenopausal estrogen replacement.

C. Pharmacology

1. Naturally occurring estrogens and their esterified or conjugated derivatives are readily absorbed through the gastrointestinal tract, skin, and mucous membranes. Estrogen is also quickly absorbed when administered intramuscularly. Estrogen administered orally is rapidly metabolized (and partially inactivated) by the microsomal enzymes of the liver.

2. The synthetic estrogen analogs (e.g., *ethinyl estradiol* [ETH in il ess tra DYE ole] and *mestranol* [MES tra nole]) are well absorbed after oral administration (or through the skin or mucous membranes) and are metabolized more slowly than the naturally occurring estrogens by the liver and peripheral tissues. They are also generally fat soluble and are stored in adipose tissue from which they are slowly released. The synthetic estrogen analogs therefore have a prolonged action and potency when compared to natural estrogens. Delivery of *ethinyl estradiol* by transdermal patch is effective in treating postmenopausal symptoms.

3. Estrogens are hydroxylated in the liver to derivatives that can be glucuronidated or sulfated. These final derivatives are inactive as estrogens and are excreted in the urine. [Note: In individuals with liver damage, serum estrogen levels may increase, causing feminization in males or signs of estrogen excess in females.]

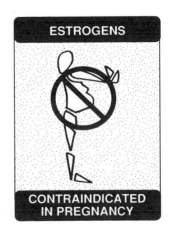

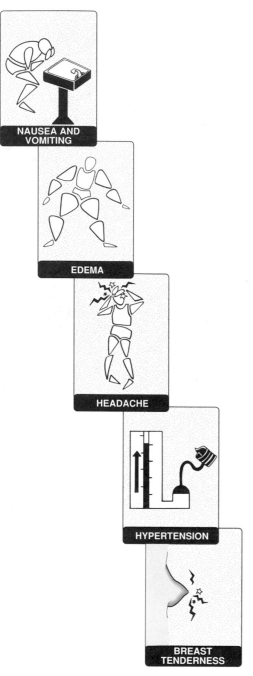

Figure 27.3
Some adverse effects associated
with estrogen therapy.

D. Adverse effects

1. Nausea and vomiting are the most common adverse effects of estrogen therapy (Figure 27.3).

2. Breast tenderness, endometrial hyperplasia, and postmenopausal bleeding may occur, all of which can be minimized by using the smallest effective dose of estrogen.

3. Hyperpigmentation, an increased frequency of migraine headaches, and hypertension can also result from estrogen therapy.

4. Estrogens can cause edema through retention of water and sodium.

5. Estrogens are contraindicated in patients with carcinoma of the breast and in patients with estrogen-dependent neoplasms (e.g., carcinoma of the endometrium). [Note: See exception, p.244.]

6. Estrogen therapy decreases bile flow and therefore can cause an increased frequency of cholestasis and gallbladder disease.

7. *Diethylstilbestrol* has been implicated as the possible cause of a rare, clear cell cervical or vaginal adenocarcinoma observed among the daughters of women who took the drug during early pregnancy.

E. Antiestrogens

Antiestrogens, which modify or oppose the action of estrogens, include hormones, such as the progestins and androgens. Other nonsteroidal antiestrogenic compounds, such as *clomiphene* [KLOE mi feen] and *tamoxifen* [ta MOX i fen], inhibit the action of estrogens by interfering with their access to cytoplasmic receptor sites. They are considered "competitive antagonists" or "weak agonists" of the natural estrogens. *Clomiphene* also interferes with the negative feedback of estrogens on the hypothalamus and pituitary and therefore causes an increase in the secretion of GnRH and gonadotropins. This results in a stimulation of ovarian function. The drug has been used successfully to treat infertility associated with anovulatory cycles. *Tamoxifen* is currently used in the treatment of advanced breast cancer in postmenopausal women (p.354). [Note: Normal breast growth is stimulated by estrogens. It is therefore not surprising that some breast tumors regress following treatment with antiestrogens.] The nonsteroidal antiestrogenic compounds are equally effective when given by mouth or by injection. The most prominent adverse effect caused by these drugs is ovarian enlargement, which is reversible once the drug is withdrawn.

III. PROGESTINS

Progesterone is the most important natural progestin. It is produced both in females (secreted by the corpus luteum, primarily during the second half of the menstrual cycle [Figure 27.4], and by the placenta) and in males (secreted by the testes) in response to LH. It is also synthesized by the adrenal cortex in both sexes. Progesterone helps to promote the development of a secretory endometrium that can accommodate implantation of a newly forming embryo. The high levels of progesterone released during the second half of the menstrual cycle (the luteal phase) inhibit the production of gonadotropin, and therefore, further ovulation. If conception takes place, progesterone continues to be secreted, maintaining the endometrium in a favorable state for the continuation of the pregnancy and decreasing uterine contractions. If conception does not take place, the release of progesterone from the corpus luteum ceases abruptly. This decline stimulates the onset of menstruation. (See Figure 27.4 for a summary of the hormones produced during the menstrual cycle.)

A. Mechanism of action

Progesterone, like estrogen, acts on target tissues by first interacting with a specific receptor protein in the cytoplasm of target cells. The progesterone-receptor complex is transported into the nucleus where it interacts with nuclear chromatin, stimulating the synthesis of specific RNAs.

B. Therapeutic uses of progestins

The major clinical use of progestins is in contraception, where they are generally used with estrogens, either in combination or in a sequential manner. Natural progesterone is not used widely as a therapeutic agent because of the problems associated with its rapid metabolism and hence its low bioavailability. Synthetic progestins used in contraception are not rapidly inactivated by first-pass metabolism and can be administered orally. These agents include *medroxyprogesterone acetate* [me DROX ee proe JESS ter one], *norethindrone* [nor eth IN drone], *hydroxyprogesterone acetate* [hye drox ee proe JESS ter one], and *norgestrel* [nor JESS trel]. Other clinical uses of the progestins are in the control of dysfunctional uterine bleeding, the treatment of dysmenorrhea, suppression of postpartum lactation, and the management of endometriosis. They are also used to treat endometrial carcinomas.

C. Pharmacology

Progesterone is rapidly absorbed after its administration by any route. It has a short half-life in the plasma, since it is almost completely metabolized in one passage through the liver. The glucuronidated metabolite (pregnanediol glucuronide) is excreted by the kidney. Synthetic progestins are less rapidly metabolized.

D. Adverse effects

The major adverse effects associated with the use of progestins are weight gain, edema, and depression. Thrombophlebitis and pulmonary embolism may occur.

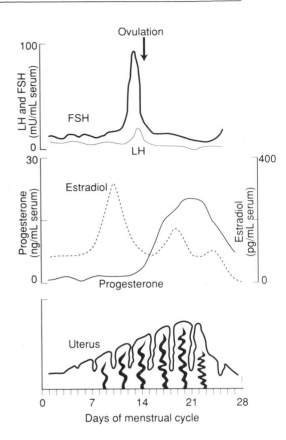

Figure 27.4
Menstrual cycle showing plasma levels of pituitary and ovarian hormones, and a schematic representation of changes in the morphology of the uterine lining.

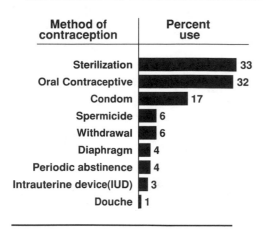

Figure 27.5
Comparison of contraceptive use among U.S. women ages 15 to 44 years.

E. Antiprogestin

Mifepristone (also designated RU 486) binds to the cytoplasmic progestin receptor and thereby acts as a progestin antagonist. Administration of this drug to females early in pregnancy, in most cases (85%) results in abortion of the fetus. The major adverse effects are significant uterine bleeding and the possibility of an incomplete abortion. *Mifepristone* can also be used as a contraceptive, which is given once a month during the midluteal phase of the cycle when progesterone is normally high.

IV. ORAL CONTRACEPTIVES

Drugs have been identified that decrease fertility by a number of different mechanisms, for example, preventing ovulation, impairing gametogenesis or gamete maturation, or interfering with gestation. Currently, interference with ovulation is the most common pharmacological intervention for preventing pregnancy (Figure 27.5).

A. Major classes of oral contraceptives

1. **Combination pills:** Products containing a combination of estrogen and progestin are the most common type of oral contraceptives. The estrogen component suppresses ovulation while the progestin prevents implantation in the endometrium and makes the cervical mucus impenetrable to sperm. Combination pills contain a constant low dose of estrogen given over 21 days plus a concurrent low but increasing dose of progestin given over 3 successive 7-day periods (called the "triphasic regimen"). The pills are taken for 21 days followed by a 7-day withdrawal period to induce menses. [Note: Estrogens that are commonly present in the combination pills are *ethinyl estradiol* and *mestranol*.] These preparations are highly effective in achieving contraception (Figure 27.6).

2. **Progestin pills:** Products containing a progestin only, usually *norethindrone* or *norgestrel* (called a "mini-pill"), are taken daily on a continuous schedule. Progestin-only pills deliver a low, continuous dosage of drug. These preparations are less effective than the combination pill (Figure 27.6) and may produce irregular menstrual cycles more frequently than the combination product. The progestin-only pill has limited patient acceptance because of anxiety over the increased possibility of pregnancy and the frequent occurence of menstrual irregularities.

3. **Progestin implants:** Subdermal capsules containing *levonorgestrel* offer long term contraception. Six capsules, each the size of a match stick, are placed subcutaneously in the upper arm. The progestin is slowly released from the capsules providing contraceptive protection for approximately 5 years. The implant is cheaper than oral contraceptives, nearly as reliable as sterilization, and totally reversible if the implants are surgically removed. Principal side effects are irregular menstrual bleeding and headaches. Once the progestin-containing capsules are implanted,

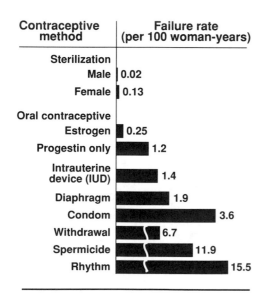

Figure 27.6
Comparison of failure rate for various methods of contraception.

this method of contraception does not rely on patient compliance.

4. **Postcoital contraception:** A fourth type of contraceptive strategy uses high-dose estrogen administered within 72 hours of coitus and continued twice daily for 5 days. This is the so-called ''morning-after'' pill. *Diethylstilbestrol* is currently used for this purpose.

B. Mechanism of action

The mechanism of action of these contraceptives is not completely understood. It is likely that the combination of estrogen and progestin administered over approximately a 3-week period inhibits ovulation. [Note: The estrogen provides a negative feedback on the release of LH and FSH by the pituitary gland, thus preventing ovulation. The progestin stimulates normal bleeding at the end of the menstrual cycle.]

C. Adverse effects

Most adverse effects are believed to be due to the estrogen component, but cardiovascular effects reflect the action of both estrogen and progestin. The incidence of side effects with oral contraceptives is relatively low and is determined by the specific compounds and combinations used.

1. **Major adverse effects:** The major side effects are breast fullness, depression, dizziness, edema, headache, nausea, and vomiting.

2. **Cardiovascular:** The most serious side effects are cardiovascular effects that are most common among women who smoke and who are over 35 years of age, although they may affect women of any age. These effects include thromboembolism, thrombophlebitis, hypertension, and increased incidences of myocardial infarction, and of cerebral and coronary thrombosis.

3. **Carcinogenic:** Oral contraceptives may cause an increased incidence of certain cancers, including carcinoma of the vagina and uterus, and the production of benign tumors of the liver that may rupture and hemorrhage.

4. **Metabolic:** Decreased dietary carbohydrate absorption by the intestine is sometimes associated with oral contraceptives, along with an increased incidence of abnormal glucose tolerance tests (similar to the changes seen in pregnancy).

5. **Serum lipids:** The combination pill causes a change in the serum lipoprotein profile: estrogen causes an increase in HDL and a decrease in LDL (a desirable occurence), whereas progestins have the opposite effect. [Note: The potent progestin, *norgestrel,* causes the greatest increase in the LDL/HDL ratio.] Therefore, estrogen-dominant preparations are best for individuals with elevated serum cholesterol.]

6. **Contraindications:** Oral contraceptives are contraindicated in the presence of cerebrovascular disease, thromboembolic disease, estrogen-dependent neoplasms, liver disease, and migraine headache.

V. ANDROGENS

The androgens are a group of steroids that have anabolic and/or masculinizing effects in both males and females. Testosterone is the most important androgen in humans, and is synthesized by Leydig's cells in the testes, and, in smaller amounts, by cells in the ovary of the female and in the adrenal gland. Androgens are necessary during embryonic development of the male phenotype and, specifically, for the virilization of the urogenital tract. They play an essential role in FSH-initiated spermatogenesis. During puberty in males, androgens are necessary for sexual development, namely they stimulate enlargement of the testes, growth of the scrotum and penis, and appearance of pubic hair. Androgens are also responsible for the anabolic growth of skeletal musculature, growth spurt, and closing of epiphyseal plates of the long bones at puberty. [Note: This causes a problem when androgens (anabolic steroids) are given to athletes at too young an age.] Deepening of the voice and the sexual behavior and aggressiveness of males are also stimulated by androgens.

In adult males, testosterone secretion by Leydig's cells is controlled by hormonal signals from the hypothalamus (GnRH), by way of the pituitary gland (FSH and LH). LH was originally known as interstitial cell-stimulating hormone, ICSH in males. [Note: LH stimulates steroidogenesis in the Leydig's cells, whereas FSH is necessary for the initiation of spermatogenesis.] Testosterone or its metabolite 5-α-dihydrotestosterone (DHT, see later) inhibits production of these specific tropic hormones and thus regulates testosterone production (Figure 27.7). Synthetic modifications of the androgen structure are designed to (1) modify solubility and susceptibility to enzymatic breakdown (thus prolonging the half-life of the hormone) and (2) separate anabolic and androgenic effects.

A. Mechanism of action

Like the estrogens and progestins, androgens bind to a specific cytoplasmic receptor in a target cell. The hormone/receptor complex enters the nucleus where it binds to DNA and stimulates the synthesis of specific mRNAs. In muscle and liver, testosterone itself is the active compound. However, transformation of testosterone to DHT is important in reproductive tissues, including the prostate, and in stimulating hair growth. [Note: Testosterone analogs that cannot be converted to DHT have less effect on the reproductive system than they do on the skeletal musculature.]

B. Therapeutic uses

1. **Androgenic effects:** Androgenic steroids are used in patients with inadequate testicular function. [Note: This hypogonadism can be caused by problems with the testes themselves or be secondary to failure of the pituitary gland.]

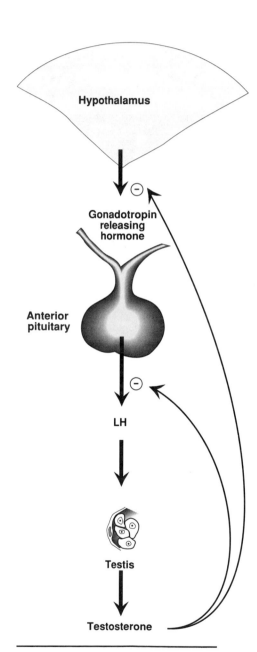

Figure 27.7
Regulation of secretion of testosterone.

Hypothalamus

Gonadotropin releasing hormone

Anterior pituitary

LH

Testis

Testosterone

2. **Anabolic effects:** Anabolic steroids can be used to treat senile osteoporosis and severe burns, to speed recovery from surgery or from chronic debilitating diseases, and to counteract the catabolic effects of externally administered adrenal cortical hormones.

3. **Growth:** Androgens are used in conjunction with other hormones to promote skeletal growth in pituitary dwarfism.

4. **Advanced or metastatic breast cancer:** This is the most common reason for large-dose, long-term androgen therapy in women. The treatment causes virilizing side effects. [Note: Newer testosterone derivatives such as *testolactone* cause less virilization.]

5. **Endometriosis:** *Danazol* [DA na zole], a mild androgen, is used in the treatment of endometriosis (ectopic growth of the endometrium).

6. **Unapproved use:** To increase lean body mass and muscle strength in athletes and "body builders" (see "Adverse Effects" later).

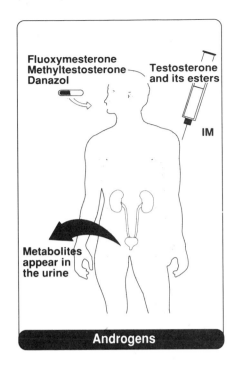

Androgens

C. Pharmacology

1. Testosterone cannot be given orally because of inactivation by first-pass metabolism. As with the other sex steroids, testosterone is rapidly absorbed by the liver and other tissues, and metabolized to relatively or completely inactive compounds that are excreted primarily in the urine but also in the feces. Testosterone and its C-17-esters (e.g., *testosterone cyprionate* [tess TOSS ter one] are administered intramuscularly. [Note: The addition of the esterified lipid makes the hormone more lipid-soluble, thereby increasing its duration of action.] Testosterone and its esters demonstrate a 1 : 1 relative ratio of androgenic to anabolic activity.

2. Testosterone derivatives (e.g., *fluoxymesterone* [floo ox ee MESS te rone] and *danazol*) also have a longer half-life in the body than does the naturally occurring androgen. *Fluoxymesterone* is effective when given orally, and it has a 1 : 2 androgenic to anabolic ratio. Because it is not readily converted to DHT, it is less active than testosterone in the reproductive system and does not induce puberty. It has a longer half-life than does testosterone.

D. Adverse effects

1. In females, androgens can cause masculinization with acne, growth of facial hair, deepening of the voice, male pattern baldness, and excessive muscle development. Menstrual irregularities may also occur. Testosterone should not be used by pregnant women, because of the possible virilization of the female fetus.

2. In males, excess androgens can cause priapism, impotence, decreased spermatogenesis, and gynecomastia.

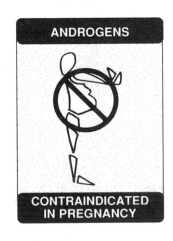

ANDROGENS

CONTRAINDICATED IN PREGNANCY

3. In children, androgens can cause growth disturbances resulting from premature closing of the epiphyseal plates and abnormal sexual maturation.

4. Androgens increase serum LDL and lower serum HDL levels; therefore they increase the LDL/HDL ratio and potentially increase the risk for premature coronary heart disease.

5. Androgens can cause fluid retention leading to edema.

6. Use of anabolic steroids by athletes can cause premature closing of the epiphysis of the long bones, which interrupts development. The high doses taken by these athletes may also result in hepatic abnormalities, increased aggression ('' 'roid rage''), and psychotic episodes, as well as the other adverse effects just described.

E. Antiandrogens

Antiandrogens, such as *cyproterone acetate* [si PROE ter one] and *flutamide* [FLOO ta mide], act as competitive inhibitors of androgens. They inhibit the action of the androgens at the target cell. These drugs have been used to treat hirsutism in females and prostatic carcinoma in males.

VI. ADRENAL CORTICOSTEROIDS

The adrenal cortex is divided into three zones (Figure 27.8). The outer zone (zona glomerulosa) produces mineralocorticoids (e.g., aldosterone), which are responsible for regulating salt and water metabolism. Production of aldosterone is regulated primarily by the renin-angiotensin system (p.176). The middle zone (zona fasciculata) secretes glucocorticoids (e.g., *cortisol* [KOR ti sol]), which are concerned with normal metabolism and resistance to stress. The inner zone (zona reticularis) secretes adrenal androgens. Secretion by the two inner zones, and to some extent, the outer zone, are controlled by pituitary ACTH, which is stimulated in turn by corticotropin-releasing factor (CRF), that is produced by the hypothalamus. Adrenal glucocorticoids serve as feedback inhibitors of ACTH and CRF secretion (Figure 27.8).

A. Mechanism of action

Like the other steroid hormones previously discussed, the adrenocorticoids bind to specific intracellular receptors in target tissues. The receptor-hormone complex is then transported into the nucleus where the complex interacts with the DNA causing an increase in the synthesis of specific RNAs.

B. Actions

Some normal actions and some selected mechanisms of adrenocorticoids are described in this section. Understanding these actions aids the reader in better comprehending the results of

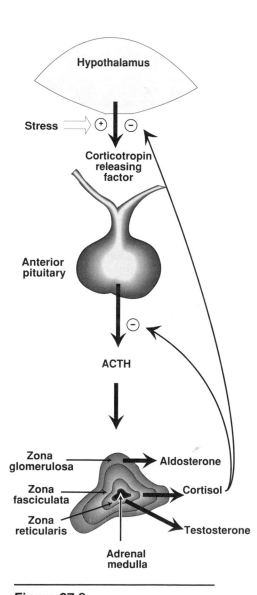

Figure 27.8
Regulation of corticosteroid secretion.

adrenal insufficiency and the uses of adrenocorticoids as therapeutic agents in a variety of disorders.

1. Glucocorticoids

a. **Promote normal metabolism**: Glucocorticoids stimulate gluconeogenesis by both increasing amino acid uptake via the liver and kidney and promoting increased activity of gluconeogenic enzymes. They stimulate protein catabolism and lipolysis, thereby providing the building blocks and energy needed for glucose synthesis. [Note: Glucocorticoid insufficiency may result in hypoglycemia, for example, during stressful periods or fasting.]

b. **Increase resistance to stress**: By raising plasma glucose levels, glucocorticoids provide the body with the energy it requires to combat stress caused by, for example, trauma, fright, infection, bleeding, or debilitating disease. Glucocorticoids also cause a rise in blood pressure, apparently by enhancing the vasoconstrictor action of adrenergic stimuli on small vessels. [Note: Individuals with adrenal insufficiency may also respond to severe stress by becoming hypotensive.]

c. **Alter blood cell levels in plasma**: Glucocorticoids cause a decrease in eosinophils, basophils, monocytes, and lymphocytes. In contrast, they increase the blood levels of hemoglobin, erythrocytes, and polymorphonuclear leukocytes. [Note: The decrease in circulating lymphocytes and macrophages results in a decreased ability of the body to fight infections.]

d. **Anti-inflammatory action**: Glucocorticoids can dramatically reduce the inflammatory response because of their abilities to lower peripheral lymphocyte levels and to inhibit the enzyme phospholipase A_2—the enzyme that releases arachidonic acid, the precursor of the prostaglandins and leukotrienes, from membrane-bound phospholipid (p.363).

e. **Affect other components of the endocrine system**: Feedback inhibition of ACTH production by elevated glucocorticoids causes inhibition of further glucocorticoid synthesis as well as thyroid-stimulating hormone production (p. 229), whereas growth hormone production is increased.

2. Mineralocorticoids

Water and electrolyte homeostasis: Mineralocorticoids help control the body's water volume and concentration of electrolytes, especially sodium and potassium. Aldosterone acts on kidney tubule cells, causing a reabsorption of sodium, bicarbonate, and water. Conversely, aldosterone decreases reabsorption of potassium, which is then lost in the urine. [Note: Elevated aldosterone levels may cause alkalosis and hypokalemia, whereas retention of sodium and water leads to an increase in blood volume and blood pressure (p.220).]

C. Therapeutic uses of the adrenal corticosteroids

Several semisynthetic derivatives of the glucocorticoids have been developed that vary in their anti-inflammatory potency, the degree to which they cause sodium retention, and the length of time of activity. These are summarized in Figure 27.9.

1. **Replacement therapy for primary adrenocortical insufficiency (Addison's disease):** This disease is caused by adrenal cortex dysfunction (as diagnosed by the lack of patient response to administration of ACTH). *Hydrocortisone* [hye droe KOR ti sone], which is identical to the natural *cortisol,* is given to correct the deficiency. Failure to do so results in death. The dosage of *hydrocortisone* is divided so that two thirds of the normal daily dose is given in the morning, and one third in the afternoon. [Note: The goal of this regimen is to approximate the daily hormone levels resulting from the circadian rhythm exhibited by cortisol, which causes plasma levels to be maximal around 8 A.M. and then to decrease throughout the day to their lowest level around 1 A.M.] Administration of *fludrocortisone* [floo droe KOR ti sone], a synthetic mineralocorticoid with some glucocorticoid activity, may also be necessary to raise the mineralocorticoid activity to normal levels.]

2. **Replacement therapy for secondary or tertiary adrenocortical insufficiency:** These deficiencies are caused by a defect either in CRF production by the hypothalamus or ACTH production by the pituitary. [Note: Under these conditions, the adrenal cortex synthesis of mineralocorticoids is less impaired than that of glucocorticoids.] The adrenal cortex responds to ACTH administration by synthesizing and releasing the adrenal corticosteroids. *Hydrocortisone* is also used for these deficiencies.

3. **Diagnosis of Cushing's syndrome:** Cushing's syndrome is caused by a hypersecretion of glucocorticoids that is due to either excessive release of ACTH by the anterior pituitary or to an adrenal tumor. The *dexamethasone* suppression test is used to diagnose the cause of an individual's case of Cushing's syndrome. This synthetic glucocorticoid suppresses cortisol release in individuals with pituitary-dependent Cushing's syndrome, but it does not suppress glucocorticoid release from adrenal tumors.

4. **Replacement therapy for congenital adrenal hyperplasia** (CAH): This is a group of diseases resulting from an enzyme defect in the synthesis of one or more adrenal steroid hormones. Treatment of this condition requires administration of sufficient corticosteroids to normalize the patient's hormone levels. Choice of replacement hormone depends on the site of the lesion.

5. **Relief of inflammatory symptoms :** Glucocorticoids dramatically reduce the manifestations of inflammations (e.g., rheumatoid and osteoarthritis inflammations, inflammatory conditions of the skin), including the redness, swelling, heat, and tenderness that are commonly present at the inflammatory site. The effect of glucocorticoids on the inflammatory process is the result of their

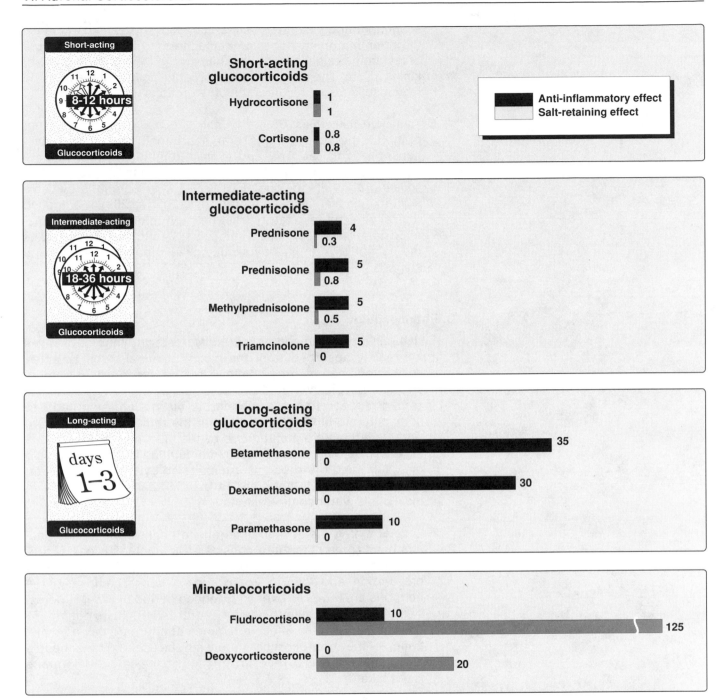

Figure 27.9
Pharmacological properties of some commonly used natural and synthetic corticosteroids; activities are all relative to hydrocortisone =1. Time refers to duration of action.

effects on the distribution, concentration, and function of leukocytes. These effects include an increase in the concentration of neutrophils; a decrease in the concentrations of lymphocytes (T and B cells), basophils, eosinophils, and monocytes; and an inhibition of the ability of leukocytes and macrophages to respond to mitogens and antigens. Glucocorticoids also influence the inflammatory response by their abilities to reduce the amount of histamine released by basophils and to inhibit the activity of kinins. [Note: The ability of glucocorticoids to inhibit the immune response is also a result of the other actions just described.]

6. **Treatment of allergies:** Glucocorticoids are useful in the treatment of the symptoms of drug, serum, and transfusion allergic reactions, bronchial asthma, and allergic rhinitis. These drugs are not, however, curative. [Note: The introduction of *beclomethasone dipropionate* [be kloe METH a sone] as an aerosol provided a significant advance in the therapy of asthma (p.209). It is applied topically to the respiratory tract through inhalation from a metered dose dispenser. This minimizes systemic effects and allows the patient to significantly reduce or eliminate the use of oral steroids.]

D. Pharmacology

1. Naturally occurring adrenal corticosteroids and their derivatives are readily absorbed from the gastrointestinal tract. Selected compounds can also be administered intravenously, intramuscularly, or topically (Figure 27.10). Greater than 90% of the absorbed glucocorticoids are bound to plasma proteins: most to corticosteroid-binding globulin, and the remainder to albumin. Corticosteroids are metabolized by the liver microsomal oxidizing enzymes. The metabolites are conjugated to glucuronic acid or sulfate, and the products are excreted by the kidney. [Note: The half-life of adrenal steroids may increase dramatically in individuals with hepatic dysfunction.]

2. In determining the dosage of adrenocortical steroids, many factors need to be taken into consideration, including glucocorticoid versus mineralocorticoid activity, duration of action, type of preparation, and so forth. For example, when large doses of the hormone are required over an extended period of time, suppression of the hypothalamic-pituitary-adrenal (HPA) axis occurs. To prevent this adverse effect, a regimen of alternate-day administration of the adrenocortical steroid may be useful. This schedule allows the HPA axis to recover/function on the days the hormone is not taken.

E. Adverse effects

1. Osteoporosis, impaired synthesis of collagen (leading to impaired wound healing), and myopathy that results from protein catabolism are caused by glucocorticoids. [Note: Impaired growth in children is probably caused by the same action.]

2. Edema, hypertension, and congestive heart failure due to salt and water retention can occur.

3. The CNS effects range from euphoria to psychoses including suicidal tendencies. These drugs may cause a psychological dependency.

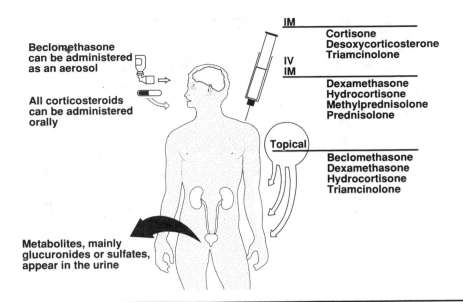

Figure 27.10
Routes of administration and elimination of corticosteriods.

4. Corticosteroids may cause stimulation of peptic ulcers.

5. Corticosteroids may cause development of iatrogenic Cushing's syndrome, including redistribution of body fat, puffy face, increased body hair growth, acne, insomnia and increased appetite.

6. Withdrawal from the drugs can be a serious problem, because if the patient has experienced hypothalamic-pituitary-adrenal suppression, abrupt removal of the drugs causes an acute adrenal insufficiency syndrome that can be lethal. This fact, coupled with the possibility of psychological dependence on the drug and the fact that withdrawal might cause an exacerbation of the disease, means that the individual schedule for withdrawal may be based on trial and error. The patient must be carefully monitored.

F. Inhibitors of adrenocorticoid biosynthesis

Three substances have proven to be useful as inhibitors of the secretion of adrenocortical substances: *metyrapone* [me TEER a pone], *aminoglutethimide* [a mee noe glu TETH i mide], and *ketoconazole* [kee toe KON a zole].

1. *Metyrapone* interferes with corticosteroid synthesis and has been used for the treatment of Cushing's syndrome. It is most commonly used in tests of adrenal function. The adverse effects encountered with *metyrapone* include salt and water retention, hirsutism, transient dizziness, and gastrointestinal disturbances.

2. *Aminoglutethimide* acts by inhibiting the conversion of cholesterol to pregnenolone. As a result, the synthesis of all hormonally active steroids is reduced. *Aminoglutethimide* has been used

therapeutically in the treatment of breast cancer to reduce or eliminate androgen and estrogen production. In these cases it is used in conjunction with *dexamethasone. Aminoglutethimide* may also be useful in the treatment of malignancies of the adrenal cortex to reduce the secretion of steroids.

3. *Ketoconazole* (an antifungal agent, see p.309) strongly inhibits all gonadal and adrenal steroid hormone synthesis. It is used in the treatment of patients with Cushing's syndrome.

Study Questions (see p.426 for answers).

Choose the ONE best answer.

27.1 All of the following statements about glucocorticoids are correct EXCEPT:

A. They may produce peptic ulcers.
B. They are useful in the treatment of refractory asthma.
C. They are contraindicated in glaucoma.
D. They are used in the treatment of Addison's disease.
E. They exert their effect by binding to receptors in the cell membrane.

27.2 Which one of the following statements is true?

A. Diethylstibestrol enhances fertility by blocking the inhibitory effect of estrogen on the pituitary.
B. Tamoxifen is an estrogen antagonist.
C. Dexamethasone has weak anti-inflammatory properties.
D. Estrogens are mainly excreted unchanged in the urine.
E. Tamoxifen is used to treat infertility.

27.3 All of the following are adverse effects associated with the used of oral contraceptive agents EXCEPT:

A. Edema.
B. Breast tenderness.
C. Nausea.
D. Increased frequency of migraine headache.
E. Increased risk of ovarian cancer.

27.4 Estrogen replacement therapy in menopausal women

A. restores bone loss accompanying osteoporosis.
B. may induce "hot flashes".
C. may cause atrophic vaginitis.
D. is most effective if instituted at the first signs of menopause.
E. require higher doses of estrogen than are required with oral contraceptive therapy.

27.5 Progestins

A. are not produced in males.
B. increase HDL and decrease LDL.
C. attenuate the increased risk of endometrial cancer associated with estrogen-only oral contraceptive agents.
D. such as progesterone are widely used in oral contraceptives.
E. commonly induce weight loss.

27.6 Which one of the following is a synthetic estrogen used in oral contraceptives?

A. Mestranol.
B. Norgestrel.
C. Clomiphene.
D. Estradiol.
E. Norethindrone.

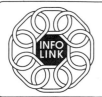

[1]See *steroid hormones, synthesis* in **Biochemistry** for a description of the enzyme deficiencies involved in the congenital adrenal hyperplasias (see index).

Principles of Antimicrobial Therapy

28

I. OVERVIEW

Antimicrobial drugs are effective in the treatment of infections because of their selective toxicity—the ability to kill an invading microorganism without harming the cells of the host. In most instances, the selective toxicity is relative, rather than absolute, requiring that the concentration of the drug be carefully controlled to attack the microorganism while still being tolerated by the host. Selective antimicrobial therapy takes advantage of the biochemical differences that exist between microorganisms and human beings.

II. SELECTION OF ANTIMICROBIAL AGENTS

Selection of the most appropriate antimicrobial agent depends on (1) the identity of the organism and its sensitivity to a particular agent, (2) the site of the infection, (3) the safety of the agent, and (4) patient factors.

A. Identification and sensitivity of the organism

Characterization of the organism is central to the selection of the proper drug. It is essential to obtain a sample culture of the organism prior to initiating treatment if possible.

1. **Laboratory methods of identification**

   a. A rapid assessment of the nature of the organism can sometimes be made on the basis of differential stains, such as the Gram stain, but it is generally necessary to culture the infective organism in order to arrive at a conclusive diagnosis.

   b. The most commonly used method to test susceptibility to antibiotics is disk diffusion (Figure 28.1).

2. **Empiric therapy prior to organism identification**

   a. **The acutely ill patient:** Ideally the selection of an antimicrobial agent occurs after the drug sensitivity of the infecting organ-

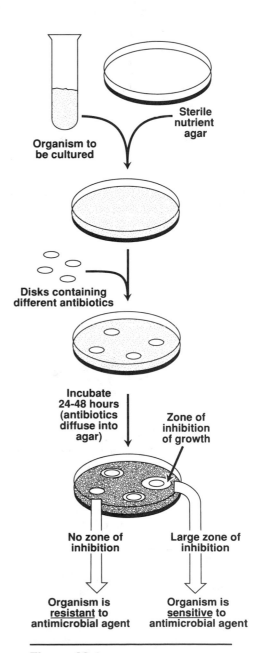

Figure 28.1
Disk diffusion method for determining the sensitivity of bacteria to antimicrobial agents.

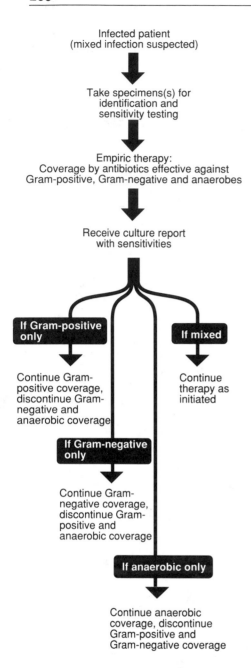

Figure 28.2
Therapeutic strategy in treating patients with an infection of unknown origin.

ism has been established. However, acutely ill patients usually require immediate treatment that is initiated after specimens for laboratory analyses are obtained but before the results of the culture are available.

  b. **Selecting a drug:** The choice of drug in the absence of sensitivity data is influenced by patient history (e.g.,travel, age), location of the infection, and results of the Gram stain. One may also initiate empiric therapy with a combination of antibiotics covering infections by both gram-positive and gram-negative microorganisms. Figure 28.2 summarizes a typical therapeutic strategy for a patient with an infection of unknown origin.

B. The site of the infection

1. **Effect of vascular perfusion:** Effective levels of the antibiotic must reach the infection site; therefore any change that diminishes access of the drug to the infected area may alter the effectiveness of the treatment. For example, poor perfusion of an anatomic area, like the lower limbs of the diabetic, make infections in these regions notoriously difficult to treat.

2. **Blood-brain barrier:** Treatment of infections of the central nervous system, such as meningitis, depends on the ability of a drug to penetrate into the cerebrospinal fluid. The blood-brain barrier (p.7) ordinarily excludes many antibiotics. However, inflammation enhances penetrability and allows sufficient levels of many (but not all) antibiotics to enter the cerebrospinal fluid.

C. The safety of the agent

1. **Inherent toxicity of the drug:** Many of the antibiotics, such as the penicillins, are among the least toxic of all drugs because they interfere with a site unique to the growth of microorganisms. Other antimicrobial agents (for example, *chloramphenicol*) are less specific and are reserved for life-threatening infections because of the drug's potential for serious toxicity.

2. **Patient factors:** Safety is not only related to the inherent nature of the drug but also to patient factors that can predispose to toxicity (see Section D).

D. Status of the patient

1. **Immune system:** Elimination of infecting organisms from the body depends on an intact immune system (Figure 28.3). Antibacterial drugs decrease the microbial population (bactericidal, p.261), or inhibit further bacterial growth (bacteriostatic), but the host defenses must ultimately eliminate the invading organisms. Immunocompromised patients have weakened immune defenses, and higher than usual doses of bactericidal agents are required to eliminate the infective organism.

2. **Renal dysfunction:** Poor kidney function (10% or less of normal) causes accumulation of antibiotics that are ordinarily eliminated by this route. This may lead to serious adverse effects that can be

controlled by adjusting the dose or the dosage schedule of the antibiotic. [Note: The number of functioning nephrons decreases with age, making elderly patients particularly vulnerable.]

3. **Hepatic dysfunction:** Antibiotics that concentrate in the liver (for example, *erythromycin, tetracycline*) are contraindicated in treating patients with liver disease.

4. **Pregnancy:** All antibiotics cross the placenta. Adverse effects to the fetus are rare, except for tooth dysplasia and inhibition of bone growth encountered with the tetracyclines. However, some anthelmintics are embryotoxic and teratogenic (p.325).

5. **Lactation:** A nursing infant can receive antibiotics (as well as other drugs) administered to the mother via the breast milk. Even though the concentration of an antibiotic in breast milk is usually low, the total dose may be enough to cause problems.

III. BACTERIOSTATIC VERSUS BACTERICIDAL DRUGS

Antimicrobial drugs are classified as either bacteriostatic or bactericidal. (See Figure 28.4 for examples of drugs in these categories.) Bacteriostatic drugs arrest the growth and replication of bacteria at serum levels achievable in the patient, thus limiting the spread of infection while the body's immune system attacks, immobilizes, and eliminates the pathogens. If the drug is removed before the immune system has scavenged the organisms, enough viable organisms may remain to begin a second cycle of infection. Bactericidal agents kill bacteria (Figure 28.5).

IV. CHEMOTHERAPEUTIC SPECTRA

The chemotherapeutic spectrum of a particular drug refers to the species of microorganisms affected by that drug. In this book, bacteria that are commonly encountered as infectious agents are presented in pie charts in which each segment represents a general class of microorganisms, e.g., gram-positive cocci (Figure 28.6A). In each section of the text covering a particular antibiotic agent, the microbial classes that are "generally" treated with that agent are highlighted. [Note: One section of the pie chart is labeled "Other" and represents any of several microorganisms defined in different chapters.]

A. Narrow spectrum

Chemotherapeutic agents acting only on a single or a limited group of microorganisms are said to have a narrow spectrum. For example, *isoniazid* is active only against mycobacteria (Figure 28.6B).

B. Extended spectrum

Extended spectrum is the term applied to antibiotics that are effective against gram-positive organisms and also against a significant number of gram-negative bacteria. For example, *ampicillin* is con-

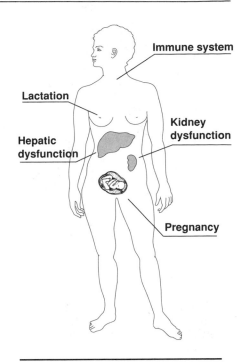

Figure 28.3
Patient factors that influence selection of antimicrobial agents.

Bactericidal

> **Aminoglycosides**
> **Bacitracin**
> **Carbapenems**
> **Cephalosporins**
> **Colistin**
> **Methenamine**
> **Monobactams**
> **Penicillins**
> **Polymyxin B**
> **Quinolones**
> **Vancomycin**

Bacteriostatic

> **Chloramphenicol**
> **Clindamycin**
> **Erythromycin**
> **Lincomycin**
> **Nitrofurantoin**
> **Sulfonamides**
> **Tetracyclines**
> **Trimethoprim**

Figure 28.4
Classification of antimicrobial agents as either bactericidal or bacteriostatic.

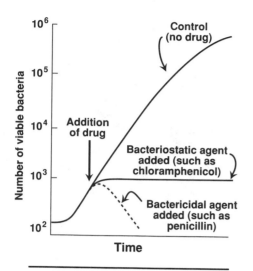

Figure 28.5
Effects of bactericidal and bacteriostatic drugs on the growth of bacteria in vitro.

sidered to have an extended spectrum because it acts against gram-positive and gram-negative bacteria.

C. Broad spectrum

Drugs such as *tetracycline* and *chloramphenicol* affect a wide variety of microbial species and are referred to as broad spectrum antibiotics (Figure 28.6C). Administration of broad spectrum antibiotics can drastically alter the nature of the normal bacterial flora and can precipitate a superinfection of an organism, such as candida whose growth is normally kept in check by the presence of other microorganisms.

V. COMBINATIONS OF ANTIMICROBIAL DRUGS

It is therapeutically advisable to treat with the single agent that is most specific for the infecting organism. This strategy reduces the possibility of superinfection and decreases the occurrence of resistant organisms (see section VI). However, situations in which combinations of drugs are employed do exist, for example, the treatment of tuberculosis involves drug combinations. Treatment with a combination of drugs may lead to the emergence of superinfections, antagonism between the drugs, or an increased incidence of toxicity.

VI. DRUG RESISTANCE

Bacteria are said to be resistant if their growth is not halted by the maximum level of an antibiotic that is tolerated by the host. Microbial species that are normally responsive to a particular drug may develop

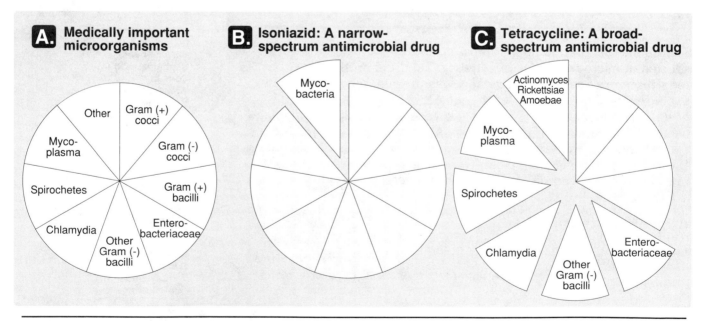

Figure 28.6
A. Medically important bacterial species. B. Isoniazid, a narrow-spectrum antimicrobial agent. C. Tetracycline, a broad-spectrum antimicrobial agent.

strains that are resistant to that agent. This is usually accomplished through an alteration of their chromosomal or extrachromosomal (plasmid) DNA, followed by selection for resistant strains. Furthermore, these special plasmids (R-factors), which carry genes for resistance to one or more antimicrobial drugs, can be transferred from one organism to another either by transduction or conjugation. Multiple drug resistance spread by this mechanism has become a clinically significant problem. For example, methicillin-resistant Staphylococcus aureus is also resistant to all antibiotics except *vancomycin* and possibly *ciprofloxacin, rifampin* and *imipenem/cilastatin*.

VII. PROPHYLACTIC ANTIBIOTICS

Certain clinical situations require the use of antibiotics for the prevention rather than the treatment of infections. Since the indiscriminate use of antimicrobial agents can result in bacterial resistance and superinfection, prophylactic use is restricted to clinical situations where benefits outweigh the potential risks.

A. Therapeutic uses

Therapeutic uses include the following:
1. prevention of streptococcal infections in patients with a history of rheumatic heart disease.

2. pretreatment of patients undergoing dental extractions who have implanted prosthetic devices, such as artificial heart valves.

3. prevention of tuberculosis or meningitis among individuals who are in close contact with infected patients.

4. presurgical treatment in gastrointestinal procedures, vaginal hysterectomy, cesarean section, joint replacement, and open fracture surgery.

VIII. COMPLICATIONS OF ANTIBIOTIC THERAPY

Selective toxicity to the invading organism does not insure the host against adverse effects, since the drug may produce an allergic response or be toxic in ways unrelated to the drug's antimicrobial activity.

A. Hypersensitivity

Hypersensitivity reactions to antimicrobial drugs or their metabolic products frequently occur. For example, the penicillins, despite their almost absolute selective microbial toxicity, can cause serious hypersensitivity problems, ranging from rashes (urticaria) to anaphylactic shock.

B. Direct toxicity

High serum levels of antibiotic may cause toxicity by affecting cellular processes in the host. For example, aminoglycosides can cause ototoxicity by interfering with membrane function in the hair cells of the organ of Corti.

C. Superinfections

Drug therapy, particularly with broad spectrum antimicrobials or combinations of agents, can lead to alterations of the normal microbial flora of the upper respiratory, intestinal and genitourinary tracts, permitting the overgrowth of opportunistic organisms, especially fungi. These infections can involve resistant organisms and are often difficult to treat.

Study Questions   (see p.426 for answers).

Choose the ONE best answer.

28.1 Which of the following statements is correct?

A. Isoniazid is a broad spectrum antibiotic.
B. Chloramphenicol is a narrow spectrum antibiotic.
C. Ampicillin is a narrow spectrum antibiotic.
D. Tetracycline is a broad spectrum antibiotic.
E. Initial treatment usually combines a broad spectrum and a narrow spectrum antibiotic.

28.2 All of the following clinical indications require a combination of antibiotics (rather than a single agent) EXCEPT:

A. Mixed infections.
B. Infections with clinical outcomes that depend on drug synergism.
C. Infections that involve a risk of developing resistant organisms.
D. Emergency situations involving an infection of unknown cause.
E. Viral infections.

28.3 Which one of the following patients is least likely to require antimicrobial treatment tailored to the individual's condition?

A. Patient undergoing cancer chemotherapy.
B. Patient with kidney disease.
C. Elderly patient.
D. Patient with hypertension.
E. Patient with liver disease.

28.4 In which one of the following clinical situations is the prophylactic use of antibiotics NOT warranted?

A. Prevention of meningitis among individuals in close contact with infected patients.
B. Patient with a heart prosthesis having a tooth removed.
C. Presurgical treatment for implantation of a hip prosthesis.
D. Patient who complains of frequent respiratory illness.
E. Presurgical treatment in gastrointestinal procedures.

28.5 Broad spectrum antibiotics

A. increase the frequency of occurence of superinfections.
B. are appropriate for the ill patient requiring treatment before the sensitivity of the infective agent can be determined.
C. include isoniazid.
D. are as effective against sensitive organisms in immunocompromised patients as they are against these organisms in immunocompetent individuals.
E. have little effect on the nature of the normal intestinal flora.

28.6 Which one of the following anti-infective agents is bactericidal?

A. Erythromycin.
B. Penicillin.
C. Tetracycline.
D. Clindamycin.
E. Sulfonamide.

Folate Antagonists

29

I. OVERVIEW

All sulfonamides in clinical use are structurally related to p-aminobenzoic acid (PABA). Because of the emergence of resistant bacteria and the availability of *penicillin,* their use had diminished. The introduction of *trimethoprim* (p.267) in combination with *sulfamethoxazole* (generic name *co-trimoxazole*) in the mid-1970s has led to a renewed interest in sulfonamides. The drugs discussed in this chapter are shown in Figure 29.1.

II. SULFONAMIDES

A. Mechanism of action

Bacteria cannot absorb folic acid and rely on their ability to synthesize folate from PABA and pteridine. In contrast, human beings cannot synthesize folic acid but obtain preformed folate as a vitamin in their diet. Because of their structural similarity to PABA, the sulfonamides compete with this substrate for the enzyme dihydropteroate synthetase, thus preventing the synthesis of bacterial folic acid.[1] This deprives the cell of an essential cofactor for purine, pyrimidine, and amino acid synthesis (Figure 29.2, see also Figure 29.5).

B. Antibacterial spectrum

The sulfas, including the combination of *sulfamethoxazole* with *trimethoprim* (see p. 269), are bacteriostatic. These drugs are active against selected enterobacteriaceae, chlamydia, and nocardia. Typical clinical applications are shown in Figure 29.3. In addition, *sulfadiazine* [sul fa DYE a zeen] in combination with the folate reductase inhibitor *pyrimethamine* is the only effective form of chemotherapy for toxoplasmosis (p.320).

C. Resistance

Bacterial resistance to the sulfas can arise from plasmid transfers or random mutations. The resistance is generally irreversible and may be due to any of the following three possibilities.

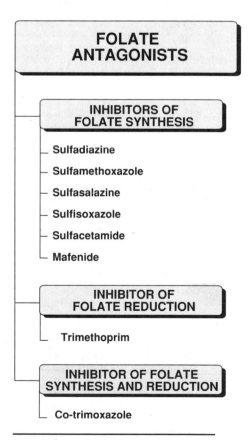

FOLATE ANTAGONISTS

INHIBITORS OF FOLATE SYNTHESIS
- Sulfadiazine
- Sulfamethoxazole
- Sulfasalazine
- Sulfisoxazole
- Sulfacetamide
- Mafenide

INHIBITOR OF FOLATE REDUCTION
- Trimethoprim

INHIBITOR OF FOLATE SYNTHESIS AND REDUCTION
- Co-trimoxazole

Figure 29.1
Summary of folate antagonists.

H₂N —⟨ ⟩— COOH

p-Aminobenzoic acid (PABA)

Pteridine precursor

dihydro-
pteroate
synthetase

Sulfanilamide
(and other
sulfonamides)

Folic acid

Figure 29.2
Competitive inhibition of folic
acid synthesis by sulfonamides.

1. **Altered enzyme:** Bacterial dihydropteroate synthetase can undergo alterations resulting in a decreased affinity for the sulfa drug. The drug therefore becomes a less effective competitor of PABA.

2. **Increased drug inactivation:** The bacterial capacity to inactivate the drug may be increased.

3. **Increased PABA synthesis:** Production of the natural substrate, PABA, by the microorganism may be enhanced through selection or mutation.

D. Pharmacology

1. **Administration:** Most sulfa drugs are well absorbed after oral administration. *Sulfasalazine* [sul fa SAL a zeen], when administered orally or as a suppository, is reserved for treatment of chronic inflammatory bowel disease (e.g., Crohn's disease or ulcerative colitis), because it is not absorbed. Intravenous sulfonamides are generally reserved for patients who are unable to take oral preparations.

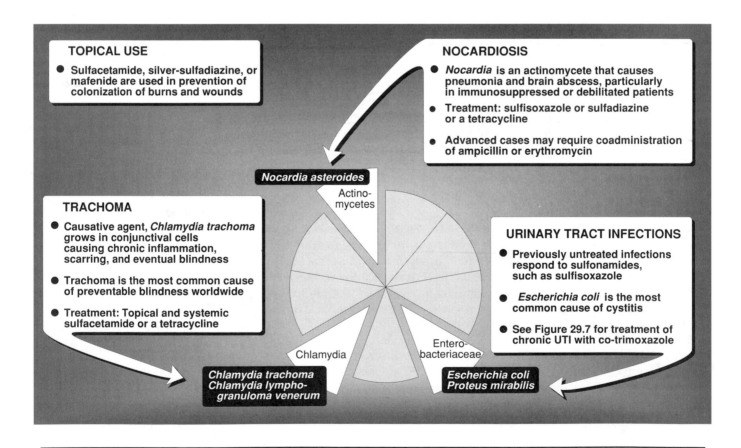

Figure 29.3
Typical therapeutic applications of sulfonamides. UTI= urinary tract infection.

2. **Distribution:**

   a. Sulfa drugs are distributed <u>throughout body water</u> and <u>penetrate well into cerebrospinal fluid</u> even in the absence of inflammation. They can also <u>pass the placental barrier.</u>

   b. Sulfa drugs are partially bound to serum albumin; the extent of binding depends on the particular agent.

3. **Metabolism:** The sulfas are <u>acetylated at N4</u>, primarily in the liver. The product is <u>devoid of antimicrobial activity, but it retains the toxic potential to precipitate at neutral or acidic pH, causing crystalluria ("stone formation")</u> and therefore potential damage to the kidney (Figure 29.4).

4. **Excretion:** Elimination of sulfas is by glomerular filtration. Therefore, depressed kidney function causes accumulation of both the parent compounds and their metabolites.

E. Adverse effects

1. **Crystalluria:** Nephrotoxicity develops as a result of crystalluria. Newer agents, such as *sulfisoxazole* [sul fi SOX a zole] and *sulfamethoxazole* [sul fa meth OX a zole] are more soluble at urinary pH than are the older sulfonamides (e.g., *sulfadiazine*) and are less liable to cause crystalluria. Adequate hydration and alkalinization of urine prevent the problem.

2. **Hypersensitivity:** Hypersensitivity reactions, such as rashes, angioedema, and Stevens-Johnson syndrome, are fairly common.

3. **Hemopoietic disturbances:** Hemolytic anemia is encountered in patients with glucose 6-phosphate dehydrogenase deficiency (p.322). Granulocytopenia and thrombocytopenia can also occur.

4. **Kernicterus:** This disorder may occur in newborns because of the displacement of bilirubin from its binding site on serum albumin and its subsequent penetration into the central nervous system.

5. **Drug potentiation:** Transient potentiation of the hypoglycemic effect of *tolbutamide* (p.10 and p.242)) or the anticoagulant effect of *warfarin* or of *bishydroxycoumarin* (p.191) results from their displacement from binding sites on serum albumin.

6. **Contraindications:** Sulfonamides form complexes with formaldehyde and therefore should not be given to patients receiving *methenamine* (p.300).

III. TRIMETHOPRIM

Trimethoprim [trye METH oh prim], a <u>potent inhibitor of bacterial dihydrofolate reductase</u>, exhibits an antibacterial spectrum similar to

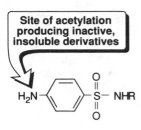

Figure 29.4
Structural features of sulfonamides.

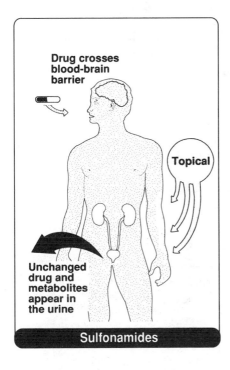

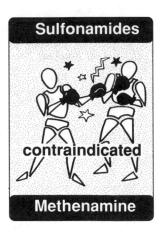

Sulfonamides

contraindicated

Methenamine

the sulfonamides. However, *trimethoprim* is most often compounded with *sulfamethoxazole* (p.269).

A. Mechanism of action

The active form of folate is the tetrahydro-derivative that is formed through reduction by dihydrofolate reductase. This enzymatic reduction (Figure 29.5) is inhibited by *trimethoprim,* causing the folate coenzymes to be unavailable for purine, pyrimidine, and amino acid synthesis.[2] The inhibitory action of *trimethoprim* is much stronger for the bacterial reductase than for the mammalian enzyme, which accounts for its selective toxicity. [Note: Examples of other folate reductase inhibitors include *pyrimethamine,* which is used with sulfonamides in parasitic infections (p.320), and *methotrexate,* which is used in cancer chemotherapy (p.341).]

B. Antibacterial spectrum

The antibacterial spectrum of *trimethoprim* is similar to that of *sulfamethoxazole* (p.266); however, *trimethoprim* is 20 to 50 times more potent than the sulfonamide. *Trimethoprim* may be used alone in acute urinary tract infections.

C. Resistance

Resistance in gram-negative bacteria is due to the presence of a dihydrofolate reductase that is altered so that it has a lower affinity for the drug.

D. Pharmacology

The pharmacologic characteristics of *trimethoprim* are similar to sulfonamides, but higher concentrations are achieved in prostatic fluid. *Trimethoprim* undergoes O-demethylation.

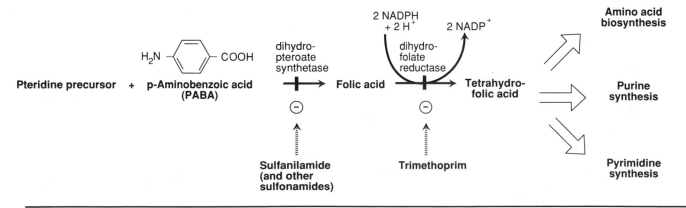

Figure 29.5
Inhibition of tetrahydrofolate synthesis by sulfonamides and trimethoprim.

E. Adverse effects

Trimethoprim can produce the effects of folate deficiency, that is, megaloblastic anemia, leukopenia, and granulocytopenia. These reactions can be reversed by the simultaneous administration of folinic acid, which does not enter bacteria.

IV. CO-TRIMOXAZOLE

Trimethoprim is most often compounded with the sulfa drug, *sulfamethoxazole.* The resulting combination, called *co-trimoxazole,* shows greater antimicrobial activity than equivalent quantities of either drug used alone. The combination was selected because of the similarity in the pharmacokinetics of the two drugs.

A. Mechanism of action

The synergistic antimicrobial activity of *co-trimoxazole* [co trye MOX a zole] results from its inhibition of two sequential steps in the synthesis of tetrahydrofolic acid: *sulfamethoxazole* inhibits the incorporation of PABA into folic acid, and *trimethoprim* prevents reduction of dihydrofolate to tetrahydrofolate (Figure 29.5). *Co-trimoxazole* exhibits more potent antimicrobial activity than *sulfamethoxazole* or *trimethoprim* alone (Figure 29.6). The most effective ratio of the drugs in the plasma is 20 parts of *sulfamethoxazole* to 1 part of *trimethoprim.*

B. Antibacterial spectrum

The combination of *trimethoprim-sulfamethoxazole* has a broader spectrum of action than the sulfas (Figure 29.7).

C. Resistance

Resistance to the *trimethoprim-sulfamethoxazole* combination is less frequently encountered than resistance to either of the drugs alone, because it requires simultaneous resistance to both drugs.

D. Pharmacology

1. **Administration and metabolism:** *Co-trimoxazole* is generally administered orally. An exception involves intravenous administration to patients with severe pneumonia caused by Pneumocystis carinii, or to patients who cannot take the drug by mouth. A nebulized (vaporized) preparation is also available.

2. **Fate:** *Trimethoprim* concentrates in the relatively acidic milieu of prostatic and vaginal fluids and accounts for the use of the *trimethoprim-sulfamethoxazole* combination in infections at these sites.

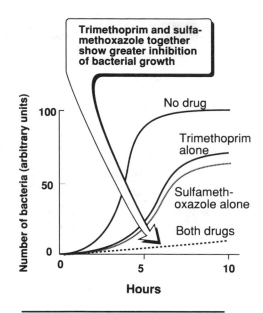

Figure 29.6
Synergism between trimethoprim and sulfamethoxazole on the inhbition of growth of *Escherichia coli.*

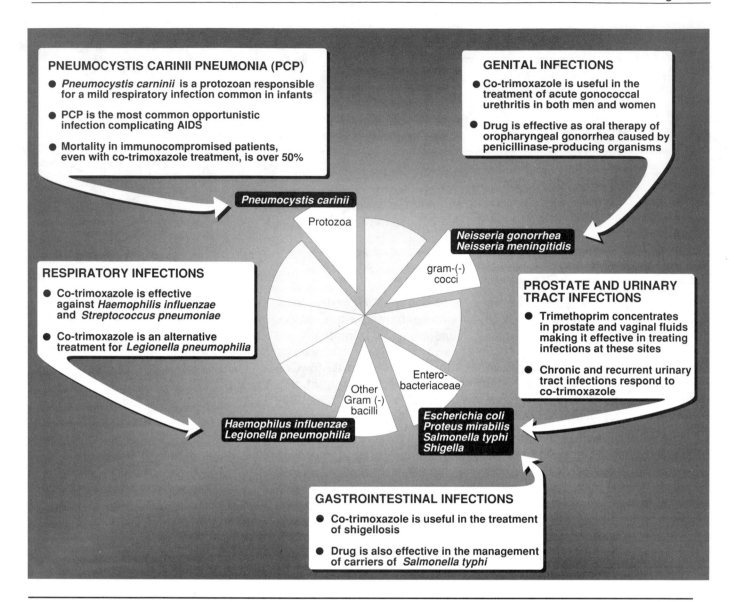

Figure 29.7
Typical therapeutic applications of co-trimoxazole (sulfamethoxazole plus trimethoprim).

E. Adverse effects

1. **Dermatological:** Reactions involving the skin are very common and may be severe in the elderly.

2. **Gastrointestinal:** Nausea, vomiting as well as glossitis, and stomatitis are not unusual.

3. **Hematological:** Megaloblastic anemia, leukopenia, and thrombocytopenia may occur; all of these effects may be reversed by the concurrent administration of folinic acid (p.342).

4. Patients with pneumocystis pneumonia frequently have drug-induced fever, rashes, diarrhea and/or pancytopenia.

Study Questions (see p.428 for answers).

Choose the ONE best answer.

29.1 Sulfonamides are useful in the treatment of which one of the following?

   A. Influenza.
   B. Gonorrhea.
   C. Most streptococcal infections.
   D. Urinary tract infections.
   E. Meningococcal infections.

29.2 Sulfonamides are agents of choice in the treatment of which one of the following?

   A. Syphilis.
   B. Cholera.
   C. Nocardiosis.
   D. Streptococcal pneumonia.
   E. Rickettsial infections.

29.3 Trimethoprim

   A. is less potent than sulfamethoxazole.
   B. inhibits the enzyme dihydropteroate synthetase.
   C. causes adverse effects that can be lessened by simultaneous administration of folinic acid.
   D. resistance has not been observed in microorganisms.
   E. stimulates purine synthesis.

29.4 All of the following statements concerning sulfonamides are correct EXCEPT:

   A. They require actively growing cultures for maximum antimicrobial activity.
   B. Allergic reactions are frequently seen adverse effects.
   C. Treatment of patients with severe renal insufficiency may lead to crystalluria.
   D. They diminish activity of warfarin.
   E. They compete with p-aminobenzoic acid for the enzyme dihydropteroate synthetase.

29.5 Sulfonamides increase the risk of neonatal kernicterus because they

   A. diminish the production of plasma albumin.
   B. increase the turnover of red blood cells.
   C. inhibit the metabolism of bilirubin.
   D. compete for bilirubin binding sites on plasma albumin.
   E. depress the bone marrow.

Questions 29.6 - 29.9: For each phrase, select the ONE drug (A-E) that is most closely associated with it. Each drug (A-E) may be selected once, more than once, or not at all.

   A. Sulfasalazine
   B. Sulfadiazine
   C. Trimethoprim-sulfamethoxazole
   D. Mafenide acetate
   E. Sulfisoxazole

29.6 It is used to prevent infections among burn patients.

29.7 It is used in the treatment of ulcerative colitis.

29.8 It is effective in treating complicated or recurrent urinary infections.

29.9 It can cause crystalluria in patients with renal insufficiency.

Answer A if 1,2 and 3 are correct.
    B if 1 and 3 are correct.
    C if 2 and 4 are correct.
    D if only 4 is correct.
    E if 1,2,3, and 4 are all correct.

29.10 Which of the following statements is/are true for the combination of trimethoprim-sulfamethoxazole?

  1. It has a broader spectrum of antimicrobial activity than either drug alone.
  2. It is used in the management of carriers of Salmonella typhi.
  3. It is effective in the treatment of pneumonia caused by Pneumocystis carinii.
  4. It is the drug of choice in treating enterococcal endocarditis.

29.11 Sulfisoxazole

  1. lowers the ratio of tetrahydrofolate to folate.
  2. is antagonized by p-aminobenzoic acid.
  3. is bactericidal.
  4. is useful in treating nocardiosis.

[1]See *folic acid* in **Biochemistry** for a discussion of the synthesis of folic acid (see index).

[2]See *tetrahydrofolic acid* in **Biochemistry** for the role of folic acid in purine and pyrimidine synthesis.

Inhibitors of Cell Wall Synthesis

30

I. OVERVIEW

Some antimicrobial drugs selectively interfere with the synthesis of the bacterial cell wall. To be maximally effective, these agents require actively proliferating microorganisms; they have little or no effect on bacteria that are not growing. The most important members of the group are the β-lactam antibiotics (Figure 30.2).

II. PENICILLINS

The penicillins [pen i SILL in] are the most widely effective antibiotics and are among the least toxic drugs known; the major adverse reaction to penicillins is hypersensitivity. The members of this family differ in their antimicrobial spectrum as well as in their stability to stomach acid and in their susceptibility to degradative enzymes. Figure 30.1 shows the main structural features of the penicillins. Figure 30.2 shows the classification of agents affecting cell wall synthesis.

A. Mechanism of action

Penicillins interfere with the last step of bacterial cell wall synthesis and thus cause cell lysis. They are therefore bactericidal. They are only effective against rapidly growing organisms that synthesize a peptidoglycan cell wall. Consequently, they are inactive against mycobacteria, fungi, and viruses.

1. **Penicillin binding proteins:** Penicillins bind to and inactivate proteins present on the bacterial cell membrane. These penicillin binding proteins (PBPs) are enzymes involved in the synthesis of the cell wall and in the maintenance of the morphological features of the bacteria. Exposure to these antibiotics can therefore lead to morphological changes or lysis of susceptible bacteria.

2. **Inhibition of transpeptidase:** PBPs catalyze formation of cross-linkages between peptidoglycan chains. Penicillin inhibits the transpeptidase step, thus hindering the formation of crosslinks essential for cell wall integrity. As a result, cell wall synthesis is blocked and the "Park peptide", UDP-acetylmuramyl-L-Ala-D-Gln-L-Lys-D-Ala-D-Ala, accumulates.

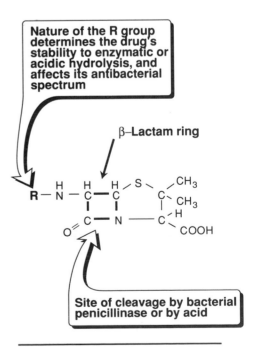

Figure 30.1
Structural features of β-lactam antibiotics.

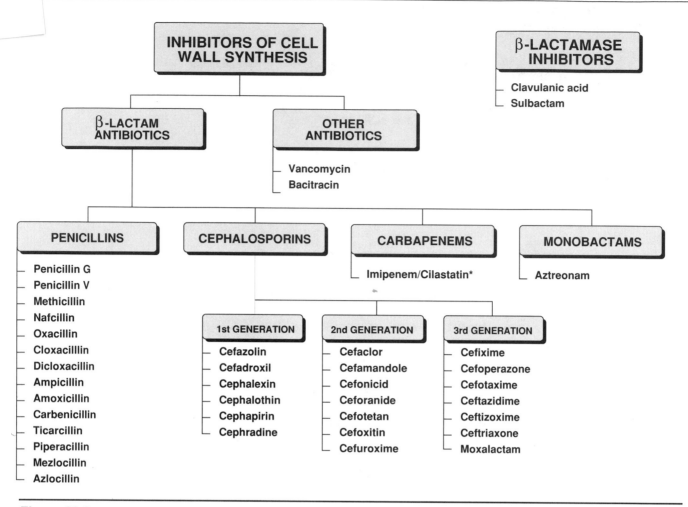

Figure 30.2
Summary of antimicrobial agents affecting cell wall synthesis *[Note: Cilastatin is not an antibiotic but an inhibitor of kidney peptidase.]

3. **Autolysins:** Many bacteria, particularly the gram-positive cocci, produce degradative enzymes (autolysins) that participate in the normal remodeling of the bacterial cell wall. In the presence of *penicillin,* the degradative action of the autolysins proceeds in the absence of cell wall synthesis. Thus, the antibacterial effect of *penicillin* is the result of both inhibition of cell wall synthesis and destruction of existing cell wall by autolysins.

B. Antibacterial spectrum

The antibacterial spectrum of the various penicillins is determined, in part, by their ability to cross the bacterial peptidoglycan cell wall and to reach the penicillin-binding proteins. In general, gram-positive microorganisms have cell walls that are easily traversed by penicillins and therefore (in the absence of resistance) are susceptible to these drugs. Gram-negative microorganisms have an outer lipid membrane surrounding the cell wall. This presents a barrier to the water-soluble penicillins that cannot reach the site of action. [Note: For this reason, penicillins have little use in the treatment of intracellular pathogens.]

1. **Natural penicillins**

   a. *Penicillin G* (*benzylpenicillin*) is the cornerstone of therapy for infections caused by a number of gram-positive and gram-negative cocci, gram-positive bacilli, and spirochetes (Figure 30.3). *Penicillin G* is susceptible to inactivation by β-lactamases (penicillinases, Figure 30.4).

   b. *Penicillin V* has a spectrum similar to *penicillin G,* but it is not used for treatment of septicemia because of its higher minimum lethal concentration (MLC, the minimum amount of the drug needed to eliminate the infection). *Penicillin V* is more acid-stable than *penicillin G.*

2. **Antistaphylococcal penicillins:** *Methicillin* [meth i SILL in], *nafcillin* [naf SILL in], *oxacillin* [ox a SILL in], *cloxacillin* [klox a SILL in], and *dicloxacillin* [dye klox a SILL in] are penicillinase-resistant penicillins. Their use is restricted to the treatment of infections caused by penicillinase-producing staphylococci. Methicillin-resistant strains are usually susceptible to *vancomycin,* and possibly to *ciprofloxacin, rifampin,* or *imipenem/cilastatin.*

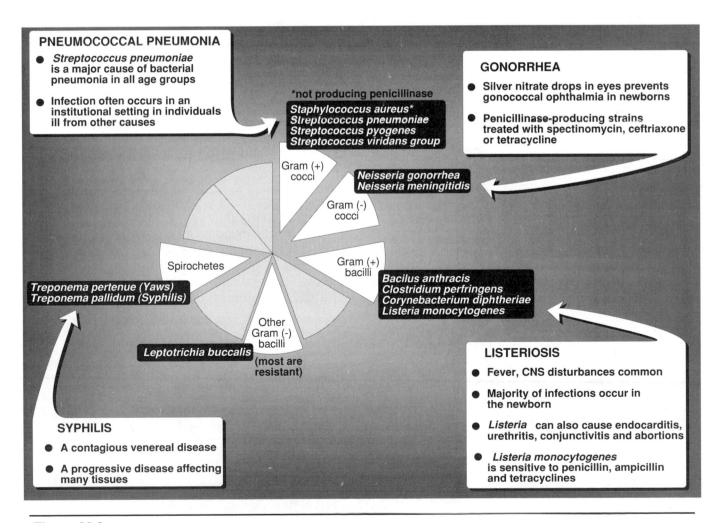

Figure 30.3
Typical therapeutic applications of penicillin G.

3. **Extended spectrum penicillins:** *Ampicillin* [am pi SIL in] and *amoxicillin* [a mox i SIL in] are less potent than *penicillin G* against gram-positive and gram-negative cocci. *Ampicillin* is the drug of choice for the gram-positive bacillus, <u>Listeria monocytogenes</u>. These drugs are called extended spectrum penicillins because of their activity against the gram-negative bacilli (Figure 30.5A). Resistance to these antibiotics is now a problem because of inactivation by plasmid-mediated penicillinase. Formulation with a β-lactamase inhibitor, such as *clavulanic acid* or *sulbactam*, can protect the penicillins from enzymatic action. (See p.282 for a discussion of these inhibitors.)

4. **Antipseudomonal penicillins:** *Carbenicillin* [kar ben i SIL in], *ticarcillin* [tye kar SILL in], and *piperacillin* [pi PER a sill in] are the antipseudomonal penicillins. *Piperacillin* is the most potent. They are effective against many gram-negative bacilli but are ineffective against klebsiella, because of its constitutive penicillinase (Figure 30.5B). Formulation of *ticarcillin* with *clavulanic acid* (see p.282) extends the antimicrobial spectrum to include penicillinase-producing organisms.

5. **Acylureido penicillins:** *Mezlocillin* [mez loe SILL in] and *azlocillin* [az loe SILL in] are also effective against <u>Pseudomonas aeruginosa</u> and a large number of gram-negative organisms.

6. **Penicillins and aminoglycosides:** The antibacterial effects of all the β-lactam antibiotics are synergistic with the aminoglycosides. Although the combination is often employed clinically, these drug types should never be placed in the same infusion fluid, because the positively charged aminoglycosides form an inactive complex with the negatively charged penicillins.

C. Resistance

Natural resistance occurs in organisms that either lack the peptidoglycan cell wall (for example, mycoplasma) or have cell wall that is impermeable to the drug. Acquired resistance to the antimicrobial actions of the penicillins by plasmid transfer has become a significant clinical problem. By obtaining a resistance plasmid, a bacterium may acquire the following abilities to withstand the β-lactamase.

1. **β-lactamase activity:** This family of enzymes hydrolyzes the cyclic amide bond of the β-lactam ring, which results in loss of bactericidal activity (see Figure 30.1). The β-Lactamases are either constitutive or, more commonly, are acquired by the transfer of plasmids. Some of the β-lactam antibiotics are poor substrates for β-lactamases and resist cleavage; thus they retain their activity against β-lactamase-producing organisms.

2. **Decreased permeability to drug:** Decreased penetration of the antibiotic through the outer cell membrane prevents the drug from reaching the target penicillin-binding proteins.

3. **Altered penicillin binding proteins:** Modified PBPs show a lower affinity for β-lactam antibiotics, requiring greater concentrations

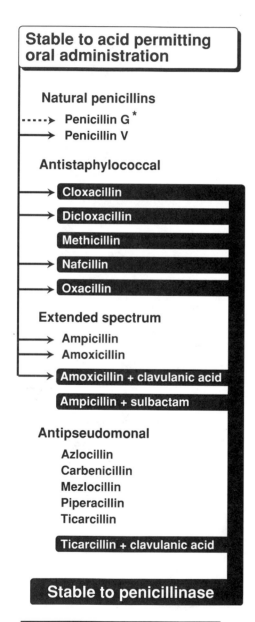

Figure 30.4
Stability of the penicillins to acid or the action of penicillinase
*[Note: Penicillin is largely inactivated by stomach acid, but doses can be adjusted so that adequate serum levels are achieved.]

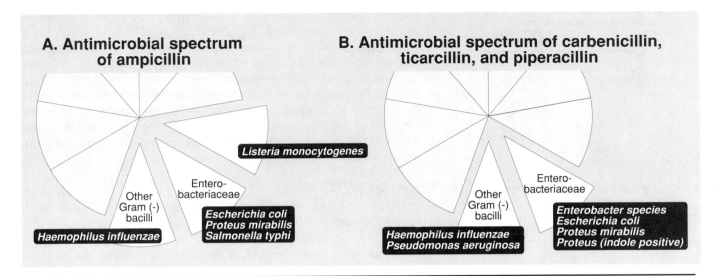

Figure 30.5
Typical therapeutic applications of ampicillin (A) and the antipseudomonal penicillins (B).

of the drug to effect binding and inhibition of bacterial growth. This mechanism may explain methicillin-resistant staphylococci.

D. Pharmacology

1. **Administration:** The route of administration is determined by the stability of the drug to gastric acid and by the severity of the infection.

   a. *Methicillin, ticarcillin, carbenicillin, mezlocillin, piperacillin, azlocillin,* and *ampicillin* plus *sulbactam* must be administered via intravenous (IV) or intramuscular (IM) pathways. *Penicillin V, amoxicillin,* and *amoxicillin* combined with *clavulanic acid* are only available as oral preparations. Others are effective by the oral, IV, or IM routes (see Figure 30.4).

   b. *Procaine penicillin G* and *benzathine penicillin G* are administered intramuscularly and serve as depot forms, as they are slowly absorbed into the circulation over a long time period.

2. **Absorption:** Most of the penicillins are incompletely absorbed after oral administration and reach the intestine in sufficient amounts to affect the composition of the intestinal flora. However, *amoxicillin* is almost completely absorbed. Consequently, it is not appropriate therapy for the treatment of salmonella-derived enteritis, since therapeutically effective levels do not reach the organisms in the intestinal crypts. Absorption of *penicillin G* and all the penicillinase-resistant penicillins is impeded by food in the stomach. Therefore, they must be administered 30-60 minutes before meals or 2-3 hours postprandially. Other penicillins are less affected by food.

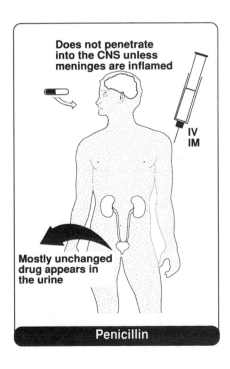

Does not penetrate into the CNS unless meninges are inflamed

IV
IM

Mostly unchanged drug appears in the urine

Penicillin

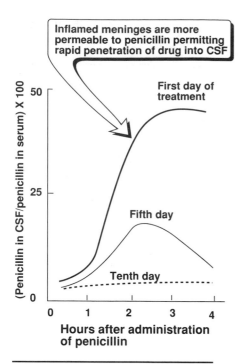

Figure 30.6
Enhanced penetration of penicillin into the cerebral spinal fluid (CSF) during inflammation.

3. **Distribution:** Distribution of the free drug throughout the body is good. All the penicillins cross the placental barrier, but none have been shown to be teratogenic. However, penetration into certain sites such as bone or cerebrospinal fluid is insufficient for therapy, unless these sites are inflamed (Figure 30.6). During the acute phase (first day), the inflamed meninges are more permeable to *penicillin,* resulting in an increased ratio in the amount of drug in the central nervous system compared to the amount in the serum. As the infection abates, inflammation subsides, and permeability barriers are reestablished.

4. **Metabolism:** Metabolism of these drugs by the host is usually insignificant, but some metabolism of *penicillin G* has been shown to occur in patients with impaired renal function.

5. **Excretion:** The primary route of excretion is through the organic acid secretory system of the kidney (p.212), as well as by glomerular filtration. Patients with impaired renal function must have dosage regimens adjusted. *Probenecid* also inhibits the secretion of penicillins.

E. Adverse reactions

Penicillins are among the safest drugs, and blood levels are not monitored, although adverse reactions do occur.

1. **Hypersensitivity:** This is the most important adverse effect of the penicillins. The major cause of *penicillin* hypersensitivity is its metabolite, penicilloic acid, which reacts with proteins and serves as a hapten to cause an immune reaction. Approximately 5% of patients have some kind of reaction, ranging from urticaria to angioedema (marked swelling of lips, tongue, periorbital area) and anaphylaxis. Cross-allergic reactions can occur among the β-lactam antibiotics. Although rashes can develop with all the penicillins, maculopapular rashes are most common with *ampicillin.* Among patients with mononucleosis who are treated with *ampicillin,* the incidence of maculopapular rash approaches 100%. A rash is also commonly seen in patients receiving both *allopurinol* (p.376) and *ampicillin.*

2. **Diarrhea:** This reaction, which is caused by a disruption of the normal balance of intestinal microorganisms, is a common problem. It occurs to a greater extent with those agents that are incompletely absorbed.

3. **Nephritis:** Acute interstitial nephritis can occur in patients receiving high doses of *methicillin.*

4. **Neurotoxicity:** The penicillins are irritating to neuronal tissue and can provoke seizures if injected intrathecally or if very high blood levels are reached. Epileptic patients are especially at risk.

5. **Platelet dysfunction:** This side effect, which involves decreased agglutination, is observed with the antipseudomonal penicillins (*carbenicillin* and *ticarcillin*) and, to some extent, with *penicillin*

G. It is generally a concern when treating patients predisposed to hemorrhage or those receiving anticoagulants.

6. **Cation toxicity:** Penicillins are generally administered as the sodium or potassium salt. Toxicities may be caused by the large quantities of sodium or potassium that may accompany the penicillin. Sodium excess may result in hypokalemic acidosis. This can be avoided by using the most potent antibiotic, which permits lower doses of drug and accompanying cations.

III. CEPHALOSPORINS

The cephalosporins and their analogs, the cephamycins, are β-lactam antibiotics that are closely related both structurally (Figure 30.7) and functionally to the penicillins. Cephalosporins have the same mode of action and mechanism of resistance as the penicillins, but they tend to be more resistant than the penicillins to β-lactamases.

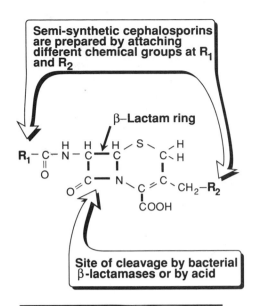

Figure 30.7
Structural features of cephalosporins.

A. Antibacterial spectrum

Cephalosporins have been classified as first, second or third generation, largely on the basis of bacterial susceptibility patterns and resistance to β-lactamases (Figure 30.8).

1. **First generation:** Cephalosporins designated first generation (Figure 30.8) include *penicillin G* substitutes that are resistant to the staphylococcal penicillinase. They also have activity against Proteus mirabilis, Escherichia coli, and Klebsiella pneumoniae (the acronym **PEcK** has been suggested).

2. **Second generation:** The second generation cephalosporins display greater activity against three additional gram-negative organisms, Haemophilus influenzae, some Enterobacter aerogenes and Neisseria species (**HENPEcK**), whereas activity against gram-positive organisms is weaker. [Note: *Cefoxitin* [se FOX i tin] is the most potent cephalosporin against Bacteroides fragilis.]

3. **Third generation:** These cephalosporins are greatly inferior to first generation cephalosporins in regard to their activity against gram-positive cocci, but third generation cephalosporins have enhanced activity against gram-negative bacilli, including those mentioned above plus most other enteric organisms and Serratia marcescens.

B. Resistance

Mechanisms of bacterial resistance to the cephalosporins are essentially the same as those described for the penicillins.

C. Pharmacology

1. **Administration:** All the cephalosporins (except for those highlighted in Figure 30.8) must be administered intravenously because of their poor oral absorption.

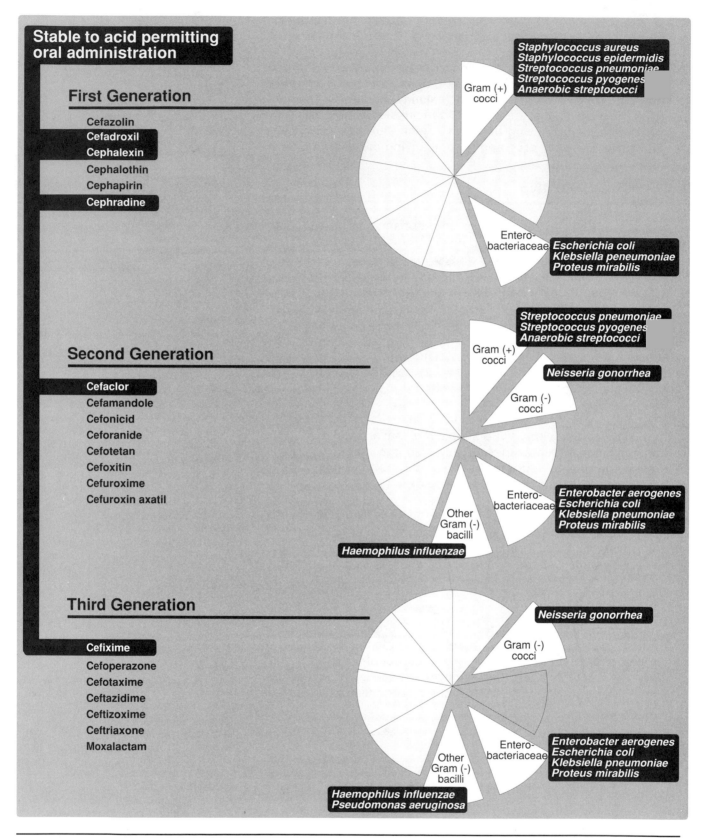

Figure 30.8
Clinically important antimicrobial spectrum of first, second, and third generation cephalosporins.

2. **Distribution:** All of these antibiotics distribute very well into body fluids. However, adequate therapeutic levels in the cerebrospinal fluid (CSF), regardless of inflammation, are achieved only with the third generation cephalosporins (for example, *cefotaxime* [sef oh TAKS eem] is the drug of choice for the treatment of meningitis caused by *Haemophilus influenzae*).

3. **Fate:** Biotransformation of cephalosporins by the host is not clinically important. Elimination occurs through tubular secretion and/or glomerular filtration; thus doses must be adjusted in the case of severe renal failure to guard against accumulation and toxicity. *Cefoperazone* and *ceftriaxone* are excreted through the bile into the feces and are frequently employed in patients with renal insufficiency.

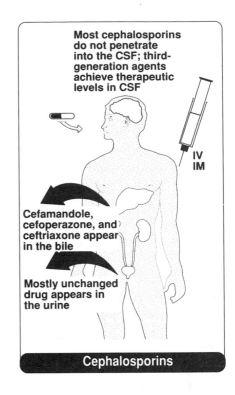

Cephalosporins

D. Adverse effects

The cephalosporins produce a number of adverse affects, some of which are unique to particular members of the group.

1. **Allergic manifestations:** The cephalosporins should be avoided or used with caution in individuals allergic to penicillins (about 15% show cross-sensitivity). In contrast, the incidence of allergic reactions to cephalosporins is 1-2% in patients without a history of penicillin allergy.

2. **A disulfiram-like effect:** When *cefamandole, cefoperazone,* and *moxalactam* [MOX a lak tam] are ingested with alcohol or alcohol-containing medications, a disulfiram-like effect is seen, because these cephalosporins block the second step in alcohol oxidation which results in the accumulation of acetaldehyde.

3. **Bleeding:** Bleeding can occur with *cefamandole, cefoperazone,* or *moxalactam,* because of anti-vitamin K effects; administration of the vitamin corrects the problem. This property of *moxalactam* has resulted in its being held in reserve.

IV. OTHER β-LACTAM ANTIBIOTICS

A. Carbapenems

Carbapenems are synthetic β-lactam antibiotics that differ from the penicillins in the sulfur atom of the thiazolidine ring (Figure 30.9). *Imipenem* [i mi PEN em] is the only drug of the group currently available.

1. **Antibacterial spectrum:** *Imipenem/cilastatin* is the broadest spectrum β-lactam antibiotic currently available. It is active against penicillinase-producing gram-positive and gram-negative organisms, anaerobes, and <u>Pseudomonas aeruginosa</u>, although other pseudomonas strains are resistant. However, resistant strains of <u>Pseudomonas aeruginosa</u> have been reported to arise during therapy. *Imipenem* resists hydrolysis by most β-lactamases. The drug plays a role in empiric therapy.

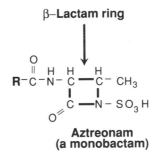

Figure 30.9
Structural features of carbapenem and monobactams.

2. **Pharmacology:** *Imipenem* is administered intravenously and penetrates well into the central nervous system. It is excreted by glomerular filtration and undergoes cleavage by a dehydropeptidase found in the brush border of the proximal renal tubule to form an inactive metabolite that is potentially nephrotoxic. Compounding the *imipenem* with *cilastatin,* a dehydropeptidase inhibitor, protects the parent drug from cleavage and thus prevents the formation of a toxic metabolite. This allows the drug to be active in the treatment of urinary tract infections. [Note: The dose must be adjusted in patients with renal insufficiency.]

3. **Adverse effects:** *Imipenem/cilastatin* can cause nausea, vomiting, and diarrhea. Eosinophilia and neutropenia are less common. High levels of these agents may provoke seizures.

B. Monobactams

The monobactams, of which *aztreonam* [az tree oh nam] is the only commercially available example, are unique because the β-lactam ring is not fused to another ring (Figure 30.9). Monobactams also disrupt cell wall synthesis. The drug's narrow antimicrobial spectrum precludes its use alone in empiric therapy (p.260). *Aztreonam* is resistant to the action of β-lactamases.

1. **Antibacterial spectrum:** The antibacterial activity of *aztreonam* is primarily directed against the enterobacteriaceae. *Aztreonam* is unique among the β-lactam group because of its effectiveness against <u>Pseudomonas aeruginosa</u> and other aerobic gram-negative bacteria, and because of its lack of activity against gram-positive organisms or anaerobes.

2. **Pharmacology:** *Aztreonam* is administered via IV or IM routes. It is excreted in the urine and can accumulate in patients with renal failure.

3. **Adverse effects:** *Aztreonam* is relatively nontoxic, but it may cause phlebitis, skin rash, and occasionally, abnormal liver function tests. *Aztreonam* has a low immunogenic potential and shows little cross-reactivity with antibodies induced by other β-lactams. Thus *aztreonam* may offer a safe alternative for treating patients allergic to *penicillin.*

V. β-LACTAMASE INHIBITORS

Hydrolysis of the β-lactam ring, either by enzymatic cleavage via a β-lactamase or by acid, destroys antimicrobial activity. β-Lactamase inhibitors, such as *clavulanic acid* and *sulbactam,* contain a β-lactam ring, but they do not have significant antibacterial activity. Instead, they bind to and inactivate β-lactamases, thereby protecting the antibiotics that are normally substrates for these enzymes. The β-lactamase inhibitors are formulated with the penicillin derivatives to protect the latter from enzymatic inactivation. Figure 30.10 shows the

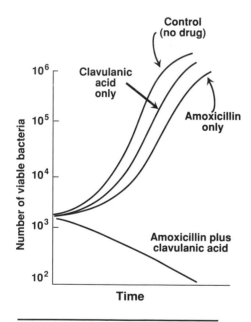

Figure 30.10
The growth of *Escherichia coli* in the presence of amoxicillin, with and without clavulanic acid.

effect of *clavulanic acid* and *amoxicillin* on the growth of a β-lactamase-producing <u>Escherichia</u> <u>coli</u>. Note that *clavulanic acid* alone is nearly devoid of antibacterial activity.

VI. OTHER AGENTS AFFECTING THE CELL WALL

A. Vancomycin

Because of the severe adverse side effects of early preparations, *vancomycin* [van koe MYE sin], a mixture of glycopeptides, was seldom used as an antibiotic. The emergence of staphylococci resistant to most antibiotics except *vancomycin* led to the reintroduction of this agent, particularly as a first line of attack against the increasing number of staphylococci and streptococci that are resistant to β-lactam antibiotics.

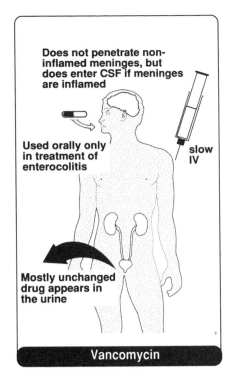

Vancomycin

1. **Mode of action:** It inhibits synthesis of bacterial cell wall phospholipids as well as peptidoglycan polymers.

2. **Antibacterial spectrum**: *Vancomycin* is bactericidal. Its present use is mainly restricted to treating infections caused by *methicillin*-resistant staphylococci, and pseudomembranous colitis caused by <u>Clostridium</u> <u>difficile</u> or staphylococci, as well as being used prophylactically in dental patients with prosthetic heart valves or in patients allergic to *penicillin* who are undergoing certain types of surgery.

3. **Resistance:** Occurring rarely, resistance is due to plasmid-mediated changes in permeability to the drug and probably is also affected by decreased binding of *vancomycin* to receptor molecules.

4. **Pharmacology**: Slow intravenous infusion is employed for treatment of systemic infections or for prophylaxis. Because *vancomycin* is not absorbed after oral administration, this route is employed for the treatment of antibiotic-induced colitis. Inflammation allows penetration into the meninges. Metabolism has not been characterized. Excretion is by glomerular filtration.

5. **Adverse effects:** Side effects are a serious problem with *vancomycin* and include fever, chills, and/or phlebitis at the infusion site; shock has occurred as a result of rapid administration. Rashes may be seen on chronic administration. Dose-related ototoxicity (cochlear damage) is associated with serum levels above 80 μg/ml. Nephrotoxicity is less frequent than with earlier preparations but may still occur.

B. Bacitracin

Bacitracin [bass i TRAY sin] is a mixture of polypeptides that inhibits bacterial cell wall synthesis. It is active against a wide variety of gram-positive organisms. Its use is restricted to topical application because of its potential for nephrotoxicity.

Study questions   (see p.429 for answers).

Choose the ONE best answer.

30.1 Which one of the following drugs is both penicillinase-resistant and effective by oral administration?

   A. Methicillin.
   B. Carbenicillin.
   C. Penicillin V.
   D. Amoxicillin plus clavulanic acid.
   E. Piperacillin.

30.2 Which one of the following antibiotics is INCORRECTLY matched with an appropriate clinical indication?

   A. Penicillin G: Pneumonia caused by Klebsiella pneumoniae
   B. Carbenicillin: Urinary tract infection caused by Pseudomonas aeruginosa
   C. Ampicillin: Bacterial meningitis caused by Haemophilus influenzae
   D. Penicillin G: Syphilis caused by Treponema pallidum
   E. Cefazolin: Osteomyelitis

30.3 Piperacillin differs from ampicillin in all of the following properties EXCEPT:

   A. Stability in gastric acid.
   B. Effectiveness as an antipseudomonal agent.
   C. Resistance to penicillinase.
   D. Spectrum of antibacterial action.
   E. The broadness of the spectrum of susceptible bacteria.

30.4 All of the following statements about penicillin G are correct EXCEPT:

   A. It is excreted from the body primarily via the hepatobiliary route.
   B. Administered orally, it is variably absorbed because of its degradation by stomach acid.
   C. It is more effective in killing growing bacteria than microorganisms in the stationary phase.
   D. It can act synergistically with aminoglycosides.
   E. Levels in the blood can be increased by administration of probenecid.

30.5 Which one of the following statements about inhibitors of cell wall synthesis is INCORRECT?

   A. The concentration of penicillin in the cerebrospinal fluid is higher when administered to patients with meningococcal meningitis than it is when given to normal patients.
   B. First generation cephalosporins are more effective against staphylococcal infections than are third generation cephalosporins.
   C. Cefoxitin is less likely to cause an allergic reaction in a patient that is hypersensitive to penicillin G than is penicillin V.
   D. The half-life of procaine penicillin administered intramuscularly is greater than the half-life of penicillin G administered orally.
   E. Third-generation cephalosporins are susceptible to β-lactamase activity.

Answer A if 1,2 and 3 are correct.
   B if 1 and 3 are correct.
   C if 2 and 4 are correct.
   D if only 4 is correct.
   E if 1,2,3 and 4 are all correct.

30.6 Cephalosporins:

   1. have the same mode of action as the penicillins.
   2. are more resistant to β-lactamases than are the penicillins.
   3. contain the β-lactam ring.
   4. as a group are all stable to stomach acid.

30.7 Third generation cephalosporins:

   1. show greater activity than first generation cephalosporins against gram-negative bacilli.
   2. include agents that are active against Pseudomonas aeruginosa.
   3. include agents that are effective in treating Serratia marcescens infections.
   4. include agents that are effective in treating meningitis.

30.8 Vancomycin:

   1. has an antibacterial spectrum similar to that of penicillin G.
   2. is effective against methicillin-resistant staphylococci.
   3. is given orally for the treatment of antibiotic-induced colitis.
   4. is inactivated by β-lactamases.

Protein Synthesis Inhibitors

31

I. OVERVIEW

Several antibiotics exert their antimicrobial effect by targeting the bacterial ribosome, which has components that differ structurally from those of the mammalian cytoplasmic ribosome (Figure 31.1). The mammalian mitochondrial ribosome, however, more closely resembles the bacterial ribosome. Thus, although drugs that interact with the bacterial site usually spare the host cells, high levels of drugs like *chloramphenicol* or the tetracyclines may cause toxic effects as a result of interaction with the mitochondrial ribosomes.

II. TETRACYCLINES

Tetracyclines [tet ra SYE kleen] are a group of closely related compounds that have small differences in clinical efficacy that reflect a variation in the pharmacokinetics of each agent.

A. Mode of action

Entry of these agents into susceptible organisms is mediated by transport proteins located in the bacterial inner cytoplasmic membrane. Binding of the drug to the 30S subunit of the bacterial ribosome is believed to block access of the amino acyl-tRNA to the mRNA-ribosome complex at the acceptor site, thus inhibiting bacterial protein synthesis.[1]

B. Antibacterial spectrum

As broad spectrum antibiotics, the tetracyclines are also effective against organisms other than bacteria. Tetracyclines are generally bacteriostatic and are the drugs of choice for infections shown in Figure 31.2.

C. Resistance

Widespread resistance to tetracyclines limits their clinical uses. The most commonly encountered naturally occurring R factor confers the inability of the organism to accumulate the drug, thus conferring resistance. Any organism resistant to one tetracycline is resistant to all. The majority of penicillinase-producing staphylococci are now also insensitive to tetracyclines.

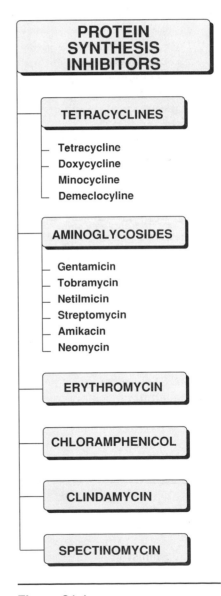

Figure 31.1
Summary of protein synthesis inhibitors.

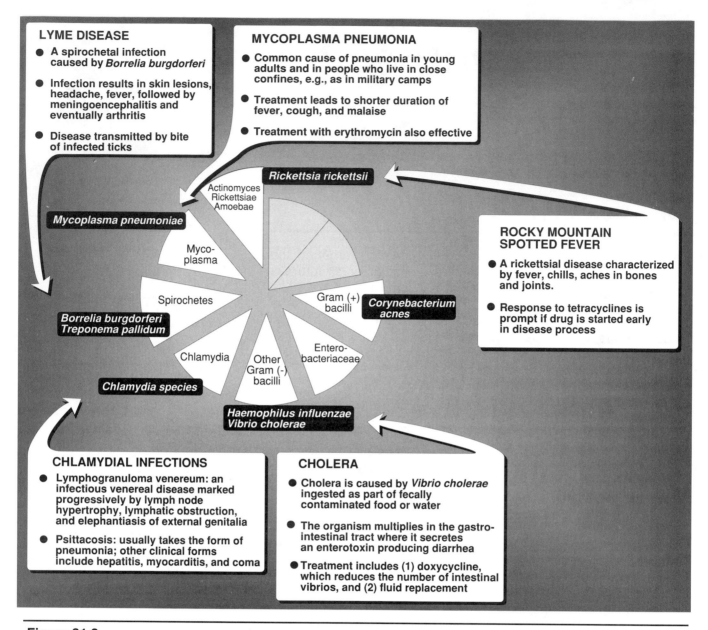

Figure 31.2
Typical therapeutic applications of tetracyclines.

D. Pharmacology

1. **Absorption:** All of the tetracyclines are adequately but incompletely absorbed after oral ingestion. Dairy foods in the diet decrease absorption because of the formation of nonabsorbable chelates of the tetracyclines with calcium ions. Nonabsorbable chelates are also formed with other divalent and trivalent cations (e.g., those found in magnesium and aluminum antacids, and in iron preparations). [Note: This presents a problem if the patient self-treats the epigastric upsets caused by tetracycline ingestion with antacids (Figure 31.3).]

2. **Distribution:** The tetracyclines concentrate in the liver, kidney, spleen, and skin and bind to tissues undergoing calcification (e.g., teeth, bones), or to tumors that have a high calcium content (e.g., gastric carcinoma). Penetration into body fluids is adequate. Though all tetracyclines enter the cerebrospinal fluid, levels are insufficient for therapeutic efficacy, except for *minocycline* [mi noe SYE kleen]. *Minocycline* not only enters the brain in the absence of inflammation, but it also appears in tears and saliva. It is therefore effective in eradicating the meningococcal carrier state. All tetracyclines cross the placental barrier and concentrate in fetal bones and dentition.

3. **Fate:** All the tetracyclines concentrate in the liver, where they are, in part, metabolized and conjugated to form soluble glucuronides. The parent drug and/or its metabolites are secreted into the bile; most tetracyclines are reabsorbed in the intestine and enter the urine by glomerular filtration. *Doxycycline* [dox i SYE kleen] is an exception, since it is preferentially excreted via the bile into the feces and therefore can be employed in treating infections in renally compromised patients.

E. Adverse effects

1. **Gastric discomfort:** Epigastric distress commonly results from irritation of the gastric mucosa (Figure 31.4). This can be controlled if the drug is taken with foods other than dairy products.

2. **Effects on calcified tissues:** Deposition in the bone and primary dentition occurs during calcification in growing children; this causes discoloration and hypoplasia of the teeth and a temporary stunting of growth. Use in pregnancy and in children younger than 8 years should be avoided.

3. **Fatal hepatotoxicity:** This side effect has been known to occur in pregnant women that received high doses of tetracyclines, especially if they are experiencing pyelonephritis.

4. **Phototoxicity:** Phototoxicity, for example, severe sunburn, occurs when the patient receiving a tetracycline is exposed to sun or ultraviolet rays. This toxicity is encountered most frequently with *doxycycline* and *demeclocycline* [dem e kloe SYE kleen].

5. **Vestibular problems:** These side effects (e.g., dizziness, nausea, vomiting) occur with *minocycline,* which concentrates in the endolymph of the ear and affects function.

6. **Superinfections:** These infections may occur with candida (for example in the vagina) or with resistant staphylococci in the intestine.

7. **Contraindications:** Renally-impaired patients should not be treated with any of the tetracyclines except *doxycycline*. Accumulation of the other tetracyclines leads to azotemia caused by diffusion of the antibiotics into the host's cells leading to disruption of the function of mitochondrial ribosomes.

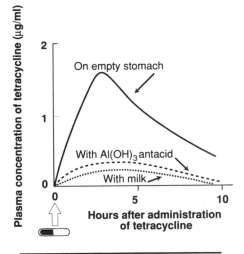

Figure 31.3
Effect of antacids and milk on the absorption of tetracyclines.

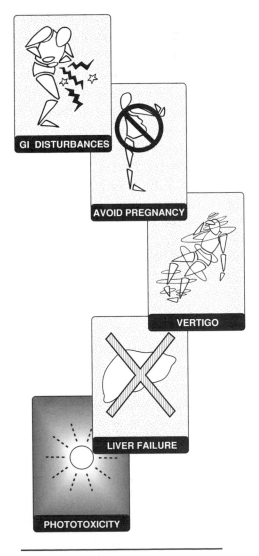

Figure 31.4
Some adverse effects of tetracycline.

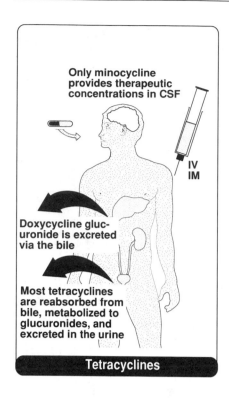

Only minocycline provides therapeutic concentrations in CSF

IV
IM

Doxycycline gluc-
uronide is excreted
via the bile

Most tetracyclines
are reabsorbed from
bile, metabolized to
glucuronides, and
excreted in the urine

Tetracyclines

III. AMINOGLYCOSIDES

Aminoglycoside antibiotics are the present mainstays of treatment of serious infections due to gram-negative bacilli. Their use is limited by the occurrence of serious toxicities, and efforts are being made to replace them with safer antibiotics. Aminoglycosides that are derived from streptomyces have "mycin" suffixes, whereas those from micro-monospora end in "micin."

A. Mode of action

All members of this family are believed to inhibit bacterial protein synthesis by the mechanism determined for *streptomycin* [strep toe MYE sin]. Susceptible organisms have an oxygen-dependent system that transports the antibiotic across the cell membrane. The antibiotic then binds to the isolated 30S ribosomal subunit, interfering with assembly of the functional ribosomal apparatus, or causing the 30S subunit of the complete ribosome to misread the genetic code. [Note: The aminoglycosides synergize with β-lactamase antibiotics (see p.276).]

B. Antibacterial spectrum

All aminoglycosides are bactericidal. They are effective only against aerobic organisms, since anaerobes lack the oxygen-requiring transport system. *Streptomycin* is commonly used to treat tuberculosis (see p.304), plague, tularemia, and in combination with *penicillin,* endocarditis caused by Streptococcus viridans. The antimicrobial spectra of four commonly used aminoglycosides, *amikacin* [am i KAY sin], *gentamicin* [jen ta MYE sin], *tobramycin* [toe bra MYE sin] and *streptomycin* are shown in Figure 31.5.

C. Resistance

Resistance can be caused by any of the three following mechanisms.

1. **Decreased uptake:** The oxygen-dependent transport system for aminoglycosides is absent.

2. **Altered receptor:** The 30S ribosomal subunit binding site has a lowered affinity for aminoglycosides.

3. **Enzymatic modification:** Plasmid-associated R factors that code for the synthesis of enzymes (e.g., acetyltransferases, nucleotidyltransferases, and phosphotransferases) modify and inactivate aminoglycoside antibiotics. Each type of enzyme has its own specificity as to substrate antibiotic; therefore, cross-resistance is not an invariable rule. *Netilmicin* and *amikacin* are less vulnerable to these enzymes than are the other antibiotics of this group.

D. Pharmacology

1. **Administration:** The highly polar, polycationic structure of the aminoglycosides prevents adequate absorption after oral admin-

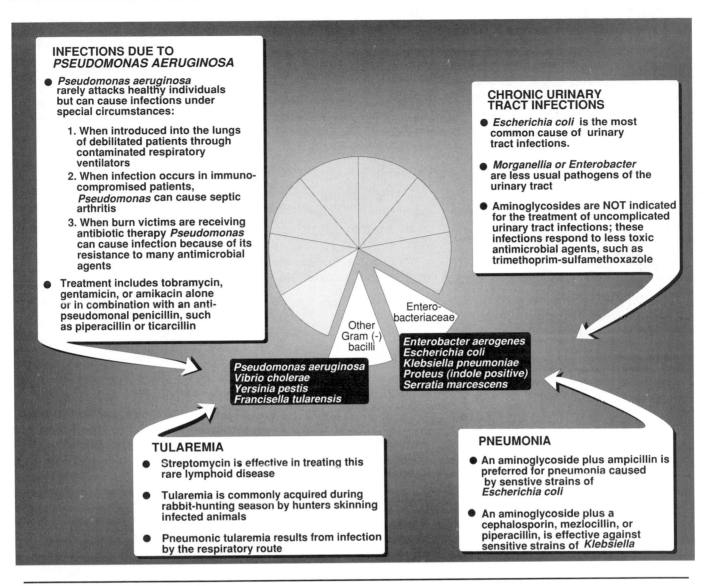

INFECTIONS DUE TO PSEUDOMONAS AERUGINOSA

● *Pseudomonas aeruginosa* rarely attacks healthy individuals but can cause infections under special circumstances:

   1. When introduced into the lungs of debilitated patients through contaminated respiratory ventilators

   2. When infection occurs in immuno-compromised patients, *Pseudomonas* can cause septic arthritis

   3. When burn victims are receiving antibiotic therapy *Pseudomonas* can cause infection because of its resistance to many antimicrobial agents

● Treatment includes tobramycin, gentamicin, or amikacin alone or in combination with an anti-pseudomonal penicillin, such as piperacillin or ticarcillin

CHRONIC URINARY TRACT INFECTIONS

● *Escherichia coli* is the most common cause of urinary tract infections.

● *Morganellia or Enterobacter* are less usual pathogens of the urinary tract

● Aminoglycosides are NOT indicated for the treatment of uncomplicated urinary tract infections; these infections respond to less toxic antimicrobial agents, such as trimethoprim-sulfamethoxazole

Other Gram (-) bacilli

Entero-bacteriaceae

Pseudomonas aeruginosa
Vibrio cholerae
Yersinia pestis
Francisella tularensis

Enterobacter aerogenes
Escherichia coli
Klebsiella pneumoniae
Proteus (indole positive)
Serratia marcescens

TULAREMIA

● Streptomycin is effective in treating this rare lymphoid disease

● Tularemia is commonly acquired during rabbit-hunting season by hunters skinning infected animals

● Pneumonic tularemia results from infection by the respiratory route

PNEUMONIA

● An aminoglycoside plus ampicillin is preferred for pneumonia caused by senstive strains of *Escherichia coli*

● An aminoglycoside plus a cephalosporin, mezlocillin, or piperacillin, is effective against sensitive strains of *Klebsiella*

Figure 31.5
Typical therapeutic applications of gentamicin, tobramycin, streptomycin and amikacin.

istration. Therefore, all aminoglycosides except *neomycin* [nee oh MYE sin], must be given parenterally to achieve adequate serum levels. The severe nephrotoxicity associated with *neomycin* precludes parenteral administration, and its current use is limited to topical application or oral treatment in hepatic coma to reduce the intestinal bacterial population.

2. **Distribution:** All of the aminoglycosides have similar pharmacokinetic properties. They penetrate most body fluids well except for the cerebrospinal fluid where penetration is poor even when the meninges are inflamed. Except for *neomycin,* they may be administered intrathecally. High concentrations accumulate in the renal cortex and in the endolymph and perilymph of the inner ear, which may account for their nephrotoxic and ototoxic

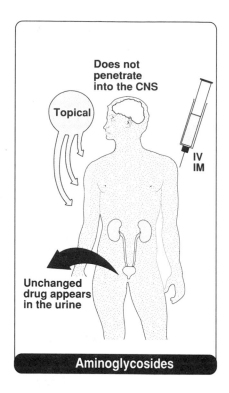

Aminoglycosides

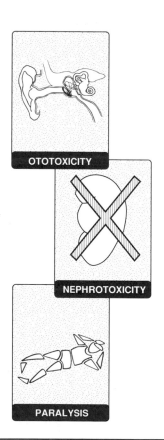

OTOTOXICITY

NEPHROTOXICITY

PARALYSIS

Figure 31.6
Some adverse effects of aminoglycosides.

potential. All cross the placental barrier and may accumulate in fetal plasma and amniotic fluid.

3. **Metabolism:** Metabolism of the aminoglycosides does not occur in the host. All aminoglycosides are rapidly excreted into the urine, predominantly by glomerular filtration. Accumulation occurs in patients with renal failure, and requires dose modification.

E. Adverse effects

It is important to monitor peak and trough plasma levels (p.18) of *gentamicin, tobramycin, netilmicin,* and *amikacin* to avoid concentrations that cause dose-related toxicities (Figure 31.6). Patient factors, such as old age, previous exposure to aminoglycosides, gender, and liver disease, tend to predispose patients to adverse reactions. The elderly are particularly susceptible to nephrotoxicity and ototoxicity.

1. **Ototoxicity:** Ototoxicity (vestibular and cochlear) is directly related to high-peak plasma levels and duration of treatment. Deafness may be irreversible, especially if the patient is simultaneously receiving another ototoxic drug such as *furosemide* (p.216), or *ethacrynic acid.* Also, lack of balance may occur because of the effects of these drugs on the vestibular apparatus.

2. **Nephrotoxicity::** Because proximal tubular cells retain the aminoglycoside, kidney damage ranging from mild renal impairment to severe acute tubular necrosis may result.

3. **Neuromuscular paralysis:** This side effect most often results after intraperitoneal or intrapleural application of large doses. The mechanism responsible is a decrease in both the release of acetylcholine from prejunctional nerve endings and the sensitivity of the postsynaptic site. This adverse effect is now relatively uncommon because of increased awareness of the toxic potential of the aminoglycosides. However, patients with myasthenia gravis are still at risk.

4. **Allergic reactions:** Contact dermatitis is a common reaction to topically-applied *neomycin.*

IV. ERYTHROMYCIN

Erythromycin [er ith roe MYE sin], a macrolide antibiotic, has a few indications where it is the drug of first choice, and a large number of applications as an alternative to *penicillin* in individuals who are allergic to β-lactam antibiotics.

A. Mode of action

Bacterial protein synthesis ceases after *erythromycin* binds irreversibly to a site on the 50S subunit of the bacterial ribosome, thus inhibiting the translocation step of protein synthesis. It is bactericidal. The binding site is either identical to or in close proximity to that for *lincomycin, clindamycin,* and *chloramphenicol.*

B. Antibacterial spectrum

Erythromycin is effective against the same organisms as *penicillin G*; therefore, it is used in patients allergic to the penicillins. In addition, it is the drug of choice for the treatment of the infections shown in Figure 31.7.

C. Resistance

Resistance to *erythromycin* is becoming a serious clinical problem. For example, most strains of staphylococci in hospital isolates are resistant to this drug. At least two mechanisms have been identified: (1) the inability of the organism to take up the antibiotic; and (2) the decreased affinity of the binding site of the 50S ribosomal subunit for the antibiotic resulting from the methylation of an adenine of 23S bacterial ribosomal RNA.

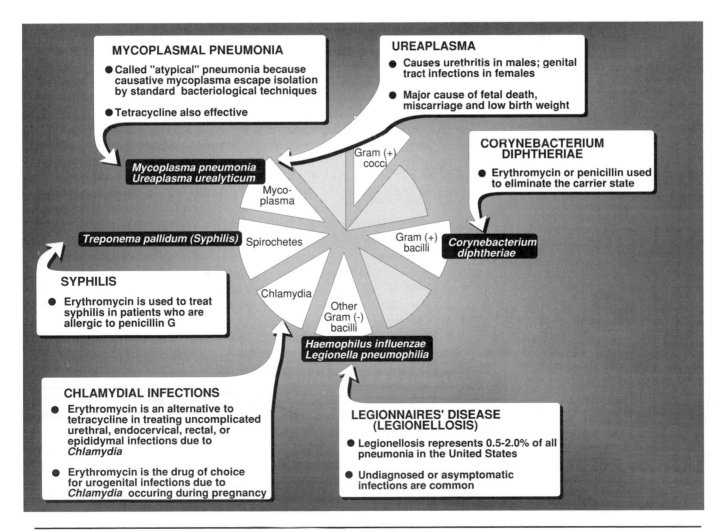

Figure 31.7
Typical therapeutic applications of erythromycin.

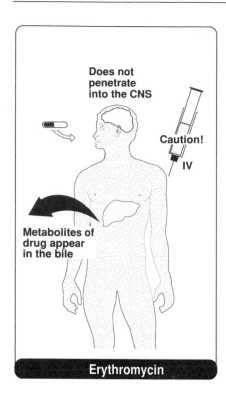

Does not penetrate into the CNS

Caution!

IV

Metabolites of drug appear in the bile

Erythromycin

D. Pharmacology

1. **Administration:** All forms of *erythromycin* are adequately absorbed on oral administration. Intravenous administration is associated with a high incidence of thrombophlebitis, and intramuscular injections are painful.

2. **Distribution:** *Erythromycin* distributes well in all body fluids except the CSF. It is one of the few antibiotics that diffuses into prostatic fluids and has the unique characteristic of accumulating in macrophages. Inflammation allows for greater tissue penetration. *Erythromycin* is concentrated in the liver.

3. **Metabolism:** The antibiotic is extensively metabolized. *Erythromycin* is known to inhibit the oxidation of a number of drugs through its interaction with the cytochrome P-450 system (p.12).

4. **Excretion:** *Erythromycin* is primarily concentrated and excreted in an active form in the bile. Partial reabsorption occurs through the enterohepatic circulation.

E. Adverse effects

1. **Epigastric distress:** This side effect is common and can lead to poor patient compliance.

2. **Cholestatic jaundice:** This side effect occurs, especially with the estolate form of *erythromycin,* presumably as the result of a hypersensitivity reaction to the estolate form (the lauryl salt of the propionyl ester of *erythromycin*).

3. **Ototoxicity:** Transient deafness has been associated with *erythromycin,* especially at high dosages.

4. **Contraindications:** Patients with hepatic dysfunction should not be treated with *erythromycin,* since the drug accumulates in the liver.

5. **Interactions:** *Erythromycin* inhibits the hepatic metabolism of *theophylline* (p.208) and *cyclosporine.* This can lead to toxic accumulations of these drugs.

V. CHLORAMPHENICOL

Chloramphenicol [klor am FEN i kole] is active against a wide range of gram-positive and gram-negative organisms, but because of its toxicity, its use is restricted to life-threatening infections.

A. Mode of action

The drug binds to the bacterial 50S ribosomal subunit and inhibits protein synthesis at the peptidyl transferase reaction. Because of the similarity of mammalian mitochondrial ribosomes to those of

Theophylline Cyclosporine Other drugs ⟹ **Serum concentration increases**

P-450 ⊖ ⟵‧‧‧‧‧‧‧‧ **Erythromycin**

Metabolites

bacteria, protein synthesis in these organelles may be inhibited at high circulating *chloramphenicol* levels.

B. Antimicrobial spectrum

Chloramphenicol, a broad spectrum antibiotic, is active not only against bacteria but also against other microorganisms, such as rickettsiae. It is either bactericidal or (more commonly) bacteriostatic, depending on the organism.

C. Resistance

Resistance is conferred by the presence of an R factor, which codes for an acetyl coenzyme A transferase that inactivates *chloramphenicol.* Another mechanism for resistance is associated with an inability of the antibiotic to penetrate the organism. This change in permeability may be the basis of multidrug resistance.

D. Pharmacology

Chloramphenicol may be administered either intravenously or orally. It is completely absorbed via the oral route because of its lipophilic nature. Excretion of the drug depends on its conversion in the liver to a glucuronide that is then secreted by the renal tubule. Only about 10% of the parent compound is excreted by glomerular filtration.

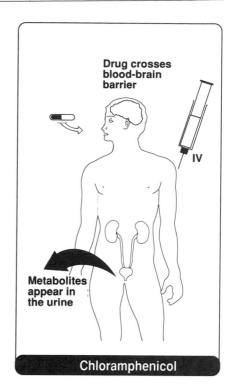

Drug crosses blood-brain barrier

IV

Metabolites appear in the urine

Chloramphenicol

E. Adverse effects

The clinical use of *chloramphenicol* is limited because of the serious adverse effects associated with its administration.

1. **Anemias:** Hemolytic anemia occurs in patients with low levels of glucose 6-phosphate dehydrogenase (p.322). Other types of anemia occurring as a side effect of *chloramphenicol* include reversible anemia, which is apparently dose-related and occurs concomitantly with therapy, and aplastic anemia, which is idiosyncratic and usually fatal. [Note: Aplastic anemia is independent of dose and may occur after therapy has ceased.]

2. **Gray baby syndrome:** This adverse effect occurs in neonates if the dosage regimen of *chloramphenicol* is not properly adjusted. Neonates have a low capacity to glucuronidate the antibiotic and they have underdeveloped renal function. They therefore have a decreased ability to excrete the drug, which accumulates to levels that interfere with the function of mitochondrial ribosomes. This leads to poor feeding, which progresses to cyanosis (hence the term "gray baby") and death.

VI. CLINDAMYCIN

A. Mode of action

Clindamycin's mode of action is the same as that of *erythromycin* (p.290).

B. Antibacterial spectrum

Clindamycin [klin da MYE sin] is employed primarily in the treatment of infections caused by anaerobic bacteria, such as <u>Bacteroides fragilis</u>, which often causes abdominal infections associated with <u>trauma</u>.

C. Resistance

Resistance mechanisms are the same as those for *erythromycin* (p.290), but cross-resistance is not a problem.

D. Pharmacology

Clindamycin is well absorbed by the oral route. It distributes well into all body fluids except the CSF. Adequate levels of *clindamycin* are not achieved in the brain, even when meninges are inflamed. Penetration into bone occurs even in the absence of inflammation. *Clindamycin* undergoes extensive oxidative metabolism to inactive products. The drug is excreted into the bile or urine by glomerular filtration, but therapeutically effective levels of the parent drugs are not achieved in the urine. Accumulation has been reported in patients with either severely compromised renal function or hepatic failure.

E. Adverse effects

In addition to skin rashes, the most serious adverse effect is potentially fatal pseudomembranous colitis caused by overgrowth of <u>Clostridium</u> <u>difficile</u>, which elaborates toxins. Oral administration of *vancomycin* (p.283) is usually effective in controlling this serious problem.

VII. SPECTINOMYCIN

Spectinomycin [spek ti noe MYE sin], an aminocyclitol, interacts with the 30S ribosomal subunit to inhibit protein synthesis. It is administered as a single intramuscular injection only for treatment of acute gonorrhea caused by penicillinase-producing <u>Neisseria</u> <u>gonorrhea</u> and/or uncomplicated gonorrhea of the genitalia or rectum, in patients who are allergic to *penicillin*. *Spectinomycin*-resistant gonococci have been reported, The resistance appears to be a chromosomal mutation but no cross-resistance to other effective agents occurs. Hypersensitivity reactions can develop.

Study questions   (see p.431 for answers).

Choose the ONE best answer.

31.1 Which one of the following diseases is NOT treated with a tetracycline derivative?

A. Cholera.
B. Lyme disease.
C. Rocky Mountain spotted fever.
D. Mycoplasma pneumonia.
E. Streptococcal infection.

31.2 Which one of the following statements about tetracycline is INCORRECT?

A. Its use is rarely contraindicated because of resistant strains.
B. It is contraindicated in pregnancy.
C. It is effective in treating infections caused by *Chlamydiae.*
D. It can form poorly absorbable complexes with calcium ions.
E. It can lead to discoloration of teeth if given to children.

31.3 Which one of the following statements about tetracyclines is INCORRECT?

A. Accumulation of tetracyclines by susceptible organisms is mediated by transport proteins located in the bacterial membrane.
B. Tetracyclines, even at high concentrations, do not affect mammalian cell metabolism.
C. Tetracyclines bind to the 30S subunit of the bacterial ribosome and block protein synthesis.
D. Phototoxicity is encountered most frequently with demeclocycline and doxycyline.
E. Doxycycline is the only tetracycline that may be used in treating patients with renal failure.

31.4 All of the following properties are exhibited by aminoglycosides EXCEPT:

A. They are poorly absorbed from gastrointestinal tract.
B. They have bactericidal properties.
C. They can achieve adequate serum levels after oral administration.
D. They bind to the 30S ribosomal subunit.
E. They are not accumulated by anaerobic microorganisms.

31.5 Which one of the following adverse effects is NOT observed with administration of aminoglycosides?

A. Anemia.
B. Nephrotoxicity.
C. Ototoxicity.
D. Respiratory paralysis.
E. Allergic reactions.

31.6 All of the following statements about erythromycin are correct EXCEPT:

A. It is often used as a penicillin substitute.
B. It binds to the 50S ribosomal subunit.
C. It is contraindicated in patients with renal failure.
D. Valid clinical uses include respiratory infections caused by Mycoplasma pneumoniae.
E. It can cause epigastric distress.

Answer A if 1,2 and 3 are correct
 B if 1 and 3 are correct.
 C if 2 and 4 are correct.
 D if only 4 is correct.
 E if 1,2,3, and 4 are all correct.

31.7 Chloramphenicol possesses which of the following properties:

1. It is useful in treating infections due to anaerobic organisms, such as Bacteroides fragilis.
2. It exhibits a broad antimicrobial spectrum.
3. It is reserved for well-defined indications in severely ill patients.
4. It may cause aplastic anemia, a usually fatal adverse effect.

31.8 Which of the following contribute(s) to gray baby syndrome when chloramphenicol is administered to neonates?

1. Decreased intestinal absorption.
2. Immature kidney function.
3. Alteration of gastrointestinal flora.
4. Low hepatic glucuronyl transferase activity.

31.9 Which of the following statements is/are characteristic of clindamycin?

1. Antibacterial activity is destroyed by a β-lactamase.
2. It may cause pseudomembranous colitis.
3. Plasma levels must be controlled to avoid deafness.
4. It is effective against anaerobic bacteria.

Questions 31.10 - 31.12: For each numbered word or phrase, select the ONE drug (A-E) that is most closely associated with it. Each drug (A-E) may be selected once, more than once, or not at all.

A. Minocycline
B. Gentamicin
C. Erythromycin
D. Doxycycline
E. Chloramphenicol

31.10 This drug is effective in eradicating the meningococcal carrier state.

31.11 This drug can potentiate the effect of theophylline.

31.12 This drug can precipitate hemolytic anemia in patients deficient in glucose 6-phosphate dehydrogenase.

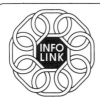

[1]See *ribosomes* in **Biochemistry** for the role of ribosomes in protein synthesis (see index).

Quinolones, Urinary Tract, and Antitubercular Agents

32

I. OVERVIEW

This chapter describes antimicrobial drugs that have specific clinical applications, for example, *isoniazid* is used in the treatment of tuberculosis. Other drugs mentioned in this chapter, such as *ciprofloxacin* and *rifampin,* have uses for more than one particular disease (Figure 32.1).

II. QUINOLONES

The older drug, *nalidixic acid* [nal i DIX ik], and the new fluoroquinolone, *norfloxacin* [nor FLOX a sin], are principally employed for recurrent urinary tract infections (UTIs, p.300). Another fluoroquinolone, *ciprofloxacin* [sip ro FLOX a sin], is effective not only for treatment of UTIs but also for systemic bacterial infections. The quinolones are bactericidal but are not effective against anaerobes.

A. Mechanism of action

The quinolones uniquely inhibit the replication of bacterial DNA by interfering with the action of DNA gyrase (topoisomerase II) during bacterial growth and reproduction. [Note: Topoisomerases are enzymes that change the configuration or topology of DNA without changing its primary structure.[1]] Since DNA gyrase is a distinct target for antimicrobial therapy, cross-resistance with other more commonly used antimicrobial drugs is rare.

B. Antimicrobial spectrum

1. *Nalidixic acid* is effective against most of the gram-negative bacteria that commonly cause UTIs, whereas most gram-positive organisms are resistant.

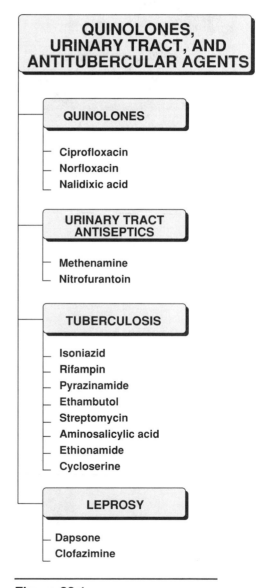

Figure 32.1
Summary of specific clinical infections.

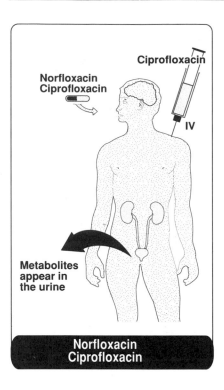

Norfloxacin
Ciprofloxacin

2. *Norfloxacin* is more potent than *nalidixic acid* and is effective against both gram-negative (including Pseudomonas aeruginosa) and gram-positive organisms. It is useful in treating complicated and uncomplicated UTIs and prostatitis.

3. *Ciprofloxacin* is more potent than *norfloxacin* and has a similar antibacterial spectrum (Figure 32.2). The serum levels achieved, however, are effective against systemic infections with the exception of enterococcal and pneumococcal infections. *Ciprofloxacin* is particularly useful in treating infections caused by multiple resistant bacteria, including many enterobacteria and gram-negative bacilli. *Ciprofloxacin* is an alternative to more toxic drugs, such as the aminoglycosides, or drugs that require parenteral administration (e.g., extended-spectrum penicillins and cephalosporins).

C. Resistance

1. **Nalidixic acid:** The drug's clinical usefulness has been limited because of the rapid emergence of resistant strains. The resistance trait is associated with the bacterial chromosome and not with a plasmid. Thus, rapid transfer of resistance is not a problem. Resistance is due either to the alteration of the A subunit of DNA gyrase or to decreased permeability of cells to the drug.

2. **Norfloxacin and ciprofloxacin:** These drugs show a less frequent emergence of resistant organisms. Organisms that are initially only marginally sensitive (for example, Pseudomonas aeruginosa and Streptococcus pneumoniae) appear to have the greatest potential for developing clinically significant resistance.

D. Pharmacology

1. **Absorption:** Despite their structural similarities, differences exist in the pharmacokinetics of quinolones. *Nalidixic acid* and *ciprofloxacin* are well absorbed after oral administration, whereas only 30-40% of an oral dose of *norfloxacin* is absorbed. An intravenous preparation of *ciprofloxacin* is now available.

2. **Distribution:** Plasma levels of free *nalidixic acid* and *norfloxacin* are insufficient for treatment of systemic infections. *Nalidixic acid* penetrates poorly throughout the body, but *ciprofloxacin* and *norfloxacin* distribute well into all tissues and body fluids. The concentration of *nalidixic acid* achieved in the urine is 10-20 times greater than that in the plasma.

3. **Metabolism:** *Nalidixic acid* undergoes metabolism to the more potent hydroxylated product, *7-hydroxynalidixic acid,* which accounts for its bactericidal effect. *Norfloxacin* and *ciprofloxacin* are metabolized to compounds with less antimicrobial activity.

4. **Excretion:** The parent drugs and their metabolites are excreted into the urine. Renal failure prolongs the half-life of each drug. *Norfloxacin* and *ciprofloxacin* are partially excreted into the bile, and this route assumes importance in renal failure.

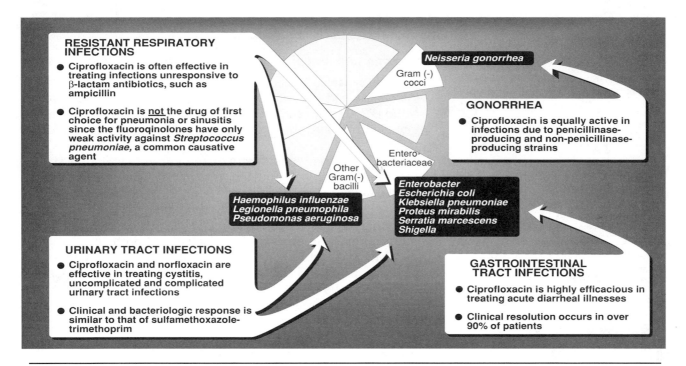

Figure 32.2
Typical therapeutic applications of ciprofloxacin.

E. Adverse reactions to nalidixic acid

The adverse effects of *nalidixic acid* include nausea, vomiting, and abdominal pain; however, reactions, such as urticaria, photosensitivity, and fever can occur. Liver function may be affected if therapy lasts longer than 2 weeks. Central nervous system (CNS) problems ranging from headache and malaise to visual disturbances are rare.

F. Adverse reactions to norfloxacin and ciprofloxacin

Toxicities similar to those for *nalidixic acid* have been reported for *norfloxacin* and *ciprofloxacin*.

1. **CNS problems:** The most prominent side effects are nausea, headache, and dizziness or lightheadedness. Thus, patients with CNS disorders should be treated cautiously with these drugs.

2. **Nephrotoxicity:** Crystalluria has been reported in patients receiving excessive doses (3-4 times normal).

3. **Contraindications:** The drugs should be avoided in pregnancy or in children (below 8 years of age), since cartilage toxicity has been found in immature experimental animals.

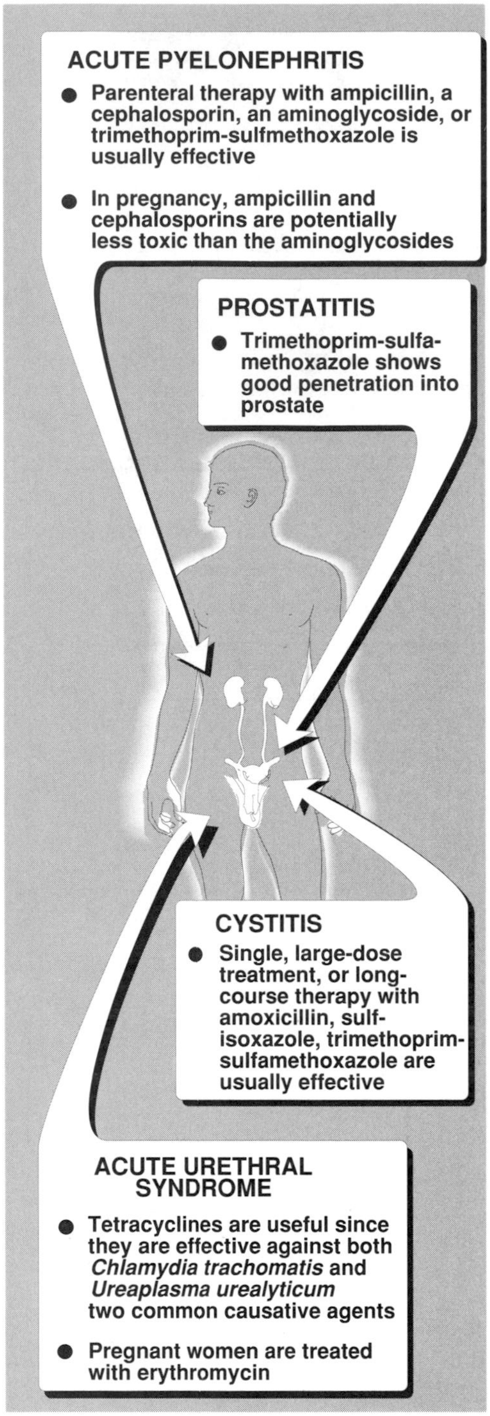

ACUTE PYELONEPHRITIS
- Parenteral therapy with ampicillin, a cephalosporin, an aminoglycoside, or trimethoprim-sulfmethoxazole is usually effective
- In pregnancy, ampicillin and cephalosporins are potentially less toxic than the aminoglycosides

PROSTATITIS
- Trimethoprim-sulfa-methoxazole shows good penetration into prostate

CYSTITIS
- Single, large-dose treatment, or long-course therapy with amoxicillin, sulf-isoxazole, trimethoprim-sulfamethoxazole are usually effective

ACUTE URETHRAL SYNDROME
- Tetracyclines are useful since they are effective against both *Chlamydia trachomatis* and *Ureaplasma urealyticum* two common causative agents
- Pregnant women are treated with erythromycin

Figure 32.3
Antimicrobial drugs commonly used in treating urinary tract infections.

III. URINARY TRACT ANTISEPTICS

A. Causes and treatment of urinary tract infections

1. **Common causes of urinary tract infections (UTI):** UTI are common in the elderly and in young women. About two thirds of uncomplicated UTI are caused by Escherichia coli; other common causes include Klebsiella pneumoniae and Proteus mirabilis infections.

2. **Treating UTI:** Agents commonly used in uncomplicated UTI include *sulfisoxazole* (p.266), *trimethoprim-sulfamethoxazole* (p.269), *amoxicillin* (p.276) or *tetracycline* (p.285 and Figure 32.3). In addition, UTI may be treated with any one of a group of agents, including *methenamine, nalidixic acid,* and *nitrofurantoin,* which are restricted to this clinical problem. The latter drugs do not achieve antibacterial levels in the circulation, but because they are concentrated in the urine, microorganisms at that site can be effectively eradicated.

B. Methenamine

1. **Mechanism of action:** In order to act, *methenamine* [meth EN a meen] must decompose at an acidic pH of 5.5 or less in the urine, thus producing formaldehyde, which is toxic to most bacteria (Figure 32.4). The reaction is slow, requiring 3 hours to reach 90% decomposition. Bacterial resistance to formaldehyde does not develop. [Note: *Methenamine* is frequently formulated with a weak acid such as mandelic acid, which lowers the pH of the urine.]

2. **Antibacterial spectrum:** *Methenamine* is primarily used for chronic suppressive therapy. Urea-splitting bacteria that alkalinize the urine, such as proteus, are usually resistant to the action of *methenamine* (p.267).

3. **Pharmacology**

   a. **Administration:** *Methenamine* is orally administered. In addition to formaldehyde, ammonium ion is produced. Because the liver rapidly metabolizes ammonia to form urea, *methenamine* is contraindicated in patients with hepatic insufficiency. Otherwise, elevated levels of circulating ammonium ions are toxic to the CNS.

   b. **Distribution and excretion:** *Methenamine* is distributed throughout the body fluids, but no decomposition of the drug occurs at pH 7.4; thus, systemic toxicity does not occur. The drug is eliminated in the urine.

4. **Adverse effects:** The side effects include gastrointestinal distress. At higher doses, albuminuria, hematuria and rashes may develop. *Methenamine mandelate* is contraindicated in treating patients with renal insufficiency, because mandelic acid may precipitate. Sulfonamides react with formaldehyde and must not be used concomitantly with *methenamine.*

C. Nitrofurantoin

Nitrofurantoin [nye troe FYOOR an toyn] is less commonly employed for treating UTIs because of its narrow antimicrobial spectrum and its toxicity.

1. **Mechanism of action:** Sensitive bacteria reduce the drug to an active agent that inhibits various enzymes and damages DNA. Activity is greater in acidic urine.

2. **Antimicrobial Spectrum:** The drug is bacteriostatic. It is useful against Escherichia coli, but other common urinary tract gram-negative bacteria may be resistant. Gram-positive cocci are susceptible.

3. **Resistance:** Resistance is constitutive. It is associated with an inability to reduce the nitrogen group in the presence of oxygen. Resistance does not develop during therapy.

4. **Pharmacology:** Absorption is complete after oral administration. The drug is rapidly excreted by glomerular filtration. The presence of the drug turns the urine brown.

5. **Adverse effects**

   a. **Gastrointestinal disturbances:** These side effects include nausea, vomiting, and diarrhea. The macrocrystalline form is better tolerated. Ingestion with food or milk ameliorates these symptoms.

   b. **Acute pneumonitis:** This is a serious complication. Other pulmonary effects, such as interstitial pulmonary fibrosis, can occur in patients being chronically treated.

   c. **Neurological problems:** Neurological side effects such as headache, nystagmus, and polyneuropathies with demyelination (footdrop) may develop.

   d. **Hemolytic anemia:** The drug is contraindicated in patients with glucose-6-phosphate dehydrogenase deficiency, neonates, and pregnant women.

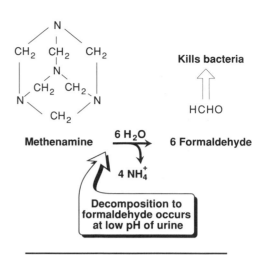

Figure 32.4
Formation of formaldehyde from methenamine at acid pH.

IV. CHEMOTHERAPY OF TUBERCULOSIS

Mycobacterium tuberculosis is one of a number of mycobacteria that can lead to serious infections of the lungs as well as the genitourinary tract, skeleton, and meninges. Tuberculosis cases are increasing chiefly among AIDS patients and the homeless (Figure 32.5).

Treating tuberculosis as well as other mycobacterial infections presents a number of therapeutic problems. The organism grows slowly, and thus the disease must be treated for up to 2 years. Patient compliance and drug toxicity are important considerations. Because resistant strains of the organism emerge during therapy, multiple drug therapy is employed to delay the emergence of resistance. *Isoniazid,*

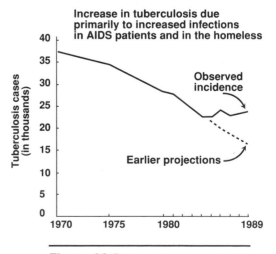

Figure 32.5
Incidence of new cases of tuberculosis.

rifampin, ethambutol, streptomycin, and *pyrazinamide* are the principal or so-called "first line" drugs because of their efficacy and acceptable degree of toxicity.

A. Isoniazid

1. **Mechanism of action:** *Isoniazid* [eye soe NYE a zid] is believed to act by inhibiting the synthesis of mycolic acids, which are unique to the mycobacterial cell walls. Mycolic acids account for the acid fastness of the mycobacteria; this property is lost after exposure to *isoniazid.*

2. **Antibacterial spectrum:** For bacilli in the stationary phase, the drug is bacteriostatic, but for rapidly dividing organisms, it is bactericidal. *Isoniazid* is specific for treatment of Mycobacterium tuberculosis, although Mycobacterium kansasii may be susceptible.

3. **Resistance**: Resistance is associated with the constitutive inability of the organism to accumulate the drug. No cross-resistance exists between *isoniazid* and other tuberculostatic drugs.

4. **Pharmacology**

   a. **Administration:** The drug is readily absorbed orally. Absorption is impaired if taken with aluminum-containing antacids.

   b. **Fate:** *Isoniazid* diffuses into all body fluids, cells, and caseous material, but levels in the central nervous system are much lower than those in the plasma. Infected tissue tends to retain the drug longer. The drug readily penetrates host cells and is effective against bacilli growing intracellularly.

   c. **Metabolism:** *Isoniazid* undergoes N-acetylation and hydrolysis, resulting in inactive products. Acetylation is genetically regulated; the fast acetylator trait is autosomally dominant. A bimodal distribution of fast and slow acetylators exists (Figure 32.6).

   d. **Excretion:** Excretion is through glomerular filtration, predominantly as metabolites. Slow acetylators excrete more of the parent compound. Depressed renal function results in accumulation of the drug, primarily in slow acetylators.

5. **Adverse effects:** The incidence of adverse effects is fairly low. They are related to the dosage and duration of administration.

   a. **Peripheral neuritis:** Peripheral neuritis (paresthesia) is the most common adverse effect; it results from pyridoxal deficiency, which is caused by *isoniazid* and *pyridoxal's* combining chemically to produce a derivative with no vitamin activity (Figure 32.7). The deficiency is corrected by pyridoxine (vitamin B_6) supplementation. [Note: *Isoniazid* can achieve levels in breast milk that are high enough to cause a pyridoxine deficiency in the infant unless the mother is supplemented with the vitamin.]

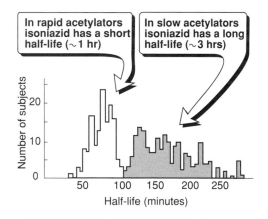

In rapid acetylators isoniazid has a short half-life (~1 hr)

In slow acetylators isoniazid has a long half-life (~3 hrs)

Number of subjects

Half-life (minutes)

Figure 32.6
Bimodal distribution of isoniazid half-lives caused by rapid and slow acetylation of drug.

b. **Hepatitis:** This is the most severe side effect associated with *isoniazid.*

c. **Hypersensitivity:** These reactions include rashes and fever.

d. **Idiosyncratic hepatotoxicity:** This adverse effect, which may be fatal has been reported. Its incidence increases among patients with increasing age, among patients who also take *rifampin,* or among those who imbibe alcohol daily.

e. **Drug interactions:** *Isoniazid* can potentiate the adverse effects of *phenytoin* (e.g., nystagmus, ataxia, p.147) because the *isoniazid* inhibits metabolism of *phenytoin.* Slow acetylators are particularly at risk.

f. **Other neurological problems:** These adverse effects include mental abnormalities, convulsions in patients prone to seizures, and optic neuritis.

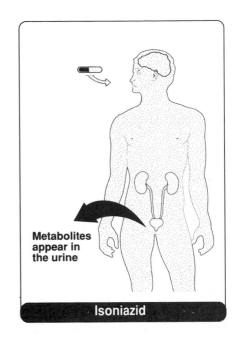

Metabolites appear in the urine

Isoniazid

B. Rifampin

Rifampin [RIF am pin] has a broader antimicrobial activity than *isoniazid* and has found application in the treatment of other bacterial infections. Because resistant strains rapidly emerge during therapy, it is never given as a single agent in the treatment of tuberculosis.

1. **Mechanism of action:** *Rifampin* interacts with the β-subunit of bacterial DNA-dependent RNA polymerase. It inhibits RNA synthesis by suppressing the initiation step. The drug is specific for prokaryotes.

2. **Antimicrobial spectrum:** *Rifampin* is bactericidal for both intracellular and extracellular mycobacteria, including M. tuberculosis, atypical mycobacteria, and M. leprae. It is frequently used prophylactically for household members exposed to meningitis caused by meningococci or Haemophilus influenzae.

3. **Resistance:** Resistance is caused by a change in the affinity of the DNA-dependent RNA polymerase for the drug.

4. **Pharmacology**

   a. **Absorption:** Absorption is adequate after oral administration.

   b. **Distribution:** Distribution occurs to all body fluids and organs. Adequate levels are attained in the cerebrospinal fluid even in the absence of inflammation. The drug is taken up by the liver and undergoes enterohepatic cycling.

   c. **Metabolism:** Oxidative deacetylation is catalyzed by the mixed function oxidases of the liver, resulting in a product that retains antitubercular activity. *Rifampin* itself can induce the hepatic mixed function oxidases, leading to a shortened half-life.

Isoniazid   **Pyridoxal**

Hydrazone derivative (inactive)

Figure 32.7

Reaction of isoniazid with pyridoxal (vitamin B$_6$).

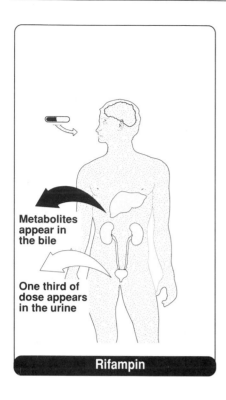

Metabolites appear in the bile

One third of dose appears in the urine

Rifampin

d. **Excretion:** Elimination is via the bile into the feces and the urine as metabolites and parent drug. Urine and feces as well as other secretions have an orange-red color; patients should be forewarned.

5. **Adverse effects:** Adverse effects are a minor problem with *rifampin.*

   a. **Common effects:** Nausea and vomiting, rash, and fever are most common.

   b. **Jaundice:** The drug should be used judiciously in patients with hepatic failure because of the jaundice that occurs rarely.

   c. **Drug interactions:** Because *rifampin* can induce the cytochrome P-450 enzymes, it can decrease the half-lives of other drugs that are coadministered and metabolized by this system (p.12). This may lead to higher dosage requirements for these agents.

C. Pyrazinamide

Pyrazinamide [peer a ZIN a mide] is an orally effective bactericidal anti-tubercular agent used for short-term, initial therapy, along with *isoniazid* and *rifampin.* It is bactericidal to actively dividing organisms. It distributes throughout the body and undergoes extensive metabolism. About 1-5% of patients taking *isoniazid, rifampin,* and *pyrazinamide* may experience liver dysfunction. Urate retention can also occur and may precipitate a gouty attack.

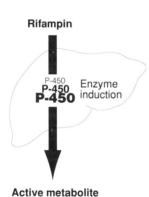

Rifampin

P-450
P-450
P-450 Enzyme induction

Active metabolite

D. Ethambutol

Ethambutol [e THAM byoo tole] is bacteriostatic and specific for most strains of Mycobacterium tuberculosis and Mycobacterium kansasii. Resistance is not a serious problem if the drug is employed with other antituberculous agents. *Ethambutol* can be used in combination with *pyrazinamide, isoniazid,* and *rifampin* to treat tuberculosis. Its mechanism of action is unknown. Absorbed on oral administration, *ethambutol* is well distributed throughout the body. It is concentrated in erythrocytes. Penetration into the central nervous system is therapeutically adequate in tuberculous meningitis. Both parent drug and metabolites are excreted by glomerular filtration and tubular secretion. The most important adverse effect is optic neuritis, which results in diminished visual acuity and loss of ability to discriminate between red and green. Visual acuity should be periodically examined. Discontinuation of the drug results in reversal of the toxic symptoms. In addition, urate excretion is decreased by the drug, thus gout may be exacerbated.

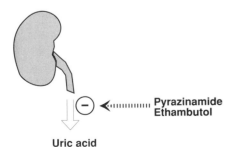

   ⊖ ⬅┈┈┈┈ **Pyrazinamide Ethambutol**

Uric acid

E. Streptomycin

Streptomycin, the first antibiotic effective in the treatment of tuberculosis, has been previously discussed with the aminoglycosides (p.288). The remaining agents employed in the therapy of this disease are secondary, and their properties are summarized very briefly.

F. Aminosalicylic acid

Aminosalicylic acid [a mee noe sal i sil ik], a bacteriostatic agent, acts as a competitive inhibitor for p-aminobenzoic acid (PABA) in folate biosynthesis. Oral absorption is adequate, and the drug is distributed throughout the body except for the cerebrospinal fluid. *Aminosalicylic acid* undergoes acetylation and inhibits acetylation of *isoniazid* to prolong the half-life of *isoniazid*. Elimination depends on urinary excretion; crystalluria can result unless the urine is alkaline. The drug may accumulate in renal failure. *Aminosalicylic acid* is associated with a high incidence of gastrointestinal problems causing poor patient compliance. Acute hemolytic anemia may be seen in patients with a glucose 6-phosphate dehydrogenase deficiency. Hypersensitivity may also occur.

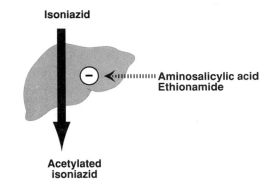

G. Ethionamide

Ethionamide [e thye on AM ide], a structural analog of *isoniazid,* is believed not to act by the same mechanism. Its oral administration is effective, and the drug is widely distributed throughout the body, including the cerebrospinal fluid. Metabolism is extensive. *Ethionamide* can inhibit acetylation of *isoniazid*. The urine is the main route of excretion. Adverse effects include gastric irritation, hepatotoxicity, peripheral neuropathies, and optic neuritis.

H. Cycloserine

Cycloserine [sye kloe SER een] is an orally effective tuberculostatic agent that distributes well throughout body fluids, including the CSF. It is metabolized, and both parent and metabolite are excreted in urine. Accumulation occurs with renal insufficiency. Adverse effects involve CNS disturbances; epileptic seizure activity may be exacerbated. Peripheral neuropathies are also a problem.

V. CHEMOTHERAPY OF LEPROSY

Leprosy (Hansen's disease) is caused by Mycobacterium leprae. Bacilli from skin lesions or nasal discharges of infected patients enter susceptible individuals via the skin or respiratory tract. The World Health Organization recommends the triple drug regimen, *dapsone, clofazimine,* and *rifampin* (p.303).

A. Dapsone

Dapsone [DAP sone] is bacteriostatic for Mycobacterium leprae, but resistant strains are encountered. It acts by inhibiting folate biosynthesis. The drug is well absorbed from the gastrointestinal tract and is distributed throughout the body. It is concentrated in the liver and undergoes acetylation. The parent drug enters the enterohepatic circulation. Both parent drug and metabolites are eliminated through the urine. Adverse reactions include hemolysis and methemoglobinemia, peripheral neuropathy, and the possibility of exacerbating leprosy.

B. Clofazimine

Clofazimine [kloe FA zi meen] is a phenazine dye that binds to DNA and inhibits template function. It is bactericidal to <u>Mycobacterium leprae</u> and has some activity against <u>Mycobacterium avium-intracellulare</u>. On oral absorption, it accumulates in tissues, allowing for intermittent therapy. Patients may develop a red discoloration of the skin. Eosinophilic enteritis has been reported as an untoward effect. The drug also has some anti-inflammatory activity.

Study Questions   (see p.432 for answers).

Choose the ONE best answer.

32.1 All of the following statements about methenamine are true EXCEPT:

A. It is used in chronic suppressive therapy of urinary tract infections.
B. It has its major antibacterial effect at alkaline pH.
C. It is contraindicated in renal insufficiency.
D. It may cause gastric disturbances.
E. Its antimicrobial activity is confined to the urinary tract.

32.2 All of the following statements about nalidixic acid are true EXCEPT:

A. Nalidixic acid is only effective against infections located in the urinary tract.
B. Children are more susceptible to nalidixic acid-induced CNS toxicities than are adults.
C. Nalidixic acid interferes in the replication of bacterial DNA by interacting with DNA gyrase (topoisomerase II) during bacterial growth and reproduction.
D. Nalidixic acid is more potent than ciprofloxacin.
E. Nalidixic acid should not be used in patients with compromised renal function.

32.3 All of the following statements about rifampin are true EXCEPT:

A. It is frequently used prophylactically for household members exposed to meningitis caused by meningococci or <u>Haemophilus</u> <u>influenzae</u>.

B. It colors body secretions red.
C. It disrupts bacterial lipid metabolism as its major mechanism of action.
D. Although rare, it can cause serious hepatotoxicity.
E. When used alone, there is a high risk of the emergence of resistant strains of mycobacteria.

32.4 All of the following statements about isoniazid are true EXCEPT:

A. It produces age dependent hepatotoxicity.
B. It readily penetrates into infected cells.
C. It inhibits mycolic acid synthesis in susceptible mycobacteria.
D. It may induce the symptoms of cyanocobalamin (vitamin B_{12}) deficiency.
E. It potentiates the adverse effects of phenytoin when the patient receives both medications concurrently.

32.5 Multiple-drug regimens are used for treatment of tuberculosis because:

A. administration of two drugs results in better penetration of cavitary lesions.
B. lower doses may be used.
C. multiple-drug regimens usually exhibit a potent synergistic effect.
D. multiple-drug regimens markedly delay the appearance of drug-resistant organisms.
E. the organism grows rapidly and therefore must be treated aggressively over a short period of time.

[1]See *topoisomerases* in **Biochemistry** for a discussion of the role of these enzymes in DNA synthesis (see index).

Antifungal Drugs

33

I. OVERVIEW

Unlike bacteria, fungi are eukaryotic and have rigid cell walls containing chitin as well as polysaccharides. Fungal infections are generally resistant to antibiotics used in the treatment of bacterial infections. Conversely, bacteria are resistant to the antifungal agents (Figure 33.1).

II. DRUGS FOR SUBCUTANEOUS AND SYSTEMIC MYCOTIC INFECTIONS

Infectious diseases caused by fungi are called mycoses and are often chronic in nature. Many common mycotic infections are superficial and only involve the skin. Fungi may also invade the skin to cause subcutaneous infections. The most serious and difficult to treat are the systemic mycoses. Immunosuppressed or debilitated patients often suffer from so-called opportunistic fungal infections (e.g., candidiasis, aspergillosis). Some mycotic infections are endemic to certain geographic regions.

A. Amphotericin B

Amphotericin B [am foe TER i sin] is a polyene antibiotic. In spite of its toxic potential, *amphotericin B* is the major drug used in the treatment of the systemic mycoses. It is sometimes used in combination with *flucytosine* so that lower levels of *amphotericin* are required.

1. **Mode of action:**

   a. Several polyene molecules bind to ergosterol present in cell membranes of sensitive fungal cells to form pores or channels that involve hydrophobic bonds between the lipophilic segment of the polyene antibiotic and the sterol (Figure 33.2). This disrupts membrane function, allowing electrolytes (particularly potassium) and small molecules to leak from the cell, resulting in cell death.

   b. Since the polyene antibiotics bind preferentially to ergosterol rather than cholesterol, the sterol found in mammalian membranes, a relative (but not absolute) specificity is conferred.

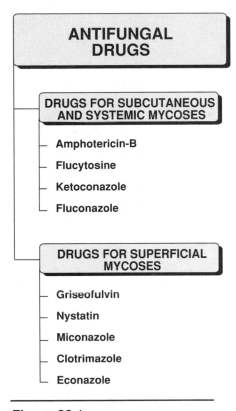

ANTIFUNGAL DRUGS

DRUGS FOR SUBCUTANEOUS AND SYSTEMIC MYCOSES

— Amphotericin-B

— Flucytosine

— Ketoconazole

— Fluconazole

DRUGS FOR SUPERFICIAL MYCOSES

— Griseofulvin

— Nystatin

— Miconazole

— Clotrimazole

— Econazole

Figure 33.1
Summary of antifungal drugs.

307

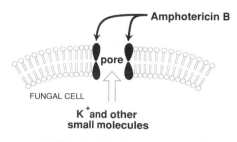

Figure 33.2
Model of pore formed by amphotericin in lipid bilayer membrane.

2. **Antifungal spectrum**: *Amphotericin B* is either fungicidal or fungistatic, depending on the organism and the concentration of the drug. It is effective against candida species, Histoplasma capsulatum, Cryptococcus neoformans, Coccidioides immitis, many strains of aspergillus, and Blastomyces dermatitidis.

3. **Resistance:** Fungal resistance, though infrequent, is associated with decreased ergosterol content of the membrane.

4. **Pharmacology:** *Amphotericin B* is administered by intravenous infusion. The intrathecal route is chosen for the treatment of meningitis caused by fungi that are sensitive to *amphotericin B*. *Amphotericin B* is distributed throughout the body becoming highly tissue-bound. Inflammation favors penetration into various body fluids, but little is found in the cerebrospinal fluid, vitreous humor, or amniotic fluid. However, *amphotericin B* does cross the placenta. Bile is the major route of excretion, although low levels of the drug, mostly metabolites, appear in the urine over a long period of time. Adjustment of dose is not required in patients with compromised renal or hepatic function.

5. **Adverse effects:** *Amphotericin B* has a low therapeutic index. Usually small test doses are administered to assess the degree of a patient's response, for example, anaphylaxis or convulsions. Other toxic manifestations include the following.

   a. **Fever and chills:** These appear with intravenous administration but usually subside with repeated administration of the drug.

   b. **Renal impairment:** Despite the low levels of the drug excreted in the urine, over 80% of patients exhibit impaired renal function. Normal renal function usually returns on suspension of the drug, but residual damage is likely at high doses. Azotemia is exacerbated by other nephrotoxic drugs, although adequate hydration can decrease its severity.

   c. **Hypotension:** A shock-like fall in blood pressure accompanied by hypokalemia may occur, requiring potassium supplementation. Care must be exercised in patients taking *digitalis*.

   d. **Anemia:** Normochromic, normocytic anemia caused by a reversible suppression of erythrocyte production may occur. This may be exacerbated in patients with human immunodeficiency virus HIV who are taking *zidovudine*.

   e. **Neurological effects:** Intrathecal administration can cause a variety of neurological problems.

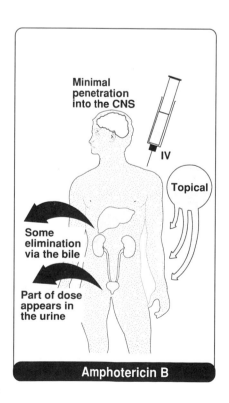

B. Flucytosine

Flucytosine [floo SYE toe seen] is a synthetic pyrimidine antimetabolite used in the treatment of systemic mycoses only in combination with *amphotericin B* except for the treatment of subcutaneous chromomycosis where the drug is used singly.

1. **Mode of action:** The drug enters fungal cells via a cytosine-specific permease. It is then converted by a series of steps to 5-fluorodeoxyuridylic acid (5-FdUMP); this acid inhibits thymidylate synthetase, thus depriving the organism of an essential DNA component (Figure 33.3). The unnatural pyrimidine is also metabolized to the nucleotide (5-FUTP) and incorporated into fungal RNA, causing disruption of its function in protein synthesis. The combination of *flucytosine* and *amphotericin B* is synergistic. [Note: The *amphotericin B* affects cell permeability, allowing more of the *flucytosine* to penetrate the cell.]

2. **Antifungal spectrum**: *Flucytosine* is fungistatic and effective in treating candidiasis, cryptococcosis, aspergillosis, and chromomycosis.

3. **Resistance:** Resistance can develop during therapy and is the reason that *flucytosine* is not used as a single antimycotic drug. The rate of emergence of resistant fungal cells is lower with the combination of *amphotericin B* and *flucytosine* than it is with *flucytosine* alone.

4. **Pharmacology:** *Flucytosine* is well absorbed by the oral route, distributes throughout the body water, and penetrates well into CSF. 5-Fluorouracil is detectable in patients and probably is due to metabolism of *flucytosine* by intestinal bacteria. Excretion of both the parent drug and its metabolites is by glomerular filtration, and the dose must be adjusted in patients with compromised renal function.

5. **Adverse effects**

   a. **Hematological toxicity:** *Flucytosine* causes reversible neutropenia, thrombocytopenia, and occasional bone marrow depression. Caution must be exercised in patients undergoing radiation or chemotherapy with drugs that depress bone marrow.

   b. **Hepatic dysfunction:** Reversible hepatic dysfunction with elevation of serum transaminases and alkaline phosphatase may occur.

   c. **Gastrointestinal disturbances:** Nausea, vomiting, diarrhea and severe enterocolitis may occur.

C. Ketoconazole

Ketoconazole [kee toe KON a zole], a substituted imidazole, is useful in treating systemic mycoses. In addition to its antifungal activity, *ketoconazole* also inhibits gonadal and adrenal steroid synthesis in humans by blocking C17-20 lyase, 11β-hydroxylase, and cholesterol side-chain cleavage; thus, it suppresses *testosterone* and *cortisol* synthesis.[1]

1. **Mode of action**: *Ketoconazole* blocks cytochrome P-450 mediated lanosterol demethylation to ergosterol, the principal sterol of

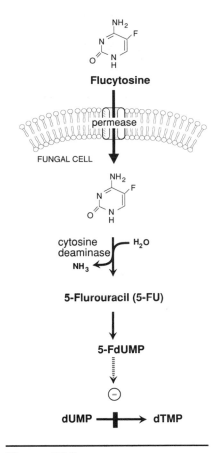

Figure 33.3
Mode of action of flucytosine.

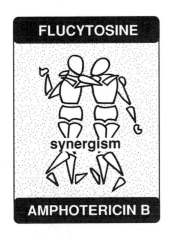

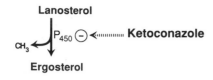

Figure 33.4
Mode of action of ketoconazole.

fungal membranes (Figure 33.4). This inhibition disrupts membrane function and increases permeability. *Ketoconazole* acts in an additive manner with *flucytosine* against candida, but antagonizes *amphotericin B*'s antifungal activity.

2. **Antifungal spectrum**: *Ketoconazole* is either fungistatic or fungicidal, depending on the dose. Although active against the same fungi as *amphotericin B,* it is most useful in the treatment of histoplasmosis. *Ketoconazole* is also effective against nonmeningeal cryptococcosis and blastomycosis. candida, and various dermatophytic infections, including those resistant to *griseofulvin* are also susceptible.

3. **Resistance:** No resistance has been observed.

4. **Pharmacology:** *Ketoconazole* is only administered orally. It dissolves in the acidic gastric contents and is absorbed through the gastric mucosa. Food, antacids, *cimetidine,* and *rifampin* impair absorption. Although penetration into tissues is limited, it is effective in the treatment of histoplasmosis in lung, bone, skin, and soft tissues. It does not enter the CSF. Extensive metabolism occurs in the liver. Induction of the cytochrome P-450 system enzymes (p.12) in the liver shortens the half-life of *ketoconazole.* Excretion is primarily through the bile. Levels of parent drug are too low to be effective against urinary tract mycotic infections.

5. **Adverse effects:** These effects are primarily gastrointestinal. In addition to allergies, other toxicities include the following effects.

   a. **Gynecomastia:** This results from blocking of androgen and adrenal steroid synthesis by *ketoconazole.*

   b. **Hepatic dysfunction:** Although the incidence is low, hepatic dysfunction, with elevation of serum transaminase levels, is a serious toxic manifestation. *Ketoconazole* may accumulate in patients with hepatic dysfunction. Plasma concentrations of the drug should be monitored in these individuals.

   c. **Contraindications:** *Ketoconazole* and *amphotericin B* should not be used together.

   d. **Drug interaction:** *Ketoconazole* can potentiate the toxicity of *cyclosporine* because it inhibits the latter's metabolism.

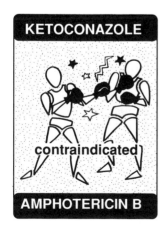

D. Fluconazole

Fluconazole [floo KON a zole] has recently become available and has made an important clinical impact. It is not structurally related to *ketoconazole,* but it does inhibit the synthesis of fungal membrane sterols. The drug is administered orally or intravenously. Its importance lies in its ability to penetrate the cerebrospinal fluid of normal and inflamed meninges. *Fluconazole* is the agent of choice for the treatment of cryptococcal meningoencephalitis, disseminated histoplasmosis, and coccidioidomycosis, conditions that appear in immunocompromised patients. These infections are characterized by a high rate of relapse, and *fluconazole* has proved effective in ambulatory treatment. The drug is excreted via the kidney. Its adverse effects are less of a problem than with *ketoconazole*; *fluconazole* has no endocrinological effects.

III. DRUGS FOR SUPERFICIAL MYCOTIC INFECTIONS

Fungi that cause superficial skin infections are called dermatophytes. Common dermatomycoses, also called tinea infections, are often referred to as ringworm, which is a misnomer, since fungi rather than worms cause the disease.

A. Griseofulvin

1. **Mode of action**: *Griseofulvin* [gri see oh FUL vin] enters susceptible fungal cells by an energy-dependent process and interacts with the microtubules within the dermatophyte to disrupt the mitotic spindle and inhibit mitosis (Figure 33.5). It accumulates in the infected, newly synthesized, keratin-containing tissues, making them unsuitable for the growth of the fungi. Therapy must be continued until normal tissue replaces infected tissue. This usually requires long-term therapy.

2. **Antifungal spectrum:** The drug is principally fungistatic. It is effective only against the dermatophytes—Trichophyton, Microsporum, and Epidermophyton. It is used in the treatment of severe tinea infections that do not respond to other antifungal agents.

3. **Resistance:** Resistance is due to the lack of the energy-dependent uptake system.

4. **Pharmacology:** Ultra-fine crystalline preparations are absorbed adequately from the gastrointestinal tract. Absorption is promoted if ingested with a high fat diet. *Phenobarbital* can interfere with the absorption of *griseofulvin*. The drug is ineffective topically. *Griseofulvin* distributes chiefly to infected keratinized tissue where it becomes bound; therefore, it is uniquely suited for the treatment of dermatophytic infections. Concentrations in other tissues and body fluids are much lower. *Griseofulvin* is extensively metabolized to the demethylated and glucuronidated form. *Griseofulvin* induces hepatic cytochrome P-450 activity and can increase the rate of metabolism of a number of drugs including oral anticoagulants (p.192). Excretion of the drug occurs via the kidney, primarily as metabolites.

5. **Adverse effects:** Toxicity is not generally a clinical problem although allergic reactions and a number of adverse effects (e.g., headache, nausea) have been reported. *Griseofulvin* may cause hepatotoxicity and is contraindicated in patients with acute intermittent porphyria due to elevated heme synthesis. The drug potentiates the intoxicating effects of alcohol. *Griseofulvin* is teratogenic.

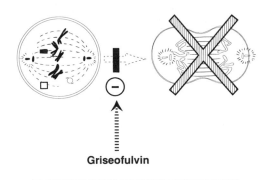

Griseofulvin

Figure 33.5
Inhibition of mitosis by griseofulvin.

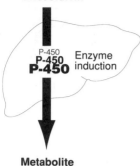

Griseofulvin

P-450
P-450 **Enzyme**
P-450 induction

Metabolite

B. Nystatin

Nystatin [nye STAT in] is a polyene antibiotic; its structure, chemistry, mode of action, and resistance resemble those of *amphotericin B.* Its use is restricted to topical treatment of candidiasis because of its systemic toxicity. The drug is negligibly absorbed from the gastrointestinal tract, and it is never used parenterally. It is administered orally for the treatment of oral and intestinal candidiasis. Excretion in the feces is nearly quantitative. Adverse effects are rare because of its lack of absorption, but occasionally nausea and vomiting occur.

C. Miconazole and other topical agents

Miconazole [mi KON a zole], *clotrimazole* [kloe TRIM a zole], and *econazole* [e KON a zole] are topically active drugs and are only rarely administered parenterally because of their severe toxicity. Their mechanism of action, antifungal spectrum, distribution, and type of metabolism are the same as *ketoconazole.*

Study Questions   (see p.433 for answers).

Questions 33.1 - 33.3: For each numbered phrase, select the ONE drug (A-E) that is most closely associated with it. Each drug (A-E) may be selected once, more than once, or not at all.

    A. Flucytosine
    B. Griseofulvin
    C. Penicillin G
    D. Amphotericin-B
    E. Ketoconazole

33.1 Binds to ergosterol present in cell membranes of sensitive fungal cells, thereby disrupting membrane function.

33.2 Blocks lanosterol demethylation to ergosterol, thus disrupting fungal membrane integrity.

33.3 Is metabolized to a product that inhibits thymidylate synthetase and thus prevents DNA synthesis.

Choose the ONE best answer.

33.4 Which one of the following drugs is not used for the treatment of systemic fungal infections?

    A. Amphotericin B.
    B. Flucytosine.
    C. Ketoconazole.
    D. Griseofulvin.
    E. Fluconazole.

33.5 All of the following statements correctly describe ketoconazole EXCEPT:

    A. It inhibits the conversion of lanosterol to ergosterol.
    B. It may produce gastrointestinal upsets.
    C. It can cause gynecomastia in males.
    D. It penetrates into the cerebrospinal fluid.
    E. It should not be combined with amphotericin B.

33.6 All of the following statements concerning griseofulvin are correct EXCEPT:

    A. It is only effective against dermatophytic infections.
    B. It exacerbates acute intermittent porphyria.
    C. It induces the hepatic cytochrome P-450 system.
    D. It enhances CNS depressant effects of ethanol.
    E. Its use in therapy for superficial mycotic infections is usually short term (several days).

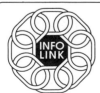

[1]See *steroid hormones, synthesis* in **Biochemistry** for the reactions of steroid biosynthesis (see index).

Antiprotozoal Drugs

34

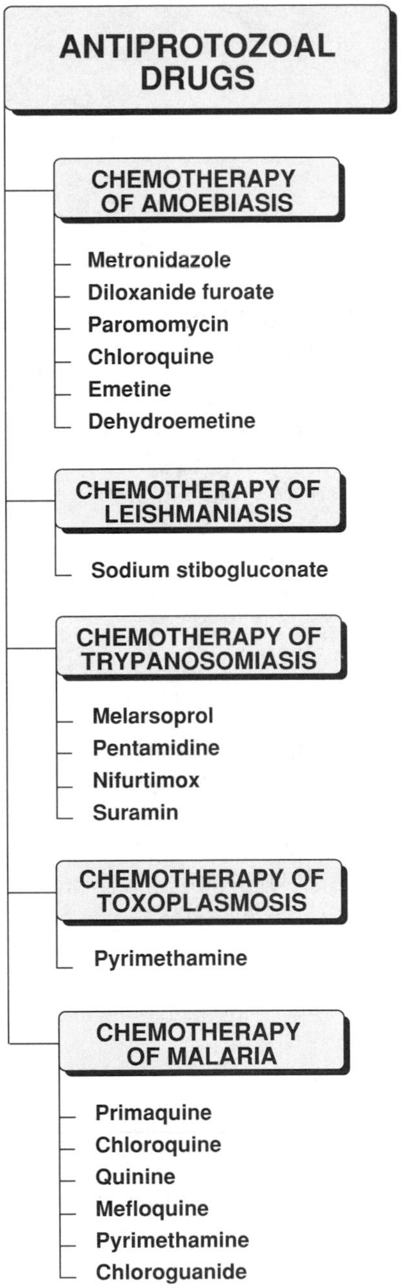

I. OVERVIEW

Protozoal infections are particularly common among people in under-developed countries where sanitary conditions, hygienic practices, and control of the vectors of transmission are inadequate. However, with increased world travel, protozoal diseases such as malaria, amebiasis, leishmaniasis, trypanosomiasis, trichomoniasis, and giardiasis are no longer confined to specific geographic locales.

Many of the antiprotozoal drugs cause toxic effects, and most of these drugs have not proved safe for pregnant patients. Furthermore, many drugs used to treat protozoan infections are not available commercially in the United States, although they can be obtained from the Center for Disease Control, Atlanta, Georgia. Drugs used to treat protozoan infections are summarized in Figure 34.1

II. CHEMOTHERAPY OF AMEBIASIS

Amebiasis (also called amebic dysentery) is an infection of the intestinal tract caused by Entamoeba histolytica. A summary of the life cycle of this organism is presented in Figure 34.2.

A. Therapeutic strategy

1. Therapy is aimed not only at the acutely ill patient but also at those who are asymptomatic carriers since dormant Entamoeba histolytica in these individuals may cause future infections in the carrier and may be a potential source of infection of others.

2. Intestinal amebae feed on normal intestinal flora. Therefore, one strategy for treating luminal amebiasis is to treat it with antibiotics, such as *tetracycline,* that eliminate intestinal flora and therefore the ameba's major food source. However, antibiotics are not highly effective when used alone; thus, they are usually combined with other antiprotozoal agents.

ANTIPROTOZOAL DRUGS

CHEMOTHERAPY OF AMOEBIASIS
- Metronidazole
- Diloxanide furoate
- Paromomycin
- Chloroquine
- Emetine
- Dehydroemetine

CHEMOTHERAPY OF LEISHMANIASIS
- Sodium stibogluconate

CHEMOTHERAPY OF TRYPANOSOMIASIS
- Melarsoprol
- Pentamidine
- Nifurtimox
- Suramin

CHEMOTHERAPY OF TOXOPLASMOSIS
- Pyrimethamine

CHEMOTHERAPY OF MALARIA
- Primaquine
- Chloroquine
- Quinine
- Mefloquine
- Pyrimethamine
- Chloroguanide

Figure 34.1
Summary of antiprotozoal agents.

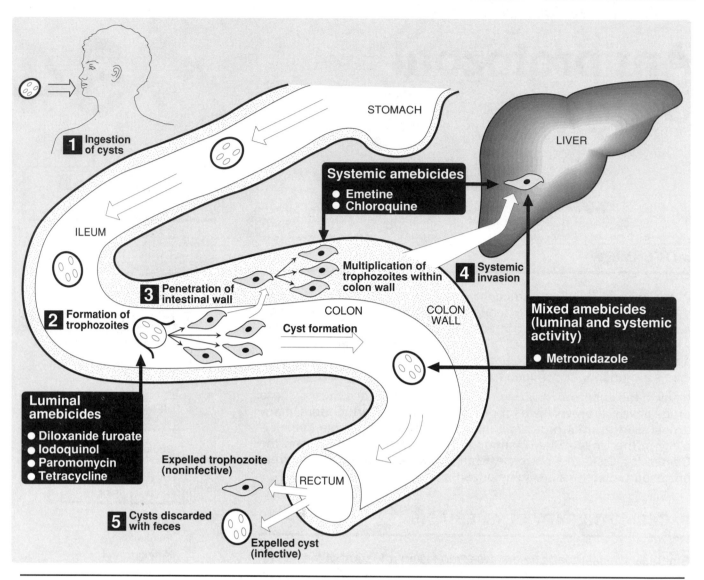

Figure 34.2
Life cycle of *Entamoeba histolytica* showing sites of action of amebicidic drugs.

B. Classification of antiprotozoal drugs

Therapeutic agents are classified as mixed, luminal, or systemic amebicides.

1. **Mixed amebicides:** These amebicides, including *metronidazole*, are effective against both the luminal and systemic forms of the disease.

2. **Luminal amebicides:** Luminal amebicides such as *diloxanide furoate*, *tetracycline*, and *paromomycin*, act on the parasite in the lumen of the bowel.

3. **Systemic amebicides:** These amebicides, including *emetine*, *dehydroemetine*, and *chloroquine*, are effective against amebae in the intestine and the liver.

C. Mixed amebicide: metronidazole

Amebiasis is generally treated with a combination of *metronidazole* [me troe NYE da zole] plus a luminal amebicidal drug, such as *diloxanide furoate.* This combination provides cure rates of greater than 90%. Moreover, *metronidazole* has many other clinical applications.

1. **Mode of action:** *Metronidazole* is selectively toxic not only for amebae but also for anaerobic organisms (including bacteria), and for anoxic or hypoxic cells. Some anaerobic protozoan parasites (including amebae) possess ferrodoxinlike, low-redox potential, electron transport proteins that participate in metabolic electron removal reactions. The nitro group of *metronidazole* is able to serve as an electron acceptor, forming a reduced cytotoxic compound that binds to proteins and DNA and results in cell death.

2. **Antimicrobial spectrum**

    a. *Metronidazole* is the agent of choice for treating infections caused by <u>Entamoeba histolytica</u>, <u>Giardia lamblia</u>, and <u>Trichomonas vaginalis</u> in both males and females.

    b. *Metronidazole* finds extensive use in the treatment of infections caused by anaerobic cocci and anaerobic gram-negative bacilli (for example, bacteroides species). Anaerobic grampositive bacilli, such as clostridia, are also sensitive. The drug is effective in the treatment of brain abscesses caused by these organisms.

3. **Resistance:** Resistance is not a therapeutic problem, although strains of trichomonads resistant to *metronidazole* have been reported.

4. **Pharmacology**

    a. **Administration and distribution:** *Metronidazole* is completely and rapidly absorbed after oral administration and is usually administered with a luminal amebicide, such as *diloxanide furoate.* It distributes well throughout body tissues and fluids. Therapeutic levels can be found in vaginal and seminal fluids, saliva, and cerebrospinal fluid.

    b. **Fate:** Metabolism depends on hepatic oxidation of the *metronidazole* side-chain by mixed function oxidase, followed by glucuronidation (p.12). Therefore, concomitant treatment with inducers of this enzymatic system, such as *phenobarbital* (p.97), enhance the rate of metabolism.

5. **Adverse effects:** The most common adverse effects are those associated with the gastrointestinal tract—nausea, vomiting, epigastric distress, and abdominal cramps. An unpleasant metallic taste is often experienced. Other effects include oral moniliasis (yeast infection of the mouth) and neurotoxicological problems, such as dizziness, vertigo, and numbness or paresthesias in the peripheral nervous system. [Note: These are reasons for

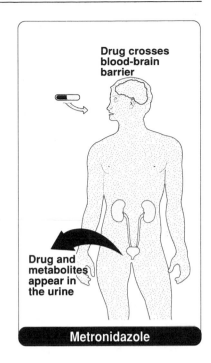

Drug crosses blood-brain barrier

Drug and metabolites appear in the urine

Metronidazole

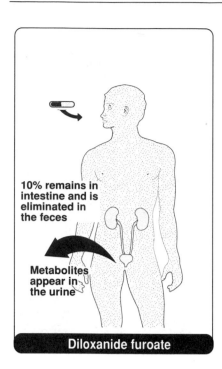

10% remains in intestine and is eliminated in the feces

Metabolites appear in the urine

Diloxanide furoate

discontinuing the drug.] If taken with alcohol, a *disulfiram*-like effect occurs (p.96).

D. Luminal amebicide: Diloxanide furoate

Diloxanide furoate [dye LOX an ide] is the drug of choice in the treatment of asymptomatic passers of cysts. Its only indication is in the treatment of intestinal amebiasis. After oral administration, *diloxanide furoate* is hydrolyzed in the intestinal mucosa, and the diloxanide is about 90% absorbed. However, the unabsorbed drug is the active amebicide. Adverse effects are mild. They include flatulence, dryness of the mouth, pruritus, and urticaria. The drug is contraindicated among pregnant women and children under 2 years of age.

E. Luminal amebicide: Paromomycin

Paromomycin [par oh moe MYE sin], an aminoglycoside antibiotic, is only effective against the intestinal (luminal) forms of amebiasis and tapeworm, since it is not significantly absorbed from the gastrointestinal tract. It is an alternate agent for amebiasis. Although directly amebicidal, *paromomycin* also exerts its antiamebic actions by reducing the population of the intestinal flora (an essential food source needed for proliferation of the amebae). Its direct amebicidal action is probably due to the effects it has on the cell membrane to cause leakage. In other microorganisms, it inhibits protein synthesis, as described earlier for the aminoglycoside antibiotics (p.288). Resistance may be due to the same mechanisms that cause resistance to the aminoglycosides (p.288). Gastrointestinal distress and diarrhea are the principal adverse effects.

F. Systemic amebicide: Chloroquine

Chloroquine [KLOR oh kwin] is used in conjunction with *metronidazole* and *diloxanide furoate* to treat and prevent amebic liver abscess. *Chloroquine* is also effective in the treatment of malaria. It eliminates trophozoites in liver abscesses, but it is not useful in treating luminal amebiasis. Administration, distribution, and adverse effects of *chloroquine* are described in the malaria section (p.320).

G. Systemic amebicides: Emetine and dehydroemetine

Emetine [EM e teen] and *dehydroemetine* [de hi dro EM e teen] are alternate agents for the treatment of amebiasis. Their use is limited by their toxicities. *Dehydroemetine* is probably less toxic than *emetine*. Close clinical observation is necessary when these drugs are used. Among the untoward effects are pain at the site of injection, transient nausea, cardiotoxicity (e.g., arrhythmias, congestive heart failure), neuromuscular weakness, dizziness, and rashes.

III. CHEMOTHERAPY OF LEISHMANIASIS

The treatments of leishmaniasis and trypanosomiasis (see next section, p.317) are difficult, because the drugs employed are limited by their toxicities and failure rates. Pentavalent antimonials, such as *sodium stibogluconate,* are the conventional therapy used in the treatment of leishmaniasis, with *pentamidine* (p.318) and *amphotericin B* (p.307) as back-up agents. *Allopurinol* (p.376) has also been reported to be effective.

A. Life cycle of the causative organism, *Leishmania*

Leishmaniasis is transmitted from animal to humans (and between humans) by the bite of infected sandflies. The sandfly transfers the flagellated promastigote form of the protozoa, which is rapidly phagocytized by macrophages. In the macrophage, the promastigotes rapidly change to nonflagellated amastigotes and multiply, killing the cell. The newly released amastigotes are again phagocytized, and the cycle continues.

B. Sodium stibogluconate

Stibogluconate [stib o GLOO koe nate] is not effective *in vitro,* therefore it has been proposed that reduction to the trivalent antimony compound is essential for activity. The exact mechanism of action has not been determined. Evidence for inhibition of glycolysis in the parasite at the phosphofructokinase reaction[1] has been found. Because it is not absorbed on oral administration, *sodium stibogluconate* must be administered parenterally. It is distributed in the extravascular compartment. Metabolism is minimal, if at all, and the drug is excreted into the urine. Adverse effects include pain at the injection site, gastrointestinal upsets, and cardiac arrhythmias. Renal and hepatic function should also be periodically monitored.

IV. CHEMOTHERAPY OF TRYPANOSOMIASIS

Trypanosomiasis refers to two chronic and eventually fatal diseases caused by species of trypanosomes: African sleeping sickness and American sleeping sickness (Figure 34.3). In African sleeping sickness, the causative organism initially lives and grows in the blood. In later stages, the parasite invades the central nervous system, causing an inflammation of the brain and spinal cord that produces the characteristic lethargy and eventually continuous sleep.

A. Melarsoprol

Melarsoprol [me LAR soe prole] is a derivative of *mersalyl oxide,* a trivalent arsenical.

1. **Mode of action:** The drug reacts with sulfhydryl groups of various substances including enzymes in both the organism and host. Parasitic enzymes may be more sensitive than are those of the host. There is some evidence that mammalian cells may be less permeable to the drug and thus are protected from its toxic effects.

2. **Antimicrobial spectrum:** *Melarsoprol* is limited to the treatment of trypanosomal infections and is lethal for these parasites.

3. **Resistance:** Resistance may be due to decreased permeability to the drug.

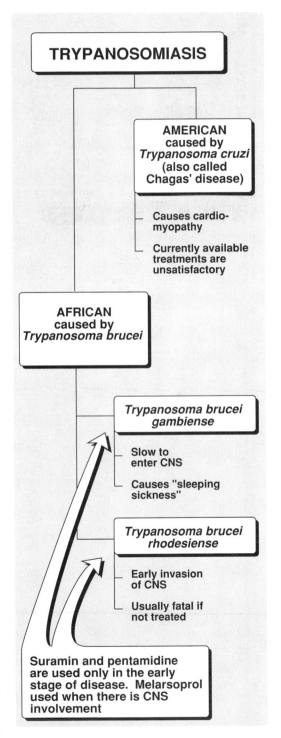

Figure 34.3
Summary of trypanosomiasis.

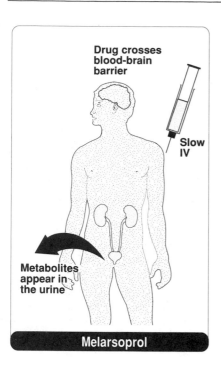

Drug crosses blood-brain barrier

Slow IV

Metabolites appear in the urine

Melarsoprol

4. **Pharmacology**

   a. **Administration and distribution:** *Melarsoprol* is usually slowly administered intravenously through a fine needle, even though it is absorbed from the gastrointestinal tract. Because it is very irritating, care should be taken not to infiltrate surrounding tissue. Adequate trypanocidal concentrations appear in the cerebrospinal fluid, which contrasts with *pentamidine* (see later), which does not enter the cerebrospinal fluid. *Melarsoprol* is therefore the agent of choice in the treatment of Trypanosoma rhodesiense, which rapidly invades the central nervous system, as well as for meningoencephalitis caused by Trypanosoma brucei gambiense.

   b. **Fate:** The host readily oxidizes the drug to the relatively nontoxic pentavalent arsenic compound. The drug has a very short half-life and is rapidly excreted into the urine.

5. **Adverse effects:**

   a. **Central nervous system toxicities:** These side effects are the most serious. Encephalopathy may appear soon after the first course of treatment but usually subsides. It may, however, be fatal.

   b. **Hypersensitivity reactions:** Such reactions may also occur. Fever may follow injection.

   c. **Gastrointestinal disturbance:** Severe vomiting and abdominal pain can be minimized if the patient is in the fasting state during drug administration and for several hours thereafter.

   d. **Contraindications:** *Melarsoprol* is contraindicated in patients with influenza. Hemolytic anemia has been seen in patients with glucose 6-phosphate dehydrogenase deficiency.

B. Pentamidine

Pentamidine [pen TAM i deen] is active against protozoal infections, including those caused by Pneumocystis carinii (p.336). [Note: Because of the increased incidence of pneumonia caused by the latter organism in immunocompromised patients such as those infected with human immunodeficiency virus (HIV), *pentamidine* has assumed an important place in chemotherapy.] *Pentamidine* is the drug of choice for the prevention and treatment of the nematolologic stage of T. brucei gambiense.

1. **Structure:** *Pentamidine isethionate* (or *methanesulfonate*) is an aromatic diamidine with a low solubility in water. It is important to promptly use prepared solutions of this drug and to protect them from light in order to guard against formation of hepatotoxic compounds.

2. **Mode of action:** T. brucei concentrates the drug by an energy-dependent, high-affinity uptake system. Although its mode of action has not been defined, evidence exists that the drug binds to the parasite's DNA, and/or that it interferes with glycolysis.

3. **Antimicrobial spectrum**: *Pentamidine* is not effective against all trypanosomes, for example, *T. cruzi* is resistant. However, *pentamidine* is effective in the treatment of systemic blastomycosis. *Pentamidine* is also effective against Pneumocystis carinii, but *trimethoprim-sulfamethoxazole* is preferred. *Pentamidine* is the drug of choice in treating patients with pneumonia caused by Pneumocystis carinii who have failed to respond to *trimethoprim-sulfamethoxazole* (p.269), or in treating individuals who are allergic to sulfonamides.

4. **Resistance**: Resistance is associated with an inability of the trypanosome to concentrate the drug.

5. **Pharmacology:**

   a. **Administration and distribution**: Fresh solutions are administered intramuscularly or as an aerosol. [Note: The intravenous route is associated with severe adverse reactions, such as a sharp fall in blood pressure and tachycardia.] The drug is concentrated and stored in the liver and kidney for a long period of time. Because it does not enter the CSF, it is ineffective against the meningoencephalitic stage of the disease.

   b. **Fate:** The drug is not metabolized and is excreted very slowly into the urine.

6. **Adverse effects**: Serious renal dysfunction may occur, which reverses on discontinuation of the drug.

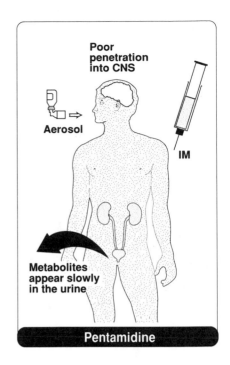

C. Nifurtimox

Nifurtimox [nye FYOOR ti mox], an experimental drug, has found use only in the treatment of acute T. cruzi infections (Chagas' disease) although treatment of the chronic stage of such infections has led to variable results. [Note: *Nifurtimox* is suppressive not curative.] *Nifurtimox* forms intracellular oxygen radicals in both the amastigote and trypomastigote of T. cruzi). These highly reactive radicals, such as superoxide radicals and hydrogen peroxide, are toxic to the organism. Mammalian cells are partially protected from such substances by the presence of enzymes such as catalase, glutathione peroxidase, and superoxide dismutase. The drug is administered orally and is rapidly absorbed and metabolized to unidentified products, which are excreted in the urine. Adverse effects are common following chronic administration, particularly among the elderly. Major toxicities include immediate hypersensitivity reactions, such as anaphylaxis; delayed hypersensitivity reactions, for example, dermatitis and icterus; and gastrointestinal problems that may be so severe as to cause weight loss. Peripheral neuropathy is relatively common, and disturbances in the CNS may also occur. In addition, cell-mediated immune reactions may be suppressed.

D. Suramin

Suramin [SOO ra min] is used primarily in the treatment and especially in the prophylaxis of African trypanosomiasis. Inhibition of enzymes involved in energy metabolism (e.g., glycerol phosphate dehydrogenase) appears to be the mechanism most closely correlated with trypanocidal activity. *Suramin* is also the drug of choice in treatment of patients with the adult forms of the filarial parasite, Onchocerca volvulus. The severity of the adverse reactions demands that the patient be carefully followed, especially if the patient is debilitated. Although infrequent, these reactions include nausea and vomiting (which causes further debilitation of the patient), shock and loss of consciousness, acute urticaria, and neurological problems that include paresthesia, photophobia, palpebral edema, and hyperesthesia of the hands and feet. Albuminuria tends to be common, but when cylindruria (the presence of renal casts in the urine) and hematuria occur, treatment should cease.

V. CHEMOTHERAPY OF TOXOPLASMOSIS

One of the most common infections in man is caused by the protozoan, Toxoplasma gondii, which is transmitted to humans when they consume raw or inadequately cooked, infected meat. Infected pregnant women can transmit the organism to the fetus. Cats are the only animals that shed oocysts that can infect other animals as well as man. The treatment of choice for this condition is the antifolate drug, *pyrimethamine* [peer i METH a meen] (p.323). A combination of *sulfadiazine* (p.265) and *pyrimethamine* is also efficacious. However, other inhibitors of folate biosynthesis, such as *trimethoprim* (p.267) and *sulfamethoxazole* (p.265) are without therapeutic efficacy in toxoplasmosis.

VI. CHEMOTHERAPY OF MALARIA

A. Parasites that cause malaria

1. **Resistant parasite:** Malaria is caused by members of the protozoal genus plasmodium that are transmitted to humans through the bite of female anopheles mosquitoes. Resistance acquired by the mosquito to insecticides and by the parasite to drugs has led to new therapeutic challenges, particularly in the treatment of Plasmodium falciparum.

2. **Clinically important species:** Four species of plasmodium have been identified with malaria; the most dangerous is Plasmodium falciparum. It causes an acute, rapidly fulminating disease that can lead to death if treatment is not instituted promptly. P. vivax causes a milder form of the disease. P. malariae is common to many tropical regions but P. ovale is rarely encountered.

3. **Life cycle of malaria parasites:** The effectiveness of a drug treatment is related to the particular species of infecting plasmodium and the stage of its life cycle. A summary of the life cycle of the parasite and the sites of therapeutic interventions are presented in Figure 34.4.

B. Tissue schizonticide: Primaquine

Primaquine [PRIM a kwin] eradicates primary exoerythrocytic forms of P. falciparum and P. vivax and the secondary exoerythrocytic

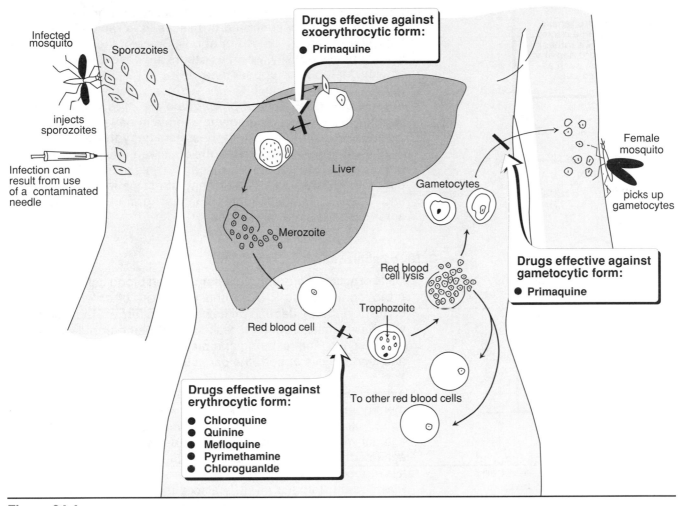

Figure 34.4
Life cycle of the malarial parasite showing the sites of action of antimalarial drugs.

forms of recurring malarias (P. vivax and P. ovale). In addition, the sexual (gametocytic) forms of all four plasmodia are destroyed in the blood or are prevented from maturing later in the mosquito. Because of its lack of activity against the erythrocytic schizonts, *primaquine* is often used in conjunction with a schizonticide.

1. **Mode of action:** This is not completely understood. Intermediates are believed to act as oxidants that are responsible for the schizonticidal action as well as for hemolysis and methemoglobinemia encountered as toxicities.

2. **Antimicrobial spectrum:** In spite of structural similarity to the 4-aminoquinolines (e.g. *chloroquine*), the 8-aminoquinolines are effective only against the exoerythrocytic stages and not the erythrocytic stage of malaria. It is therefore a tissue (exoerythrocytic) schizonticide. It is the only agent that can lead to radical cures of the P. vivax and P. ovale malarias, which may remain in the liver after the erythrocytic form of the disease is eliminated. Because *primaquine* is also gametocidal for all four plasmodia species, transmission of the disease can be interrupted.

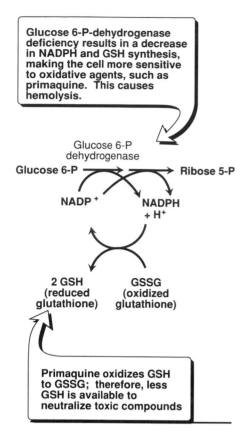

Glucose 6-P-dehydrogenase deficiency results in a decrease in NADPH and GSH synthesis, making the cell more sensitive to oxidative agents, such as primaquine. This causes hemolysis.

Glucose 6-P
dehydrogenase

Glucose 6-P → Ribose 5-P

NADP⁺   NADPH + H⁺

2 GSH (reduced glutathione)   GSSG (oxidized glutathione)

Primaquine oxidizes GSH to GSSG; therefore, less GSH is available to neutralize toxic compounds

Figure 34.5
Mechanism of primaquine-induced hemolytic anemia. GSH- reduced glutathione, GSSG- oxidized glutathione.

3. **Pharmacology:** *Primaquine* is well absorbed on oral administration and is not concentrated in tissues. It is rapidly oxidatively biotransformed to many compounds. Some of these possess the schizonticidal activity, whereas others are devoid of antimalarial activity. Metabolites appear in urine.

4. **Adverse effects:** Effects of *primaquine* are of low incidence except for drug-induced hemolytic anemia in patients with genetically low levels of glucose-6-phosphate dehydrogenase (Figure 34.5).[2] Other toxic manifestations observed after large doses of the drug include abdominal discomfort, especially in combination with *chloroquine,* (which may affect patient compliance), and occasional methemoglobinemia; granulocytopenia and agranulocytosis are rarely seen.

C. Blood schizonticide: Chloroquine

1. **Mode of action:** *Chloroquine* enters the red blood cells and blocks protozoal DNA and RNA synthesis. Uptake of *chloroquine* into erythrocytes may depend on its binding to ferriprotoporphyrin IX which is formed from the breakdown of hemoglobin in infected erythrocytes. The resulting complex may damage the membrane and lead to lysis of both the parasite and the red blood cell.

2. **Antimicrobial spectrum:** The primary therapeutic agent in the treatment of erythrocytic *falciparum* malaria is *chloroquine* [KLOR oh kwin], except in resistant strains. *Chloroquine* is less effective against *vivax* malaria. As an antimalarial, *chloroquine* is effective against only the erythrocytic stage of infection (see Figure 34.4). It is highly specific for the asexual form of Plasmodium vivax and Plasmodium falciparum. It is also effective in the treatment of extraintestinal amebiasis. The anti-inflammatory action of *chloroquine* explains its occasional use in rheumatoid arthritis and discoid lupus erythematosus.

3. **Resistance:** Resistance of plasmodia to available drugs has become a medical problem throughout Asia and some areas of Central and South America. The nature of the resistance has been suggested to be increased efflux of the drug from the resistant schizonts.

4. **Pharmacology:**

   a. **Administration and distribution:** *Chloroquine* is rapidly and completely absorbed via oral administration. Usually 4 days of therapy suffice to cure the disease. The drug concentrates in erythrocytes, liver, spleen, kidney, lung, and melanin-containing tissues as well as leukocytes. The drug also penetrates into the central nervous system and crosses the placenta.

   b. **Fate:** *Chloroquine* is extensively dealkylated by the mixed function oxidases, but some metabolic products retain antimalarial activity. Both parent drug and metabolites are excreted predominantly in the urine. Excretion rate is enhanced as urine is acidified.

5. **Adverse effects:** Side effects are minimal at low doses used in the chemosuppression of malaria. At higher doses, many more toxic effects occur, such as gastrointestinal upset, pruritus, headaches, and visual disturbances (an ophthalmological examination should be routinely performed). Discoloration of the nail beds and mucous membranes may be seen on chronic administration. *Chloroquine* should be used cautiously in patients with hepatic dysfunction or severe gastrointestinal problems, or in patients with neurological or blood disorders. *Chloroquine* can cause electrocardiographic changes, since it has a *quinidine*-like effect. It may also exacerbate dermatitis produced by *gold* or *phenylbutazone* therapy. [Note: Patients with psoriasis or porphyria should not be treated with *chloroquine* because an acute attack may be provoked.]

D. Blood schizonticide: Quinine

Quinine [KWYE nine] is now reserved for malarial strains resistant to other agents. When a *chloroquine*-resistant organism is encountered, therapy usually consists of a combination of *quinine, pyrimethamine,* and a *sulfonamide,* all administered orally. The major adverse effect of *quinine* is cinchonism, a syndrome causing nausea, vomiting, tinnitus, and vertigo. These effects are reversible and are not considered reason to suspend therapy. However, *quinine* should be suspended if a positive result to a Coombs' test for hemolytic anemia occurs.

E. Blood schizonticide: Mefloquine:

Mefloquine [MEF lo kween] appears promising as an effective single agent for suppressing and curing multidrug-resistant forms of Plasmodium falciparum. Its exact mechanism of action remains to be determined, but it apparently can damage the parasite's membrane as much as *quinine* does. Resistant strains have been identified. *Mefloquine* is absorbed well after oral administration and concentrates in the liver and lung. It has a long half-life (17 days) because of concentration in various tissues and because of its continuous circulation through the enterohepatic and enterogastric systems. The drug undergoes extensive metabolism. Its major excretory route is the feces. Adverse reactions at high doses range from nausea, vomiting, and dizziness to disorientation, hallucinations, and depression.

F. Blood schizonticide and sporontocide: Pyrimethamine

The antifolate agent, *pyrimethamine,* is frequently employed as a blood schizonticide to effect a radical cure. It also acts as a strong sporonticide in the mosquito's gut when the mosquito ingests it with the blood of the human host. *Pyrimethamine* inhibits plasmodial dihydrofolate reductase at much lower concentrations than those that inhibit the mammalian enzyme. The inhibition deprives the protozoan of tetrahydrofolate, a cofactor required in the de novo biosynthesis of purines and pyrimidines, and interconversions of certain amino acids.[3] *Pyrimethamine* alone is effective against P. falciparum. In combination with a sulfonamide, it is also used against P. malariae and Toxoplasma gondii (p.320).

G. Sporontocide: Chloroguanide

Chloroguanide [klor oh GWAN ide], another antifolate drug, acts as a blood schizonticide; it is also employed as a prophylactic and a suppressant. The rapid emergence of resistant strains has limited its place in the chemotherapy of malaria.

Study Questions   (see p.434 for answers).

Questions 34.1 - 34.3: For each numbered phrase, select the ONE drug (A-E) that is most closely associated with it. Each drug (A-E) may be selected once, more than once, or not at all.

    A. Sodium stibogluconate
    B. Diloxanide furoate
    C. Pyrimethamine
    D. Emetine
    E. Metronidazole

34.1 A systemic amebicide.

34.2 Used in the treatment of toxoplasmosis.

34.3 Used in the treatment of leishmaniasis.

Choose the ONE best answer.

34.4 All of the following statement about chloroquine are true EXCEPT:

    A. It blocks protozoal DNA and RNA synthesis.
    B. Infected cells can concentrate the drug to a greater extent than can uninfected cells.
    C. It is the drug of choice for the treatment of an acute attack of falciparum or vivax malaria.
    D. Chronic administration may cause discoloration of nail beds and mucous membranes.
    E. Only exoerythrocytic forms of plasmodium are susceptible.

34.5 All of the following statements about metronidazole are true EXCEPT:

    A. It is administered intravenously because it is poorly absorbed after oral administration.
    B. It is effective against a wide variety of anaerobic bacteria.

    C. It produces a disulfiram-like effect on the ingestion of alcohol.
    D. Dosage should be reduced in patients with hepatic dysfunction.
    E. Therapeutic levels can be found in the cerebral spinal fluid.

34.6 All of the following statements about melarsoprol are true EXCEPT:

    A. It reacts with sulfhydryl groups of various cellular substances, including enzymes.
    B. It is equally effective against African and American trypanosomiasis.
    C. Adequate trypanocidal concentrations of the drug appear in the cerebral spinal fluid.
    D. It can cause serious encephalopathy.
    E. It has a very short half-life in the body.

Answer A if 1,2, and 3 are correct.
    B if 1 and 3 are correct.
    C if 2 and 4 are correct.
    D if only 4 is correct.
    E if 1,2,3, and 4 are all correct.

34.7 Which of the following statements about primaquine is/are correct?

    1. It is effective against erythrocytic forms of malaria.
    2. It is used to effect a cure of relapsing vivax malaria.
    3. High (toxic) doses may produce corneal opacities.
    4. Glucose 6-phosphate dehydrogenase deficient individuals are at risk for hemolytic anemia.

34.8 Metronidazole is effective against:

    1. Trichomonas vaginalis.
    2. Entamoeba histolytica.
    3. Bacteroides fragilis.
    4. Aspergillus.

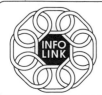

[1]See *phosphofructokinase* in **Biochemistry** for a further discussion of this enzyme (see index).

[2]See g*lucose 6-phosphate dehydrogenase deficiency* in **Biochemistry** for a more detailed discussion of this inherited disease

[3]See *tetrahydrofolic acid* in **Biochemistry** for the role of folic acid in purine and pyrimidine synthesis.

Anthelmintic Drugs

35

I. OVERVIEW

Three major groups of helminths (or worms) infect humans, the nematodes, trematodes, and cestodes. As in all antibiotic regimens, the anthelmintic drugs (Figure 35.1) are aimed at metabolic targets that are present in the parasite but are either absent from or have different characteristics than those of the host. Figure 35.2 illustrates the incidence of helminthic infections.

II. DRUGS FOR THE TREATMENT OF NEMATODES

Nematodes are elongated roundworms that possess a complete digestive system, including both a mouth and an anus. They cause infections of the intestine as well as the blood and tissues.

A. Mebendazole

Mebendazole [me BEN da zole] a synthetic benzimidazole compound, is effective against a wide spectrum of nematodes. It is a drug of choice in the treatment of infections by whipworm (Trichuris trichiura), pinworm (Enterobius vermicularis), and hookworm (Necator americanus and Ancylostoma duodenale). *Mebendazole* acts by binding to and interfering with the synthesis of the parasite's microtubules and also by decreasing glucose uptake. Affected parasites are expelled with the feces. *Mebendazole* is nearly insoluble in aqueous solution, and little of an oral dose (which is chewed) is absorbed by the body. Therefore, this drug is relatively free of toxic effects. However, it is contraindicated in pregnant women, because it has been shown to be embryotoxic and teratogenic in experimental animals.

B. Pyrantel pamoate

Pyrantel pamoate [pi RAN tel] along with *mebendazole* is effective in the treatment of infections caused by roundworm (Ascaris lumbricoides), pinworm, and hookworm. *Pyrantel pamoate* is poorly absorbed orally and exerts its effects in the intestinal tract. It acts as a depolarizing neuromuscular blocking agent, causing persistent activation of nicotinic receptors. This results in paralysis of the worm,

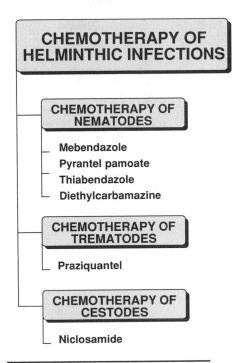

Figure 35.1
Summary of anthelmintic agents.

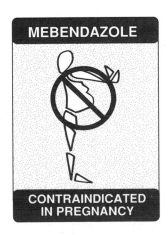

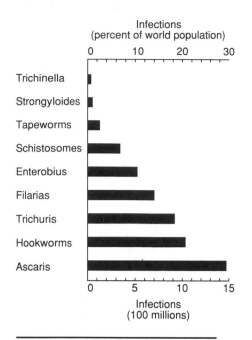

Infections
(percent of world population)

0   10   20   30

Trichinella

Strongyloides

Tapeworms

Schistosomes

Enterobius

Filarias

Trichuris

Hookworms

Ascaris

0   5   10   15

Infections
(100 millions)

Figure 35.2
Relative incidence of helminth
infections worldwide.

which is then expelled from the host's intestinal tract. Adverse effects are mild, and include nausea, vomiting, and diarrhea.

C. Thiabendazole

Thiabendazole [thye a BEN da zole], another synthetic benzimidazole, is effective against strongyloidiasis cutaneous larva migrans (or creeping eruption) and trichinosis (caused by Trichinella spiralis), as well as against infections due to Strongyloides stercoralis (threadworm). Despite its structural similarity to *mebendazole, thiabendazole* has a more limited usefulness because of its potential toxicity. Though nearly insoluble in water, the drug is readily absorbed on oral administration. The adverse effects most often encountered are dizziness, anorexia, nausea, and vomiting. There have been reports of central nervous system symptomatology. Among the cases of erythema multiforme and Stevens-Johnson syndrome there have also been a number of fatalities.

D. Diethylcarbamazine

Diethylcarbamazine [dye eth il kar BAM a zeen] is the drug of choice in the treatment of filariasis (caused by Wuchereria bancrofti or Brugia malayi). Following treatment, the organisms become immobilized. Their surface membranes then undergo alterations that render them more susceptible to host defense mechanisms. However, the precise mechanism of action is unknown. The drug is rapidly absorbed from the gastrointestinal tract, partially metabolized, and is then excreted in the urine. The side effects of the medication are mild. However, some reactions occur because of the dying parasites. They usually affect the skin (e.g., pruritus, wheals) but can also be systemic.

III. DRUGS FOR THE TREATMENT OF TREMATODES

The trematodes (flukes) are leaf-shaped flatworms that are generally characterized by the tissues they infect. For example, they may be categorized as liver, lung, intestinal, or blood flukes.

A. Praziquantel

Trematode (fluke) infections are generally treated with *praziquantel* [pray zi KWON tel]. This drug is an agent of choice for the treatment of all forms of schistosomiasis. Permeability of the cell membrane to calcium is increased, causing contracture and paralysis of the parasite. *Praziquantel* is rapidly absorbed after oral administration and distributes into the cerebrospinal fluid. High levels occur in the bile. The drug is extensively metabolized oxidatively, resulting in a short half-life. The metabolites are inactive and are excreted through the urine. Common adverse effects include drowsiness, dizziness, malaise, and anorexia, as well as gastrointestinal upsets. The drug is not recommended for pregnant women or nursing mothers.

IV. DRUGS FOR THE TREATMENT OF CESTODES

The cestodes, or "true tapeworms," typically have a flat, segmented body and attach to the host's intestine. Like the trematodes, the tapeworms lack a mouth and a digestive tract throughout their life cycle.

A. Niclosamide

Niclosamide [ni KLOE sa mide] is the drug of choice for most cestode (tapeworm) infections. Its action has been ascribed to inhibition of the parasite's mitochondrial anaerobic phosphorylation of ADP which produces usable energy in the form of ATP. The drug is lethal for the cestode's scolex and segments of cestodes but not for the ova. A laxative is administered prior to oral administration of *niclosamide.* This is done to purge the bowel of all dead segments in order to preclude digestion and liberation of the ova, which may lead to cysticercosis.

Figure 35.3 summarizes the infections caused by nematodes and the common therapy used for these infections.

Study Questions (see p.435 for answers).

Questions 35.1 - 35.4: For each numbered phrase, select the ONE drug (A-E) that is most closely associated with it. Each drug (A-E) may be selected once, more than once, or not at all.

A. Mebendazole
B. Praziquantel
C. Niclosamide
D. Pyrantel pamoate
E. Thiabendazole

35.1 A drug of choice for the treatment of infections caused by roundworm, pinworm, and hookworm.

35.2 Acts as a depolarizing neuromuscular blocking agent.

35.3 A drug of choice for the treatment of all forms of schistosomiasis.

Choose the ONE best answer.

35.4 A drug of choice for the treatment of most tapeworm infections.

35.5 All of the following statements about mebendazole are correct EXCEPT:

A. It is contraindicated in pregnant women.
B. It is the drug of choice in the treatment of whipworm infections.
C. It is effective by oral administration.
D. It is active against cestodes.
E. It interferes with glucose uptake by the parasite.

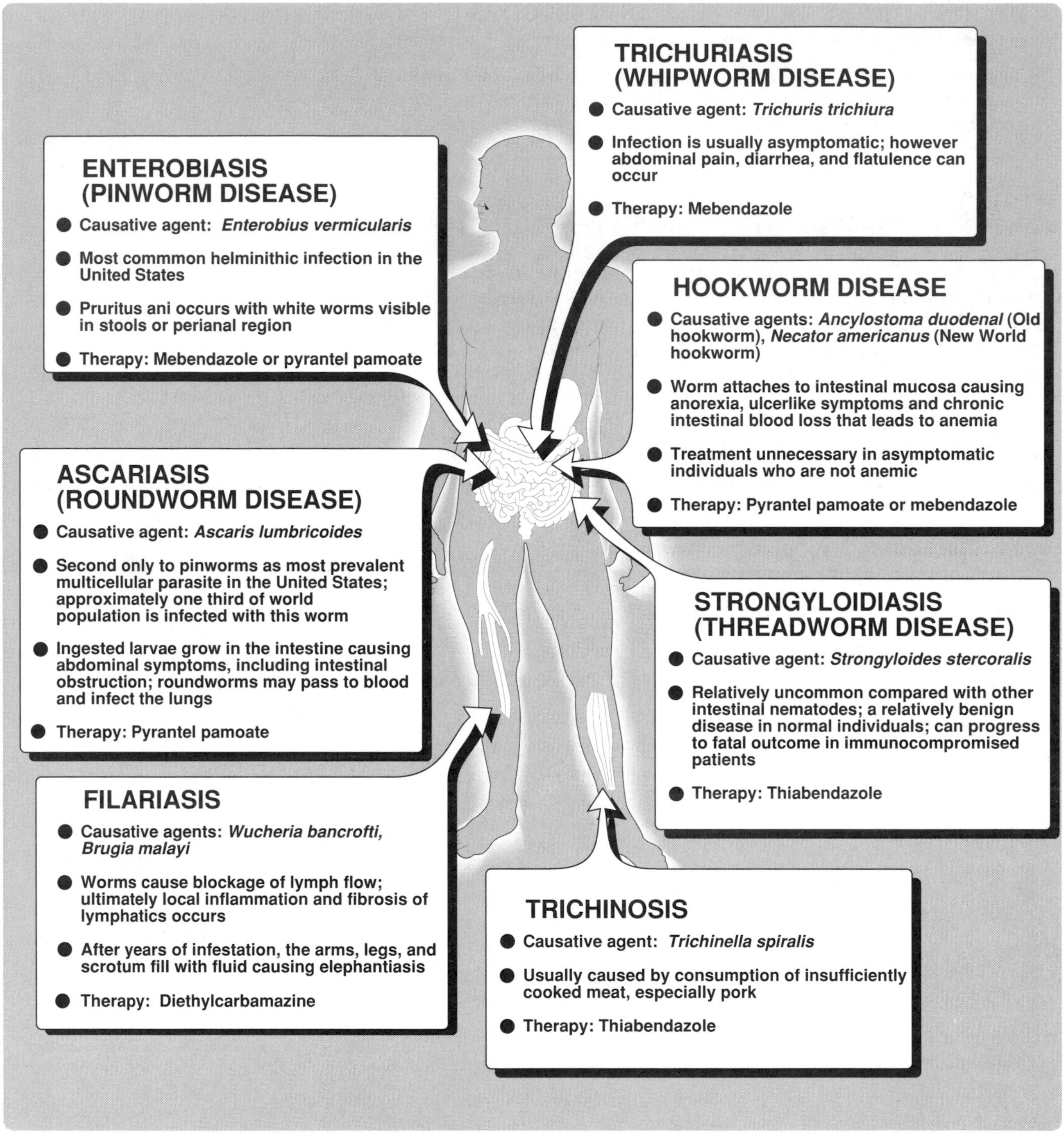

Figure 35.3
Characteristics and therapy for commonly encountered nematode infections.

Antiviral Drugs

36

I. OVERVIEW

Viruses are obligate intracellular parasites. Viruses lack both a cell wall and a cell membrane and do not carry out metabolic processes. They are not affected by antimicrobial agents. Viral reproduction uses many of the host's metabolic processes, and few drugs are selective enough to prevent viral replication without injury to the host. Nevertheless, some drugs sufficiently discriminate between cellular and viral reactions to be effective and yet nontoxic (Figure 36.1).

II. TREATMENT OF RESPIRATORY VIRUSES

Respiratory tract viruses include the influenza A type and the respiratory syncytial virus (RSV). The drugs used in these diseases are variably effective.

A. Amantadine and rimantadine

In many viral infections the clinical symptoms appear late in the course of the disease at a time when most of the virus particles have replicated. [Note: This contrasts with bacterial diseases in which the clinical symptoms are usually coincident with bacterial proliferation.] At this late, symptomatic stage of the viral infection, administration of drugs that block viral replication have limited effectiveness. However, some antiviral agents are useful as prophylactic agents. For example, *amantadine* [a MAN ta deen] has been shown to be very effective in preventing influenza A infections. The drug is also effective in the treatment of some cases of Parkinson's disease (p.89).

1. **Mode of action:** The precise antiviral mechanism of *amantadine* remains to be established, but it is presumed to interfere with uncoating of the virus. After binding to the cell membrane, the virus is engulfed by endocytosis, forming an endosome. Acidification of the endosome is required for uncoating of the virus before the viral nucleic acid enters the cytosol. It has been suggested that *amantadine,* which is a weak base, buffers the acid in the endosome, thereby preventing viral uncoating.

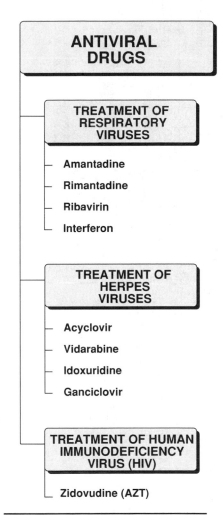

Figure 36.1
Summary of antiviral drugs.

329

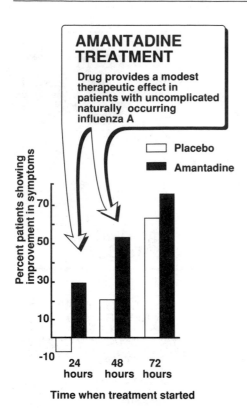

Figure 36.2
Improvement in symptoms of individuals with naturally occurring influenza infection treated with amantadine.

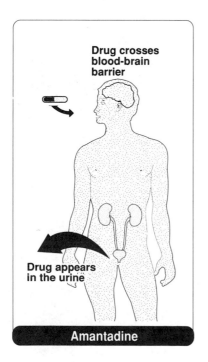

2. **Resistance**: Influenza A resistance to *amantadine* is not a clinical problem as yet; however, more recent viral isolates have shown a higher incidence of resistance.

3. **Antiviral spectrum**: *Amantadine's* therapeutic antiviral spectrum is limited to influenza A virus. Its effectiveness is directly related to its administration relative to infection. The drug is 70-90% effective in preventing infection if treatment is begun at the time of exposure to the virus. *Amantadine* does not impair the immune response to influenza A vaccine and can be administered as a supplement to vaccination, thus providing protection until antibody response occurs (usually 2 weeks in healthy adults). Treatment is particularly useful in high risk patients who have not been vaccinated or during epidemics. In individuals with influenza A infection, *amantadine* reduces the duration and severity of systemic symptoms if started within the first 48 hours after exposure to the virus (Figure 36.2).

4. **Pharmacology:**

   a. **Absorption and distribution:** The drug is well absorbed on oral administration. It distributes throughout the body and readily penetrates into the central nervous system (CNS).

   b. **Fate:** *Amantadine* is not extensively metabolized. It is excreted into the urine and may accumulate to toxic levels in patients with renal failure.

5. **Adverse effects:** Side effects are mainly associated with the CNS. Minor neurological symptoms include insomnia, dizziness, and ataxia. More serious side effects have been reported (e.g., hallucinations, seizures). The drug should be employed cautiously in patients with psychiatric problems, cerebral atherosclerosis, renal impairment, or epilepsy. *Rimantadine* [ri MAN ta deen], an investigational analog of *amantadine,* is equally as effective as amantadine, but it does not cause CNS reactions, since it does not cross the blood-brain barrier. *Amantadine* should be used with caution in pregnant and nursing mothers, because the drug has been found to be embryotoxic and teratogenic in rats.

B. Ribavirin

Ribavirin [rye ba VYE rin] is a synthetic guanosine analog. It is effective against a broad spectrum of RNA and DNA viruses.

1. **Mode of action:** The mode of action has been studied only for the influenza viruses. *Ribavirin* is first converted to the 5'-phosphate derivative, the major product being the compound, ribavirin-triphosphate (RTP), which has been postulated to exert its antiviral action by any or all of three possible mechanisms: (1) decreasing the intracellular concentration of GTP as a result of competitive inhibition of IMP dehydrogenase; (2) inhibiting 5'-cap formation of mRNAs; and/or (3) inhibiting the function of virus-coded RNA polymerases necessary to initiate and elongate viral mRNAs. [Note: Rhinoviruses and enteroviruses, which contain

preformed mRNA and do not synthesize mRNA in the host cell, are relatively resistant to the action of *ribavirin*.]

2. **Antiviral spectrum:** *Ribavirin* is used in treating infants and young children infected with severe RSV infections. Favorable responses of acute hepatitis A virus and influenza A infections have also been reported. *Ribavirin* may reduce the mortality and viremia of Lassa fever.

3. **Pharmacology:**

   a. **Route of administration:** *Ribavirin* is effective orally and intravenously, and it is also effective as an aerosol in certain respiratory viral conditions, such as in the treatment of influenza and RSV infection.

   b. **Distribution:** Studies of drug distribution in primates showed retention in all tissues, except brain. Metabolism beyond the triphosphate analog is practically nonexistent. The drug is eliminated in the urine.

4. **Adverse effects:** Side effects reported for oral or parenteral use have included dose-dependent transient anemia in Lassa fever victims. Elevated bilirubin has been reported. The aerosol may be safer, since no adverse effects have been reported after its use. Because of teratogenic effects in experimental animals, *ribavirin* is contraindicated in pregnancy.

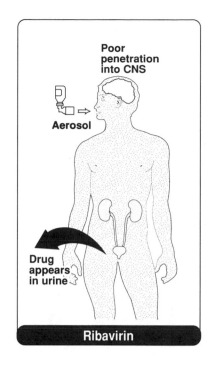

Ribavirin

C. Interferon

Interferon [in ter FEER on] is a family of naturally occurring glycoproteins that interfere with the ability of viruses to infect cells. Although *interferon* inhibits the growth of many viruses in vitro, its activity in vivo against viruses causing respiratory infection has been disappointing.

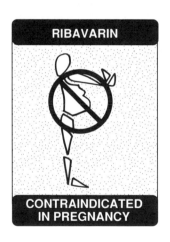

RIBAVARIN

CONTRAINDICATED IN PREGNANCY

III. TREATMENT OF HERPES VIRUS INFECTIONS

Herpes viruses are associated with a broad spectrum of diseases, e.g., cold sores, viral encephalitis, and genital infections that are particularly dangerous to the newborn. The drugs that are effective against these viruses exert their actions on the acute phase of viral infections and are without effect on the latent phase. They are all purine or pyrimidine analogs that inhibit DNA synthesis.

A. Acyclovir

1. **Mode of action:** *Acyclovir* [ay SYE kloe ver], a guanine analog that lacks a sugar moiety, is monophosphorylated in the cell by the herpes virus-coded enzyme, thymidine kinase. Therefore virus-infected cells are most susceptible. The monophosphate analog is converted to the di- and triphosphate forms by the host cells. Acyclovir triphosphate is incorporated into the viral DNA, causing premature DNA-chain termination (Figure 36.3). Irreversible

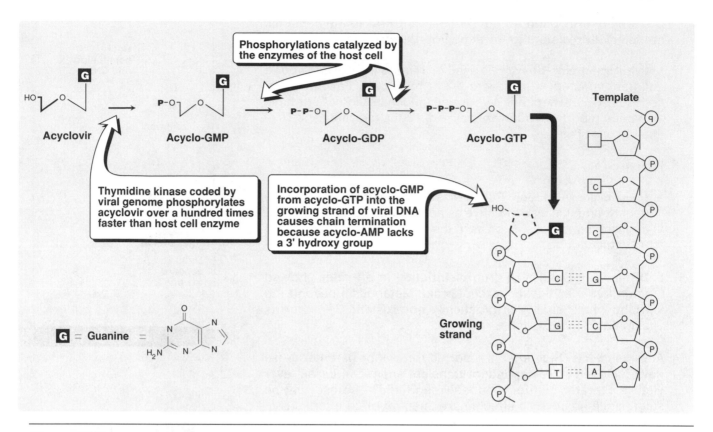

Figure 36.3
Conversion of acyclovir to acyclovir triphosphate and the subsequent incorporation into viral DNA, causing chain termination.

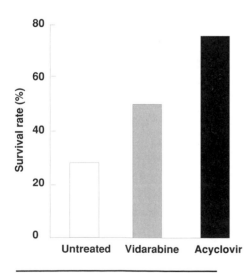

Figure 36.4
Acyclovir increases the rate of survival in patients with herpes-simplex encephalitis.

binding of the acyclovir-containing template primer to viral DNA polymerase inactivates the enzyme. It is less effective against the host enzyme.

2. **Resistance:** Altered thymidine kinase and DNA polymerases have been found in some resistant viral strains.

3. **Antiviral spectrum**: *Acyclovir* has a greater specificity than *vidarabine* against herpes viruses. Herpes simplex virus-1 (HSV-1), HSV-2, and varicella-zoster virus (VZV) are sensitive to *acyclovir*, but Epstein-Barr virus (EBV) and cytomegalovirus (CMV) are resistant because of the lack of thymidine kinase. *Acyclovir* is the treatment of choice in herpes simplex encephalitis, and is more efficacious than *vidarabine* in increasing the rate of survival (Figure 36.4). The most common use of *acyclovir* is in therapy of genital herpes infections. [Note: In all cases, *acyclovir* inhibits only actively replicating viruses and has no effect on latent viruses.]

4. **Pharmacology**:

   a. **Administration and distribution:** Administration can be by an intravenous, oral or topical route. The drug distributes well throughout the body, including the cerebrospinal fluid.

b. **Fate:** *Acyclovir* is partially metabolized to 9-carboxymethoxy-guanine, an inactive product. Excretion into the urine occurs both by glomerular filtration and tubular secretion. *Acyclovir* accumulates in patients with renal failure.

5. **Adverse effects:** Side effects depend on the mechanism of administration. For example, local irritation may occur from topical application; headache, diarrhea, nausea, and vomiting may result after oral administration; transient renal dysfunction may occur at high doses or in a dehydrated patient receiving the drug intravenously.

B. Vidarabine (ara-A)

Vidarabine [vye DARE a been] (*arabinosyl adenine, ara-A*) is the most effective of the nucleoside analogs and is also the least toxic.

1. **Mode of action:** *Vidarabine,* an adenosine analog, is converted to its 5'-triphosphate analog in the cell. *Vidarabine* is postulated to inhibit viral DNA by one or more of the following mechanisms at concentrations below those that affect host DNA synthesis: (1) inhibition of virus-specific DNA polymerase, (2) inhibition of virus-specific ribonucleotide reductase, and/or (3) direct incorporation into viral DNA.

2. **Resistance:** Some resistant herpes virus mutants have been detected that have altered DNA polymerase.

3. **Antiviral spectrum:** *Vidarabine* is active against herpes simplex virus type 1 (HSV-1), HSV-2, and varicella-zoster virus (VZV). Its use is limited to treatment of herpes simplex keratitis, encephalitis, and herpes zoster and varicella infections in immunocompromised patients.

4. **Pharmacology:**

a. **Administration and distribution:** To be effective systemically, *vidarabine* must be administered intravenously over a prolonged time, usually 12 hours. Because of its poor solubility, the drug must be administered in large volumes of fluid that can be hazardous to patients. Because of these requirements, *vidarabine* can be difficult to use in seriously ill patients. *Vidarabine* penetrates into the brain and is effective in the treatment of herpes simplex encephalitis. *Vidarabine* ointment is effective in the treatment of herpetic and vaccinial keratitis and in herpes simplex keratoconjunctivitis.

b. **Fate:** *Vidarabine* undergoes deamination to arabinofuranosyl hypoxanthine. The parent drug and its metabolites are found in the urine. Adverse effects during short-term use are not serious. The CNS disturbances, however, can be a problem in patients with impaired hepatic or renal function.

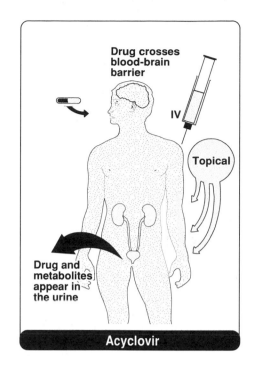

Drug crosses blood-brain barrier

IV

Topical

Drug and metabolites appear in the urine

Acyclovir

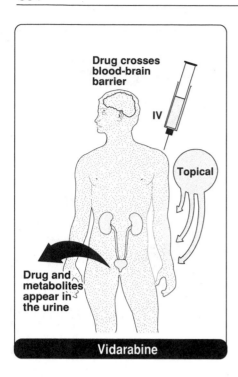

Drug crosses blood-brain barrier

IV

Topical

Drug and metabolites appear in the urine

Vidarabine

C. Idoxuridine

The first antiviral compound demonstrated to be clinically effective was *idoxuridine* [eye dox YOOR i deen]. *Idoxuridine,* a thymidine analog, is phosphorylated to the triphosphate within the cell. It is incorporated into both viral and mammalian DNA. Presence of the analog in the DNA makes it more susceptible to breakage, potentially leading to mutations. *Idoxuridine* is restricted to topical use against herpes simplex keratitis because of its toxicity. It is applied topically either as a solution or as an ointment. Adverse effects are associated with application to the conjunctiva—irritation, pruritus, pain, and photophobia.

D. Ganciclovir (DHPG)

The lack of effect of available nucleoside analogs on cytomegalovirus (CMV) infection led to the synthesis of the *acyclovir* analog, *ganciclovir* [gan SYE kloe ver]. It is the only drug currently available for treatment of CMV infections in immunocompromised patients. *Ganciclovir* is activated through conversion to the nucleoside triphosphate by cellular enzymes. The nucleotide form inhibits viral DNA polymerase and can also become incorporated into the DNA chain. Resistant CMV strains have been detected, but the mechanism of resistance is not yet known. *Ganciclovir* is administered intravenously and distributed throughout the body, including the cerebrospinal fluid. Excretion into the urine occurs through glomerular filtration and tubular secretion. Like *acyclovir, ganciclovir* accumulates in patients with renal failure. Adverse effects include severe, dose-dependent neutropenia. [Note: Combined treatment with *zidovudine* can result in additive neutropenia.]

IV. TREATMENT FOR ACQUIRED IMMUNODEFICIENCY DISEASE (AIDS)

A. Zidovudine (3'-Azido-3'-Deoxythymidine, AZT)

One of the most effective drugs currently approved for treatment of human immunodeficiency virus (HIV) infection and AIDS is the pyrimidine analog, *3'-azido-3'-deoxythymidine* (*AZT*); other pyrimidine analogs, for example, *2',3'-dideoxycytidine* (*DDC*) and *2',3'-dideoxyinosine* (*DDI*), are undergoing trials. *AZT* has the generic name of *zidovudine* [zye DOE vyoo deen]. Although not curative, these agents can interfere in the multiplication of the virus and slow progression of the disease to prolong survival rate. *AZT* is presently employed in patients shown to have documented HIV antibodies. Improvement both in immunological status (increase in absolute number of helper-induced T cells) and survivability has been reported.

1. **Mode of action:** *AZT* must be converted to the corresponding nucleotide to exert its antiviral activity. Mammalian thymidine kinase metabolizes *AZT* to the various phosphorylated products. AZT-triphosphate is then incorporated into the growing chain of viral (but not mammalian nuclear) DNA by reverse transcriptase. Because *AZT* lacks a hydroxyl at the 3' position, another 5'-3' phosphodiester linkage cannot be formed. Thus, synthesis of the DNA chain is terminated, and replication of the virus cannot take

place. The relative lack of discrimination of the viral reverse transcriptase is believed to favor the introduction of the *AZT* into the viral-catalyzed process; the cellular DNA polymerase is more selective. In addition, the phosphorylation of deoxythymidylic acid (dTMP) to the corresponding diphosphate is inhibited by the *azido-thymidine monophosphate (AZT-MP)*.

2. **Resistance:** Effectiveness decreases with time, but the mechanism for this is not known.

3. **Antiviral spectrum:** Presently the only clinical use for *AZT* is in the treatment of patients infected with HIV.

4. **Pharmacology:** The drug is well absorbed after oral administration. Penetration across the blood-brain barrier is excellent. The drug has a half-life of 1 hour, and most of it is excreted as the glucuronide.

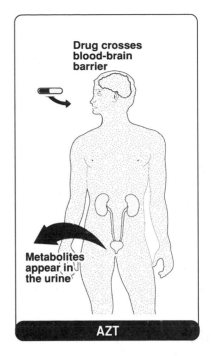

5. **Adverse effects:** In spite of its seeming specificity, *AZT* is toxic to bone marrow, for example, anemia and leukopenia occur in patients receiving high doses. Headaches are also common. Seizures have been reported in patients with advanced disease. *AZT's* toxicity is potentiated if glucuronidation is decreased by coadministration of drugs like *probenecid, acetaminophen, lorazepam, indomethacin,* and *cimetidine.* [Note: These drugs are themselves glucuronidated and thus can interfere with the glucuronidation of *AZT.* These drugs should be avoided or used with caution in patients receiving *AZT.*] *DDI* is less toxic to bone marrow than is *AZT,* but it has caused fatal pancreatitis; *DDC* causes neurological problems.

6. **Opportunistic infections:** Infection with the HIV virus leads to destruction of the T4 lymphocyte, a cell that is vital to the cellular immune systems. Thus, many infections that are normally combatted with cellular immune mechanisms occur with increased frequency in AIDS patients. Opportunistic infections (Figure 36.5) are the predominant causes of life-threatening illness in this group of patients.

Study Questions   (see p.435 for answers).

Choose the ONE best answer.

36.1 All of the following statements about acyclovir are correct EXCEPT:

 A. It is the treatment of choice for influenza infections.
 B. It is incorporated into the viral DNA causing premature DNA chain termination.
 C. It is the treatment of choice in herpes simplex encephalitis.
 D. It reduces the duration of lesions associated with genital herpes infections.
 E. It inhibits only actively replicating viruses, not latent ones.

36.2 All of the following statements about amantadine are correct EXCEPT:

 A. It is effective in the prophylaxis of influenza A infections.
 B. It causes CNS disturbances at high doses.
 C. It reduces the duration and severity of systemic symptoms of active influenza A.
 D. It is extensively metabolized.
 E. It is effective in the treatment of some cases of Parkinson's disease.

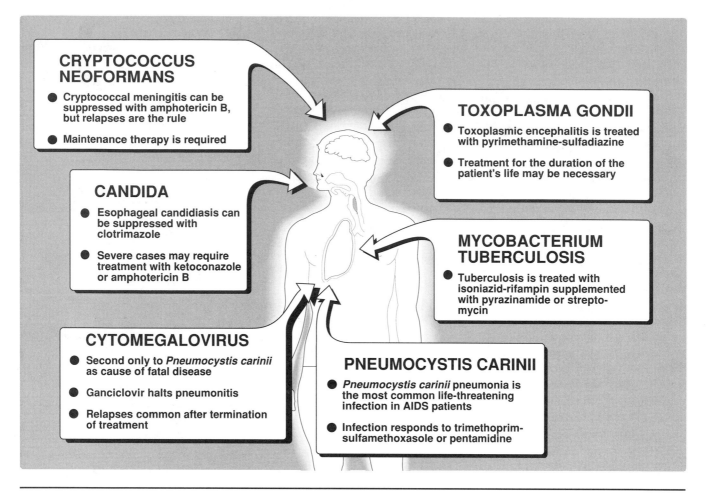

Figure 36.5
Treatment of secondary infections in patients with depressed immune system.

36.3 Which one of the following antiviral agents exhibits the greatest selective toxicity for the invading virus?

A. Idoxuridine.
B. Amantadine.
C. Acyclovir.
D. Zidovudine.
E. Ribavirin.

36.4 All of the following statements about zidovudine (AZT) are correct EXCEPT:

A. It must be converted to the nucleotide form to express its antiviral activity.
B. It is incorporated into growing viral but not mammalian nuclear DNA.
C. It is currently used to treat severe herpes virus and respiratory syncytial virus infections as well as AIDS.
D. It is toxic to bone marrow and causes adverse hematological effects.
E. It penetrates the CNS.

Questions 36.5 - 36.8: For each numbered phrase, select the ONE drug (A-E) that is most closely associated with it. Each drug (A-E) may be selected once, more than once, or not at all.

A. Amantadine
B. Zidovudine (AZT)
C. Idoxuridine
D. Vidarabine
E. Ganciclovir

36.5 It is restricted to the topical treatment of herpes simplex keratitis.

36.6 It is used solely in the treatment of influenza A infections.

36.7 It is an adenosine analog that is active against all members of the herpes virus group that infects humans.

36.8 It is used in the treatment of cytomegalovirus infections in immunocompromised patients.

Anticancer Drugs

37

I. OVERVIEW

It is estimated that 25% of the population of the United States will face a cancer diagnosis during their lifetime. Less than a quarter of these patients will be cured solely by surgery and/or local radiation. Most of the remainder will receive systemic chemotherapy at some time during their illness. (See Figure 37.1 for a summary of anticancer agents.) In a small fraction (approximately 10%) of cancer patients representing selected diseases, the chemotherapy will result in a cure or a prolonged remission. However, in most cases, the drug therapy will produce only a regression of the disease, and relapse may eventually lead to death. Thus, the overall 5-year survival for cancer patients is about 40%, ranking cancer second only to cardiovascular disease as a cause of mortality.

II. PRINCIPLES OF CANCER CHEMOTHERAPY

A. Treatment strategies

1. **Goal of treatment:** The ultimate goal of chemotherapy is a cure, that is, long-term, disease-free survival. Cure requires the eradication of every neoplastic cell. If a cure is not attainable, then the goal becomes palliation (i.e., alleviation of symptoms and avoidance of life-threatening toxicity), which allows the individual to maintain a "normal" existence. In either case, the neoplastic cell burden is initially reduced either by surgery (debulking) and/or radiation, followed by chemotherapy, immunotherapy, or a combination of these treatment modalities (Figure 37.2).

2. **Indications for treatment:** Chemotherapy is indicated when neoplasms are disseminated and not amenable to surgery. Chemotherapy is also used as a supplement to surgery, and radiation treatment is used to reduce the number of micrometastases.

3. **Tumor susceptibility and the growth cycle:** The fraction of tumor cells that are in the replicative cycle influences their susceptibility to most cancer chemotherapeutic agents.

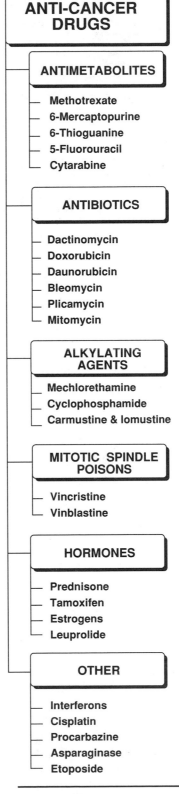

Figure 37.1
Summary of cancer chemotherapy agents.

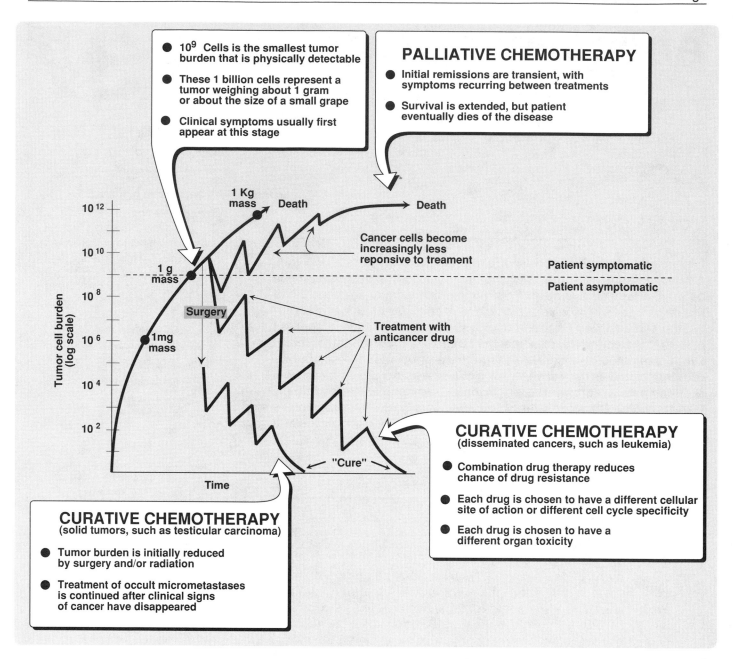

Figure 37.2
Effects of various treatments on the cancer cell burden in a hypothetical cancer patient

a. Both normal cells and tumor cells go through the same growth cycle (Figure 37.3). However, normal and neoplastic tissue may differ in the number of cells that are in the various stages of the cycle. Chemotherapeutic agents that are effective only in replicating cells, that is those cells that are cycling, are said to be cell-cycle specific (Figure 37.3), whereas other agents are cell cycle nonspecific. The nonspecific agents, although generally more toxic in cycling cells, are also useful against tumors with a low percentage of replicating cells.

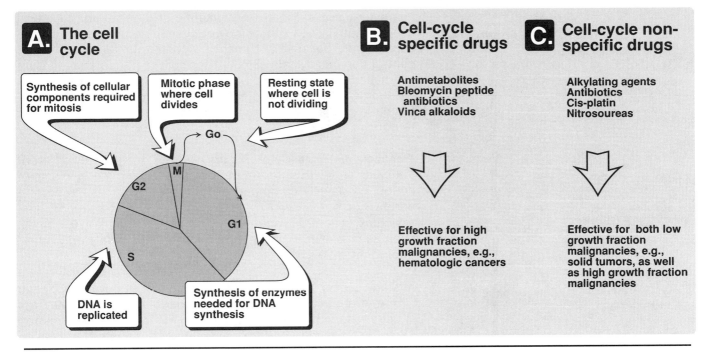

Figure 37.3
Effects of chemotherapeutic agents on the growth cycle of mammalian cells.

b. The growth rate of most tumors in vivo is initially rapid, but it decreases as the tumor size increases because of the unavailability of adequate vascularization, which leads to a lack of nutrients and oxygen (see Figure 37.2). Reducing the tumor burden through surgery or radiation promotes the recruitment of the remaining cells into active proliferation and increases their susceptibility to chemotherapeutic agents.

4. **Effect of treatment on normal cells:** Therapy aimed at killing rapidly proliferating cells also affects normal cells undergoing proliferation—for example, buccal mucosa, bone marrow, gastrointestinal (GI) mucosa, and hair cells—contributing to the toxic manifestations of such therapy.

B. Treatment regimens and scheduling

1. **Log kill:** Destruction of cancer cells by chemotherapeutic agents follows first order kinetics, that is, a given dose of drug destroys a constant fraction of cells. The term "log kill" is used to describe this phenomenon. For example, a diagnosis of leukemia is generally made when there are about 10^9 (total) leukemic cells. Consequently, if treatment leads to a 99.999% kill, then 0.001% of 10^9 cells (or 10^4 cells) would remain; this is equivalent to a 5-log kill. At this point the patient appears asymptomatic, that is, the patient is in remission (see Figure 37.2). For most bacterial infections, a 5-log (100,000-fold) reduction in the number of microorganisms results in a cure, since the immune system can eradicate the residual bacterial cells. However, tumors cells are not as readily eliminated, and additional treatment is required to totally eradicate the leukemic cell population.

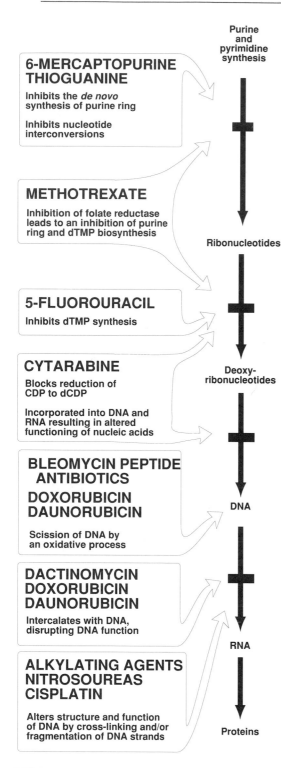

6-MERCAPTOPURINE THIOGUANINE

Inhibits the *de novo* synthesis of purine ring

Inhibits nucleotide interconversions

METHOTREXATE

Inhibition of folate reductase leads to an inhibition of purine ring and dTMP biosynthesis

5-FLUOROURACIL

Inhibits dTMP synthesis

CYTARABINE

Blocks reduction of CDP to dCDP

Incorporated into DNA and RNA resulting in altered functioning of nucleic acids

BLEOMYCIN PEPTIDE ANTIBIOTICS DOXORUBICIN DAUNORUBICIN

Scission of DNA by an oxidative process

DACTINOMYCIN DOXORUBICIN DAUNORUBICIN

Intercalates with DNA, disrupting DNA function

ALKYLATING AGENTS NITROSOUREAS CISPLATIN

Alters structure and function of DNA by cross-linking and/or fragmentation of DNA strands

Purine and pyrimidine synthesis

Ribonucleotides

Deoxy-ribonucleotides

DNA

RNA

Proteins

Figure 37.4
Target sites for cancer chemo-therapeutic agents

2. **Pharmacological sanctuaries:** Leukemic or other tumor cells find sanctuary in tissues into which certain chemotherapeutic agents cannot enter because of transport constraints, for example, the central nervous system (CNS). Therefore, a patient may require irradiation of the craniospinal axis or require intrathecal administration of drugs to eliminate the leukemic cells at that site. Similarly, drugs may be unable to penetrate certain areas of solid tumors.

3. **Treatment protocols:** Cytotoxic agents with qualitatively different toxicities and with different molecular sites and mechanisms of action are usually combined at full doses. This results both in <u>additive</u> or <u>potentiated</u> cytotoxic effects and in reduced host toxicities. In contrast, agents with similar dose-limiting toxicities, such as myelosuppression, can be combined safely only by reducing the doses of each.

   a. Many cancer treatment protocols have been developed; each one is applicable to a particular neoplastic state. They are usually identified by an acronym. For example, a common regimen called POMP for the treatment of acute lymphocytic leukemia (ALL) consists of **P**rednisone (p.353), **O**ncovin (*vincristine,* p.352), **M**ethotrexate (p.341) and **P**urinethol (*mercaptopurine,* p.343).

   b. Therapy is scheduled intermittently to allow recovery of the patient's immune system, thereby reducing the potential side effect of serious infection.

C. Target sites for chemotherapeutic agents

The aim of cancer chemotherapy is to cause a lethal cytotoxic lesion that can arrest the tumor's progression. The attack is directed against metabolic sites essential to cell replication, for example, the availability of purine and pyrimidine precursors for DNA or RNA synthesis (Figure 37.4).

D. Problems associated with chemotherapy

1. **Resistance:** Some tumor types may be inherently resistant to certain chemotherapeutic drugs. Other tumor types may acquire resistance to the cytotoxic effects of the medication, particularly after prolonged administration of low drug doses. The development of drug resistance is minimized by short-term, intensive, intermittent therapy with combinations of drugs. Drug combinations are effective against a broader range of resistant cell lines in the tumor population. A variety of mechanisms are responsible for drug resistance; each is considered separately under the particular drug.

2. **Toxicity:**

   a. **Common adverse effects:** Most chemotherapeutic agents have a narrow therapeutic index. Rapidly dividing normal tissues are most susceptible to toxic reactions. Severe vomiting, stomatitis, and alopecia occur to a lesser or greater extent during therapy with all antineoplastic agents. Vomiting can sometimes be controlled by administration of cannabinoids (p.107) or phenothiazines (p.127). Some toxicities, such as myelosuppression, are common to many agents, whereas other adverse reactions are confined to specific agents, for example, cardiotoxicity with *doxorubicin* and pulmonary fibrosis with *bleomycin*.

b. **Duration of adverse effects:** The duration of the side effects varies widely. For example, alopecia is transient, but the cardiac, pulmonary, and bladder toxicities are irreversible.

c. **Minimizing adverse effects:** Some toxic reactions may be ameliorated by interventions, such as perfusing the tumor locally (e.g., a sarcoma of the arm), removing some of the patient's marrow prior to intensive treatment, then reimplanting it, or promoting intensive diuresis to prevent bladder toxicities. The megaloblastic anemia that occurs with *methotrexate* can be effectively counteracted by administering *folinic acid* (*leucovorin, 5-formyltetrahydrofolic acid*, p.342).

3. **Treatment-induced tumors:** Since most antineoplastic agents are mutagens, neoplasms (e.g., acute nonlymphocytic leukemia) may arise 10 or more years after the original cancer was cured. Treatment-induced neoplasms are especially a problem after therapy with alkylating agents (p.349).

III. ANTIMETABOLITES

Antimetabolites are structurally related to normal cellular components. They generally interfere with the availability of normal purine or pyrimidine nucleotide precursors by inhibiting their synthesis or by competing with them in DNA or RNA synthesis. Their maximal cytotoxic effects are S-phase (and therefore cell-cycle) specific.

A. Methotrexate

Methotrexate [meth oh TREX ate] is structurally related to folic acid and acts as an antagonist of that vitamin. Folate plays a central role in a variety of metabolic reactions involving the transfer of one-carbon units. These are key in replicating cells for the biosynthesis of methionine; the purine nucleotides adenine and guanine; and the pyrimidine nucleotide, deoxythymidylic acid (dTMP, Figure 37.5). It is no wonder that *methotrexate* adversely affects cell survival.[1]

1. **Site of action:**

a. After absorption of folic acid from dietary sources or from that produced by intestinal flora, the vitamin undergoes reduction to the tetrahydrofolate form (FH_4) by the intracellular NADPH-dependent dihydrofolate reductase. *Methotrexate* enters the cell by an active transport process, which normally mediates

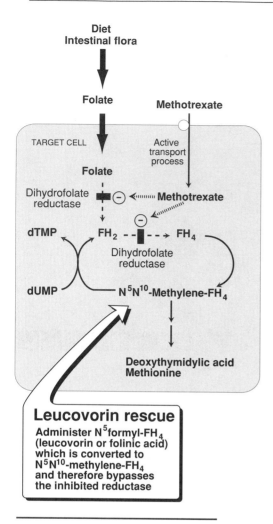

Figure 37.5
Mechanism of action of methotrexate
and the effect of administration
of leucovorin [FH_2=dihydrofolate;
FH_4 =tetrahydrofolate]

the entry of N^5-methyl FH_4. At high *methotrexate* concentrations, the drug enters the cell by diffusion. *Methotrexate* has an unusually strong affinity for dihydrofolate reductase, and its inhibition can only be reversed by a thousand-fold excess of the natural substrate, dihydrofolate (FH_2, Figure 37.5) or by administration of *leucovorin,* which bypasses the blocked enzyme and replenishes the folate pool. [Note: *Leucovorin,* or *folinic acid,* is the N^5-formyl group carrying form of FH_4.][2]

b. Decreased biosynthesis of thymidylic acid, methionine, and the purines (adenine and guanine) leads to depressed DNA and RNA synthesis and to cell death.

2. **Resistance:** Resistance to *methotrexate* is characteristic of non-proliferating cells. The following mechanisms of resistance in neoplastic cells have been detected.

a. **Increased enzyme:** Amplification of the gene that codes for dihydrofolate reductase results in higher levels of this enzyme. Higher doses of the drug are then required to be effective and therefore increased toxicity ensues.

b. **Modified enzyme:** In some instances the enzymatic affinity for *methotrexate* is diminished.

c. **Less drug pumped into the cell:** Decreased concentration of the drug in neoplastic cells resulting from decreased influx has also been observed, which is apparently caused by a change in the carrier-mediated transport involved in pumping *methotrexate* into the cell.

3. **Therapeutic applications:** *Methotrexate* is effective against acute lymphocytic leukemia, choriocarcinoma, Burkitt's lymphoma in children, breast cancer, head and neck carcinomas, and also in nonneoplastic diseases, for example, severe psoriasis and rheumatoid arthritis. High dose *methotrexate* is of particular importance in the treatment of osteogenic sarcoma; it should be followed by administration of *leucovorin* to rescue the bone marrow (see the discussion of its adverse effects, later).

4. **Pharmacology:**

a. **Administration and distribution:** *Methotrexate* is readily absorbed from the GI tract, but it can also be administered by the intramuscular (IM), intravenous (IV), and intrathecal routes. Because *methotrexate* does not penetrate the blood-brain barrier, it is administered intrathecally to destroy neoplastic cells in the central sanctuary sites.

b. **Fate:** Although folates found in the blood have a single terminal glutamate, most intracellular folates are converted to polyglutamates. These are preferentially retained inside the cells and are usually more efficient cofactors than are the monoglutamates. *Methotrexate* is also metabolized to polyglutamate derivatives. This property is important, because the polyglutamates remain within the cell even in the absence of extracellular drug, in contrast to *methotrexate per se,* which rapidly leaves the cell after the extracellular drug disappears. The polyglutamates also inhibit dihydrofolate reductase. *Methotrexate* undergoes hydroxylation at the 7 position. The 7-OH derivative is less water soluble, and at high doses, it may lead to crystalluria. Therefore, it is important to keep the urine alkaline and the patient well hydrated to avoid renal toxicity caused by crystalluria. Excretion of the parent drug and the 7-OH metabolite occurs via the urinary tract.

5. **Adverse effects:**

a. Most frequent toxicities are stomatitis, myelosuppression, erythema, rash, urticaria, alopecia, nausea, vomiting, and diarrhea. Some of these can be prevented by administering *leucovorin,* which is taken up more readily by normal cells than by tumor cells (Figure 37.5). Doses of *leucovorin* must be kept minimal to avoid interference with the antitumor action of the *methotrexate.*

b. **Renal damage:** Although uncommon during conventional therapy, renal damage is a complication of high dose *methotrexate.*

c. **Hepatic function:** Hepatic function should be monitored. Long-term use may lead to fibrosis.

d. **Neurologic toxicities:** Neurologic toxicities, which are associated with intrathecal administration, include subacute meningeal irritation, stiff neck, headache, and fever. Seizures, encephalopathy, or paraplegia occur rarely. Long-lasting effects, such as learning disabilities, have been seen in children who received the drug by this route.

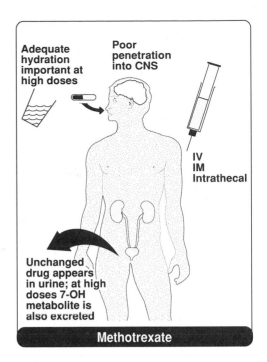

Adequate hydration important at high doses

Poor penetration into CNS

IV IM Intrathecal

Unchanged drug appears in urine; at high doses 7-OH metabolite is also excreted

Methotrexate

B. 6-Mercaptopurine

The drug *6-mercaptopurine* [mer kap toe PYOOR een] (*6-MP*) is the thiol analog of the purine, hypoxanthine. Of all the purine analogs tested, only *6-mercaptopurine* and *thioguanine* (*6-TG*) have proved beneficial for treating neoplastic disease.

1. **Site of action:**

a. To exert its antileukemic effect, *6-mercaptopurine* must penetrate target cells and be converted to the corresponding nucleotide, 6-mercaptopurine ribose phosphate (6-MPRP—also known as 6-thioinosinic acid, or thio-IMP). The addition of the ribose phosphate is catalyzed by the salvage pathway enzyme, hypoxanthine-guanine phosphoribosyl transferase (HGPRT).[3]

b. Although the nature of the exact cytotoxic step is not known, the unnatural nucleotide, 6-MPRP, can inhibit the first step of *de novo* purine ring biosynthesis as well as formation of AMP and xanthinylic acid (XMP) from inosinic acid (IMP).[4]

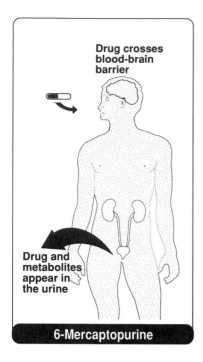

6-Mercaptopurine

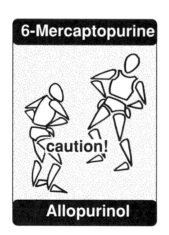

2. **Resistance:** Resistance is associated with either an inability to biotransform *6-MP* to the corresponding nucleotide because of decreased levels of HGPRT (e.g., in Lesch-Nyhan syndrome where patients are deficient in this enzyme), or it is associated with increased metabolism of the drug to thiouric acid, which is excreted in the urine.

3. **Therapeutic applications:** The agent, *6-MP,* is used principally in the maintenance of remission in ALL.

4. **Pharmacology:**

   a. **Administration and metabolism:** Absorption by the oral route is erratic. The *6-MP* undergoes metabolism in the liver to the S-CH$_3$ derivative or to thiouric acid. The latter reaction is catalyzed by xanthine oxidase. Because *allopurinol,* a xanthine oxidase inhibitor,[5] is frequently administered to cancer patients receiving chemotherapy to reduce hyperuricemia, it is important to decrease the dose of *6-MP* in these individuals to avoid accumulation of the drug and exacerbation of toxicities.

   b. **Excretion:** The parent drug and its metabolites are excreted by the kidney.

5. **Adverse effects:** Side effects include nausea, vomiting, diarrhea, mild myelotoxicity, and thrombocytopenia.

C. 6-Thioguanine

6-Thioguanine [thye oh GWAH neen] (*6-TG*), another purine analog, is primarily used in the treatment of acute myelocytic leukemia (AML) in combination with *daunorubicin* and *cytarabine.* Like *6-MP, 6-TG* must first be converted to the nucleotide form, which then inhibits the biosynthesis of the purine ring and the phosphorylation of GMP to GDP. *6-TG* can also be incorporated into DNA. Unlike *6-MP, allopurinol* does not potentiate *6-TG* action. Otherwise, toxicities are the same as those for *6-MP.*

D. 5-Fluorouracil

5-Fluorouracil [flure oh YOOR a sil] (*5-FU*), a pyrimidine analog, has a stable fluorine atom at position 5 of the uracil ring in place of a hydrogen atom. The fluorine interferes with the conversion of deoxyuridylic acid to thymidylic acid, thus depriving the cell of one of the essential precursors for DNA synthesis.

1. **Site of action:** *5-FU per se* is devoid of antineoplastic activity and must be converted to the corresponding deoxynucleotide (5-FdUMP, Figure 37.6), which competes with deoxyuridine monophosphate (dUMP) for the enzyme thymidylate synthetase. DNA synthesis decreases leading to imbalanced cell growth and cell death.

2. **Resistance:** Resistant cells are encountered that have lost the ability to convert *5-FU* into its active form or have altered or

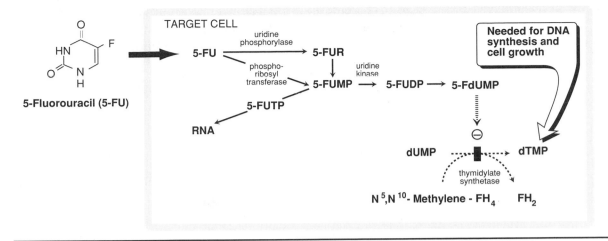

Figure 37.6
Mechanism of 5-fluorouracil's cytotoxic action. 5-Fluorouracil is converted to 5-FdUMP which competes with deoxyuridine monophosphate (dUMP) for the enzyme thymidylate synthetase

increased thymidylate synthetase or have increased the rate of *5-FU* catabolism.

3. **Therapeutic applications:** *Fluorouracil* is employed primarily in the treatment of slowly growing, solid tumors (e.g., colon, breast, ovarian, pancreatic, and gastric carcinomas). It is also effective for the treatment of superficial basal cell carcinomas when applied topically.

4. **Pharmacology:** Because of its severe toxicity to the GI tract, *5-FU* is given intravenously or, in the case of skin cancer, topically. The drug penetrates well into all tissues including the central nervous system (CNS). *5-FU* is metabolized in the liver largely to CO_2, which is expired. The dose must be adjusted in the case of impaired hepatic function.

5. **Toxicities:** In addition to nausea, vomiting, diarrhea, and alopecia, severe ulceration of the oral and GI mucosa, bone marrow depression, and anorexia are frequently encountered.

E. Cytarabine

Cytarabine [sye TARE a been] (*cytosine arabinoside, ara-C*) is an analog of 2'-deoxycytidine in which the natural ribose residue is replaced by D-arabinose. It acts as a pyrimidine antagonist.

1. **Site of action:** *Ara-C* enters cells by a carrier-mediated transport process. Like the other purine and pyrimidine antagonists, *ara-C* must be sequentially phosphorylated to the corresponding nucleotide, cytosine arabinoside triphosphate (ara-CTP), in order to be cytotoxic. The exact cytotoxic locus is unknown. The false nucleotide functions as an antagonist of deoxycytidine triphosphate (dCTP) and competitively inhibits DNA polymerase. It is

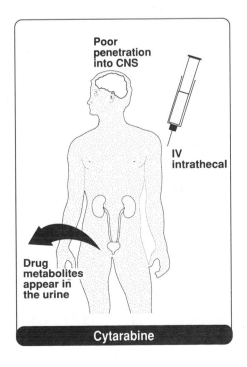

Poor penetration into CNS

IV
intrathecal

Drug metabolites appear in the urine

Cytarabine

thus S-phase (and therefore cell-cycle) specific. *Ara-C* is also incorporated into nucleic acids to form DNA and RNA with strand breaks and altered functions. It can also inhibit the reduction of CDP to dCDP.

2. **Resistance:** Resistance to *ara-C* may result from a defect in the transport process, a change in participating enzymes, or an increased pool of the natural dCTP nucleotide.

3. **Therapeutic indications:** The major clinical use is in acute myelogenous leukemia in combination with *6-TG* and *daunorubicin.*

4. **Pharmacology:** *Ara-C* is not effective when given orally because of its deamination to the noncytotoxic uracil arabinoside (ara-U) by cytidine deaminase in the intestinal mucosa. It distributes throughout the body, but it does not penetrate the CNS in sufficient amounts to be effective against meningeal leukemia. However, it may be injected intrathecally. *Ara-C* undergoes extensive oxidative deamination in the body to ara-U. Both *ara-C* and ara-U are excreted by the kidney.

5. **Adverse effects:** Nausea, vomiting, diarrhea, and severe myelosuppression are the major toxicities. Hepatic dysfunction is also occasionally encountered. *Ara-C* may cause seizures or altered mental states on intrathecal injection.

IV. ANTIBIOTICS

These drugs owe their cytotoxic action to their interactions with DNA, leading to disruption of DNA function. Except for *bleomycin,* they are cell cycle nonspecific, but they have a greater effect in cycling cells.

A. Dactinomycin

Dactinomycin [dak ti noe MYE sin], known to biochemists as *actinomycin D,* was the first antibiotic to find therapeutic application in tumor chemotherapy.

1. **Site of action:** The drug intercalates into the small groove of the double helix and binds to deoxyguanylic acid moieties, forming a stable *dactinomycin*-DNA complex. The complex interferes primarily with DNA-dependent RNA polymerase, although at high doses, *dactinomycin* also interferes in DNA synthesis. The drug may also cause strand breaks like *doxorubicin.*

2. **Resistance:** Resistance is believed to be due to DNA repair and/or to increased efflux of the antibiotic from the cell.

3. **Therapeutic applications:** *Dactinomycin* is used in combination with surgery and *vincristine* (p.352) for the treatment of Wilm's tumor. With *methotrexate* (p.341) it is effective in the treatment of gestational choriocarcinoma and is used to treat some soft tissue sarcomas.

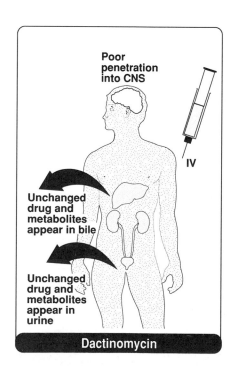

Poor penetration into CNS

IV

Unchanged drug and metabolites appear in bile

Unchanged drug and metabolites appear in urine

Dactinomycin

4. **Pharmacology:** The drug, administered intravenously, is concentrated in the liver where it undergoes some metabolism. Most of the parent drug and metabolites are excreted via the biliary tract, the remainder via the urine.

5. **Adverse effects:** The major dose-limiting toxicity is bone marrow depression. Other adverse reactions include nausea, vomiting, diarrhea, stomatitis, and alopecia. Extravasation produces serious problems. Another toxicity associated with *dactinomycin* is sensitization to radiation; inflammation at sites of prior radiation therapy may occur.

B. Doxorubicin and daunorubicin

Doxorubicin [dox oh ROO bi sin] and *daunorubicin* [daw noe ROO bi sin] are classified as anthracycline antibiotics. *Doxorubicin* is frequently referred to by its trade name *adriamycin.*

1. **Site of action:** The anthracyclines have three major activities, all of which are maximal in the S phase:

   a. **Intercalation in the DNA:** The drug inserts between adjacent base pairs and binds to the sugar-phosphate backbone of DNA, thus blocking DNA and RNA synthesis.

   b. **Binding of the drug to cell membranes:** This action alters the function of transport processes coupled to phosphatidyl inositol activation.

   c. **Generation of oxygen radicals through lipid peroxidation:** Cytochrome P-450 reductase (present in cell nuclear membranes) catalyzes reduction of some of the anthracyclines to semiquinone free radicals. These, in turn, reduce molecular O_2-producing superoxide ions and hydrogen peroxide, which mediate single strand scission of DNA (Figure 37.7). Tissues with ample superoxide dismutase (SOD) activity are protected. Tumors as well as the heart are generally low in SOD. In addition, cardiac tissue lacks catalase and thus cannot dispose of hydrogen peroxide. This may explain the cardiotoxicity of *doxorubicin* as compared to the other anthracyclines, which cannot be reduced and are found to be less toxic to the heart.

2. **Resistance:** Resistance has been ascribed to decreased cellular uptake, increased efflux via the transport glycoprotein (P-glycoprotein), and, possibly, decreased cytochrome P-450 reductase and DNA repair.

3. **Therapeutic applications:** Applications for these two agents differ despite their structural similarity and their apparently similar mechanisms of action. *Doxorubicin* is one of the most important and widely used anticancer drugs. It is used for treatment of a variety of carcinomas and sarcomas, including acute lymphocytic leukemia, breast and lung cancer, and Hodgkin's disease. *Daunorubicin* is used in the treatment of acute myelocytic leukemia.

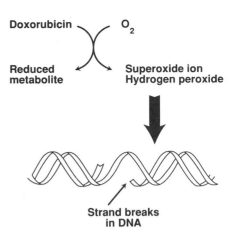

Figure 37.7
Doxorubicin interacts with molecular oxygen producing superoxide ions which cause single strand breaks in DNA

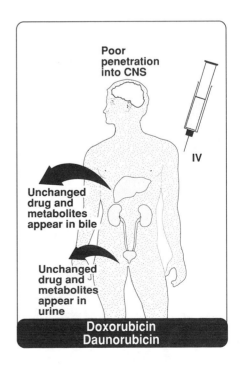

4. **Pharmacology:**

   a. **Absorption and distribution:** Both drugs must be administered intravenously. Extravasation is a serious problem that can lead to tissue necrosis. They bind to plasma proteins as well as to tissues where they are widely distributed. They do not penetrate into the central nervous system.

   b. **Fate:** Both drugs undergo metabolism to products that are also cytotoxic. The liver (through the bile) is the major route of excretion, and the dose must be modified in patients with impaired hepatic function. Some renal excretion also occurs, but the dose generally need not be adjusted in patients with renal failure. The drug imparts a red color to the urine.

5. **Adverse effects:** Irreversible, dose-dependent cardiotoxicity is the most serious adverse reaction. As with *dactinomycin,* both *doxorubicin* and *daunorubicin* also cause a transient bone marrow suppression, stomatitis, and GI tract disturbances. Alopecia is usually severe. Irradiation of the thorax increases the risk of cardiotoxicity.

C. Bleomycin

1. **Site of action:** *Bleomycin* [blee oh MYE sin] is a mixture of different copper chelating glycopeptides that, like the anthracycline antibiotics, cause scission of DNA by an oxidative process. A DNA-*bleomycin*-Fe(II) complex appears to undergo oxidation; the liberated electrons react with oxygen to form superoxide or hydroxide radicals, which in turn attack the phosphodiester bonds resulting in strand breakage and chromosomal aberrations (Figure 37.8). *Bleomycin* is cell-cycle specific, and causes cells to accumulate in the G_2 phase.

2. **Resistance:** These mechanism(s) have not been elucidated, but DNA repair seems likely.

3. **Therapeutic applications:** *Bleomycin* is primarily employed in the treatment of testicular tumors in combination with *vinblastine.* Response rates are about 90% and are even higher if *cisplatin* is added to the regimen. *Bleomycin* is also effective, although not curative, for squamous cell carcinomas and lymphomas.

4. **Pharmacology:**

   a. **Administration and distribution:** *Bleomycin* is effectively administered by a number of routes, including subcutaneous, intramuscular, intravenous, and intracavitary. The drug is localized in epithelial organs, such as skin, lung, peritoneum, and lymphatic tissue.

   b. **Fate:** Most of the parent drug is excreted unchanged into the urine by glomerular filtration, necessitating dose adjustment in patients with renal failure.

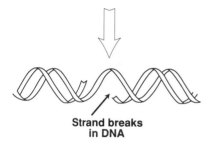

Bleomycin-Fe $^{++}$

Strand breaks
in DNA

Figure 37.8
Bleomycin causes breaks in
DNA by an oxidative process

5. **Adverse effects:** Pulmonary toxicity is the most serious adverse effect, progressing from rales, cough, and infiltrate to potentially fatal fibrosis. Other toxic effects include anaphylactoid reactions and a high incidence of fever. Mucocutaneous reactions and alopecia are common. Hypertrophic skin changes and hyperpigmentation of the hands are prevalent.

D. Plicamycin and mitomycin

Plicamycin (*mithramycin*) and *mitomycin* also exert their cytotoxicity through restriction of DNA function.

1. *Plicamycin* [plik a MI cin] has a relative toxic specificity for osteoclasts and lowers plasma calcium concentration in hypercalcemic patients—especially those with bone tumors. Toxicities include hemorrhage as well as effects on the bone marrow, liver, and kidneys.

2. *Mitomycin* [mye toe MYE sin] is employed in the treatment of a variety of solid tumors, but its effectiveness is limited by myelosuppression. It potentiates the cardiotoxic effects of *doxorubicin*.

V. ALKYLATING AGENTS

Alkylating agents exert their cytotoxic effects by binding to various cell constituents. Alkylation of DNA is probably the crucial cytotoxic reaction that is lethal to the tumor cell. These agents are often said to be radiomimetic (i.e., they imitate the action of radiation), because similar effects are produced by certain kinds of ionizing radiations. Alkylating agents do not discriminate between cycling and resting cells but are most toxic for rapidly dividing cells. They are used to treat a wide variety of lymphatic and solid cancers in combination with other agents.

A. Mechlorethamine

Mechlorethamine [me klor ETH a meen] (nitrogen mustard) was developed during Word War I for use in chemical warfare. Its potential as an antileukemic agent was recognized after it was found to produce profound lymphocytopenia. The nitrogen mustards are called ''bifunctional'' alkylating agents, because they can bind to two separate sites.

1. **Site of action:** *Mechlorethamine* is transported into the cell by the choline uptake system. Alkylation of the N7 nitrogen of guanine in DNA linkage is considered responsible for its cytotoxic effect (Figure 37.9).

   a. Consequences of this alkylation reaction include crosslinkages between chains and a depurination, which leads to a nick in the DNA chain and facilitates strand breaks. It can also cause miscoding mutations.

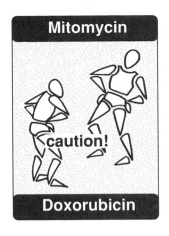

Figure 37.9
Alkylation of guanine bases in DNA is responsible for the cytotoxic effect of mechlorethamine

b. Though the alkylating reactions can occur in both cycling and resting cells (and are therefore cell-cycle nonspecific), proliferating cells are more sensitive, especially in G_1 and S phases.

2. **Resistance:** Resistance has been ascribed to DNA repair as well as to decreased permeability of the drug.

3. **Therapeutic applications:** *Mechlorethamine* is used primarily in the treatment of Hodgkin's disease as part of the MOPP regimen (**M**echlorethamine, **O**ncovin, **P**rednisone, **P**rocarbazine), but it is also useful in the treatment of some solid tumors.

4. **Pharmacology:** *Mechlorethamine* is very unstable; solutions must be made up just prior to administration. The drug is administered only intravenously; the drug can cause severe tissue damage if extravasation occurs.

5. **Adverse effects:** Its adverse effects include severe vomiting (centrally mediated). Severe bone marrow depression limits extensive use. Latent viral infections (e.g., Herpes zoster) may appear because of immunosuppression. Extravasation is a serious problem.

B. Cyclophosphamide

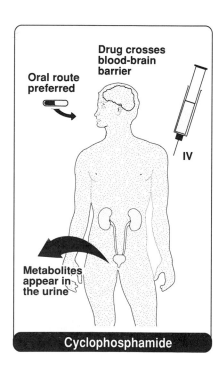

Cyclophosphamide

1. **Site of action:** *Cyclophosphamide* [sye kloe FOSS fa mide], a nitrogen mustard, is first biotransformed to its hydroxylated intermediate by the cytochrome P-450 system. The hydroxylated intermediates undergo breakdown to form the active phosphoramide mustard and acrolein. Interaction of the phosphoramide mustard with DNA is considered to be the cytotoxic action.

2. **Resistance:** Resistance is probably a result of DNA repair and decreased permeability.

3. **Therapeutic applications:** *Cyclophosphamide* has a broad clinical spectrum; it is used either alone or as part of a regimen in treatment of a wide variety of neoplastic diseases, e.g., Burkitt's lymphoma and breast cancer. Nonneoplastic disease entities, such as nephrotic syndrome and intractable rheumatoid arthritis, are also effectively treated with *cyclophosphamide*.

4. **Pharmacology:** Unlike most of the alkylating agents, *cyclophosphamide* is preferentially administered by the oral route. After hydroxylation takes place in the liver via the P-450 system, the precursor of the active phosphoramide mustard is transported to target tissues where it is further transformed to the active alkylating agent. Minimal amounts of the parent drug are excreted into the feces (after biliary transport) or into the urine by glomerular filtration.

5. **Adverse effects:** The most prominent toxicities (after nausea, vomiting, and diarrhea) are bone marrow depression and hemor-

rhagic cystitis, which can lead to fibrosis of the bladder. The latter toxicity has been attributed to acrolein in the urine. Adequate hydration and mannitol-induced diuresis as well as installation into the bladder of N-acetylcysteine or MESNA (sodium 2-mercaptoethane sulfonate) to trap the offending agent minimize this problem. A complication is the increased secretion of antidiuretic hormone (ADH), which occurs with therapy so that hydration must be carefully monitored to avert possible water intoxication. *Furosemide* (p.215) can prevent the water retention. Other toxicities include effects on the germ cells resulting in amenorrhea, testicular atrophy, and sterility. Secondary malignancies may appear years after therapy.

C. Nitrosoureas

Lomustine [loe MUS teen] is the methylated derivative of *carmustine* [kar MUS teen]. They are classified as alkylating agents.

1. **Site of action:** The *nitrosoureas* exert cytotoxic effects by an alkylating mechanism that inhibits DNA replication and, eventually, RNA and protein synthesis. Although they alkylate resting cells, cytotoxicity is expressed only on cell division; therefore nondividing cells can escape if DNA repair occurs.

2. **Resistance:** Although the nature of resistance to *nitrosoureas* is unknown, it probably results from DNA repair.

3. **Therapeutic applications:** These applications are limited. Because of their ability to penetrate into the CNS, the *nitrosoureas* are employed in the treatment of malignant glioma.

4. **Pharmacology:** In spite of the similarities in their structure, *carmustine* is administered intravenously, whereas *lomustine* is given orally. Their most striking property is their ability to readily penetrate into the CNS, because of their lipophilicity. The drugs undergo extensive metabolism. *Phenobarbital* reduces their cytotoxicity, suggesting that the mixed-function oxidases are responsible for their detoxification. The kidney is the major excretory route.

5. **Adverse effects:** These include delayed hematopoietic depression, which may be due to metabolic products. An aplastic marrow may develop on prolonged use. Renal toxicity related to duration of therapy is also encountered.

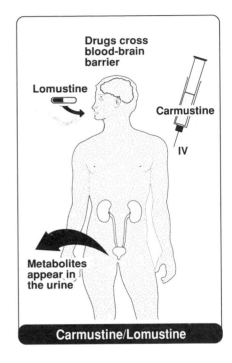

Carmustine/Lomustine

VI. MITOTIC SPINDLE POISONS

The mitotic spindle is part of a larger intracellular skeleton (cytoskeleton) that is essential for the internal movements occurring in the cytoplasm of all eukaryotic cells. The mitotic spindle consists of a system of microtubules, and it is essential for the equal partitioning of DNA in the two new cells formed when a eukaryotic cell divides.

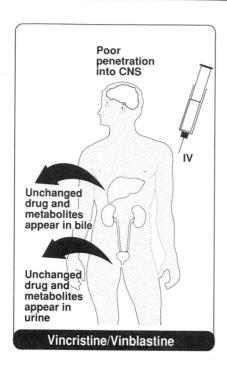

Poor penetration into CNS

IV

Unchanged drug and metabolites appear in bile

Unchanged drug and metabolites appear in urine

Vincristine/Vinblastine

A. Vincristine and vinblastine

Vincristine [vin KRIS teen] and *vinblastine* [vin BLAST een] are structurally-related compounds derived from the periwinkle plant, *Vinca rosea*. They are therefore referred to as the vinca alkaloids.

1. **Site of action:** *Vincristine* and *vinblastine* are both cycle specific and phase specific, since they block mitosis in metaphase. Their binding to the microtubular protein, tubulin, disrupts the spindle apparatus and causes termination of assembly of the cytoskeletal protein. Their binding also causes depolymerization of the microtubules. This in turn prevents chromosomal segregation and cell proliferation (Figure 37.10).

2. **Resistance:** Resistant cells have been shown to have enhanced binding of *vinblastine* to a single membrane protein that is absent in drug-sensitive cells. The protein is probably the P-glycoprotein (for "permeability" glycoprotein), which is responsible for the efflux of *vincristine* and *vinblastine* in cells resistant to the drug.

3. **Therapeutic applications:** Although *vincristine* and *vinblastine* are structurally very similar, their therapeutic indications are different. They are generally administered in combination with other drugs. *Vincristine* is used in the treatment of acute lymphoblastic leukemia in children, Wilm's tumor, Ewing's soft tissue sarcoma, and Hodgkin's disease, as well as some other rapidly proliferating neoplasms. [Note: *Vincristine* (whose trade name is *Oncovin*) is the "O" in the MOPP regimen for Hodgkin's disease.] *Vinblastine* is administered with *bleomycin* (p.348) and *cisplatin* (p.356) for the treatment of metastatic testicular carcinoma. It is also used in the treatment of systemic Hodgkin's disease and other lymphomas.

4. **Pharmacology:**

   a. **Administration:** Intravenous administration of *vincristine* or *vinblastine* leads to rapid cytotoxic effects and cell destruction. This leads to the release and degradation of purines producing uric acid and hyperuricemia, which is ameliorated by administration of the xanthine oxidase inhibitor, *allopurinol* (p.376).

   b. **Fate:** The metabolism of the vinca alkaloids has not been described. The agents are concentrated in the liver and are excreted into bile and feces. Dose must be modified in patients with impaired hepatic function or biliary obstruction.

5. **Adverse effects:**

   a. *Vincristine* and *vinblastine* have certain toxicities in common. These include phlebitis or cellulitis, if the drugs extravasate during injection, as well as nausea, vomiting, diarrhea, and alopecia.

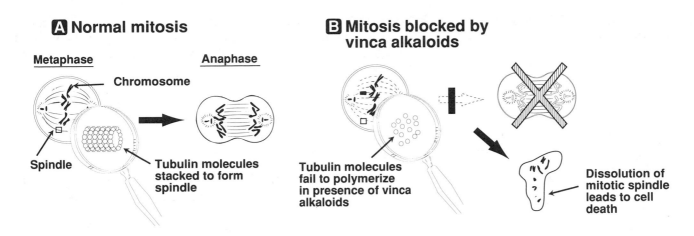

A Normal mitosis

Metaphase   Anaphase

Chromosome

Spindle

Tubulin molecules
stacked to form
spindle

**B Mitosis blocked by
vinca alkaloids**

Tubulin molecules
fail to polymerize
in presence of vinca
alkaloids

Dissolution of
mitotic spindle
leads to cell
death

Figure 37.10
Mechanism of action of the mitotic spindle poisons.

b. However, their toxicities also differ. *Vinblastine* is a more potent myelosuppressant, whereas peripheral neuropathy (paresthesias, loss of reflexes, foot-drop, and ataxia) is associated with *vincristine.*

VII. HORMONES

Hormones act by controlling proliferation and function of several tissue types, including the mammary and prostate glands. For a hormone to have an influence on a cell, that cell must have receptors that are specific for that hormone. Some do not consider drugs such as *prednisone* or *tamoxifen* to be true cytotoxic agents, since they physiologically antagonize hormone-stimulated processes necessary for cell proliferation rather than causing a cytotoxic lesion.

A. Prednisone

Prednisone [PRED ni sone] is a potent synthetic anti-inflammatory corticosteroid with less mineralocorticoid activity than cortisol. The use of this compound in the treatment of lymphomas stems from the observation that patients with Cushing's syndrome (a syndrome associated with hypersecretion of cortisol) have lymphocytopenia and decreased lymphoid mass. These result from corticosteroid action on lymphocyte formation and distribution (i.e., movement from the circulation to lymphoid tissue).

1. **Site of action:** The steroid binds to a receptor that triggers the production of specific proteins (see Figure 37.11). The specific mechanism for its lymphocytopenic action after interaction with DNA remains to be elucidated.

2. **Resistance:** Resistance is associated with an absence of or a decreased affinity for the receptor protein.

A Mechanism of steroid hormone action

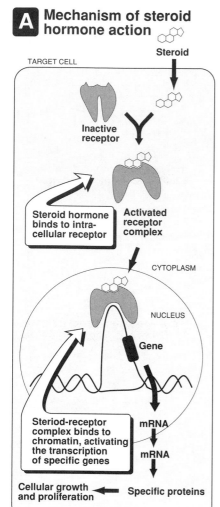

B Actions of anti-estrogen drugs

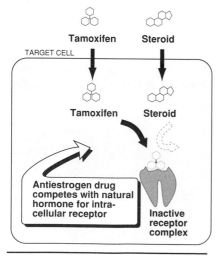

Figure 37.11
Action of antiestrogen agents.

3. **Therapeutic applications:** *Prednisone* is primarily employed to induce remission in patients with acute lymphocytic leukemia and in the treatment of both Hodgkin's and non-Hodgkin's lymphomas.

4. **Pharmacology:** See p.256 for a discussion of the pharmacological aspects of *prednisone* and its toxic actions.

B. Tamoxifen

Tamoxifen [ta MOX i fen] is an estrogen antagonist, structurally related to the synthetic estrogen, *diethylstilbestrol.*

1. **Site of action:** *Tamoxifen* binds to the estrogen receptor but the complex is not productive (i.e., RNA synthesis does not ensue). The result is a depletion of estrogen receptors, and the growth-promoting effects of the natural hormone are suppressed. Its action is not related to any specific phase of the cell cycle. Estrogen competes with *tamoxifen*; therefore, the drug is not effective in premenopausal women.

2. **Resistance:** Resistance is associated either with a decreased affinity for the receptor or a decreased number of receptors.

3. **Therapeutic applications:** Its clinical use is confined to the treatment of estrogen-dependent breast and endometrial cancers.

4. **Pharmacology:** *Tamoxifen* is effective on oral administration. It is partially metabolized by the liver. Unchanged drug and its metabolites are excreted predominantly through the bile into feces.

5. **Adverse effects:** Side effects are similar to those of natural estrogen, that is, hot flashes, nausea, vomiting, skin rash, and vaginal bleeding and discharge (due to some slight estrogenic activity of the drug). *Tamoxifen* can also lead to increased pain if the tumor has metastasized to bone.

C. Estrogens

Estrogens, such as *estrone* or *diethystilbestrol,* are used to treat prostatic cancer. Estrogens inhibit the growth of prostatic tissue by competing with androgens for intracellular receptors sites, thus blocking the effects of androgens in androgen-dependent prostatic tumors. Estrogens are also used in the treatment of metastatic mammary carcinoma in women who are more than 5 years postmenopausal. Estrogen treatment can cause serious complications, such as thromboemboli, myocardial infarction, strokes, and hypercalcemia. In women, loss of libido may accompany menstrual changes. Men taking estrogens may show gynecomastia and impotence.

D. Leuprolide

A synthetic nonapeptide, *leuprolide* [loo PROE lide] is an analog of gonadotropin-releasing hormone. It acts to inhibit the release of

FSH and LH, and thus, reduces androgen synthesis (p.230). It is effective subcutaneously against metastatic carcinoma of the prostate. Its adverse effects are minimal compared to estrogen. A depot formulation has been approved for monthly administration.

VIII. OTHER CHEMOTHERAPEUTIC AGENTS

A. Interferons

Interferons [in ter FEER on] are glycoproteins that can be synthesized by most mammalian cell types. Initially, these compounds were found to interfere in the replication of various viruses, hence the name, *interferon*. However, subsequent investigations have shown that they also affect cell motility and proliferation, and modulate immunological responses, such as antibody formation, delayed hypersensitivity, graft rejection, natural killer cell recruitment, and macrophage activation.

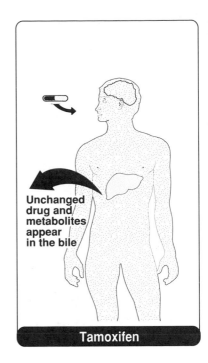

Tamoxifen

1. **Classification:** Human interferons have been classified into three type's, α, β, and γ, on the basis of their antigenicity. The α interferons are primarily leukocytic, whereas the β and γ interferons are produced by connective tissue fibroblasts and T lymphocytes, respectively. Recombinant DNA techniques in bacteria have made available large quantities of α *interferon/species A*—designated $\alpha2(A)$ *interferon*—which has the advantage of being purer than previous preparations derived from leukocytes.

2. **Site of action:** The exact mechanism by which *interferon* is cytotoxic is unknown. *Interferon* secreted from producing cells interacts with surface receptors on other cells, at which site they exert their effects. The bound *interferon* is not internalized nor is it degraded. The α and β interferons compete for binding and presumably bind at the same receptor or in close proximity; g interferons bind at different receptors.

3. **Therapeutic indications:** $\alpha2(A)$ *Interferon* is presently approved for the management of hairy cell leukemia. More than 90% of patients treated with α *interferon* have shown resolution of cytopenia, reduction in the incidence of serious infection, and reduction in the need for transfusions. *Interferon* is also being tested in the treatment of various tumors, including squamous cell carcinoma, melanoma, multiple myeloma, among others.

4. **Pharmacology:** *Interferon* is well absorbed after intramuscular injections. Being a protein, it is probably degraded by proteases.

5. **Adverse effects:** Fever with chills occurs during the first few days of treatment. Dose-related toxicity includes leukopenia and possibly thrombocytopenia. Fatigue, malaise, anorexia, weight loss, alopecia, and transient elevation of liver enzymes have also been reported. Transient and reversible nephrotoxicity with proteinuria has been seen at high doses.

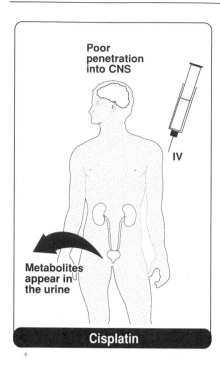

Poor penetration into CNS

IV

Metabolites appear in the urine

Cisplatin

B. Cisplatin

Cisplatin [SIS pla tin] (cis-diaminedichloroplatinum II) is a member of a new class of anticancer drugs, namely the platinum coordination complexes. Only the *cis* configuration is effective as a cytotoxic agent. *Cisplatin* has synergistic cytotoxicity with radiation and other chemotherapeutic agents.

1. **Site of action:** Its mechanism of action is similar to that of the alkylating agents. The complex binds to DNA to form inter- and intra-strand crosslinks, resulting in inhibition of both DNA and RNA synthesis. *Cisplatin* can also bind to proteins and SH groups. Cytotoxicity can occur at all stages of the cell cycle, but the cell is most vulnerable to its actions in G_1 and S.

2. **Resistance:** No mechanism has been elucidated, but DNA repair has been proposed.

3. **Therapeutic applications:** *Cisplatin* has found application in the treatment of many solid tumors, such as metastatic testicular carcinoma in combination with *vinblastine* and *bleomycin,* ovarian carcinoma in combination with *cyclophosphamide,* and alone for bladder carcinoma.

4. **Pharmacology:** *Cisplatin* is administered IV in saline solution. Over 90% of the drug is bound to serum proteins. It concentrates in the liver, kidney, intestinal, and ovarian cells, but it does not penetrate into the cerebral spinal fluid (CSF). The renal route is the main avenue for excretion.

5. **Adverse effects:** Severe, persistent vomiting occurs 1 hour after administration and may continue for as long as 5 days. The major limiting toxicity is dose-related nephrotoxicity, which can be ameliorated by aggressive hydration and diuresis with *mannitol.* The nephrotoxicity involves the distal convoluted tubule and collecting ducts. Hypomagnesemia and hypocalcemia usually occur concurrently; it is important to correct calcium levels before correcting magnesium levels. Other toxicities include ototoxicity, with high frequency hearing loss and tinnitus; mild bone marrow suppression; some neurotoxicity, characterized by paresthesia and loss of proprioception; and hypersensitivity reactions, ranging from skin rashes to anaphylaxis. Patients receiving aminoglycosides (p.288) concomitantly are at a greater risk for nephrotoxicity and ototoxicity.

C. Procarbazine

Procarbazine [proe KAR ba zeen] is a methylhydrazine compound that is structurally unrelated to any of the other anticancer agents.

1. **Site of action:** Its mechanism of action may be similar to that of the alkylating agents, because strand scission of DNA is observed, and DNA and RNA synthesis are inhibited. However, metabolism of *procarbazine* leads to the formation of hydrogen peroxide and formaldehyde, so that oxidative processes involving free radicals may be responsible for the altered function of the genome.

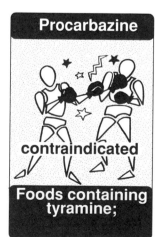

Procarbazine

contraindicated

Foods containing tyramine;

2. **Resistance:** The mechanism for resistance is unknown.

3. **Therapeutic application:** *Procarbazine* is used in the treatment of Hodgkin's disease, as part of the "MOPP" regimen.

4. **Pharmacology:** *Procarbazine* rapidly equilibrates between the plasma and the CSF after oral or parenteral administration. It is metabolized oxidatively to an azo derivative and hydrogen peroxide. Metabolites and the parent drug are excreted through the kidney.

5. **Adverse effects:** Besides the usual nausea, vomiting, diarrhea, and myelosuppression, the drug can cause psychic disturbances, since it inhibits monoamine oxidase. It is important that the patient be warned against ingesting foods that contain tyramine (e.g., aged cheeses, beer, and wine). Ingestion of alcohol leads to a disulfiram-type reaction. *Procarbazine* is both mutagenic and teratogenic. Nonlymphocytic leukemia has developed in patients treated with the drug.

D. L-Asparaginase

L-Asparaginase [a SPAR a gi nase] catalyzes the deamination of asparagine to aspartic acid and ammonia. The form of the enzyme used chemotherapeutically is derived from bacteria.

1. **Site of action:** Some neoplastic cells require an external source of asparagine, because of their limited capacity to make sufficient L-asparagine to support growth and function. *L-Asparaginase* hydrolyzes blood asparagine and thus deprives the tumor cells of this nutrient required for protein synthesis (Figure 37.12).

2. **Resistance:** Resistance is partially due to inactivation of the enzyme protein by a protease.

3. **Therapeutic application:** *L-Asparaginase* is used to treat acute lymphocytic leukemia in combination with *vincristine* and *prednisone*.

4. **Pharmacology:** The enzyme must be administered either IV or IM because it is destroyed by gastric enzymes. Disposition remains undefined.

5. **Adverse effects:** Toxicities include a range of hypersensitivity reactions (since it is a foreign protein), a decrease in clotting factors and liver abnormalities, as well as pancreatitis, seizures, and coma.

E. Etoposide (VP-16)

Etoposide [e toe POE side] is a semisynthetic derivative of a plant alkaloid. It blocks cells in the late S-G$_2$ phase of the cell cycle. Several mechanisms have been suggested to account for its cytotoxic effect. These include degradation of DNA, inhibition of nucleoside transport, and/or inhibition of mitochondrial oxidation.

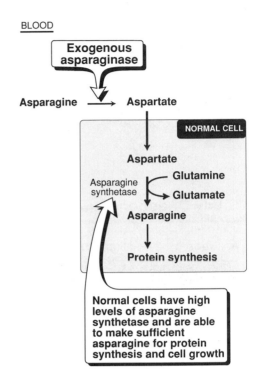

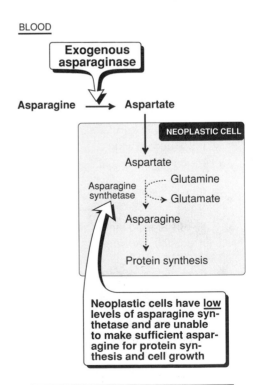

Figure 37.12
Mechanism of action of L-asparaginase.

No mechanism for resistance has been described. *Etoposide* finds its major clinical use in the treatment of oat cell carcinoma of the lung and refractory testicular carcinoma. It is currently being tested in other therapeutic protocols. *Etoposide* may be administered either IV or orally. It is highly bound to plasma proteins and distributes throughout the body, but it enters the CSF poorly. Metabolites are converted to glucuronide and sulfate conjugates and are excreted in the urine. A small fraction of the drug is eliminated in the bile. Dose-limiting myelosuppression is the major toxicity. Other toxicities are alopecia, anaphylactic reactions, nausea, and vomiting. Hypotension may occur if the drug is injected rapidly. The drug is teratogenic in experimental animals.

The anticancer agents are summarized in Figure 37.13

Study Questions   (see p.436 for answers).

Answer A if 1,2 and 3 are correct.
   B if 1 and 3 are correct.
   C if 2 and 4 are correct.
   D if only 4 is correct.
   E if 1,2,3 and 4 are all correct.

37.1 Which of the following agents show(s) cytotoxicity that is cell-cycle specific?

   1. Methotrexate.
   2. Dactinomycin.
   3. Bleomycin.
   4. Mechlorethamine.

37.2 Which of the following drugs is/are metabolized to a cytotoxic product?

   1. 6-Mercaptopurine.
   2. Dactinomycin.
   3. 5-Fluorouracil.
   4. Lomustine.

Choose the ONE best answer.

37.3 All of the following agents cause their cytotoxic effects by interference in DNA transcription EXCEPT:

   A. Doxorubicin.
   B. Tamoxifen.
   C. Cyclophosphamide.
   D. Mechlorethamine.
   E. Cisplatin.

37.4 Myelosuppression is a particularly serious toxicity with all of the following EXCEPT:

   A. Vinblastine.
   B. Cyclophosphamide.
   C. Cytarabine.
   D. Mechlorethamine.
   E. L-Asparaginase.

37.5 Cells resistant to methotrexate may

   A. have higher than normal levels of dihydrofolate reductase.
   B. have higher levels of formyl tetrahydrofolate.
   C. metabolize the drug to inactive products.
   D. have a decreased metabolic need for folate.
   E. show an increased uptake of methotrexate.

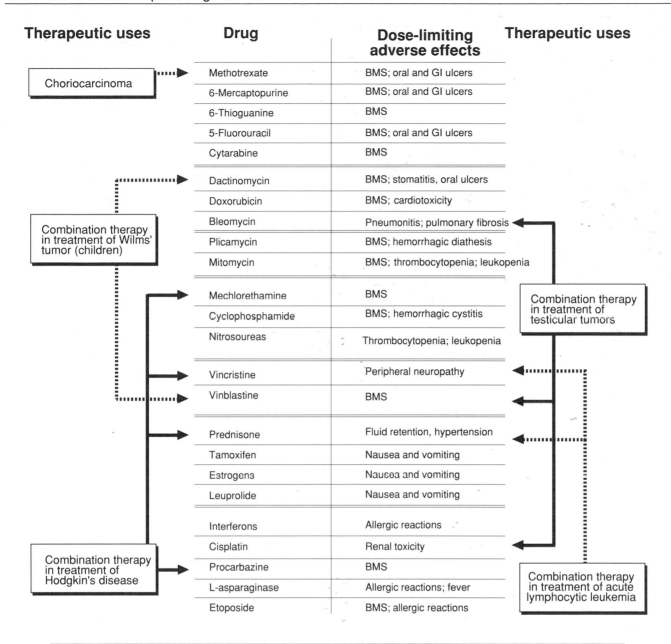

Therapeutic uses	Drug	Dose-limiting adverse effects	Therapeutic uses
Choriocarcinoma	Methotrexate	BMS; oral and GI ulcers	
	6-Mercaptopurine	BMS; oral and GI ulcers	
	6-Thioguanine	BMS	
	5-Fluorouracil	BMS; oral and GI ulcers	
	Cytarabine	BMS	
	Dactinomycin	BMS; stomatitis, oral ulcers	
	Doxorubicin	BMS; cardiotoxicity	
Combination therapy in treatment of Wilms' tumor (children)	Bleomycin	Pneumonitis; pulmonary fibrosis	
	Plicamycin	BMS; hemorrhagic diathesis	
	Mitomycin	BMS; thrombocytopenia; leukopenia	
	Mechlorethamine	BMS	Combination therapy in treatment of testicular tumors
	Cyclophosphamide	BMS; hemorrhagic cystitis	
	Nitrosoureas	Thrombocytopenia; leukopenia	
	Vincristine	Peripheral neuropathy	
	Vinblastine	BMS	
	Prednisone	Fluid retention, hypertension	
	Tamoxifen	Nausea and vomiting	
	Estrogens	Nausea and vomiting	
	Leuprolide	Nausea and vomiting	
	Interferons	Allergic reactions	
	Cisplatin	Renal toxicity	
Combination therapy in treatment of Hodgkin's disease	Procarbazine	BMS	Combination therapy in treatment of acute lymphocytic leukemia
	L-asparaginase	Allergic reactions; fever	
	Etoposide	BMS; allergic reactions	

Adverse effects and precautions commonly observed with anticancer drugs

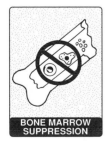
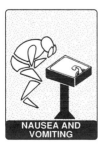
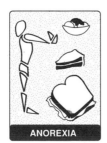
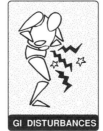
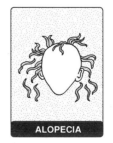
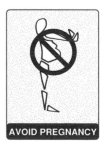

BONE MARROW SUPPRESSION

NAUSEA AND VOMITING

ANOREXIA

GI DISTURBANCES

ALOPECIA

AVOID PREGNANCY

Figure 37.13
Summary of cancer chemotherapy agents. BMS= bone marrow suppression.

37.6 All of the following statements are true EXCEPT:

A. Patients with Hodgkin's disease being treated with procarbazine should be cautioned against ingesting food derived from fermentative sources.

B. Vincristine is effective in inducing remission in childhood acute lymphocytic leukemia.

C. X-irradiation of the craniospinal axis is an effective adjuvant therapy in the treatment of acute lymphocytic leukemia.

D. Treatment with alkylating agents can induce secondary tumors.

E. Tamoxifen complexes with DNA to inhibit RNA synthesis.

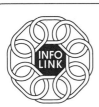

[1]See *methotrexate* in **Biochemistry** for role of this drug in preventing cell division (see index).

[2]See *one-carbon pool* in **Biochemistry** for a more detailed discussion of tetrahydrofolate metabolism

[3]See *hypoxanthine-guanine phosphoribosyl transferase* in **Biochemistry** for a summary of this pathway.

[4]See *purines, nucleotide synthesis* in **Biochemistry** for a summary of this pathway

[5]See *xanthine oxidase* in **Biochemistry** for the role of this enzyme in purine degradation.

Anti-inflammatory Drugs

I. OVERVIEW

Inflammation is a normal, protective response to tissue injury that is caused by physical trauma, noxious chemicals, or microbiological agents. Inflammation is the body's effort to inactivate or destroy invading organisms, remove irritants, and set the stage for tissue repair. When healing is complete, the inflammatory process usually subsides. However, inflammation is sometimes inappropriately triggered by an innocuous agent, such as pollen, or by an autoimmune response, as in some asthmas or rheumatoid arthritis. In such cases, the defense reactions themselves may cause progressive tissue injury, and anti-inflammatory or immunosuppressive drugs may be required to modulate the inflammatory process.

Inflammation is triggered by the release of chemical mediators from injured tissues and migrating cells. The specific chemical mediators vary with the type of inflammatory process and include amines, such as histamine and 5-hydroxytryptamine; lipids, such as the prostaglandins; small peptides, such as bradykinin; and larger peptides, such as interleukin-1. Discovery of such a variety of chemical mediators has clarified the apparent paradox that different drugs are effective in treating one form of inflammation but not others. Thus, a drug may interfere with the action of a particular mediator important in one type of inflammation but be without effect in inflammatory processes not involving the target mediator. The drugs described in this chapter are summarized in Figure 38.1. [Note: The use of corticosteroids in the treatment of inflammation is discussed on p.252.]

II. PROSTAGLANDINS

Many of the nonsteroidal anti-inflammatory drugs (NSAIDs) act by inhibiting the synthesis of prostaglandins. Thus, an understanding of NSAIDs requires a description of the actions and biosynthesis of prostaglandins—unsaturated fatty acid derivatives containing 20 carbons

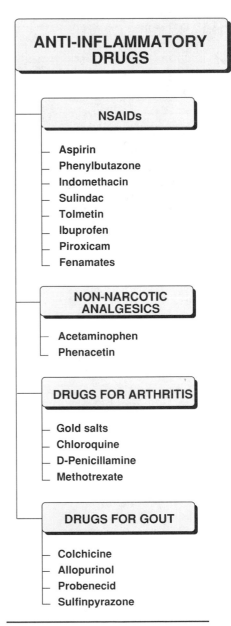

ANTI-INFLAMMATORY DRUGS

NSAIDs
- Aspirin
- Phenylbutazone
- Indomethacin
- Sulindac
- Tolmetin
- Ibuprofen
- Piroxicam
- Fenamates

NON-NARCOTIC ANALGESICS
- Acetaminophen
- Phenacetin

DRUGS FOR ARTHRITIS
- Gold salts
- Chloroquine
- D-Penicillamine
- Methotrexate

DRUGS FOR GOUT
- Colchicine
- Allopurinol
- Probenecid
- Sulfinpyrazone

Figure 38.1
Summary of nonsteroidal anti-inflammatory drugs.

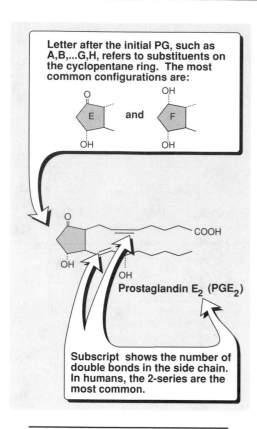

Figure 38.2
Structural features of
prostaglandins.

and a cyclic ring structure. Figure 38.2 shows the important structural features of the prostaglandins.

A. Role of prostaglandins as local mediators

1. Prostaglandins and related compounds are produced in minute quantities by virtually all tissues. They generally act on the tissues in which they are synthesized and are rapidly metabolized to inactive products at their site of action. Therefore, the prostaglandins do not circulate in the blood at significant concentrations.

2. Thromboxanes, leukotrienes, and the hydroperoxyeicosatetraenoic and hydroxyeicosatetraenoic acids (HPETEs and HETEs) are related lipids; they are synthesized from the same precursors as are the prostaglandins, using interrelated pathways (Figure 38.3).

B. Synthesis of prostaglandins

1. **Arachidonic acid:** This 20-carbon fatty acid is the primary precursor of the prostaglandins and related compounds (Figure 38.3). Arachidonic acid is present as a component of the phospholipids of cell membranes (primarily in phosphatidyl inositol and other complex lipids). Free arachidonic acid is released from tissue phospholipids by the action of phospholipase A_2 and other acyl hydrolases, via a process controlled by hormones and other stimuli (Figure 38.3).

2. **Cyclooxygenase and lipoxygenase pathways:** There are two major pathways in the synthesis of the eicosanoids from arachidonic acid (Figure 38.3). All eicosanoids with ring structures, that is, the prostaglandins, thromboxanes, and prostacyclins, are synthesized via the cyclooxygenase pathway. The leukotrienes, HETE, and HPETE are hydroxylated derivatives of straight-chain fatty acids and are synthesized via the lipoxygenase pathway (Figure 38.3).[1]

C. Actions of prostaglandins

1. **Mechanism of action:** Many of the actions of prostaglandins are mediated by their binding to membrane receptors, causing the subsequent activation or inhibition of adenyl cyclase. In some tissues, however, prostaglandins appear to act by mechanisms that do not involve cAMP. $PGF2\alpha$, the leukotrienes, and thromboxane A_2 (TXA_2) mediate certain actions by causing the increase of intracellular Ca^{++}.

2. **Functions in the body:** Prostaglandins produced endogenously in the tissues act as local chemical signals that fine tune the response of a specific cell type. For example, the release of thromboxane from platelets is a signal to initiate recruitment of new platelets for aggregation (i.e., the first step in clot formation). However, in other tissues, elevated levels of thromboxane convey a different signal; for example, in certain smooth muscles, thromboxane induces contraction. Prostaglandins are one of the

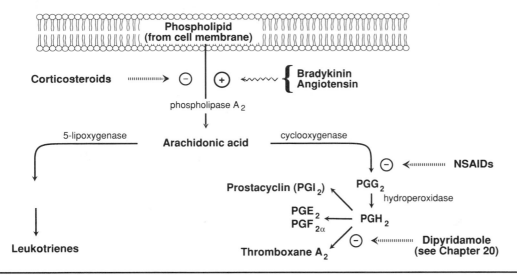

Figure 38.3
Synthesis of prostaglandins and leukotrienes.

chemical mediators that are released in allergic and inflammatory processes (p.208).[2]

III. NSAIDs

The nonsteroidal anti-inflammatory drugs (NSAIDs) are a group of chemically dissimilar agents that have as their primary effect the inhibition of prostaglandin synthesis. *Aspirin* is the prototype of this group; it is the drug to which all other anti-inflammatory agents are compared. About 15% of patients show an intolerance to *aspirin*. Therefore, it is primarily for these individuals that the other NSAIDs are useful. In addition, some of the newer NSAIDs are marginally superior to *aspirin* in certain patients, because they have greater anti-inflammatory activity and/or cause less gastric irritation, thus permitting easier administration and better patient compliance. However, the newer NSAIDs are as much as 15 times more expensive than *aspirin,* and some have proved to be more toxic in other ways.

A. Aspirin and other salicylates

Aspirin [AS pir in] is unique among the NSAIDs in irreversibly acetylating (and thus inhibiting) cyclooxygenase (Figure 38.4). The other NSAIDs are all reversible inhibitors of cyclooxygenase. *Aspirin* is also rapidly deacetylated by esterases in the body, producing salicylate, which itself has anti-inflammatory, antipyretic, and analgesic effects.

1. **Mechanism of action:** The antipyretic and anti-inflammatory effects of the salicylates are due primarily to inhibition of prostaglandin synthesis at the thermoregulatory centers in the hypothalamus and at peripheral target sites. The blockade of prostaglandin synthesis prevents the sensitization of pain receptors to both mechanical and chemical stimuli. *Aspirin* may also

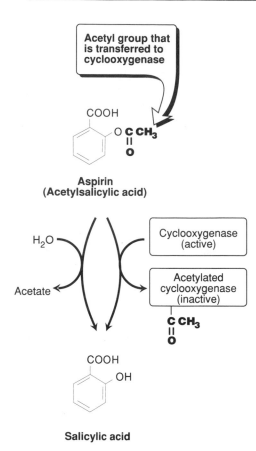

Figure 38.4
Acetylation of cyclooxygenase
by aspirin.

depress pain stimuli at subcortical sites (i.e., the thalamus and hypothalamus).

2. **Actions:**

The NSAIDs, including *aspirin,* have three major therapeutic actions, namely they reduce inflammation (anti-inflammatory), reduce pain (analgesic), and diminish fever (antipyretic, see Figure 38.5). However, as described later in this section, not all of the NSAIDs are equally potent in each of these actions.

a. **Anti-inflammatory actions:** *Aspirin* inhibits cyclooxygenase activity (see Figure 38.3). This leads to inhibition of prostaglandin synthesis and modulates those aspects of inflammation in which the prostaglandins act as mediators. *Aspirin* inhibits inflammation but neither arrests the progress of the disease nor induces remission. [Note: *Acetaminophen,* although a useful analgesic and antipyretic, has *weak* anti-inflammatory activity and is therefore not useful in the treatment of inflammation such as those seen with rheumatoid arthritis (Figure 38.5). *Acetaminophen* is therefore discussed separately (p.371).]

b. **Analgesic action:** Prostaglandin E$_2$ (PGE$_2$) is thought to sensitize the nerve endings to the action of bradykinin, histamine, and other chemical mediators released locally by the inflammatory process. Thus, by decreasing prostaglandin synthesis, *aspirin* and other NSAIDs inhibit the sensation of pain. The salicylates are used mainly for the management of pain of low to moderate-intensity that arises from integumental structures rather than that arising from the viscera.

c. **Antipyretic action:** Fever occurs when an endogenous fever-producing agent (pyrogen) is released from white cells that are activated by infection, hypersensitivity, or inflammation. The salicylates appear to lower body temperature in patients with fever by inhibition of PGE$_2$ synthesis and release by the thermoregulatory centers of the anterior hypothalamus in response to an endogenous pyrogen. *Aspirin* is effective in rapidly reducing the body temperature of febrile patients through increased heat dissipation as a result of peripheral vasodilation. *Aspirin* has little effect on normal body temperature.

d. **Respiratory actions:** *Aspirin* at therapeutic doses increases alveolar respiration. Higher doses work directly on the respiratory center, resulting in hyperventilation and respiratory alkalosis, which is adequately compensated by the kidney.

e. **Gastrointestinal effects:** Normally, prostacyclin (PGI$_2$) inhibits gastric acid secretion, whereas PGE$_2$ and PGF2α stimulate synthesis of protective mucus in both the stomach and small intestine. In the presence of *aspirin,* prostaglandins and prostacyclins are not synthesized, resulting in increased acid secretion and diminished mucous protection. This may cause epigastric distress, ulceration, and/or hemorrhage. [Note: The prostaglandin derivative, *misoprostol,* is used in the treatment of aspirin-induced ulcer (p.380).]

f. **Effect on platelets:** Thromboxane A_2 enhances platelet aggregation, whereas PGI_2 decreases it. Low doses (60-80 mg daily) of *aspirin* can irreversibly inhibit thromboxane production in platelets without markedly affecting production in the endothelial cells of the blood vessel. This results in reduced platelet aggregation (the first step in thrombus formation) and, hence, produces an anticoagulation effect with a prolongation of bleeding time. The acetylation of cyclooxygenase is irreversible and, therefore, persists for the lifetime (3-7 days) of the platelet, since no new proteins are synthesized in platelets that are without nuclei. This contrasts with the endothelial cells, which can synthesize new molecules of cyclooxygenase. [Note: The actions of *aspirin* as an antithrombotic drug are described on p.188.]

g. **Actions on the kidney:** Cyclooxygenase inhibitors prevent the synthesis of PGE_2 and PGI_2, which are responsible for maintaining renal blood flow, particularly in the presence of circulating vasoconstrictors (Figure 38.6). Decreased synthesis of prostaglandins can result in retention of sodium and water and may cause edema and hyperkalemia in some patients. Interstitial nephritis can also occur with all of the NSAIDs except *aspirin.*

3. **Therapeutic uses:**

a. *Sodium salicylate, choline salicylate* (in the liquid formulation), *choline magnesium salicylate,* and *aspirin* are used as

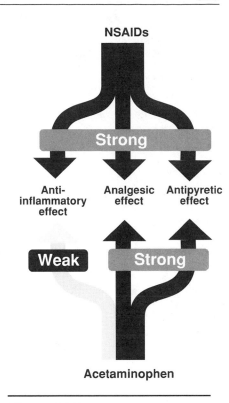

Figure 38.5
Actions of NSAIDs and acetaminophen.

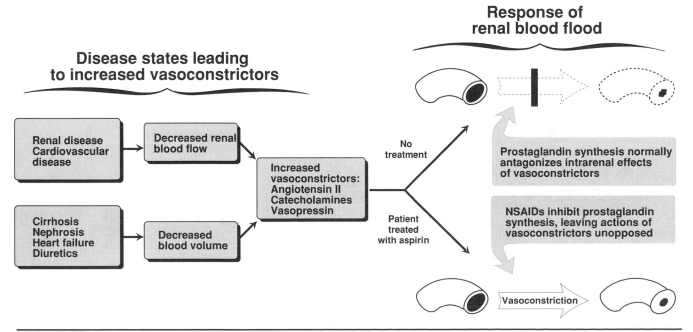

Figure 38.6
Renal effect of aspirin inhibition of prostaglandin synthesis.

antipyretics, and analgesics; in the treatment of gout, rheumatic fever, and rheumatoid arthritis; and to inhibit platelet aggregation. The analgesic and the anti-inflammatory action of salicylates make these compounds the drugs of choice in the treatment of rheumatoid arthritis. Commonly treated conditions requiring analgesia include headache, arthralgia, and myalgia.

b. *Salicylic acid* is used topically to treat corns, calluses, and epidermophytosis (an eruption caused by fungi).

c. *Salicylamide* is included in the formulations of several over-the-counter analgesic and sedative preparations. However, the effect of *salicylamide* is not reliable.

d. *Methyl salicylate* ("oil of wintergreen") is used externally as a cutaneous counterirritant in liniments.

e. *Diflunisal,* a diflurophenyl derivative of salicylic acid, is not metabolized to salicylate and therefore cannot cause salicylism (salicylate intoxication, p.368). *Diflunisal* is 3-4 times more potent than *aspirin* as an analgesic and an anti-inflammatory agent, but it does not have antipyretic properties. [Note: *Diflunisal* does not enter the central nervous system (CNS) and therefore cannot relieve fever.]

f. Low doses of *aspirin* decrease the incidence of transient ischemic attack and unstable angina in humans (see p.188 for a further discussion of this phenomenon).

4. **Pharmacology:**

a. **Administration and distribution:** Salicylates, especially methyl salicylate, are absorbed through intact skin. After oral administration, salicylates are absorbed from the stomach and the small intestine. Rectal absorption of the salicylates is slow and unreliable, but it is a useful route for administration to vomiting children. Salicylates cross both the blood-brain barrier and the placenta.

b. **Dosage:** The salicylates exhibit analgesic activity at low doses; only at higher doses do these drugs show anti-inflammatory activity (Figure 38.7). For example, two 300 mg *aspirin* tablets administered 4 times a day produce analgesia, whereas 12 to 20 tablets per day produce both analgesic and anti-inflammatory activity. Low dosages of *aspirin* (160 mg every other day) have been shown to reduce the incidence of recurrent myocardial infarction and to reduce mortality in postmyocardial infarction patients. Further, *aspirin* in a dose of 160 to 325 mg/day appears to be beneficial in the prevention of a first myocardial infarction, at least in men over the age of 50 years. Thus, prophylactic aspirin therapy is advocated in patients with clinical manifestations of coronary disease if no specific contraindications are present.

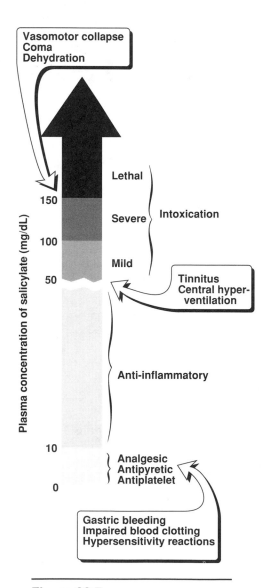

Figure 38.7
Dose-dependent effects of salicylate.

c. **Metabolism:** At normal low dosages (600 mg/day), *aspirin* is hydrolyzed to salicylate and acetic acid by esterases present in tissues and blood (see Figure 38.4). Salicylate is converted by the liver to water-soluble conjugates that are rapidly cleared by the kidney, resulting in elimination with first-order kinetics and a serum half-life of 3.5 hours. At anti-inflammatory dosages (4g/day), the hepatic metabolic pathway becomes saturated, and zero-order kinetics are observed, with the drug having a half-life of 15 hours or more (Figure 38.8). The saturation of the hepatic enzymes requires treatment for from several days to 1 week.

5. **Adverse effects:**

a. **GI:** The most common GI effects of the salicylates are epigastric distress, nausea, and vomiting. Microscopic GI bleeding is almost universal in patients treated with salicylates. [Note: *Aspirin* is an acid. At stomach pH, *aspirin* is uncharged; consequently it readily crosses into the mucosal cells where it ionizes (becomes negatively charged) and becomes trapped (see p.4 for discussion of ion trapping), thus potentially causing direct damage to the cells. *Aspirin* should be taken with food and large volumes of fluids to diminish GI disturbances.]

b. **Blood:** The irreversible acetylation of platelet cyclooxygenase reduces the level of platelet TXA_2, resulting in inhibition of platelet aggregation and a prolonged bleeding time. For this reason *aspirin* should not be taken for at least 1 week prior to surgery. When salicylates are administered, anticoagulants may have to be given in reduced dosage.

c. **Respiration:** In toxic doses, salicylates cause respiratory depression and a combination of uncompensated respiratory and metabolic acidosis.

d. **Metabolic processes:** Large doses of salicylates uncouple oxidative phosphorylation.[3] The energy normally used for the production of ATP is dissipated as heat, which explains the pyretic effect of salicylates when given in toxic quantities.

e. **Hypersensitivity:** Approximately 15% of patients taking *aspirin* experience hypersensitivity reactions. Symptoms of true allergy include urticaria, bronchoconstriction, or angioneurotic edema. Fatal anaphylactic shock is rare.

f. **Reye's syndrome:** *Aspirin* given during viral infections has been associated with an increased incidence of Reye's syndrome. Therefore, *acetaminophen* should be substituted for *aspirin* in children requiring medication. Reye's syndrome is an often fatal, fulminating hepatitis with cerebral edema.

g. **Drug interactions:** Concomitant administration of salicylates with many classes of drugs may produce undesirable side effects (Figure 38.9).

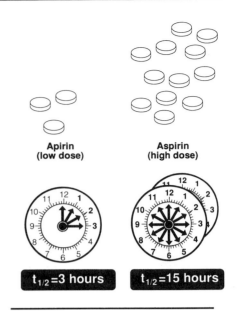

Figure 38.8
Effect of dose on the half-life of aspirin.

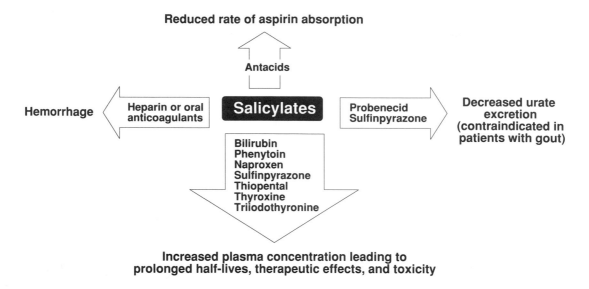

Figure 38.9
Drugs interacting with salicylates.

6. **Toxicity:**

   a. **Salicylism:** Salicylate intoxication may be mild or severe. The mild form is called *salicylism* and is characterized by nausea, vomiting, marked hyperventilation, headache, mental confusion, dizziness, and tinnitus (ringing or roaring in the ears). When large doses of salicylate are administered, severe salicylate intoxication may result. The symptoms listed above are followed by restlessness, delirium, hallucinations, convulsions, coma, respiratory and metabolic acidosis, and death from respiratory failure. Children are particularly prone to salicylate intoxication. Ingestion of as little as 10 g of *aspirin* (or 5 g of methyl salicylate, the latter being used as a counterirritant in liniments) can cause death in children. [Note: *Diflunisal* does not cause salicylism.]

   b. **Treatment of salicylism:** Treatment should include measurement of serum salicylate concentrations and of pH to determine the best form of therapy. In mild cases, symptomatic treatment is usually sufficient. Increasing the pH of the urine enhances the elimination of salicylate. In serious cases, mandatory measures include the intravenous (IV) administration of fluid, dialysis (hemodialysis or peritoneal dialysis), and the frequent measurement and correction of acid-base and electrolyte balances.

B. Phenylbutazone

   1. **Actions:** *Phenylbutazone* [fen ill BYOO ta zone] has powerful anti-inflammatory effects but weak analgesic and antipyretic activities.

2. **Therapeutic uses:** *Phenylbutazone* is prescribed chiefly in short-term therapy of acute gout and in acute rheumatoid arthritis when other NSAID agents have failed. The usefulness of *phenylbutazone* is limited by its toxicity. *Aspirin* and newer NSAIDs are superior to *phenylbutazone* in most applications.

3. **Pharmacology:** *Phenylbutazone* is rapidly and completely absorbed after oral or rectal administration.

4. **Adverse effects:** *Phenylbutazone* is poorly tolerated by many patients; adverse effects occur in nearly one half of those treated. Because of these effects, the drug should be given for short periods of time—up to 1 week only. Patients should be observed closely, and frequent blood tests should be taken.

   a. The most common adverse effects of *phenylbutazone* are nausea, vomiting, skin rashes, and epigastric discomfort (Figure 38.10).

   b. Other side effects include fluid and electrolyte (sodium and chloride) retention, with resulting edema and decreased urine volume. Also, diarrhea, vertigo, insomnia, blurred vision, euphoria, nervousness, and hematuria may occur.

   c. *Phenylbutazone* reduces the uptake of iodine by the thyroid glands, sometimes resulting in goiter and myxedema.

   d. The most serious adverse effects are agranulocytosis and aplastic anemia.

C. Indomethacin

1. **Actions:** *Indomethacin* [in doe METH a sin] has anti-inflammatory, antipyretic, and analgesic properties. Although *indomethacin* is more potent than *aspirin* as an anti-inflammatory agent, it is inferior to the salicylates at doses tolerated by rheumatoid arthritic patients. In certain instances, however (for example, with acute gouty arthritis, ankylosing spondylitis, and osteoarthritis of the hip), *indomethacin* is more effective than *aspirin* or any of the other NSAIDs.

2. **Therapeutic uses:** Although *indomethacin* is a potent anti-inflammatory agent, it is quite toxic and should therefore be used only for the treatment of the conditions just described. *Indomethacin* is also beneficial as an agent to control pain associated with uveitis and postoperative ophthalmic pain as well as an antipyretic for Hodgkin's disease when the fever is refractory to other agents.

3. **Pharmacology:** *Indomethacin* is rapidly and almost completely absorbed from the upper GI tract after oral administration. It is metabolized by the liver; unchanged drugs and metabolites are excreted in bile and urine.

4. **Adverse effects:** Adverse effects with *indomethacin* occur in up to 50% of patients treated; approximately 20% find the adverse

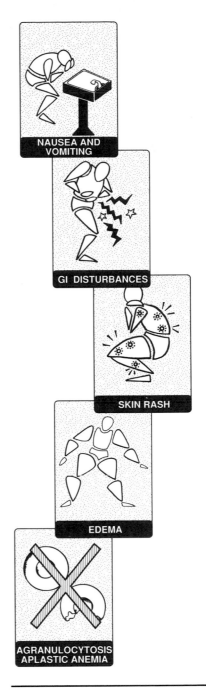

Figure 38.10
Some adverse effects of phenylbutazone.

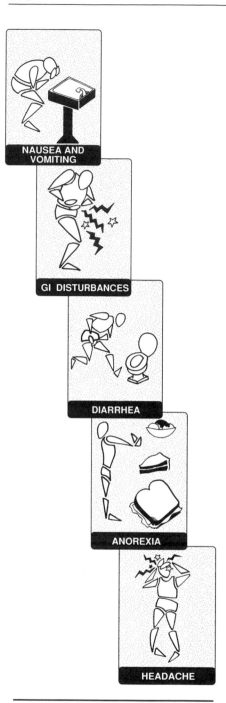

NAUSEA AND VOMITING

GI DISTURBANCES

DIARRHEA

ANOREXIA

HEADACHE

Figure 38.11
Some adverse effects of
indomethacin.

effects to be intolerable and discontinue use of the drug. Most adverse effects are dose related.

a. **GI:** GI complaints consist of nausea, vomiting, anorexia, diarrhea, and abdominal pain (Figure 38.11). Ulceration of the upper GI tract can occur, sometimes with perforation and hemorrhage.

b. **CNS:** Of the effects on the CNS, the most severe and frequent is frontal headache, which occurs in 25-50% of patients who chronically use *indomethacin.* Other frequent CNS effects are dizziness, vertigo, light-headedness, and mental confusion.

c. **Acute pancreatitis:** Acute pancreatitis has been known to occur. Hepatic effects are rare, but some fatal cases of hepatitis and jaundice have been reported.

d. **Hematopoietic reactions:** Hematopoietic reactions reported with *indomethacin* include neutropenia, thrombocytopenia, and (rarely) aplastic anemia.

e. **Hypersensitivity reactions:** These side effects include rashes, urticaria, itching, acute attacks of asthma, and 100% cross-reactivity with *aspirin.*

D. Sulindac

Sulindac [sul IN dak] is an inactive pro-drug that is closely related to *indomethacin. Sulindac* itself has little pharmacological activity. Metabolism by hepatic microsomal enzymes produces the active form of the drug. *Sulindac* has analgesic and anti-inflammatory activities. The drug is less potent than *indomethacin. Sulindac* has a long duration of action. The drug is useful in the treatment of rheumatoid arthritis, ankylosing spondylitis, osteoarthritis, and acute gout. The therapeutic applications and the adverse reactions are similar to but less severe than those of the other NSAIDs.

E. Ibuprofen

Ibuprofen [eye BYOO proe fen] and the related drugs, *naproxen, ketoprofen,* and *fenoprofen,* have anti-inflammatory, analgesic, and antipyretic activities. *Ibuprofen* has the same anti-inflammatory potency as *aspirin.* These drugs can cause hypersensitivity reactions and GI disturbances, but they are better tolerated than *aspirin.*

F. Piroxicam

Piroxicam [peer OX i kan] has a half-life of 45 hours, which permits administration once a day. GI disturbances are encountered in approximately 20% of patients. *Piroxicam* is used to treat rheumatoid arthritis, ankylosis spondylitis, and osteoarthritis. (See Figure 38.12 for a summary of the therapeutic advantages and disadvantages of members of the NSAID family.)

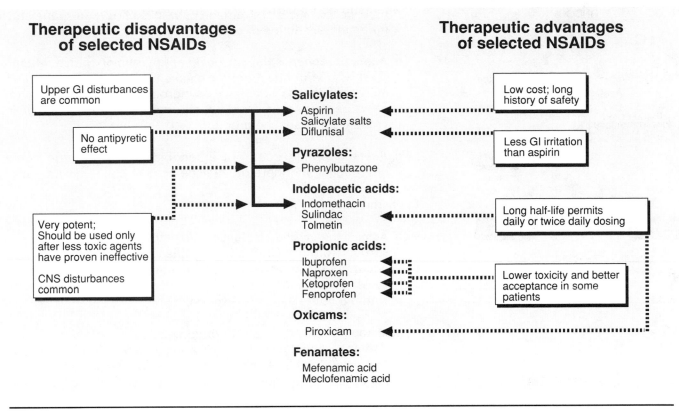

Figure 38.12
Summary of nonsteroidal anti-inflammatory agents (NSAIDs).

IV. NON-NARCOTIC ANALGESICS

Non-narcotic analgesics, unlike the NSAIDs, have little or no anti-inflammatory activity. They have a therapeutic advantage over narcotic analgesics in that they do not cause physical dependence or tolerance.

A. Acetaminophen and phenacetin

1. **Actions:** *Acetaminophen* [a seat a MEE noe fen] and *phenacetin* [fe NASS e tin] act by inhibiting prostaglandin synthesis in the CNS. This explains their antipyretic and analgesic properties. They have less effect on cyclooxygenase in peripheral tissues, which accounts for their weak anti-inflammatory activity. *Acetaminophen* and *phenacetin* do not affect platelet function or increase blood clotting time, and they lack many of the side effects of *aspirin.*

2. **Therapeutic uses:**

   a. *Acetaminophen* is a suitable substitute for the analgesic and antipyretic effects of *aspirin* in those patients with gastric complaints and in those for whom prolongation of bleeding

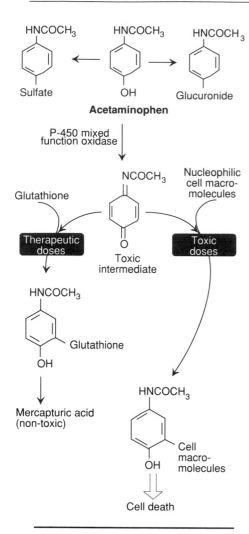

Figure 38.13
Metabolism of acetaminophen.

time would be a disadvantage or who do not require the anti-inflammatory action of *aspirin*.

b. *Acetaminophen* is the analgesic-antipyretic of choice for children with viral infections or chicken pox (recall that *aspirin* increases the risk of Reye's syndrome, p. 367). *Acetaminophen,* because of its lower toxicity, has replaced *phenacetin* in virtually all headache products.

c. *Acetaminophen* does not antagonize the uricosuric agent *probenecid* and therefore may be used in patients with gout.

3. **Pharmacology:**

a. **Administration and distribution:** *Acetaminophen* is rapidly absorbed from the GI tract. A significant first-pass metabolism occurs in the luminal cells of the intestine and in the hepatocytes. *Phenacetin* is largely converted to *acetaminophen* within 3 hours of administration.

b. **Metabolism:** Under normal circumstances, *acetaminophen* is conjugated in the liver to form inactive glucuronylated or sulfated metabolites. A portion of *acetaminophen* is hydroxylated to form N-acetyl-benzoquinoneimine—a highly reactive and potentially dangerous metabolite that reacts with sulfhydryl groups. At normal doses of *acetaminophen,* the N-acetyl-benzoquinoneimine reacts with the sulfhydryl group of glutathione, forming a nontoxic substance (Figure 38.13).

c. **Toxicity:** At large doses the available glutathione in the liver becomes depleted and N-acetyl-benzoquinoneimine reacts with the sulfhydryl groups of hepatic proteins, forming covalent bonds (Figure 38.13). Hepatic necrosis, a very serious and potentially life-threatening condition, can result. Renal tubular necrosis may also occur. *Acetaminophen* and its metabolites are excreted in the urine.

4. **Adverse effects:**

a. With normal therapeutic doses, *acetaminophen* is virtually free of any significant adverse effects. Skin rash and minor allergic reactions occur infrequently. There may be minor alterations in leukocyte count, but these are generally transient. Renal tubular necrosis and hypoglycemic coma are rare complications of prolonged large-dose therapy.

b. An overdose of 10 g or more in an adult may result in the potentially fatal hepatic necrosis discussed above. However, administration of *N-acetylcysteine,* which contains sulfhydryl groups to which the toxic metabolite can bind, can be life-saving if administered within 12 to 20 hours of ingestion of the overdose.

V. SLOW-ACTING, ANTI-INFLAMMATORY AGENTS

In contrast to the NSAID drugs described earlier, remittive (remission-inducing) arthritis drugs are slow-acting. They do not act by inhibiting cyclooxygenase and have no analgesic or primary anti-inflammatory activity. These drugs are used primarily for rheumatic disorders, especially in cases where the inflammation does not respond to cyclooxygenase inhibitors. They slow the course of the disease and may also induce a remission, preventing further destruction of the joints and involved tissues.

A. Gold salts

Gold compounds, like the other drugs in this group, cannot repair existing damage. Rather, they can only prevent further injury. The currently available gold preparations are *gold sodium thiomalate, aurothioglucose,* and *auranofin.*

1. **Mechanism of action:** It is believed that gold salts are taken up by macrophages and suppress phagocytosis and lysosomal enzyme activity. This mechanism retards the progression of bone and articular destruction.

2. **Therapeutic uses:** The major use of gold salts is in the treatment of rheumatoid arthritis that does not respond to salicylates or other nonsteroidal anti-inflammatory therapy. They are the most effective agents for the rapidly progressive types of the disease, particularly if given in the early stages of the disease.

3. **Pharmacology**: *Gold sodium thiomalate* and *aurothioglucose* are water-soluble salts that are administered intramuscularly. *Auranofin,* the newest gold preparation, may be taken by mouth. If a favorable response is achieved without serious toxic reaction, the drug can be continued indefinitely.

4. **Adverse effects:**

   a. About one third of those patients receiving treatment with gold salts experience some adverse effects. The most common adverse effect is dermatitis of the skin or of the mucous membranes (especially in the mouth), which occurs in up to 20% of patients.

   b. Other possible adverse effects include proteinuria and nephrosis (5-8% of patients) and rare, severe blood disorders, such as agranulocytosis and aplastic anemia.

B. Chloroquine and hydroxychloroquine

The pharmacology of these drugs which are also used in the treatment of malaria, is presented on p.322. The mechanism of their anti-inflammatory activity is unclear. In treating inflammatory disorders, they are reserved for rheumatoid arthritis that has been unresponsive to the NSAIDs or else they are used in conjunction with an NSAID, allowing a lower dose of *chloroquine* [KLOR oh kwin] or *hydrochloroquine* to be administered. These drugs have been shown to slow progression of erosive bone lesions and may induce remission. They do cause serious adverse effects as described on pp.322 and 323.

C. D-Penicillamine

Penicillamine [pen i SILL a meen] is an analog of the amino acid cysteine. It slows the progress of bone destruction and rheumatoid arthritis; its mechanism of action is unknown. Prolonged treatment with *penicillamine* has serious side effects, which are not tolerated by many patients; therefore it is used primarily in the treatment of rheumatoid arthritis after use of gold salts has failed but before use of corticosteroids has been attempted. [Note: Penicillamine is also used as a chelating agent in the treatment of poisoning by heavy metals.]

D. Methotrexate

Methotrexate [meth oh TREX ate] was recently approved by the FDA for treatment of patients with severe rheumatoid arthritis who have not responded adequately to NSAIDs and at least one other slow-acting agent. Response to *methotrexate* occurs sooner than is usual for other slow-acting agents—often within 3 to 6 weeks of starting treatment. Doses of *methotrexate* required for this treatment are much lower than those needed in cancer chemotherapy; therefore the adverse effects (p.343) are minimized. The most common side effects observed after *methotrexate* treatment of rheumatoid arthritis are cytopenias (particularly depression of the white blood cell count), cirrhosis of the liver, and an acute pneumonialike syndrome.

VI. DRUGS EMPLOYED IN THE TREATMENT OF GOUT

Gout is a metabolic disorder characterized by high levels of uric acid in the blood. This hyperuricemia results in the deposition of crystals of sodium urate in the tissue, especially in the kidney and joints. Hyperuricemia does not always lead to gout, but gout is always preceded by hyperuricemia. In humans, sodium urate is the endproduct of purine metabolism.[4]

The deposition of urate crystals initiates an inflammatory process involving the infiltration of granulocytes which phagocytize the urate crystals. In addition, there is an increase in lactate production in the synovial tissues. The resulting local decrease in pH fosters further deposition of urate crystals. (See Figure 38.14 for a summary of this process.)

A. Treating acute gout

The cause of hyperuricemia is an overproduction of uric acid relative to the patient's ability to excrete it. Most therapeutic strategies for gout involve lowering the uric acid level below the saturation

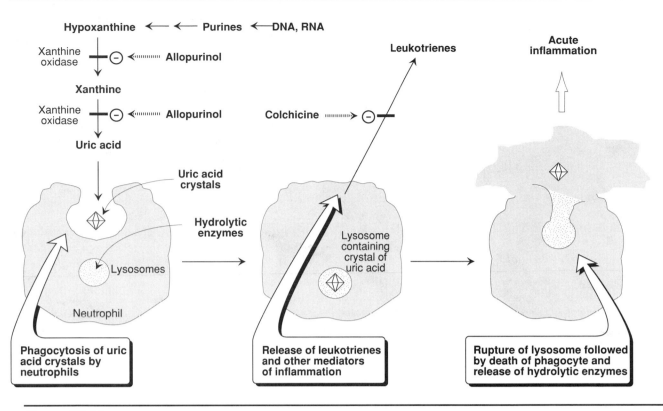

Figure 38.14
Role of uric acid in the inflammation of gout.

point, thus preventing the deposition of urate crystals. Acute gouty attacks can result from a number of conditions, including excessive alcohol consumption, a diet rich in purines, or kidney disease. Acute attacks are treated with *colchicine* to decrease movement of granulocytes into the affected area and with NSAIDs to decrease pain and inflammation. [Note: *Aspirin* is contraindicated, however, because it competes with uric acid for the organic acid secretion mechanism in the kidney proximal tubule.]

B. Treating chronic gout

Chronic gout can be caused by a genetic defect in the rate of purine synthesis or as a result of renal deficiency, Lesch-Nyhan Syndrome,[5] or excessive synthesis of uric acid associated with treatment of a malignancy. Treatment strategies for chronic gout include the use of uricosuric drugs that increase the excretion of uric acid, thereby reducing its concentration in plasma, and the use of *allopurinol,* which is a selective inhibitor of the terminal steps in the biosynthesis of uric acid.

C. Colchicine

Colchicine [KOL chi seen], a plant alkaloid, has a prophylactic, suppressive effect that helps to reduce the incidence of acute gouty attacks. It is not a uricosuric agent nor is it an analgesic, although it relieves pain in acute attacks of gout. *Colchicine* does not prevent

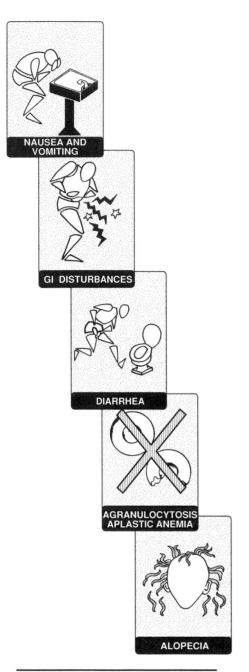

Figure 38.15
Some adverse effects of colchicine.

the progression of gout to acute gouty arthritis, but it does have a suppressive, prophylactic effect that reduces the number of acute attacks and relieves residual pain.

1. **Mechanism of action:** *Colchicine* binds to microtubular protein, causing its depolymerization. This inhibits cell functions, such as the mobility of granulocytes, thus decreasing their migration into the affected area. Furthermore, *colchicine* blocks cell division by binding to mitotic spindles. *Colchicine* also inhibits the lipoxygenase pathway, thus decreasing the synthesis of the leukotrienes.

2. **Therapeutic uses:** *Colchicine* is prophylactically effective in the treatment of acute attacks of gout, usually alleviating pain of gout within 12 hours. The anti-inflammatory activity of *colchicine* is specific for gout. It is only rarely effective in other kinds of arthritis.

3. **Pharmacology:** *Colchicine* is administered either orally, followed by rapid absorption from the GI tract, or IV, which circumvents adverse effects on the GI tract. The drug is recycled in the bile and is excreted unchanged by the liver or kidney.

4. **Adverse effects:** *Colchicine* treatment may cause nausea, vomiting, abdominal pain, and diarrhea (Figure 38.15). Chronic administration may lead to myopathy, agranulocytosis, aplastic anemia, and alopecia.

D. Allopurinol

1. **Mechanism of action:** *Allopurinol* [al oh PURE i nole] is a purine analog. It reduces the production of uric acid by competitively inhibiting the last two steps in uric acid biosynthesis, which are catalyzed by xanthine oxidase. [Note: Uric acid is less water-soluble than its precursors. Therefore, if xanthine oxidase is inhibited, the circulating purine derivatives become more soluble and therefore are less likely to precipitate].[6]

2. **Therapeutic uses:** *Allopurinol* is effective in the treatment of primary hyperuricemia of gout and hyperuricemia secondary to other conditions, including hyperuricemia associated with certain malignancies (those in which large amounts of purines are produced) or renal disease.

3. **Pharmacology:**

   a. **Administration:** *Allopurinol* is completely absorbed after oral administration. The primary metabolite is alloxanthine (oxypurinol) which is also a xanthine oxidase inhibitor. The pharmacological effect of administered *allopurinol* results from the combined activity of these two compounds.

   b. **Metabolism:** The plasma half-life of *allopurinol* is short (2 hours), whereas the half-life of oxypurinol is long (15 hours). Thus, effective inhibition of xanthine oxidase can be maintained with once daily dosage.

5. **Adverse effects:** *Allopurinol* is well tolerated by most patients.

  a. Hypersensitivity reactions are the most common adverse reaction, occurring among approximately 3% of patients. The reactions may occur even after months or years of chronic administration.

  b. Acute attacks of gout may occur more frequently during the first several weeks of therapy; therefore *colchicine* and NSAIDs should be administered concurrently.

  c. *Allopurinol* may interfere with the metabolism of anti-cancer agents, such as *6-thioguanine* and *6-mercaptopurine* (p.344).

E. Uricosuric agents: probenecid and sulfinpyrazone

Probenecid [proe BEN e sid], a general inhibitor of the tubular secretion of organic acids, and *sulfinpyrazone* [sul fin PEER a zone], a derivative of *phenylbutazone* (p.368), are the two most commonly used uricosuric agents. At therapeutic doses, they block proximal tubular resorption of uric acid. [Note: At low dosage, these agents block proximal tubular secretion of uric acid.] These drugs have few adverse effects. Probenecid blocks the tubular secretion of penicillin and is sometimes used to increase levels of the antibiotic.

Study Questions   (see p.437 for answers).

Choose the ONE best answer.

38.1 In which of the following conditions would aspirin be contraindicated?

  A. Myalgia.
  B. Fever.
  C. Peptic ulcer.
  D. Rheumatoid arthritis.
  E. Unstable angina.

38.2 Overdoses of salicylates lead to all of the following EXCEPT:

  A. Nausea and vomiting.
  B. Tinnitus (ringing or roaring in the ears).
  C. Marked hyperventilation.
  D. Increased metabolic rate.
  E. Increase in blood pH.

38.3 Acetaminophen has all of the following properties EXCEPT:

  A. It is a weaker anti-inflammatory agent than aspirin.
  B. It reduces fever of viral infections in children.
  C. It is an aspirin substitute in patients with peptic ulcer.
  D. It exacerbates gout.
  E. It causes hepatotoxic effects at high doses.

38.4 Which of the following statements concerning gold salts is correct?

  A. They may provide immediate relief of arthritic pain.
  B. They act by inhibiting prostaglandin synthesis.
  C. They frequently cause dermatitis of the skin or mucous membranes.
  D. They are drugs of first choice in treating arthritis.
  E. They must all be given intramuscularly.

Answer A if 1,2 and 3 are correct.
    B if 1 and 3 are correct.
    C if 2 and 4 are correct.
    D if only 4 is correct.
    E if 1,2,3 and 4 are all correct.

38.5 Which of the following are correctly paired?

1. Indomethacin: Causes frontal headaches
2. Sulindac: Long half-life permits daily or twice daily dosing
3. Naproxen: Better tolerated than aspirin in some patients
4. Phenylbutazone: Less toxic than aspirin

38.6 Colchicine:

1. is used prophylactically to reduce the number of acute gouty attacks.
2. can cause serious GI problems.
3. inhibits microtubule function.
4. has general use as an anti-inflammatory drug.

38.7 Allopurinol:

1. decreases uric acid in the blood.
2. increases excretion of uric acid.
3. produces increased excretion of xanthine.
4. is a toxic compound with a high frequency of adverse effects.

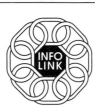

[1]See *prostaglandin synthesis* in **Biochemistry** for a more detailed discussion of the cyclooxygenase and lipoxygenase pathways (see index).

[2]See *prostaglandins, biological actions* in **Biochemistry** for a summary of the bewildering range of physiological responses elicited by these potent chemicals.

[3]See *oxidative phosphorylation* in **Biochemistry** for a summary of this pathway.

[4]See *purines, degradation* in **Biochemistry** for a summary of this pathway.

[5]See *gout* in **Biochemistry** for a description of this disease.

[6]See *uric acid* in **Biochemistry** for a description of the biosynthesis of this compound.

Autacoids and Autacoid Antagonists

39

I. OVERVIEW

The word autacoid comes from the Greek: autos (self) and akos (medicinal agent, or remedy). The autacoids are a variety of substances of widely differing structures and pharmacological activities. They all have the common feature of being formed by the tissues on which they act; thus, they function as local hormones. The autacoids also differ from circulating hormones in that they are produced by many tissues rather than in specific endocrine glands. The drugs described in this chapter (Figure 39.1) are either autacoids (both naturally occurring and synthetic analogs) or autacoid antagonists (i.e., compounds that inhibit the synthesis of certain autacoids or interfere with their interactions with receptors).

II. PROSTAGLANDINS

Prostaglandins are unsaturated fatty acid derivatives that act on the tissues in which they are synthesized and are rapidly metabolized to inactive products at the site of action. The biosynthesis and actions of the prostaglandins are presented on p. 361.

A. Compounds that affect the synthesis of prostaglandins

1. **Nonsteroidal anti-inflammatory drugs (NSAIDs):** Many drugs exert their therapeutic effects by inhibiting the endogenous synthesis of prostaglandins or thromboxanes (see Figure 38.3, p.363).

2. **Corticosteroids:** Corticosteroids cause inhibition of the action of the phospholipases that release arachidonic acid from tissue phospholipids. This inhibition limits the availability of arachidonic acid and all subsequent products, thereby reducing inflammation.

3. **Vasoactive compounds:** Vasoactive compounds, such as bradykinin and angiotensin II, activate the release of arachidonic acid, resulting in increased synthesis of the prostaglandins and related compounds.

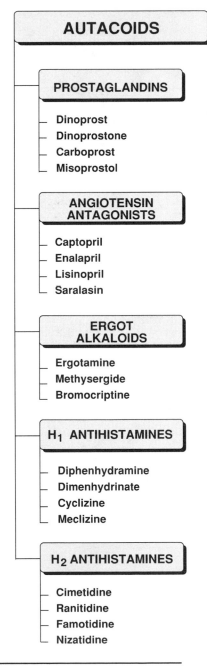

AUTACOIDS

PROSTAGLANDINS
- Dinoprost
- Dinoprostone
- Carboprost
- Misoprostol

ANGIOTENSIN ANTAGONISTS
- Captopril
- Enalapril
- Lisinopril
- Saralasin

ERGOT ALKALOIDS
- Ergotamine
- Methysergide
- Bromocriptine

H$_1$ ANTIHISTAMINES
- Diphenhydramine
- Dimenhydrinate
- Cyclizine
- Meclizine

H$_2$ ANTIHISTAMINES
- Cimetidine
- Ranitidine
- Famotidine
- Nizatidine

Figure 39.1
Summary of drugs affecting the autacoids.

Dinoprost, dinoprostone, carboprost

● Act directly on myometrium to induce contractions and labor

● Administration is by intraamnionic or intravaginal instillation from the 12th week through the second trimester of pregnancy

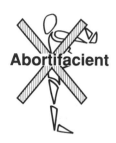

Abortifacient

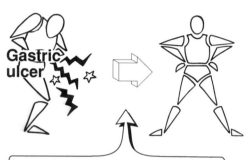

Gastric ulcer

Misoprostol

● Inhibits secretion of HCl and pepsin and enhances mucosal resistance

● Useful in patients with gastric ulcer who chronically take aspirin

Figure 39.2
Therapeutic applications of prostaglandin derivatives.

B. Prostaglandins as drugs

Systemic administration of prostaglandins evokes a bewildering array of effects, a fact that limits the therapeutic usefulness of these agents. However, several of the naturally occurring prostaglandins, such as *dinoprost* [DYE noe prost], *dinoprostone* [dye noe PROST one], and *carboprost* [KAR boe prost], find use as abortifacients (i.e., agents causing abortions, Figure 39.2). *Misoprostol* [MIZ o prost ol] is a recently approved, synthetic prostaglandin E_1 analog used to inhibit the secretion of hydrochloric acid in the stomach. It produces inhibition of gastric acid and pepsin secretion and enhances mucosal resistance to injury. *Misoprostol* is particularly useful in patients with gastric ulcer who are chronically taking nonsteroidal anti-inflammatory agents (see p.224 for a more complete discussion of this drug).

III. ANGIOTENSINS

The angiotensins are a group of peptides of known structure that have several pharmacological actions. They are best known for their vasoconstrictor activity, which leads to an elevation of blood pressure. Pharmacological agents that inhibit the synthesis of certain angiotensins or compete with the binding of angiotensins to appropriate receptor sites are useful in the treatment of hypertension (p.175). Angiotensin itself has no approved therapeutic applications.

A. Synthesis and degradation of the angiotensins

1. **Renin release:** The angiotensins are derived from angiotensinogen, a plasma α_2 globulin, originating primarily in the liver (Figure 39.3). Baroreceptors in the kidney, acting in response to reduced arterial pressure (or to a reduction in the sodium supply in the renal distal tubule), release the enzyme renin. This peptidase converts angiotensinogen to angiotensin I, a 10-amino acid peptide with limited intrinsic pharmacological activity. The rate of renin secretion is controlled by a variety of factors, including the sympathetic nervous system. Therefore, a number of drugs that interfere with the sympathetic nervous system, such as *propranolol* (p.74) and *clonidine* (p.182), inhibit the secretion of renin.

2. **Angiotensin converting enzyme:** Angiotensin I is converted to angiotensin II in the presence of angiotensin converting enzyme (ACE), also known as peptidyl dipeptidase (Figure 39.3). Angiotensin II, an octapeptide, is the most active of the angiotensins and is the body's most potent circulating vasoconstrictor and stimulator of aldosterone secretion. ACE is localized in the endothelium of the blood vessels of the lungs, kidneys, and other organs. [Note: ACE also converts bradykinin and other kinins to inactive fragments (p.384).]

3. **Inactivation of angiotensin II:** Angiotensin II is enzymatically converted to angiotensin III, which is rapidly destroyed by being converted into inactive peptide fragments.

B. Actions of the angiotensins

Angiotensin II receptors are located on the plasma membrane of target cells in a variety of tissues. The wide range of physiological responses to angiotensin II are thus determined by the tissue type to which it binds.

1. **Vasoconstriction:** Angiotensin is a vasoconstrictor that is 40 times more potent than norepinephrine. It causes direct contraction of vascular smooth muscle, especially that of the arterioles (Figure 39.3).

2. **Increased release of aldosterone:** Angiotensin stimulates the synthesis and secretion of aldosterone by the zona glomerulosa of the adrenal cortex. Aldosterone in turn promotes sodium and water retention and potassium wasting. Thus, activation of the renin-angiotensin-aldosterone system leads to increased peripheral vascular resistance and intravascular volume (Figure 39.3).

3. **Activation of sympathetic nervous system:** Angiotensins have several other activities (such as, positive inotropic and chronotropic effects on the heart, an increased release of catecholamine, an increased secretion of antidiuretic hormone, and increased thirst), which complement actions on the vascular system and contribute to an elevation in blood pressure (Figure 39.3).

IV. ANGIOTENSIN ANTAGONISTS

Two types of agents modify angiotensin levels and activity. The first group inhibits the activity of ACE. Three currently available ACE inhibitors are *captopril, enalapril,* and *lisinopril.* The second group, angiotensin analogs, blocks angiotensin receptors.

A. Captopril

1. **Mechanism of action:** *Captopril* [KAP toe pril] inhibits the action of ACE and, therefore, decreases the conversion of inactive angiotensin I to the potent angiotensin II. The drug also diminishes the rate of bradykinin inactivation (see Figure 39.5). Thus, vasodilation occurs as a result of the combined effects of diminished levels of angiotensin II, which lowers vasoconstriction, and increased levels of bradykinin, which promote the vasodilatory effect.

2. **Actions:**

   a. **Decreased blood pressure:** *Captopril* lowers peripheral vascular resistance by vasodilation, indirectly causing a decrease in blood pressure (p.181).

   b. **Decreased aldosterone levels:** The drug decreases circulating levels of aldosterone, causing decreased retention of sodium and fluid and increased retention of potassium.

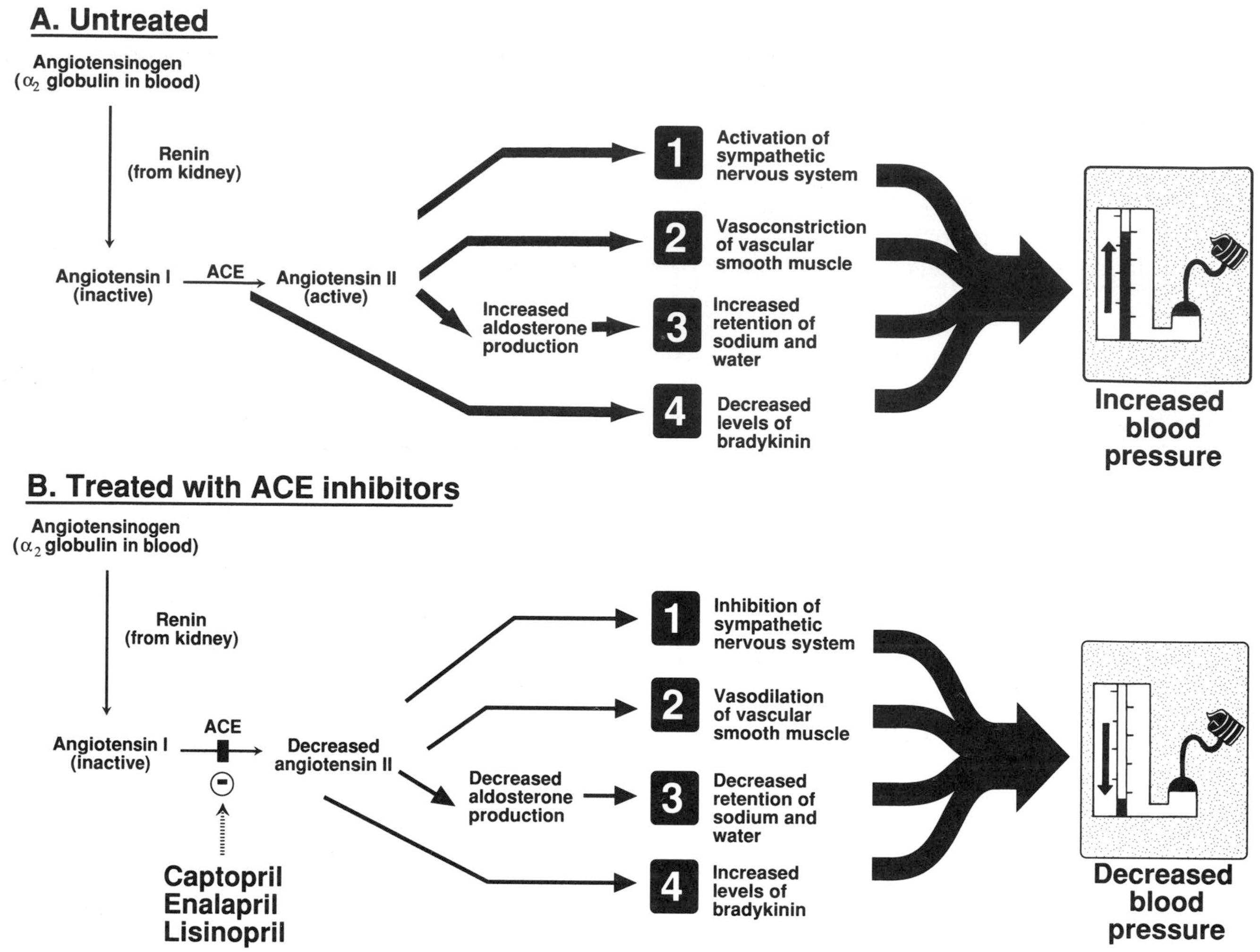

A. Untreated

B. Treated with ACE inhibitors

Figure 39.3
A. Effects of angiotensin converting enzyme (ACE); B. Effects of ACE inhibitors.

c. **Increased bradykinin:** *Captopril* increases levels of circulating bradykinin, causing vasodilation and elevated plasma concentrations of prostaglandins. (See p.363 for the action of bradykinin on prostaglandin synthesis.)

d. **Increased cardiac performance:** As a result of the changes just described, stroke and cardiac output are improved.

3. **Therapeutic uses:**

a. **Mild-to-moderate hypertension:** *Captopril* produces a significant reduction of hypertension regardless of the degree or cause of the disorder. *Captopril* is more useful in treating hypertension than are the angiotensin analogs (see later), since *captopril* does not result in agonist activity. (See p.175 for a more complete discussion of hypertension.)

b. **Refractory hypertension:** *Captopril* treatment is effective in approximately one half of patients with chronic hypertension. The remaining 50% of patients require additional antihypertensive agents, most often a diuretic or a β blocker (p.179). Chronic use of *captopril* does not alter sympathetic reflex activity (often the cause of sedation, lethargy, orthostatic hypotension, and impotence).

c. **Congestive heart failure:** Vasodilators provide an important advance beyond the benefits obtained with *digitalis* (p.155) and diuretics (p.211). *Captopril* is the vasodilator of choice for patients with congestive heart failure.

4. **Pharmacology:** *Captopril* is administered orally two or three times daily and is well absorbed, although absorption is reduced by food. *Captopril* undergoes some hepatic metabolism, and both the unchanged drug and its metabolites are excreted in the urine. The dosage should be reduced for patients with impaired renal function.

5. **Adverse effects:** *Captopril* is generally well tolerated. Reported side effects include dizziness, light-headedness, and fainting (because of an excessive drop in blood pressure). Less commonly observed side effects are rashes, fever, arthralgia (a severe, non-inflammatory pain in a joint), leukopenia, and proteinuria.

B. Enalapril

Enalapril [e NAL a pril], like *captopril,* is an ACE inhibitor. *Enalapril* is a pro-drug that must be converted by the liver to *enalaprilat,* which is 10-20 times more potent than *captopril* and has a longer duration of action. Its effects are similar to that of *captopril,* except that *enalapril* does not produce significant increases in bradykinin or prostaglandin levels and shows fewer adverse effects. *Enalapril* has recently been shown to increase the survival of patients with congestive heart failure.

C. Lisinopril

Structurally, *lisinopril* [lye SIN oh pril] differs from *captopril* in that it does not contain a sulfhydryl group, and it differs from *enalapril* in that it is not an ester pro-drug and thus does not require bioactivation by the liver. *Lisinopril* has a long duration of action, which allows it to be used as a single daily dose in the treatment of hypertension. *Lisinopril* is well tolerated in a manner similar to *captopril*. *Lisinopril* appears to be comparable to *captopril* for the treatment of congestive heart failure. Adverse effects associated with *lisinopril* are relatively minor and are comparable to those associated with *enalapril*. Figure 39.4 compares the three ACE inhibitors.

D. Saralasin

Saralasin [sar AL a sin], an angiotensin receptor blocker, is an angiotensin II analog in which phenylalanine is replaced by sarco-

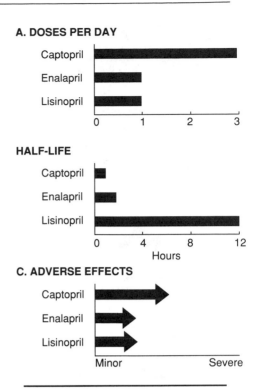

Figure 39.4
A comparison of angiotensin converting enzyme (ACE) inhibitors.

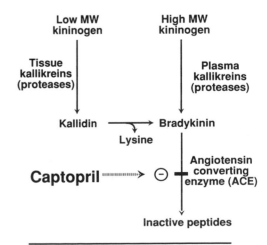

Figure 39.5
Biosynthesis and degradation of bradykinin. MW= molecular weight.

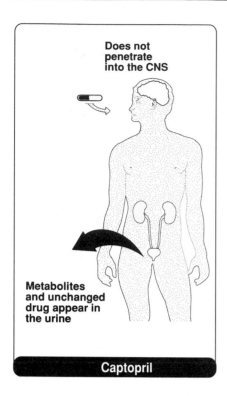

Does not penetrate into the CNS

Metabolites and unchanged drug appear in the urine

Captopril

sine. The drug is both an angiotensin antagonist and a weak agonist. In the presence of high blood levels of angiotensin II, *saralasin* functions as a competitive antagonist by blocking tissue receptors; thus it also lowers arterial blood pressure. However, at low angiotensin II levels, *saralasin* acts as an agonist, increasing blood pressure. *Saralasin* is used as an aid in the diagnosis of angiotensin II-dependent hypertension.

V. THE KININS: BRADYKININ AND KALLIDIN

The kinins are a large group of polypeptides that have vasodilator and hypotensive actions. The two best known kinins are bradykinin and kallidin.

A. Synthesis and degradation of the kinins

1. Bradykinin is a nonapeptide found in plasma formed from a class of α-2 globulins known as kininogens (Figure 39.5).

2. Bradykinin is inactivated by a group of enzymes known as kininases. The major catabolizing enzyme is kininase II, which is identical to peptidyl dipeptidase (ACE, p.380). Kininase II (ACE) is inhibited by *captopril,* resulting in increased concentrations of circulating bradykinin, which is a potent vasodilator. This may contribute to the antihypertensive effect of *captopril* (see Figure 39.3).

B. Pharmacological actions of the kinins

1. **Vasodilation and vasoconstriction:**

   a. Kinins are among the most potent vasodilators of all the autacoids, acting on arteriolar beds of the heart, liver, skeletal muscle, kidney, intestines, and ovaries (Figure 39.5). This activity may be mediated by release of vasodilator prostaglandins (Figure 38.3, p.363).

   b. In contrast, the kinins cause veins to *contract.* They also cause contraction in nonvascular smooth muscle, such as gastrointestinal and bronchiolar muscle, and in most visceral smooth muscle. [Note: Bradykinin and kallidin have similar pharmacological properties.]

2. **Increased vascular permeability:** The kinins cause increased vascular permeability and edema, which are characteristic of late stage inflammation (p.363).

3. **Pain:** The kinins are potent pain-inducing agents in both the viscera and skin.

VI. SEROTONIN AND ITS ANTAGONISTS

Serotonin (5-hydroxytryptamine, 5-HT) is an autacoid with a wide variety of pharmacological actions. Approximately 90% of the serotonin in the body is located in the enterochromaffin cells of the gastrointestinal tract. Most of the remaining serotonin is present in platelets and in the central nervous system (primarily the hypothalamus and the basal ganglia), where it is found in high concentrations.

A. Effects of endogenous serotonin

1. **Chemical mediator:** Serotonin acts as a chemical neurotransmitter (p.31). It has been implicated in many functions, such as pain perception; normal and abnormal behaviors, including affective disorders (p.122); and regulation of food intake, sleep, temperature, blood pressure, and neuroendocrine functions. The actions of serotonin are mediated by receptors located on the cell surface of target tissues. These receptors are different from those that bind histamine, acetylcholine, or the catecholamines.

2. **Regulation of pituitary gland:** Serotonin participates in the regulation of pituitary secretions. It stimulates the release of adrenocorticotropic hormone (ACTH), growth hormone, and prolactin, and it inhibits the release of luteinizing hormone (LH), follicle stimulating hormone (FSH), and thyroid stimulating hormone (TSH).

3. **Serotonin and migraine headaches:** Although the cause of migraine headaches is unknown, serotonin appears to be involved in their pathology. Normally, when platelets aggregate, they release serotonin from intracellular storage granules. Platelets from individuals with migraine headaches release their serotonin more readily than those of normal persons. Serotonin is a constrictor of arteries and may thus contribute to decreased cerebral blood flow during an episode of migraine headache. In addition, serotonin increases the sensitivity of pain receptors and increases vessel permeability, allowing pain-producing kinins to escape into the tissues surrounding the cerebral vessels. Figure 39.6 shows the drugs used to treat migraine headaches.

4. **Effects on vasculature:** Serotonin constricts most arteries and veins but dilates vessels in skeletal muscle.

B. Drugs that affect serotonin levels

Serotonin itself has no clinical applications as a drug. However, several substances can influence the endogenous levels of serotonin in the tissues.

1. **Tryptophan:** Exogenously administered tryptophan can increase serotonin levels in those tissues where it is synthesized. Tryptophan hydroxylase, the rate-limiting enzyme in the synthesis of serotonin (Figure 39.7), is generally not saturated with its substrate. Administration of additional tryptophan can, therefore increase the rate of serotonin synthesis.

2. **Inhibitors of membrane uptake:** Tricyclic antidepressants, such as *imipramine* (p.119), inhibit the receptor-mediated uptake of serotonin by the neurons, thus allowing higher levels of serotonin to

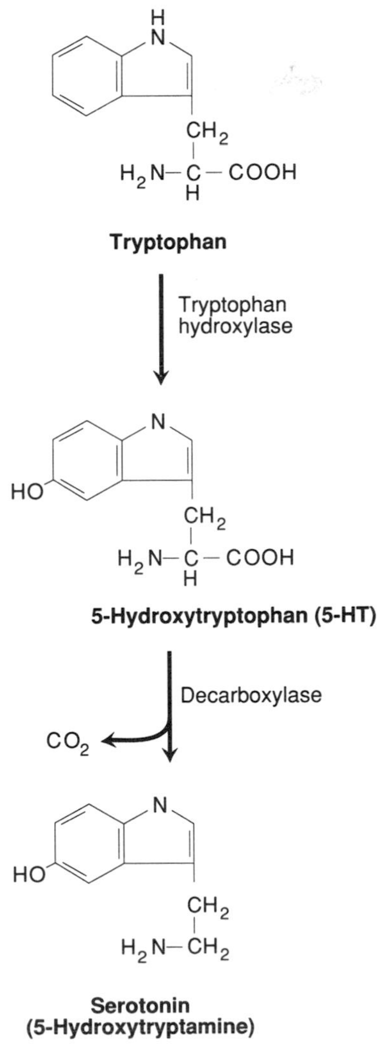

Tryptophan

Tryptophan hydroxylase

5-Hydroxytryptophan (5-HT)

Decarboxylase

CO_2

Serotonin (5-Hydroxytryptamine)

Figure 39.7
Biosynthesis of serotonin.

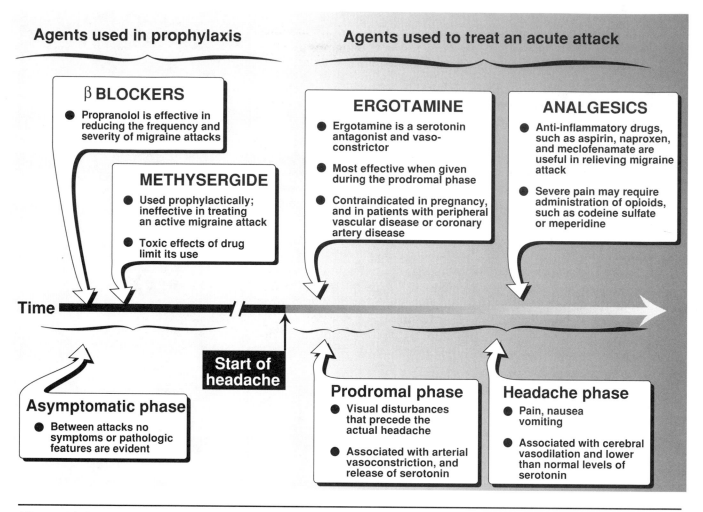

Figure 39.6
Drugs useful in the treatment and prophylaxis of migraine headaches.

remain in the synapse. Other, more potent, antidepressant drugs, such as *fluoxetine* (p.122) also act in this way.

3. **Inhibitors of serotonin degradation:** The monoamine oxidase inhibitors (MAO, p.123) are the most important group of drugs that inhibit serotonin degradation. Their use results in elevated levels of serotonin at the synapse.

4. **Inhibitors of neuron vesicle uptake and storage of serotonin:** *Reserpine* and *tetrabenazine* deplete stores of serotonin in neurons. Their use may precipitate a depressive episode (p.79).

5. **Cyproheptadine:** This drug blocks H_1-histamine receptors and serotonin receptors (p.390). It is used to treat pruritus dermatosis (itches) and smooth muscle manifestation of carcinoid tumor (a tumor that synthesizes excessive quantities of serotonin).

VII. ERGOT ALKALOIDS

Ergot alkaloids are a chemically complex group of compounds synthesized by a fungus that infects grains under damp growing conditions. The most useful therapeutic agents in this group are *ergotamine* [er GOT a meen] and the ergot derivatives, *methysergide* [meth i SER jide] and *bromocriptine* [broh moh KRIP teen].

A. Mechanism of action:

The ergot alkaloids show a complex pattern of vascular actions, including agonistic as well as antagonistic effects at α receptors and agonistic activity at dopamine and serotonin receptors.

B. Actions

1. **Central nervous system (CNS):** Ergot alkaloids cause hallucinations at high doses.

2. **Vascular smooth muscle:** Ergot derivatives cause prolonged vasospasm, which may result in severe ischemia and gangrene.

3. **Uterine smooth muscle:** Ergot alkaloids stimulate uterine muscle, which may result in abortion in pregnant women.

C. Therapeutic uses

1. **Migraine:** *Ergotamine* causes vasoconstriction, which diminishes the pulsation of the cerebral vasculature (see Figure 39.6). The drug is most effective when administered during the early phase of an attack.

2. **Hyperprolactinemia:** *Bromocriptine mesylate* is effective in reducing the elevated levels of circulating prolactin that accompany pituitary tumors.

3. **Postpartum hemorrhage:** Ergot alkaloids are used only for control of uterine bleeding after delivery. These drugs should never be given before delivery.

D. Pharmacology:

The gastrointestinal absorption of the ergot alkaloids is variable, but it can be increased by caffeine (that is, coffee increases effectiveness of ergot alkaloids).

E. Adverse effects:

The most common side effects are diarrhea, nausea, and vomiting. More serious complications can arise from prolonged vasospasm and gangrene. Hallucinations occur at high doses. *Nitroprusside,* a powerful direct-acting vasodilator (p.183), is used to treat vasoconstriction characteristic of toxic overdosage with *ergotamine.*

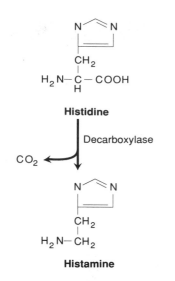

Figure 39.8
Biosynthesis of histamine.

VIII. OVERVIEW OF HISTAMINE

Histamine is a chemical messenger that mediates a wide range of cellular responses, including allergic and inflammatory reactions, gastric acid secretion, and possibly neurotransmission in parts of the brain. Histamine has no clinical applications, but agents that interfere with the action of histamine have important therapeutic applications.

A. Location, synthesis, and release of histamine

1. **Location:** Histamine occurs in practically all tissues, but it is unevenly distributed, with high amounts found in lung, skin, and the gastrointestinal (GI) tract (sites where the "inside" of the body meets the "outside"). It is found in high concentration in mast cells or basophils. Histamine also occurs as a component of venoms and in secretions from insect stings.

2. **Synthesis:** Histamine is an amine formed by the decarboxylation of the amino acid histidine (Figure 39.8). This process occurs primarily in the mast cells, basophils, and in the lungs, skin, and gastrointestinal mucosa—the same tissues in which histamine is stored. In mast cells, histamine is stored in granules as an inactive complex composed of histamine and the polysulfated anion, heparin, along with an anionic protein. If histamine is not stored, it is rapidly inactivated by MAO.

3. **Release of histamine:** The release of histamine may be the primary response to some stimuli, but most often, histamine is just one of several chemical mediators released. Stimuli causing the release of histamine from tissues include the following:

   a. The destruction of cells as a result of cold, bacterial toxins, bee sting venoms, trauma, and so forth.

   b. The dissolution of cytoplasmic granules as a result of the action of radiation or surfactants.

   c. The action of histamine liberators, which include foreign proteins, drugs (such as *curare* and *morphine*), dextran, or radiograph contrast media.

   d. Allergy and anaphylaxis.

B. Mechanism of action of histamine

Histamine released in response to the stimuli just described exerts its effects by binding to two types of receptors, designated H_1 and H_2, located on the surfaces of cells. These receptors mediate a variety of responses. For example, the H_1 receptors are important in producing smooth muscle contraction and increasing capillary permeability, whereas the H_2 receptors mediate gastric acid secretion. The two histamine receptors exert their pharmacological effects by different second messenger pathways; binding of an agonist to the H_1 receptor stimulates the intracellular activity of the polyphosphatidylinositol cycle (p.33), whereas stimulation of H_2 re-

H₁-Receptors

EXOCRINE EXCRETION

Increased production of nasal and bronchial mucus, resulting in respiratory symptoms.

BRONCHIAL SMOOTH MUSCLE

Constriction of bronchioles results in symptoms of asthma, decreased lung capacity.

INTESTINAL SMOOTH MUSCLE

Constriction results in intestinal cramps and diarrhea

SENSORY NERVE ENDINGS

Acts as local anesthetic resulting in decreased pain and itch

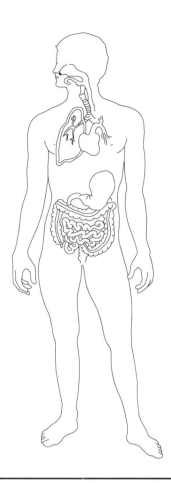

H₁- and H₂-Receptors

CARDIOVASCULAR SYSTEM

Lowers systemic blood pressure by reducing peripheral resistance, Causes positive chronotropism (mediated by H_2 receptors) and a positive inotropism (mediated by both H_1 and H_2 receptors).

SKIN

Dilation and increased permeability of the capillaries results in leakage of proteins and fluid into the tissues. In the skin this results in the classical "triple response" - wheal formation, reddening due to local vasodilation, and flare ("halo").

H₂-Receptors

Stomach

Stimulation of gastric hydrochloric acid secretion.

Figure 39.9
Actions of histamine.

ceptors enhances the production of cAMP by adenylate cyclase (p.33).

C. Actions of histamine

Histamine has a wide range of pharmacological effects (Figure 39.9). Some of these actions are mediated by both H_1 and H_2 receptors. Others are mediated by only one class of receptors.

D. Role of histamine in allergy and anaphylaxis

1. There is a similarity between the symptoms resulting from intravenous (IV) injection of histamine and those associated with anaphylactic shock and allergic reactions. These include contraction of smooth muscle, stimulation of secretions, dilation and increased permeability of the capillaries, and stimulation of sensory nerve endings.

2. Symptoms associated with allergy and anaphylactic shock result from the release of certain mediators from their storage sites. Such mediators include histamine, serotonin (p.384), leukotrienes (p.363), and the eosinophil chemotactic factor of anaphy-

laxis. In some cases, these cause a localized allergic reaction, producing, for example, actions on the skin or respiratory tract. Under other conditions, these mediators may cause a full-blown anaphylactic response. It is thought that the difference between these two situations results from differences in the sites from which mediators are released and their rates of release. If the release of histamine is slow enough to permit its inactivation before it enters the blood stream, a local allergic reaction results. However, if histamine release is too fast for inactivation to be efficient, a full-blown anaphylactic reaction occurs. (See p.207 for a more complete discussion of allergic reactions.)

IX. BLOCKERS OF HISTAMINE H₁ RECEPTORS

A. Mechanism of action

1. The term "antihistamine," without a modifying adjective, refers to the classic H₁ receptor blockers. These compounds do not influence the formation or release of histamine, but rather they block the receptor-mediated response of a target tissue. [Note: This contrasts with the action of *cromolyn* (p.208), which inhibits

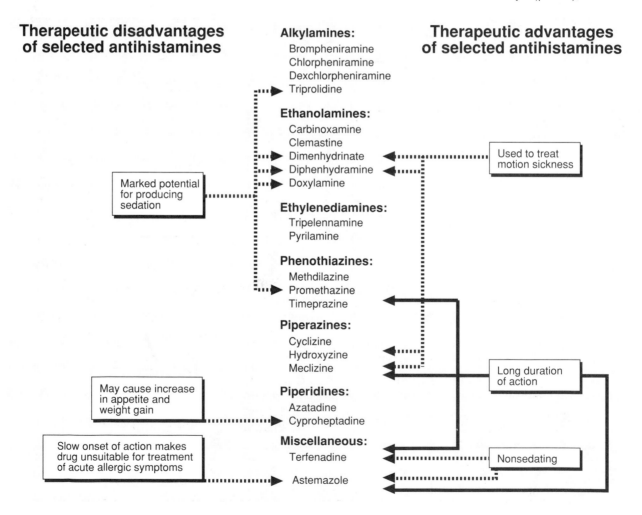

Figure 39.10
Summary of therapeutic advantages and disadvantages of the H₁-histamine receptor blocking agents.

the release of histamine from mast cells and is useful in the treatment of asthma.]

2. The H_1 receptor blockers are classified according to their chemical structures (Figure 39.10). The similarities between the structure of histamine and these antihistamines are sufficient for these compounds to compete for histamine at receptor sites on target cells. However, the differences between the structures do not permit H_1 receptor blockers to serve as histamine agonists.

3. The histamine receptors are distinct from those that bind serotonin, acetylcholine, and the catecholamines.

B. Actions

1. H_1 antihistamines antagonize all actions of histamine except for those mediated solely by H_2 receptors. The action of all of the H_1-receptor blockers is qualitatively similar. However, most of these blockers have additional effects unrelated to their blocking of H_1 receptors; these effects probably reflect binding of the H_1 antagonists to cholinergic, adrenergic, or serotonin receptors (Figure 39.11).

2. The pharmacological effects of H_1-receptor blockers are numerous. They provide almost complete protection against the symptoms produced by injected histamine.

C. Therapeutic uses

1. **Allergic conditions:** Antihistamines are the drugs of choice in controlling the symptoms of allergic rhinitis and urticaria because histamine is the principal mediator. However, the H_1-receptor blockers are ineffective in treating bronchial asthma (p.207), be-

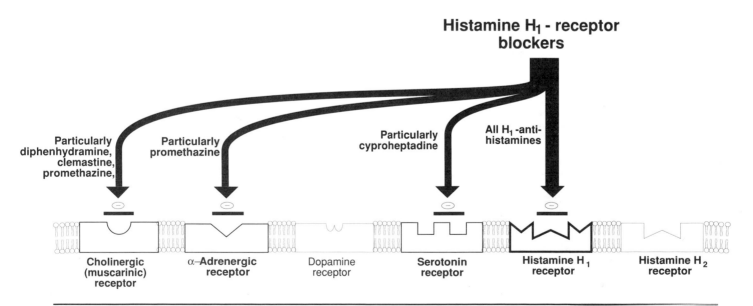

Figure 39.11
H_1-antihistamines block at histamine receptors as well as at adrenergic, cholinergic, and serotonin-binding receptors.

cause histamine is only one of several mediators. [Note: *Epinephrine* has actions on smooth muscle that are opposite to those of histamine and it acts at different receptors. Therefore, *epinephrine* is the drug of choice in treating systemic anaphylaxis and other conditions that involve massive release of histamine.]

2. **Motion sickness and nausea:** Along with the antimuscarinic agent *scopolamine* (p.48), certain H_1-receptor blockers, such as *diphenhydramine* [dye fen HYE dra meen], *dimenhydrinate* [dye men HYE dri nate], *cyclizine* [SYE kli zeen],and *meclizine* [MEK li zeen] (Figure 39.10), are the most effective agents for the prevention of the symptoms of motion sickness. The antihistamines prevent or diminish vomiting and nausea mediated by both the chemoreceptor and vestibular pathways. The antiemetic action of these substances seems to be independent of their antihistaminic and other actions. Other antiemetic agents are summarized in Figure 13.4.

3. **Somnifacients:** Some of the antihistamines, such as *diphenhydramine,* have strong sedative properties and are used in the treatment of insomnia (p.99).

D. Pharmacology

1. **Administration:** H_1-receptor blockers are well absorbed after oral administration, with maximum serum levels occurring at 1-2 hours. The average plasma half-life is 4-6 hours, except for *meclizine,* which has a half-life of 12-24 hours.

2. **Distribution:** H_1-receptor blockers have high bioavailability; they are distributed in all tissues, including the CNS.

3. **Metabolism:** The major site of biotransformation is the liver. Minute amounts of unchanged drug and most of the metabolites are excreted in the urine.

E. Adverse effects

H_1 receptor blockers have a low specificity, that is, they interact not only with histamine receptors but also with muscarinic cholinergic receptors, α-adrenergic receptors, and serotonin receptors (Figure 39.11). The extent of interaction with these receptors and, as a result, the nature of the side effects vary with the structure of the drug. Some side effects may be undesirable, and others may have therapeutic value. Furthermore, the incidence and severity of adverse reactions varies between individual subjects.

1. **Sedation:** The most frequently observed adverse reaction is sedation. Other central actions include tinnitus, fatigue, dizziness, lassitude, incoordination, blurred vision, and tremors.

2. **Dry mouth:** Oral antihistamines also exert a weak anticholinergic effects, leading not only to a drying of the nasal passage but also to a tendency to dry the oral cavity.

3. **Drug interactions:** Interaction of H_1-receptor blockers with other drugs can cause serious consequences, such as the potentiation of the effects of all other CNS depressants, including alcohol. Persons taking MAO inhibitors (p.123) should not take antihistamines, since the MAO inhibitors can exacerbate the anticholinergic effects of the antihistamines.

4. **Overdoses:** Although the margin of safety of H_1-receptor blockers is relatively high and chronic toxicity is rare, acute poisoning is relatively common, especially in young children. The most common and dangerous effects of acute poisoning are those on the CNS, including hallucinations, excitement, ataxia, and convulsions. If untreated, the patient may experience a deepening coma and collapse of the cardiorespiratory system.

X. BLOCKERS OF HISTAMINE H₂ RECEPTORS

Histamine H_2-receptor blockers have little if any affinity for H_1 receptors. Three H_2-receptor blockers available in the United States are *cimetidine, ranitidine,* and *famotidine.*

A. Cimetidine

1. **Actions:**

   a. *Cimetidine* [sye MET i deen] acts on H_2 receptors in the stomach, blood vessels, and other sites. It is a competitive antagonist of histamine and is fully reversible.

   b. *Cimetidine* completely inhibits gastric acid secretion induced by histamine, gastrin, or pentagastrin. However, it only partially inhibits gastric acid secretion induced by acetylcholine or *bethanechol* (p.40).

2. **Therapeutic uses:**

   a. *Cimetidine* is used in the treatment of those conditions that require the reduction of gastric acid secretion. These include duodenal ulcer, nonmalignant gastric ulcer, gastroesophageal reflux disease, pathological hypersecretion states associated with Zollinger-Ellison syndrome, systemic mastocytosis, and multiple endocrine adenomas.

   b. *Cimetidine* is used for the treatment of ulcers, but when treatment is discontinued, ulcer formation can recur. In such cases, small maintenance doses of *cimetidine* are effective against recurrences.

   c. By reducing gastric acidity, *cimetidine* has decreased the number of patients undergoing elective surgery for duodenal ulcer. However, it has not lowered the number of operations performed for perforations and other complications of duodenal ulcer.

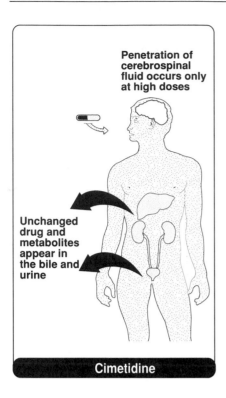

Penetration of cerebrospinal fluid occurs only at high doses

Unchanged drug and metabolites appear in the bile and urine

Cimetidine

3. **Pharmacology:**

a. **Absorption:** Almost 80% of an orally administered dose of *cimetidine* is absorbed from the GI tract. *Cimetidine* is unevenly distributed in various organs of the body. Only small amounts cross the blood-brain barrier. Less than 25% of *cimetidine* in the blood is bound to plasma proteins.

b. **Excretion:** *Cimetidine* normally has a short serum half-life. The half-life is increased in renal failure. Approximately 30% of a dose of *cimetidine* is slowly inactivated by the liver's microsomal mixed function oxygenase system (p.12). The other 70% is excreted unchanged in the urine.

4. **Adverse reactions:**

a. The adverse effects of *cimetidine* are usually minor and are associated mainly with the major pharmacological activity of the drug, namely reduced gastric acid production. Side effects occur only in a small number of patients and generally do not require discontinuation of the drug.

b. The most common side effects are headache, dizziness, diarrhea, and muscular pain. Other CNS effects (confusion, hallucinations) occur primarily in elderly patients or after prolonged administration.

c. *Cimetidine* can also have endocrine effects, since it acts as a nonsteroidal antiandrogen. These effects include gynecomastia, galactorrhea (continuous release/discharge of milk), and reduced sperm count.

5. **Drug interactions:** *Cimetidine* blocks hepatic mixed function oxygenase (p.12) and thus inhibits the microsomal metabolism of several other drugs, causing higher blood levels and enhancement of their effects.

B. Ranitidine

1. **Actions:** *Ranitidine* [ra NYE ta deen] is a new, potent, H_2 receptor blocker. Compared to *cimetidine, ranitidine* is longer acting and is five to ten times as potent.

2. **Therapeutic uses and pharmacokinetics:** *Ranitidine's* therapeutic uses and pharmacokinetics are similar to those described for *cimetidine.*

3. **Adverse effects:** *Ranitidine* has minimal side effects. It does not produce the antiandrogenic or prolactin-stimulating effects of *cimetidine.* Because it does not inhibit the mixed function oxygenase system in the liver, it does not affect the concentration of other drugs.

C. Famotidine

Famotidine [fa MOE ti deen] is similar to ranitidine in its pharmacological action, but it is 20-160 times more potent than *cimetidine* and 3-20 times more potent than *ranitidine.*

D. Nizatidine

Nizatidine [nye ZAT i deen] is similar to *ranitidine* in its pharmacological action and potency. In contrast to *cimetidine, ranitidine,* and *famotidine* (which are metabolized by the liver), *nizatidine* is eliminated principally by the kidney. Since little first-pass metabolism occurs with *nizatidine,* its bioavailability is nearly 100%.

Study Questions   (see p.438 for answers).

Choose the ONE best answer.

39.1 Which of the following are major effects of angiotensin II?

    A. Inhibition of the sympathetic nervous system.
    B. Vasodilation.
    C. Decreased blood pressure.
    D. Promotes sodium and water retention and potassium wasting.
    E. Hypotension.

39.2 Angiotensin converting enzyme (ACE) has all of the following properties EXCEPT:

    A. converts bradykinin to inactive fragments.
    B. is localized in the endothelium of the blood vessels of the lungs, kidney, and other organs.
    C. is also known as peptidyl dipeptidase.
    D. is a dipeptidase.
    E. is inhibited by saralasin.

39.3 All of the following statements are true EXCEPT:

    A. Serotonin acts through the same receptors that bind histamine.
    B. At high blood levels of angiotensin II, saralasin lowers arterial blood pressure, whereas at low blood levels of angiotensin II, saralasin increases arterial blood pressure.
    C. Phenelzine inhibits serotonin degradation.
    D. Tricyclic antidepressants, such as imipramine, increase serotonin levels in the synapse.
    E. Reserpine depletes the store of serotonin in the neurons and may precipitate a depressive episode.

39.4 Ergot alkaloids:

    A. cause vasodilation.
    B. exert their actions by binding to specific ergot amine receptors.
    C. are useful in treating acute migraine headache.
    D. are useful to maintain uterine muscle tone during pregnancy.
    E. have actions similar to those of nitroprusside.

Answer A if 1,2 and 3 are correct.
  B if 1 and 3 are correct.
  C if 2 and 4 are correct.
  D if only 4 is correct.
  E if 1,2,3 and 4 are all correct.

39.5 Histamine H_1-receptor blockers are useful in the treatment of

  1. urticaria.
  2. seasonal rhinitis.
  3. drug reactions.
  4. bronchial asthma.

39.6 Which of the following statements regarding histamine H_2-receptor blockers is/are correct?

  1. Cimetidine is more potent and longer acting than ranitidine.
  2. Cimetidine shows little or no effect because of interactions with H_1-histamine receptor.
  3. Ranitidine has endocrine effects, including gynecomastia, galactorrhea, and reduced sperm count.
  4. Cimetidine binds to hepatic mixed function oxidase and, therefore, inhibits the microsomal metabolism of certain drugs.

39.7 Which of the following statements regarding the effects of histamine is/are true?

  1. The cardiovascular effects of histamine are mediated by both H_1 and H_2 receptors.
  2. Stimulation of histamine H_1 receptors results in smooth muscle relaxation.
  3. Combination of histamine with H_2 receptors causes stimulation of gastric acid secretion.
  4. The effect of histamine on the skin is a result of the stimulation of H_1 receptors.

Glossary

Abortifacient: An agent that terminates pregnancy

Abscess: Localized accumulation of pus caused by infection

Acne: Skin disorder due to inflammation of the sebaceous gland

Adenoma: A tumor of epithelial tissue, usually benign and well circumscribed

Adipocyte: A cell from adipose tissue; a fat cell

Adjuvant: Anything that assists a process, for example, a substance that enhances the immunological response to an antigen

Aerobic: Pertaining to an organism that grows in the presence of oxygen

Afferent: Conveying inward or toward a center; e.g., sensory nerve impulse traveling toward the central nervous system

Afterload: Resistance against which the blood is expelled

Agglutination: The clumping of cells, microorganisms, and so forth, caused by antibodies or other natural or synthetic chemical factors

Agonist: A drug that can interact with specific receptors and thus initiates a response

Agranulocytosis: A marked decrease in the level of granular white blood cells (especially polymorphonuclear leukocytes)

Akathisia: The inability to remain in a sitting position due to motor restlessness and muscle quivering

Alkaloid: One of a number of bases with a nitrogen-containing heterocyclic structure that are found in plants and of which many are widely used as drugs

Allergen: An antigen (such as pollen or house dust) that causes a hypersensitivity reaction

Alopecia: Baldness; hair-loss

Amenorrhea: Absence of menstrual bleeding

Amnesia: Partial or complete memory loss

Amygdala: One of the basal ganglia; a roughly almond-shaped mass of gray matter deep inside each cerebral hemisphere

Anaerobe: An organism that grows in the absence of oxygen

Anaphylaxis: The acute or exaggerated allergic response of a previously sensitized host in response to exposure to a foreign substance (antigen)

Angina: A condition characterized by cramping or painful spasms; a sense of suffocation or suffocating pain

Ankylosis: Stiffness or immobilization of a joint caused by disease or injury

Anorexia: A lack of appetite or an aversion to food

Anovulatory: Failing to release an ovum

Antagonist: An agent that opposes or resists the action of another

Antiseptic: A substance that inhibits growth of infectious agents

Antitussive: A medication that relieves or prevents a cough

Aplastic: Incomplete or otherwise defective development or regeneration of an organ or tissue

Arrhythmia: Any variation from normal rhythm; refers especially to an irregular heart beat

Arthralgia: Severe pain in a joint, that is not caused by inflammation

Arthritis: Inflammation of a joint; may cause swelling, pain, tenderness, deformity

Arthroplasty: Creation of an artificial joint when required, e.g., in the case of ankylosis

Arthrosclerosis: Stiffness of joints

Ascites: An accumulation of watery fluid in the peritoneal cavity

Asphyxiation: Impaired or absent respiratory process due to lack of oxygen in the inspired air or to obstruction of air flow to the lungs

Asymptomatic: Being symptomless

Asystole: Absence of systolic activity in the heart

Ataxia: Incoordination of voluntary movements in the absence of paralysis

Atonic: Relaxed; lacking muscle tone

Atrioventricular: Pertaining to both the atria and ventricles of the heart

Atrophy: A wasting of a tissue, organ, or part or all of an organism

Autoimmune: Having an immunological response to the tissues or substances of ones own body

Automaticity: State of not being under voluntary control

Autosomal: Associated with a chromosome (autosome) other than the sex chromosomes

Axon: A neuronal process that conducts nervous impulses away from the cell body

Azotemia: An abnormal increase in the urea concentration (or that of other nitrogen containing substances) in blood plasma

397

Baroreceptor: Pressure receptors located in the aortic arch, cardiac auricle, vena cava, and carotid sinus that sense blood pressure by responding to the relative stretch of large vessel walls. They regulate reflex control of blood pressure and heart rate.

Basophil: Any cell whose cytoplasm can be stained with basic dyes, e.g., polymorphonuclear leukocytes with small numbers of cytoplasmic granules

Bradycardia: A slow heart rate, usually defined as a rate less than 60 beats per minute

Bradykinesia: Extremely slow voluntary movement

Buccal: Relating to the cheek

Carcinoma: A malignant epithelial tumor

Caseous: Cheesy or curdlike

Catatonia: A type of schizophrenia characterized by stupor, rigidity, agitation, or other alterations in motor reactivity and muscle tone

Cathartic: An osmotic, irritant, or stimulant agent that promotes bowel movement

Chelate: To form a complex between a metal ion and two or more polar groups of a single molecule

Chemotactic: Pertaining to a compound that provides a chemical stimulus; causing a directional movement of an organism

Chitin: A tough polysaccharide found in certain fungi and the exoskeletons of arthropods

Choriocarcinoma: Highly malignant neoplasm consisting of rapidly dividing trophoblasts that invade and multiply in maternal tissues

Chronotropism: An alteration in rate (e.g., heart rate or any recurring phenomenon)

Cinchonism: Syndrome resulting from excessive or prolonged treatment with alkaloids, such as quinine (also called quininism)

Cirrhosis: A progressive disease of the liver that is characterized by diffuse fibrosis and that is caused by parenchymal necrosis, followed by nodular regeneration of hepatic cells.

Clonic: Describing the rapid, sequential, alternating contractions and relaxations of a muscle during clonus

Cognitive: Pertaining to cognition: the ways of thinking and knowing that include remembering, reasoning, perceiving, imagining, sensing, recognizing, and judging

Congener: One of two or more substances that are related in molecular structure

Conjugate: Joined or coupled; refers to a compound formed by addition of substituents such as glucuronic acid, sulfate, etc.

Constipation: Condition in which bowel movements are delayed or incomplete

Crystalluria: Presence of crystals in the urine, e.g., sulfonamide drugs may crystallize in the urine

Cycloplegia: Paralysis of accommodation due to loss of power in the ciliary muscle of the eye

Cytopenia: An abnormal reduction in the number of cells in the circulating blood or bone marrow

Cytoskeleton: The intracellular protein scaffolding that determines the cell's shape, flexibility, and motility

Depolarize: To reduce the potential across a cell membrane

Dermatitis: Any inflammatory skin disease

Detrusor: A muscle whose contraction results in expelling a substance (e.g., the urinary bladder)

Diastole: The period of atrial and ventricular myocardial relaxation in the cardiac cycle

Dilate: To expand in size

Dilation: Enlargement of a hollow vessel or organ beyond its normal size or extent

Disseminate: Widely spread throughout an organ, a system, or the entire body

Distal: Located farther or farthest away from the center of the body (or from the beginning of a structure, or from the attached end)

Diuretic: Any drug or factor that induces a state of increased urine flow

Duodenum: The first (and widest) part of the small intestine

Dwarfism: The condition of being a markedly undersized individual or an abnormally short structure from any cause

Dyscrasia: Presence of abnormal material in the blood (e.g., blood dyscrasia is due to an abnormality of blood cells or bone marrow)

Dysentery: A disease of the bowel characterized by abdominal cramping and diarrhea, often with blood and mucus present in the watery stool

Dyskinesia: Any movement abnormality, e.g., incoordination, spasm, irregular movements. Facial dyskinesia (irregular protrusion of tongue and lip movements) may be caused by phenothiazines.

Dysmenorrhea: Painful menstruation

Dysphoria: A feeling of dissatisfaction or unpleasantness

Dysplasia: Abnormal or incomplete development of a part of the body

Dyspnea: Shortness of breath

Dysrhythmia: Abnormal rhythm

Dysuria: Painful or difficult urination

Eclampsia: In patients with preeclampsia, the occurence of one or more convulsions that are not due to other cerebral conditions such as cerebral hemorrhage or epilepsy

Ectopic: Out of place; e.g., a heart beat that arises from a focus other than the sinoatrial node or a pregnancy occurring other than within the uterus

Edema: The presence of excessive fluid in tissues

Efferent: Conveying outward or away from a center, e.g., nerve impulses traveling from the central nervous system to an organ

Electrocardiography: A recording of the potentials of the heart detected on the surface of the body

Embolism: The obstruction or occlusion of a vessel by gas or solid material that has traveled through the blood stream (e.g., a blood clot that has become dislodged)

Emetic: A substance that causes vomiting

Empirical: Based on practical experience but not proved scientifically

Encephalopathy: Any degenerative condition or disease of the brain

Endemic: Describing a disease persistently present in a given community or region

Endocarditis: Inflammation of the endocardium, the membrane lining the heart

Endogenous: Originating or produced within an organism

Endolymph: The fluid filling the membranous labyrinth of the inner ear

Endometriosis: The ectopic presence of endometrial tissue (i.e., at locations outside of the uterus)

Endothelium: A layer of cells located on the surface of connective tissue that lines the heart, blood vessels, and lymphatic channels

Enteral: Pertaining to administration of a drug either by the oral, sublingual, or rectal route

Eosinophilia: An abnormal increase in the number of eosinophilic leukocytes

Epigastric: Pertaining to or located within the epigastrium (the upper middle part of the abdomen)

Epilepsy: A neurologic disorder characterized by the tendency to suffer recurrent seizures

Epiphyseal: Pertaining to an epiphysis (the end of a long bone developed from a secondary center of ossification)

Erythema: Redness of skin due to capillary dilation

Erythrocyte: Mature red blood cell

Erythropoiesis: Formation of red blood cells

Erythropoietin: A protein that enhances erythropoiesis by stimulating formation of proerythroblasts and release of reticulocytes from bone marrow

Eukaryotic: An organism whose cells contain a nucleus enclosed by a nuclear membrane

Euphoria: A feeling of well-being, contentment, or elation, often exaggerated and not well founded

Exacerbation: An increase in the severity of a disease or its signs or symptoms

Exocrine: Secretion of a substance to the surface of the body (usually through ducts)

Exogenous: Originating or produced outside an organism

Extrapyramidal: Located outside of the corticospinal (pyramidal) tract; refers to the ganglia, nuclei, and reticular formation and to their descending connections, which modulate motor systems background activity

Extrasystole: Premature systole; a cardiac depolarization originating at a site other than at the sinoatrial node

Extravasate: To leak fluid (e.g., blood, lymph, urine) into the tissues out of the vessel that is supposed to contain it

Fasciculation: Involuntary twitchings or contractions of groups of muscle fibers (fasciculi)

Febrile: Feverish

Fibrillation: Fine, rapid contraction or twitching of fibers in cardiac or skeletal muscle

Flatulence: The presence of an excessive amount of gas in the intestines and stomach

Follicle: A small, saclike mass of cells, usually containing a cavity

Fulminating: Occurring suddenly and severely, as the onset of a pain or of an illness

Galactorrhea: Excessive or persistent discharge of milk from the breasts (of either sex)

Gallstone: A concretion composed chiefly of cholesterol and/or bile pigments, found in the gallbladder or bile duct

Gangrene: Tissue necrosis due primarily to obstruction or loss of blood supply

Genome: The total genetic information present in a cell

Gingival: Relating to the gums

Glaucoma: A disease of the eye caused by an increase in intraocular pressure sufficient to damage the structure and/or function of the eye

Glycosuria: Carbohydrates in the urine

Gonorrhea: A contagious inflammation of the genital mucous membrane due to infection by *Neisseria gonorrhoeae*

Granulocyte: A mature granular leukocyte, i.e. neutrophil, basophil, and eosinophil

Granulocytopenia: Less than the normal number of granular leukocytes in the blood

Gynecomastia: Enlargement of the male breast

Hapten: A substance, often an organic chemical with low molecular weight, that alone is unable to elicit production of an antibody but that is capable of binding to specific proteins, thereby forming an antigen

Hematuria: Condition in which urine contains blood or red blood cells

Hemodialysis: Removal of soluble substances from the blood by diffusion through a semipermeable membrane

Hemophilia: A serious, inherited hemorrhagic disease caused by a deficit in the ability of blood to coagulate

Hemopoietic: Pertaining to the process of formation and development of blood cells and other formed elements in the blood

Hemorrhage: The escape of blood from blood vessels

Hemostatic: Pertaining to an agent that arrests either hemorrhage or blood flow within vessels

Hirsutism: Presence of excessive facial and body hair, especially in women

Hyperesthesia: Exaggerated sensitivity to sound, taste, smell, sex, touch, or visual stimuli

Hyperkalemia: High concentration of potassium in plasma

Hyperkinesia: Abnormally intense motor activity

Hypernatremia: Elevated serum concentration of sodium

Hyperplasia: An increase in the number of cells in a tissue or organ (excluding a tumor), causing an increase in the bulk of the tissue or organ

Hyperpyrexia: Excessively high body temperature

Hyperreflexia: Exaggerated reflexes

Hypersensitivity: State where exposure to an antigen for a second or subsequent time produces a greater response than that produced on initial exposure

Hyperthermia: Hyperpyrexia that is usually therapeutically induced

Hypertrophy: Increase in the size of part or all of an organ due to an increase in the size of its component cells

Hyperuricemia: Elevated uric acid or urate concentration in the blood

Hypokalemia: Low plasma concentration of potassium

Hypothermia: A body temperature significantly below normal

Hypovolemia: Abnormal reduction in circulating blood volume

Hypoxia: Inadequate oxygen concentration in body tissues

Iatrogenic: An unfavorable response (e.g., complication, injury, etc.) to therapy, caused by the therapeutic effort itself

Icterus: Jaundice

Idiopathic: Pertaining to a disease or other pathologic condition having no known cause

Idiosyncratic: Pertaining to one or more properties or characteristics peculiar to an individual's physical or mental nature. Idiosyncrasies can be caused by an exaggerated response to some drugs and foods.

Impotence: Inability to achieve penile erection

Infarct: An area of tissue necrosis caused by ischemia due to an interrupted blood supply

Infarction: The process of infarct formation

Inotropic: Either enhancing or inhibiting the speed or force of muscle contraction

Intercostal: Between the ribs

Interstitium: A small gap in the structure of a tissue or organ, or a crevice between parts of the body

Intima: The innermost layer

Intrathecal: Within the meninges of the spinal cord

Intubation: The introduction of a tube into an orifice or vessel, e.g., into the trachea during anesthesia

Ischemia: Inadequate blood flow to a part or organ

Jaundice: Icterus; yellowish discoloration of the skin and mucous membrane due to hyperbilirubinemia and deposition of bile pigment

Keratinized: Having developed a horny layer

Keratitis: Inflammation of the cornea

Ketoacidosis: Acidosis due to the enhanced production of ketone bodies (i.e., acetoacetate and β-hydroxybutyrate)

Lassitude: A state of weariness

Latent: Existing, but hidden or dormant

Lethargy: A state of excessive fatigue

Leukopenia: Lymphocytopenia, lymphopenia; an abnormal decrease in the number of circulating blood leukocytes

Libido: Sexual desire

Lymphoblastic: Pertaining to the production of lymphocytes

Lymphocytic: Pertaining to or characterized by lymphocytes

Lymphocytopenic: (see leukopenia)

Lymphoma: A general term for malignant neoplasms primarily affecting the lymph nodes

Maculopapular: Marked by small, discolored, non-raised patches on the skin (macules) and small growths on the skin (papules)

Malaise: A feeling of general uneasiness or discomfort

Mania: An emotional disorder characterized by excited but unstable moods, exaltation, hyperactivity, and mental overactivity

Megaloblast: An abnormally large, nucleated erythrocyte precursor cell seen almost exclusively in pernicious anemia or other disorders of folic acid or vitamin B_{12} metabolism

Melanin: Natural pigment of the hair, skin, and retina

Melanoma: A malignant neoplasm derived from cells capable of producing melanin

Metastatic: Pertaining to metastases, i.e., movement of a malignancy from one body site to another

Micturition: Urination; the desire to urinate

Mitogen: An agent that stimulates mitosis

Morbidity: The number of sick persons (or cases of a disease) per a given population per unit time

Morbilliform: Skin rash resembling measles

Mortality: The number of deaths per a given population per unit time

Mutagen: An agent that causes an alteration in the genetic material

Myalgia: Muscular pain

Myasthenia: Muscular weakness

Mydriasis: Dilation of the pupil

Narcolepsy: A sudden, uncontrollable tendency to fall asleep at irregular intervals, involving attacks that last from minutes to hours

Natriuretic: Pertaining to or causing increased excretion of sodium in the urine

Necrosis: The morphologic changes that follow the death of one or more cells, a portion of tissue, or an organ

Neonate: An infant during the first 4 weeks after birth

Neoplasm: A tumor

Neuralgia: Severe, stabbing or throbbing pain in the area served by a sensory nerve

Neuropathy: Any disease of the nervous system

Neutropenia: An abnormally small number of neutrophils in the blood

Nociceptive: Capable of responsiveness or sensitivity to painful or injurious stimuli

Normochromic: Being normal in color; used especially to describe erythrocytes with normal hemoglobin concentration

Normocytic: Having erythrocytes of normal volume (normocytes)

Nystagmus: Rapid, spontaneous, rhythmic movement of the eye; movement may be jerky or pendular

Occipital: Pertaining to the back of the head (the occiput)

Occlude: To close off, obstruct

Opportunistic: Pertaining to a microorganism that causes a disease only in a host whose immunological status has been compromised

Orthostatic: Pertaining to an erect posture

Osteoarthritis: Degenerative joint disease

Osteoclast: A giant, multinuclear cell responsible for bone absorption and degradation

Osteomyelitis: An inflammation of all areas of bone including the marrow

Osteonecrosis: Death of bone in mass

Osteoporosis: Loss of both bone mineral and protein leading to reduction in the quantity and quality of bone

Ototoxic: Toxic to the ear

Palliation: Relieving the severity of symptoms without acting to cure the disease

Palpebral: Pertaining to the eyelids

Palpitation: Strong, rapid, or irregular heart beats that are perceptible to the patient

Palsy: Paralysis

Pancytopenia: A reduction in the number of all formed elements in the circulating blood

Paranoia: A mental disorder characterized by delusions, which are often persecutory in nature

Paraplegic: Pertaining to an individual with paralysis of both lower extremities and, often, the lower trunk

Parenteral: Introducing a substance into the body by a route other than the gastrointestinal tract, e.g., by intramuscular, intravenous, subcutaneous, or intramedullary injection

Paresthesia: A sensation such as burning, pins and needles, tickling, or tingling that occurs spontaneously without external cause

Paroxysmal: Pertaining to a sharp spasm or convulsion or to a sharp intensification of the symptoms of a disorder

Pathogen: A microorganism (including the viruses) capable of causing disease

Periorbital: Surrounding the ocular orbit

Perivascular: Surrounding a blood or lymph vessel

Pernicious: Destructive, harmful

Phenotype: The identifiable structural and functional characteristics of an organism that are determined by the combined influences of both the genotype and environment

Pheochromocytoma: A usually benign paraganglioma of the adrenal medulla, characterized by secretion of epinephrine and/or norepinephrine

Phlebitis: Inflammation of a vein

Phobia: Pathologic morbid fear or avoidance

Photophobia: An abnormal intolerance of light, especially by the eyes

Photosensitivity: A sensitivity to light

Piloerection: Erection of hair, e.g., due to cold

Pilomotor: Causing or pertaining to movement of hair

Platelet: A membrane-bound fragment of megakaryocyte cytoplasm, normally present in large numbers in blood. Platelets play an important role in blood clotting

Poikilothermy: Condition in which the temperature of an organism varies with the temperature of the surrounding environment (the normal condition for invertebrates, fish, etc.)

Preload: The degree to which the myocardium is stretched before it contracts

Priapism: A persistent, usually painful, erection of the penis, unrelated to sexual stimulation

Prophylactic: Agents that tend to or are intended to prevent the occurence of disease

Proprioception: Awareness of balance, position, and movement of parts or all of the body

Prostatectomy: Partial or total removal of the prostate

Proximal: Located nearer or nearest the center of the body (or the beginning of a structure or the attached end)

Pruritus: Itching

Psoriasis: A common inflammatory skin disease of which the characteristic lesion is a dull red or pink, scaly, well-demarcated plaque occurring on any part or proportion of the skin surface

Psychosomatic: Emotional and psychological contributors to physical disorders (e.g., peptic ulcer, hypertension)

Psychotomimetic: Hallucinogenic

Pyelonephritis: Inflammation of the renal parenchyma, usually due to bacterial infection

Pyretic: Febrile (feverish)

Pyrogen: Any substance that induces fever

Radiomimetic: Producing effects similar to those of radiation

Refractory: Unresponsive; resistant to treatment

Remission: A reduction or even the disappearance of the symptoms of a disease; the period during which this reduction occurs (may be temporary)

Resection: Surgical removal of a part of a structure

Rheumatic: Pertaining to musculoskeletal system abnormalities

Sarcolemmal: Pertaining to the sarcolemma, the plasma membrane of a muscle fiber

Sarcoplasmic: Pertaining to the sarcoplasm, the nonfibrillar cytoplasm of a muscle fiber

Septicemia: Severe, generalized infection resulting from the dissemination of pathogenic microorganisms and their toxins in the circulating blood

Sinoatrial: Of or relating to the sinus venosus and the atrium of the heart

Somatic: Pertaining to the skeleton or skeletal muscle, as distinct from the viscera of the body

Somnifacient: Promoting sleep

Somnolence: Drowsiness, sleepiness

Splanchnic: Visceral; pertaining to the viscera

Spondylitis: Inflammation of one or more vertebrae

Squamous: Scaly

Stenosis: A narrowing of the lumen of any canal, an orifice, or tubular organ

Stomatitis: Any generalized inflammation of the oral mucosa

Sublingual: Beneath the tongue

Supine: Lying on the back

Syncope: Fainting due to a global reduction in cerebral blood flow causing generalized cerebral ischemia

Syncytial: Pertaining to a syncytium, a multinucleated mass of protoplasm not subdivided into individual cells

Synergistic: Pertaining to synergism, the cooperative action by two or more drugs, muscles, organs, or other entities so that the combined action is greater than that of each separate element

Synovial: Pertaining to synovia, the viscous fluid secreted by synovial membranes that serves as a lubricant for joints, tendons, sheaths, and bursae

Tachyarrhythmia: Any disturbance of cardiac rhythm, either regular or irregular, in which the heart rate exceeds 100 beats per minute

Tachycardia: A rapid heart rate, generally greater than 100 beats per minute

Teratogenic: Causing the production of a developmentally abnormal fetus

Thrombocytopenia: A smaller than normal number of platelets in the circulating blood

Thrombophlebitis: Inflammation of a vein associated with thrombosis

Thrombosis: Formation of a thrombus (clot) within a blood vessel

Thymoleptic: Pertaining to a tendency to change or elevate mood without unnecessarily stimulating the central nervous system

Thyrotoxicosis: The condition resulting from hyperthyroidism due to any cause

Uremia: An excess of urea in the blood

Uricosuric: Pertaining to the stimulation of urinary excretion of uric acid

Urticaria: An eruption of transient, edematous, often itchy swellings of the skin; hives

Uveitis: Inflammation of the choroid, ciliary body, and iris (i.e., the entire uveal tract)

Vertigo: A hallucination of irregular or whirling motion, either of the subject itself or of his surroundings

Xerostomia: Dry mouth due to decreased salivary secretion

Answers to Study Questions

Chapter 1: ABSORPTION, DISTRIBUTION, AND ELIMINATION OF DRUGS

1.1 The correct answer is D.
Which one of the following statements is correct?

A. Weak bases are absorbed efficiently across the epithelial cells of the stomach. {**False: In the stomach a weak base is primarily in the protonated, charged form, which does not readily cross the epithelial cells of the stomach.**}

B. Coadministration of atropine speeds the absorption of a second drug. {**False: Atropine is a parasympathetic blocker and slows gastric emptying. This delays the rate of drug absorption.**}

C. Drugs showing large V_d can be efficiently removed by dialysis of the plasma. {**False: A large V_d indicates that most of the drug is outside the plasma space and dialysis would not be effective.**}

✔D. Stressful emotions can lead to a slowing of drug absorption. {**True: Both exercise and strong emotions prompt sympathetic output, which slows gastric emptying.**}

E. If the V_d for a drug is small, most of the drug is in the extraplasmic space. {**False: A small V_d indicates extensive binding to plasma proteins.**}

1.2 The correct answer is C.
Which one of the following is true for a drug whose elimination from plasma shows first-order kinetics.

A. The half-life of the drug is proportional to the drug concentration in plasma. {**False: The half-life is a constant.**}

B. The amount eliminated per unit time is constant. {**False: For first-order reactions, the fraction of the drug eliminated is constant, not the amount.**}

✔C. The rate of elimination is proportional to the plasma concentration. {**True: This is the definition of first-order metabolism.**}

D. Elimination involves a rate-limiting enzymatic reaction operating at its maximal velocity. {**False: Such a situation would show zero-order kinetics.**}

E. A plot of drug concentration versus time is a straight line. {**False: First-order kinetics show a linear plot of log drug concentration versus time.**}

1.3 The correct answer is B.
All of the following statements are true EXCEPT:

A. Aspirin (pK$_a$ = 3.5) is 90% in its lipid-soluble, protonated form at pH = 2.5. {**Incorrect choice: At one pH unit on the acid side of pKa, the [HA]/[A-] = 10, or 90% as HA, the protonated form of aspirin.**}

✔B. The basic drug promethazine (pK$_a$ = 9.1) is more ionized at pH = 7.4 than at pH = 2. {**Correct choice: As the pH of the solution becomes less than pK$_a$, the ratio [BH$^+$]/[B] increases; thus BH$^+$ is greater at pH = 2.**}

C. Absorption of a weakly basic drug is likely to be faster from the intestine than from the stomach. {**Incorrect choice: Weak bases are more charged in the acidic gastric juice and are not readily absorbed.**}

D. Acidification of the urine accelerates the secretion of a weak base, pK$_a$ = 8. {**Incorrect choice: The drug is more ionized in acidified urine and less able to be reabsorbed.**}

E. Uncharged molecules more readily cross cell membranes than charged molecules. {**Incorrect choice.**}

1.4 The correct answer is A.
A patient is treated with drug A, which has a high affinity for albumin and is administered in amounts that do not exceed the binding capacity of albumin. A second drug, B, is added to the treatment regimen. Drug B also has a high affinity for albumin but is administered in amounts that are 100 times the binding capacity of albumin. Which of the following occurs after administration of drug B?

✔A. An increase in the tissue concentrations of drug A. {**True: Drug A is largely bound to albumin and only a small fraction is free. Most of drug A is sequestered on albumin and is inert in terms of exerting pharmacological actions. If drug B is administered, it displaces drug A from albumin, leading to rapid increase in the concentration of free drug A in plasma, because almost 100% is now free. Drug A moves out of the plasma into the interstitial water and the tissues.**}

B. A decrease in the tissue concentrations of drug A. {**False: See A.**}

C. A decrease in the volume of distribution of drug A. {**False: The V_d of drug A increases.**}

D. A decrease in the half-life of drug A. {**False: A larger volume of distribution provides less drug to the organ of excretion and prolongs the overall lifetime of the drug.**}

E. Addition of more drug A significantly alters the serum concentration of unbound drug B. {**False: Since drug B is already in 100-fold excess of its albumin-binding capacity, dislodging some drug B from albumin does not significantly affect its serum concentration.**}

403

1.5 The correct answer is B.
The addition of glucuronic acid to a drug

A. decreases its water solubility. {**False: Glucuronic acid is charged, and the drug conjugate shows increased water solubility.**}

✔B. usually leads to inactivation of the drug. {**True: The addition of glucuronic acid prevents recognition of the drug by its receptor.**}

C. is an example of a Phase I reaction. {**False: Conjugation is a Phase II reaction.**}

D. is an important pathway in the newborn. {**False: Neonates are deficient in the conjugating enzymes.**}

E. involves cytochrome P-450. {**False: Cytochrome P-450 is involved in Phase I reactions.**}

1.6 The correct answer is D.
Drugs showing zero-order kinetics of elimination

A. are more common that those showing first order kinetics. {**False: In most clinical situations the concentration of a drug is much less than the Michaelis-Menten constant (K_m).**}

B. decreases in concentration exponentially with time. {**False: The decrease is linear with time.**}

C. have a half-life independent of dose. {**False: The half-life increases with dose.**}

✔D. show a plot of drug concentration versus time that is linear. {**True.**}

E. show a constant fraction of the drug is eliminated per unit time. {**False: A constant amount of drug is eliminated.**}

1.7 The correct answer is D.
A drug, given as a 100-mg single dose, results in a peak plasma concentration of 20 μg/ml. The apparent volume of distribution is (assume a rapid distribution and negligible elimination prior to measuring the peak plasma level):

A. 0.5 L. {**False**}

B. 1 L. {**False**}

C. 2 L. {**False**}

✔D. 5 L. {**True: V_d = D/C, where D = total amount of drug in the body and C = plasma concentration of drug. Thus V_d = 100 mg/20 μg/ml = 100 mg/20 mg/L = 5 L.**}

E. 10 L. {**False**}

1.8 The correct answer is D.
Which one of the following statements is correct?

A. A drug given intravenously has more potential for first-pass hepatic metabolism than the same drug given orally. {**False: Most drugs absorbed from the gastrointestinal tract enter the hepatic portal circulation and encounter the liver prior to distribution in the general circulation. With intravenous administration, the drug is not absorbed by the gastrointestinal tract; therefore, first-pass metabolism by the liver is avoided.**}

B. Inhalation has the disadvantage of very slow absorption. {**False: Inhalation provides the rapid delivery of a drug across the large surface area of the alveolar membrane and can produce actions almost as rapidly as intravenous injection.**}

C. Passive diffusion typically involves a specific carrier protein and shows saturation kinetics. {**False: These are characteristics of active transport.**}

✔D. Bioavailability of a drug administered intravenously is 100%. {**True: By definition bioavailability is 100% for drugs administered intravenously.**}

E. An exceptionally large K_d indicates that the drug is rapidly metabolized. {**False: An exceptionally large V_d indicates considerable sequestration of the drug in some organ or compartment.**}

Chapter 2: PHARMACOKINETICS AND DRUG RECEPTORS

2.1 The correct answer is D.
A drug with a half-life of 12 hours is administered by continuous intravenous infusion. How long will it take for the drug to reach 90% of its final steady-state level?

A. 18 hours. {**False**}

B. 24 hours. {**False**}

C. 30 hours. {**False**}

✔D. 40 hours. {**True: One approaches 90% of the final steady-state concentration in 3.3 $\times$ $t_{1/2}$ = 3.3 $\times$ 12.**}

E. 48 hours. {**False**}

2.2 The correct answer is A.
Which of the following results in a doubling of the steady-state concentration of a drug?

✔A. Doubling the rate of infusion. {**True: The steady-state concentration of a drug is directly proportional to the infusion rate.**}

B. Maintaining the infusion rate, but doubling the loading dose. {**False: Increasing the loading dose provides a transient increase in drug level, but the steady-state level remains unchanged.**}

C. Doubling the rate of infusion and doubling the concentration of the infused drug. {**False: This regimen leads to a 4-fold increase in the steady-state drug concentration.**}

D. Tripling the rate of infusion. {**False: This leads to a 3-fold increase in the steady-state drug concentration.**}

E. Quadrupling the rate of infusion. {**False: This regimen leads to a 4-fold increase in the steady-state drug concentration.**}

2.3 The correct answer is C.

The graded dose-response curve for a drug is shown as curve B in the above graph. Which curve best describes the response expected in the presence of a competitive antagonist?

A. Curve A. {False: A shift of the dose-response curve to the left indicates an increase in the apparent potency and is only seen in the presence of agents that act synergistically.}

B. Curve B. {False: Curve B is observed only if there is no effect of the competitive antagonist.}

✔C. Curve C. {True: A competitive agonist shifts the dose-response curve to the right, with no change in the maximal response seen at high agonist concentration.}

D. Curve D. {False: A competitive antagonist does not change the maximal response seen at high agonist concentration. Curve D is a noncompetitive agonist.}

E. Curve E. {False: A competitive antagonist does not change the maximal response seen at high agonist concentration.}

2.4 The correct answer is D.

Which of the following statements is correct?

A. If 10 mg of drug A produces the same response as 100 mg of drug B, drug A is more efficacious than drug B. {False: No information is provided about efficacy, the maximal effect that a drug can produce. Drug A is more potent than drug B.}

B. The greater the efficacy, the greater the potency of a drug. {False: Efficacy and potency can vary independently.}

C. In selecting a drug, potency is usually more important than efficacy. {False: The maximal response is often more important than the amount of drug needed to achieve the response.}

✔D. In the presence of a full agonist, a partial agonist acts like a competitive inhibitor. {True: By displacing a fully active agonist, the partial agonist decreases the maximal response.}

E. Variation in response to a drug among different individuals is most likely to occur with a drug showing a large therapeutic index. {False: Variability between patients in the pharmacokinetics of a drug is most important clinically when the effective and toxic doses are not very different, as is the case with a drug that shows a small therapeutic index.}

2.5 The correct answer is D.

Which of following most closely describes the clearance rate of a drug that is infused at a rate of 4 mg/min and produces a steady-state concentration of 6 mg/L in the plasma?

A. 67 ml/min. {False}

B. 132 ml/min. {False}

C. 300 ml/min. {False}

✔D. 667 ml min. {True: Clearance is the volume of plasma from which all drug is removed in a given time (in this case per minute). At steady state, the excretion rate = infusion rate = 4 mg/min. Thus, clearance (ml/min) = excretion rate (mg/ml)/plasma concentration (mg/ml) = (4 mg/ml)/(0.006 mg/ml) = 667 ml/min.}

E. 1200 ml/min. {False.}

2.6 The correct answer is C.

The antimicrobial drug, tetracycline, is found to be therapeutically effective when 250 mg of drug are present in the body. The $t_{1/2}$ of tetracycline is 8 hours. What is the correct rate of infusion?

A. 7 mg/min. {False}

B. 12 mg/min. {False}

✔C. 22 mg/min. {True: The correct rate of infusion is R = K_dV_dC, where K_d = $0.69/t_{1/2}$ = 0.69/8 hours = 0.086 hr⁻1; therefore, the instantaneous rate of loss of the tetracycline is 8.6 %/hr of whatever amount of drug is present in the body. V_dC = the total amount of drug in the body. When 250 mg of tetracycline are present in the body, the rate of drug loss is 250 mg × 8.6% per hour = 250 × 0.086 hr⁻1 = 21.5 mg/hr.}

D. 37 mg/min. {False}

E. 45 mg/min. {False}

2.7 The correct answer is C.

A drug has a V_d of 30 L and a clearance rate of 20 L/hr, with 50% being eliminated by the liver and 50% excreted by the kidney. A maintenance regimen is 200 mg every 12 hours. Which of the following most closely produces the same steady-state concentration in a patient with 50% renal function?

A. 25 mg every 3 hours. {False}

B. 100 mg every 6 hours. {False}

✔C. 150 mg every 12 hours. {True: The rate of drug elimination is normally 200/12 hours = 16.6 mg/hour, with 50% or 8.3 mg/hour normally being excreted by the kidney. In a patient with 50% kidney function, the liver eliminates 8.3 mg/hour and the kidney excretes 4.2 mg/hour, or 12.5 mg/hour total excretion. The maintenance regimen must therefore provide 12.5 mg/hour, or 150 mg/12 hours.}

D. 150 mg every 6 hours. {False.}

E. 200 mg every 6 hours. {False.}

2.8 The correct answer is D.

Which of the following is least likely to influence the response to a drug?

A. Affinity of receptor for drug. {**Incorrect choice: A higher affinity for a drug increases the drug-receptor concentration and creates a greater response.**}

B. Efficacy. {**Incorrect choice: Efficacy is the maximal response.**}

C. Bioavailability. {**Incorrect choice: Bioavailability influences the amount of drug that reaches the drug's receptor.**}

✔D. Therapeutic index. {**Correct choice.**}

E. Route of administration. {**Incorrect choice.**}

Chapter 3: THE AUTONOMIC NERVOUS SYSTEM

3.1 The correct answer is E (1,2,3,4).
Which of the following statements concerning the autonomic nervous system is/are correct?

✔1. The autonomic nervous system is composed entirely of efferent neurons. {**True: These visceral motor (efferent) neurons innervate smooth muscle of the viscera, cardiac muscle, and the exocrine glands.**}

✔2. The sympathetic division is activated in response to stressful situations. {**True: Conditions such as trauma, fear, hypoglycemia, cold, or exercise activate the sympathetic neurons.**}

✔3. The parasympathetic division originates from cell bodies in the central nervous system. {**True: Both sympathetic and parasympathetic neurons emerge from the brain stem or spinal cord.**}

✔4. The control of blood pressure is mainly a sympathetic activity, with essentially no participation of the parasympathetic system. {**True: Blood pressure is regulated largely by sympathetic control of vascular tone.**}

3.2 The correct answer is B (1,3).
Which of the following statements concerning the parasympathetic nervous system are correct?

✔1. The actions of the parasympathetic division usually oppose the effects of the sympathetic division. {**True**}

2. The parasympathetic system often discharges as a single, functional system. {**False: Stimulation of the entire parasympathetic division would produce massive, undesirable, and unpleasant symptoms. Instead, discrete parasympathetic fibers are activated separately.**}

✔3. The parasympathetic division is involved in accommodation of near vision, movement of food, and urination. {**True**}

4. The postganglionic fibers of the parasympathetic division are long, compared to those of the sympathetic nervous system. {**False**}

3.3 The correct answer is A (1,2,3).
Which of the following compounds function(s) as second messenger(s)?

✔1. cAMP. {**True**}
✔2. Inositol 1,4,5-triphosphate. {**True**}
✔3. Diacylglycerol. {**True**}
4. GTP. {**False**}

3.4 The correct answer is B (1,3).
Which of the following is/are characteristic of parasympathetic stimulations?

✔1. Increase in intestinal motility. {**True**}
2. Inhibition of bronchial secretion. {**False**}
✔3. Contraction of sphincter muscle in the iris of the eye (miosis). {**True**}
4. Contraction of sphincter of urinary bladder.{**False**}

3.5 The correct answer is C.
Administration of a drug that acts to dilate arterioles would cause which one of the following?

A. Increased output from the parasympathetic neurons. {**False: Dilation of arteries activates the baroreceptor reflex causing an increase in sympathetic output and a decrease in parasympathetic activity.**}

B. Bradycardia (decreased heart rate). {**False: Increased sympathetic activity increases heart rate.**}

✔C. Increased contractility of the heart. {**True: Increased sympathetic activity increases cardiac force.**}

D. No change in arterial blood pressure. {**False: Blood pressure decreases in response to arterial vasodilation.**}

E. Activation of the sympathetic and parasympathetic output to the heart. {**False**}

Questions 3.6–3.7: For the following two question use the diagram shown on page 34, which represents the parasympathetic, sympathetic, and somatic nervous systems.

3.6 The correct answer is B.
Norepinephrine acts as a neurotransmitter at which of the following sites?

A. Site A. {**False: Acetylcholine is released at this site.**}
✔B. Site B. {**True**}
C. Sites C and D. {**False: Acetylcholine is released at this site.**}
D. Site D. {**False**}
E. Sites D and E. {**False: Acetylcholine is released at these sites.**}

3.7 The correct answer is E.
Acetylcholine acts as a neurotransmitter at which of the following sites?

A. Site A only. {**False**}
B. Site B only. {**False**}
C. Sites C and D only. {**False**}
D. Sites D and B only. {**False**}
✔E. Sites A, C, D, and E only. {**True**}

Chapter 4: CHOLINERGIC AGONISTS

4.1 The correct answer is A (1,2,3).
Which of the following is/are expected symptoms of poisoning with isoflurophate?

✔1. Paralysis of skeletal muscle. {**True: Since isoflurophate inhibits acetylcholinesterase and increases the concentration of acetylcholine at the synapse, it mimics neuromuscular stimulation.**}
✔2. Increased bronchial secretions. {**True: Isoflurophate mimics parasympathetic stimulation.**}
✔3. Miosis. ({**True: See the answer above.**}
4. Tachycardia. {**False: Bradycardia and decreased cardiac output results from increased parasympathetic stimulation.**}

4.2 The correct answer Is E (1,2,3,4).
Which of the following correctly match a cholinergic agonist with its pharmacological actions?

✔1. Bethanechol: Stimulates atonic bladder. {**True**}
✔2. Carbachol: Induces release of epinephrine from the adrenal medulla. {**True: This a nicotinic action of the drug.**}
✔3. Acetylcholine: Decreases heart rate and cardiac output. {**True**}
✔4. Pilocarpine: Reduces intraocular pressure. {**True**}

4.3 The correct answer is B (1,3).
Pilocarpine:

✔1. is used to lower intraocular pressure in glaucoma. {**True: Pilocarpine is used in glaucoma where it is the treatment of choice for the acute attack.**}
2. selectively binds to nicotine receptors. {**False: Pilocarpine exhibits mainly muscarinic activity.**}
✔3. is not cleaved by acetylcholinesterase. {**True: Pilocarpine is unaffected by acetylcholinesterase.**}
4. causes profuse sweating. {**False**}

4.4 Physostigmine:
The correct answer is A (1,2,3).

✔1. acts at peripheral muscarinic and nicotinic receptors. {**True**}
✔2. produces CNS effects. {**True**}
✔3. can be used to treat an overdose of atropine. {**True**}
4. is hydrolyzed by acetylcholinesterase. {**False**}

4.5 An overdose of neostigmine.
The correct answer is B (1,3).

✔1. may result in bowel hypermotility, salivation, and sweating. {**True: Neostigmine stimulates muscarinic receptors.**}
2. has a shorter duration of action than edrophonium. {**False: Neostigmine acts for 2–4 hours, compared to a few minutes for edrophonium.**}
✔3. increases the acetylcholine concentration at the neuromuscular junction. {**True: This property makes neostigmine useful in treating myasthenia gravis.**}
4. is contraindicated in glaucoma. {**False: Neostigmine can be used to lower intraocular pressure, but pilocarpine is more effective.**}

4.6 The correct answer is C.
Which of the following statements is true?

A. Low doses of physostigmine and bethanechol have similar effects on the neuromuscular junction. {**False: Physostigmine inhibits acetylcholinesterase, resulting in an increase in the concentration of acetylcholine at both nicotinic and muscarinic sites. By contrast, bethanechol is a direct-acting agonist that is selective for muscarinic sites and shows little effect at the neuromuscular junction, which is a nicotinic synapse.**}
B. Neostigmine is superior to edrophonium in the diagnosis of myasthenia gravis. {**False: Edrophonium, because of its shorter duration of action, is preferred for diagnostic use.**}
✔C. Cholinergic agonists cause increased gastrointestinal motility. {**True**}
D. Neostigmine has a stronger effect on the CNS than does physostigmine. {**False: Neostigmine is more polar and does not enter the CNS.**}
E. Acetylcholine is used in the treatment of urinary retention. {**False: Acetylcholine has few clinical uses because of its rapid hydrolysis and non-specific actions.**}

Chapter 5: CHOLINERGIC ANTAGONISTS

5.1 The correct answer is E (1,2,3,4).
Which of the following correctly describe(s) the pharmacological actions of atropine?

✔1. Acts at peripheral and central muscarinic cholinergic receptors. {**True: Atropine competitively antagonizes the action of acetylcholine in the periphery and the CNS.**}

✔2. Acts to decrease the motility of gut. {**True: Atropine is often used as an antispasmodic to reduce activity of the GI tract.**}

✔3. Useful in treating poisoning by organophosphate insecticides. {**True: Atropine blocks the effects of excess acetylcholine resulting from inhibition of acetylcholinesterase by organophosphates.**}

✔4. Shows less CNS action than scopolamine. {**True: Atropine has less action on the CNS.**}

5.2 The correct answer is B (1,3).
Which of the following are useful in treating poisoning with an organophosphate poison such as parathion?

✔1. Atropine and pralidoxime, when administered within hours of exposure to poison. {**True: Atropine blocks the actions of the excess acetylcholine present as a result of inhibition of acetylcholinesterase by parathion; pralidoxime reactivates acetylcholinesterase if given immediately after exposure to the organophosphate.**}

2. Neostigmine. {**False: Neostigmine is a reversible anticholinesterase drug and, hence, would only serve to exacerbate the poisoning.**}

✔3. Scopolamine. {**True: Scopolamine blocks the effects of excess accumulation of acetylcholine.**}

4. Carbachol. {**False: Carbachol is a cholinergic agonist and only exacerbates the poisoning, much in the same way as neostigmine described above in 2.**}

5.3 The correct answer is A (1,2,3).
Which of the following are correctly paired?

✔1. Succinylcholine: Depolarizes neuromuscular endplate. {**True: Succinylcholine is a nicotinic agonist that depolarizes the neuromuscular junction.**}

✔2. Neostigmine: Reverses the effects of nondepolarizing blockers, such as tubocurarine. {**True: Neostigmine, by inhibiting the action of acetylcholine esterase, increases the concentration of acetylcholine in the synaptic space, permitting the natural agonist to more effectively compete with tubocurarine.**}

✔3. Tubocurarine: May cause the release of histamine. {**True: Tubocurarine releases histamine from mast cells.**}

4. Gallamine: Acts only at neuromuscular junction. {**False: Gallamine blocks at cholinergic synapses other than the neuromuscular junction; for example, this agent blocks cardiac vagus at muscarinic sites causing sinus tachycardia.**}

5.4 The correct answer is A.
Which ONE of the following drugs most closely resembles atropine in its pharmacological actions?

✔A. Scopolamine. {**True: Scopolamine has similar effects to atropine.**}

B. Trimethaphan. {**False: Trimethaphan is a ganglionic blocker affecting nicotinic receptors; atropine affects primarily muscarinic receptors.**}

C. Physostigmine. {**False: Physostigmine, an anticholinesterase drug, is the antidote for an excess of atropine.**}

D. Acetylcholine. {**False: Atropine blocks the effects of acetylcholine.**}

E. Carbachol. {**False: Atropine blocks the effects of direct-acting agonists, such as carbachol.**}

5.5 The correct answer is C.
Which one of the following drugs does NOT produce miosis (marked constriction of the pupil)?

A. Carbachol. {**Incorrect choice: Carbachol, a direct-acting cholinergic agonist, mimics the effect of parasympathetic stimulation and produces miosis.**}

B. Isoflurophate. {**Incorrect choice: Isoflurophate, an indirect-acting cholinergic agonist, mimics the effect of parasympathetic stimulation and produces miosis.**}

✔C. Atropine. {**Correct choice: On the eye, atropine blocks all cholinergic activity resulting in mydriasis (dilation of the pupil).**}

D. Pilocarpine. {**Incorrect choice: Pilocarpine, a direct-acting cholinergic agonist, mimics the effect of parasympathetic stimulation and produces miosis.**}

E. Neostigmine. {**Incorrect choice: Neostigmine, an indirect-acting cholinergic agonist, mimics the effect of parasympathetic stimulation and produces miosis.**}

5.6 The correct answer is C.
Which one of the following drugs would be useful in the long-term treatment of myasthenia gravis?

A. Edrophonium. {**False: Edrophonium, an indirect cholinergic agonist, is useful in the diagnosis of myasthenia gravis, but its duration of action is too short for effective long-term treatment.**}

B. Atropine. {**False: Atropine blocks the action of acetylcholine on the cholinergic receptors of the neuromuscular junction.**}

✔C. Neostigmine. {**True: Neostigmine provides symptomatic treatment of myasthenia gravis by inhibiting acetylcholinesterase and thereby increasing the acetylcholine.**}

D. Scopolamine. {**False: Scopolamine, like atropine, blocks the action of acetylcholine on the cholinergic receptors of the neuromuscular junction.**}

E. Bethanechol. {**False: Bethanechol is not effective at the neuromuscular junction.**}

Chapter 6: ADRENERGIC AGONISTS

6.1 The correct answer is B (1,3).
Diastolic pressure is increased after the administration of which of the following drugs?

✔1. Norepinephrine. {**True: Norepinephrine produces intense vasoconstriction and thereby increases peripheral resistance. Both systolic and diastolic blood pressures increase.**}

2. Epinephrine. {**False: Epinephrine increases cardiac output, constricts arterioles in the skin and viscera (α effects), and dilates vessels going to skeletal muscle (β_2 effects); the overall result is an increase in systolic blood pressure and a decrease in diastolic blood pressure.**}

✔3. Amphetamine. {**True: Amphetamine is an indirect-acting agonist that increases blood pressure by α-agonist action on the vasculature as well as β-stimulatory effects on the heart.**}

4. Isoproterenol. {**False: Isoproterenol is a β-specific agonist that increases cardiac output and decreases peripheral resistance; this causes a slight increase in systolic blood pressure and a significant decrease In diastolic blood pressure.**}

6.2 The correct answer is E (1,2,3,4).
Which of the following is/are end product(s) of catecholamine metabolism?

✔1. Vanillylmandelic acid. {**True**}
✔2. Metanephrine. {**True**}
✔3. Normetanephrine. {**True**}
✔4. Homovanillic acid. {**True. Homovanillic acid is a degradation product of dopamine.**}

6.3 The correct answer is E (1,2,3,4).
Which of the following is/are correct statement(s)?

✔1. Among the physiological responses caused by α-receptor stimulation are vasoconstriction, mydriasis, and increased gastrointestinal motility. {**True**}

✔2. Among the physiological responses caused by β-receptor stimulation are vasodilation, cardiac stimulation, and bronchial relaxation.{**True**}

✔3. Epinephrine acts on both α and β receptors, whereas norepinephrine acts only on α receptors and β_1 receptors. {**True**}

✔4. Administration of atropine prior to norepinephrine leads to an increase in heart rate after norepinephrine administration. {**True: Atropine blocks the compensatory vagal reflex stimulated by vasoconstriction and elevated blood pressure.**}

6.4 The correct answer is E (1,2,3,4).
Dopamine causes which of the following actions:

✔1. Increases cardiac output. {**True**}
✔2. Dilates renal vasculature. {**True**}
✔3. Increases production of urine. {**True**}
✔4. Increases blood pressure. {**True**}

6.5 The correct answer is B (1,3).
Which of the following structures is/are more responsive to β agonists in comparison to α agonist?

✔1. Bronchial smooth muscle. {**True: Bronchial muscles contain β_2 receptors.**}

2. Radial muscle of iris. {**False: The radial muscle of the iris contains predominantly α receptors; contraction produces mydriasis.**}

✔3. Vasculature of skeletal muscle. {**True: Vessels in skeletal muscle contain mostly β_2 receptors.**}

4. Vasculature of skin. {**False: Vessels in skin contain mostly α receptors.**}

6.6 The correct answer is B (1,3).
Phenylephrine:

✔1. is an α agonist that causes vasoconstriction. {**True**}
2. is a cardioselective β agonist. {**False**}
✔3. is often found in over-the-counter nasal decongestants. {**True**}
4. affects the parasympathetic nervous system. {**False**}

6.7 The correct answer is B (1,3).
Administration of which of the following drugs leads to the stimulation of both α- and β-adrenergic receptors?

✔1. Ephedrine. {**True: Ephedrine is a mixed-acting agonist, which acts on both α and β receptors.**}

2. Isoproterenol. {**False: Isoproterenol stimulates β receptors.**}

✔3. Epinephrine. {**True**}

4. Methoxamine. {**False: Methoxamine binds primarily to α receptors.**}

6.8 The correct answer is D (4).
Administration of low doses of norepinephrine produces a decrease in heart rate. Which one of the following statements best explains this observation?

1. Norepinephrine decreases the peripheral resistance. {**False: Norepinephrine interacts with α receptors to produce peripheral vasoconstriction and an increase in peripheral resistance.**}

2. Norepinephrine activates β_2 receptors. {**False: Norepinephrine has a low affinity for β_2 receptors.**}

3. Norepinephrine directly decreases the heart rate. {**False: Norepinephrine stimulates the isolated heart muscle.**}

✓4. Norepinephrine activates a vagal reflex that decreases the heart rate. {**True: Norepinephrine causes a vasoconstriction that leads to an increase in blood pressure, which triggers a parasympathetic slowing of the heart.**}

Chapter 7: ADRENERGIC ANTAGONISTS

7.1 The correct answer is B (1,3).
Which of the following drugs decrease(s) airway resistance?

✓1. Epinephrine. {**True: Epinephrine causes a powerful bronchodilating effect by direct action on β_2 receptors of bronchial smooth muscle.**}

2. Prazosin. {**False: Prazosin blocks α_1 receptors and does not have significant bronchoconstriction effects.**}

✓3. Terbutaline. {**True: Terbutaline is a selective β_2 agonist with bronchodilation properties.**}

4. Propranolol. {**False: Propranolol blocks β_2 receptors in the lung causing bronchoconstriction.**}

7.2 The correct answer is D (4).
Systolic pressure is decreased after the injection of which of the following drugs?

1. Phenylephrine. {**False: Phenylephrine is a pure vasoconstrictor and raises systolic and diastolic blood pressures.**}

2. Dopamine. {**False: Dopamine raises systolic and diastolic blood pressures by stimulating the heart and (at high doses) causing vasoconstriction.**}

3. Ephedrine. {**False: Ephedrine raises systolic and diastolic blood pressures by vasoconstriction and cardiac stimulation.**}

✓4. Reserpine. {**True: Reserpine blocks the uptake of norepinephrine into intracellular storage vesicles, resulting in depletion of norepinephrine and gradual decline in blood pressure.**}

7.3 The correct answer is B (1,3).
Which of the following no longer causes an increase in blood pressure after the chronic administration of reserpine?

✓1. Tyramine. {**True: Tyramine is an indirect-acting adrenergic agonist that releases norepinephrine from storage vesicles. Reserpine blocks the uptake of norepinephrine into intracellular storage vesicles**

resulting in depletion of norepinephrine; reserpine thus abolished the effect of tyramine.**}

2. Ephedrine. {**False: Ephedrine is a mixed-action adrenergic agent, releasing stored norepinephrine from nerve endings and stimulating α, β_1, and β_2 receptors directly. The direct-acting effects are not abolished by reserpine, and a modest increase in blood pressure is observed.**}

✓3. Amphetamine. {**True: Amphetamine, like tyramine, is an indirect-acting agonist that is without effect if intracellular storage vesicles have been deleted by reserpine.**}

4. Norepinephrine. {**False: Norepinephrine is a direct-acting agonist that is unaffected by administration of reserpine.**}

7.4 The correct answer is E (1,2,3,4).
In a cocaine abuser, which of the following drugs is ineffective in causing vascular actions?

✓1. Reserpine. {**True: Reserpine blocks the uptake of norepinephrine into intracellular storage vesicles; cocaine blocks the uptake of norepinephrine by the plasma membrane of the neuron. Thus, chronic administration of cocaine depletes the storage vesicles of norepinephrine, and the effect of reserpine is abolished.**}

✓2. Tyramine. {**True: Tyramine is an indirect-acting adrenergic agonist that releases norepinephrine from storage vesicle; cocaine blocks the uptake of norepinephrine into the neuron and abolishes the effect of tyramine.**}

✓3. Clonidine. {**True: Clonidine acts through α_2 receptors to decrease release of norepinephrine. The chronic administration of cocaine depletes the storage vesicles of norepinephrine, and the effect of clonidine is abolished.**}

✓4. Guanethidine. {**True: Guanethidine inhibits release of norepinephrine from storage vesicles. If the vesicles have been depleted by the action of cocaine, guanethidine has little additional effect.**}

7.5 The correct answer is E (1,2,3,4).
Which of the following drugs interferes with micturition in the elderly male?

✓1. Atropine. {**True: Atropine blocks parasympathetic impulses at the bladder and has the same effects as stimulation of the sympathetic system with an α-adrenergic agonist, that is, relaxation of the detrusor muscle and an increase in tone of the trigone muscle of the bladder.**}

✓2. Cocaine. {**True: Cocaine prevents uptake of catecholamines, thus prolonging their action; this can lead to relaxation of the detrusor muscle of the bladder**

(β effect) and contraction of the sphincter muscles (α effect), which in turn can lead to difficulty in urination.}

✓3. Ephedrine. {**True: Ephedrine relaxes detrusor muscle and contracts the trigone and sphincter muscles of the bladder resulting in loss of bladder tone and decreased frequency of micturition.**}

✓4. Amphetamine. {**True: Contraction of sphincter of urinary bladder is marked, causing difficulties in urination.**}

7.6 The correct answer is C (2,4).
Which of the following dilate the pupil and decrease intraocular pressure?

1. Atropine. {**False: Atropine dilates the pupil, but it has little effect on intraocular pressure, except in the patient with narrow-angle glaucoma, where the pressure may increase.**}

✓2. Timolol. {**True: Timolol is a β-adrenergic blocker that decreases the secretion of aqueous humor by the ciliary body.**}

3. Pilocarpine. {**False: Pilocarpine contracts the pupil but does decrease the intraocular pressure and is the drug of choice for treatment of glaucoma; see Chapter 2.**}

✓4. Phenylephrine. {**True: Phenylephrine dilates the pupil and lowers intraocular pressure by its local vasoconstrictor action.**}

7.7 The correct answer is C (2,4).
Reflex bradycardia occurs by the use of which of the following drugs?

1. Phentolamine. {**False: Phentolamine is an α blocker that causes hypotension, which may set off reflex tachycardia.**}

✓2. Phenylephrine. {**True: Phenylephrine is an α_1 agonist, which causes vasoconstrictor that can induce a reflex bradycardia.**}

3. Phenoxybenzamine. {**False: Phenoxybenzamine is an α blocker that causes hypotension, which may set off reflex tachycardia.**}

✓4. Norepinephrine. {**True: Norepinephrine causes an increase in peripheral resistance, which can cause a bradycardia.**}

7.8 The correct answer is B (1,3).
Which of the following drugs antagonize(s) the bronchodilating effects of isoproterenol?

✓1. Labetalol. {**True: Labetalol is a nonspecific β blocker that can compete with isoproterenol for β_2 receptors on the bronchioles.**}

2. Phentolamine. {**False: Phentolamine is an α blocker that has minimal effects on the bronchioles.**}

✓3. Propranolol. {**True: Propranolol is a nonspecific β blocker that can compete with isoproterenol for β_2 receptors on the bronchioles.**}

4. Phenylephrine. {**False: Phenylephrine is an α_1 agonist that has minimal effects on the bronchioles.**}

7.9 The correct answer is C (2,4).
Which of the following groups of drugs is/are in correct order of DECREASING affinity for β receptors?

1. Epinephrine > norepinephrine > isoproterenol. {**False: Isoproterenol is more potent at β receptors than is epinephrine or norepinephrine.**}

✓2. Isoproterenol > epinephrine > norepinephrine. {**True: see above.**}

3. Phenylephrine > epinephrine > terbutaline. {**False: Phenylephrine is an α_1-specific agonist; epinephrine acts at both α and β, whereas terbutaline is a strong β_2-specific agonist.**}

✓4. Propranolol > prazosin = phentolamine. {**True: Propranolol is a strong β blocker, whereas prazosin and phentolamine interact preferentially with α_1 receptors.**}

7.10 The correct answer is D (4).
Which of the following drugs is useful in treating tachycardia?

1. Phenoxybenzamine. {**False: Phenoxybenzamine blocks α receptors and prevents vasoconstriction of peripheral blood vessel by endogenous catecholamines. This leads to a decrease in blood pressure and peripheral resistance, which causes a reflex tachycardia.**}

2. Isoproterenol. {**False: Isoproterenol is a potent β agonist, which promotes tachycardia.**}

3. Phentolamine. {**False: Phentolamine is an α blocker that causes hypotension, which may set off reflex tachycardia.**}

✓4. Propranolol. {**True: Propranolol is a specific β blocker, which interferes with β_1 receptors on the heart, causing bradycardia, that is, a slowing of the heart rate.**}

7.11 The correct answer is E (1,2,3,4).
Which of the following statements are true?

✓1. The administration of epinephrine after pretreatment with phenoxybenzamine causes vasodilation. {**True**}

✓2. Blockage of α receptors with phentolamine can be overcome by increasing the concentration of agonist. {**True**}

✓3. Atropine causes mydriasis by blocking the parasympathetic impulses to the sphincter muscle of the iris. {**True**}

✓4. Guanethidine decreases the blood pressure response to amphetamine. {**True**}

Chapter 8: TREATMENT OF PARKINSON'S DISEASE

8.1 The correct answer is D.
Which of the following statements is correct?

A. Chlorpromazine is indicated in treating the nausea of levodopa treatment. {**False: Chlorpromazine blocks the dopamine-receptor site in the brain and therefore blocks the beneficial effects of levodopa.**}

B. Vitamin B_6 increases the effectiveness of levodopa. {**False: Vitamin B_6 (pyridoxine) enhances the peripheral decarboxylation of levodopa.**}

C. Administration of dopamine is an effective treatment of Parkinson's disease. {**False: Dopamine itself does not cross the blood-brain barrier.**}

✔D. Levodopa-induced nausea is reduced by carbidopa. {**True: Carbidopa inhibits the peripheral decarboxylation of levodopa, permitting lower dosage.**}

E. Nonspecific MAO-inhibitors, such a phenelzine, are a useful adjunct to levodopa therapy. {**False: Phenelzine inhibits the metabolism of norepinephrine and serotonin and may produce a hypertensive crisis.**}

8.2 The correct answer is A.
Which of the following statements is INCORRECT?

✔A. Parkinsonian patients are characterized by an increased ratio of dopaminergic/cholinergic activity in the neostriatum. {**Correct choice: Parkinsonian patients show a deficiency of dopaminergic neurons, without a decrease in cholinergic actions.**}

B. Overtreatment of Parkinson's disease can result in the symptoms of psychosis. {**Incorrect choice: Elevated levels of dopamine can lead to behavorial disorders.**}

C. Diets rich in protein may decrease the effects of L-dopa. {**Incorrect choice: Levodopa and large, neutral amino acids share a transport system that is needed to enter the brain. Thus, high protein diets may lead to elevated levels of circulating amino acids, resulting in a decrease in levodopa uptake.**}

D. Dyskinesia is the most important side effect of levodopa. {**Incorrect choice: Dyskinesia is usually seen with longer term therapy and is dose-related and reversible.**}

E. Treatment with deprenyl can delay the onset of parkinsonian symptoms. {**Incorrect choice: The mechanism for this effect is unclear**}

8.3 The correct answer is D.
All of the following statements are correct EXCEPT:

A. Atropine blocks cholinergic pathway in the neostriatum. {**Incorrect choice**}

B. Deprenyl inhibits monoamine oxidase B and increases dopamine levels in the brain. {**Incorrect choice**}

C. Bromocriptine directly activates dopaminergic receptors. {**Incorrect choice**}

✔D. Amantadine inhibits the metabolism of levodopa. {**Correct choice: The mechanism of action is unknown.**}

E. Antimuscarinic agents are generally less efficacious then levodopa in the treatment of Parkinson's disease. {**Incorrect choice**}

Chapter 9: ANXIOLYTIC AND HYPNOTIC DRUGS

9.1 The correct answer is D.
Which of the following statements is correct?

A. Benzodiazepines directly open chloride channels. {**False: Benzodiazepines enhance the binding of GABA, which increases the permeability of chloride.**}

B. Benzodiazepines show analgesic actions. {**False: The benzodiazepines do not relieve pain but may reduce the anxiety associated with pain.**}

C. Clinical improvement of anxiety requires 2–4 weeks of treatment with benzodiazepines. {**False: Unlike the tricyclic antidepressants and the MAO-inhibitors, the benzodiazepines are effective within hours of administration.**}

✔D. All benzodiazepines have some sedative effects. {**True: However, only selected benzodiazepines are useful as hypnotics in the treatment of sleep disorders.**}

E. Benzodiazepines, like other CNS depressants, readily produced general anesthesia. {**False: Benzodiazepines do not produce general anesthesia and are, therefore, relatively safe drugs with a high therapeutic index.**}

9.2 The correct answer is B.
All of the following respond to treatment with benzodiazepines EXCEPT:

A. Tetanus. {**Incorrect choice: Diazepam is the drug of choice in treating the skeletal muscle spasticity characteristic of tetanus.**}

✔B. Schizophrenia. {**Correct choice: Benzodiazepines have no antipsychotic activity.**}

C. Epileptic seizure. {**Incorrect choice: Diazepam is the drug of choice for terminating a seizure.**}

D. Insomnia. {**Incorrect choice: Benzodiazepines are useful in the short-term treatment of insomnia.**}

E. Anxiety. {**Incorrect choice: The benzodiazepines are the drugs of choice in treating anxiety.**}

9.3 The correct answer is D.
Which of the following is a short-acting hypnotic?

A. Phenobarbital. {**False**}

B. Diazepam. {**False**}

C. Chlordiazepoxide. {**False**}

✔D. Thiopental. {**True: Thiopental is an ultra–short-acting drug used as an adjuvant to anesthesia.**}

E. Flurazepam. {**False.**}

9.4 The correct answer is D.
Which of the following statements is correct?

A. Phenobarbital shows analgesic properties. {**False: Phenobarbital is unable to alter the pain threshold.**}

B. Diazepam and phenobarbital induce the P-450 enzyme system. {**False: Only phenobarbital strongly induces the synthesis of hepatic cytochrome P-450 drug metabolizing system.**}

C. Phenobarbital is useful in the treatment of acute intermittent porphyria. {**False: Phenobarbital is contraindicated.**}

✔D. Phenobarbital induces respiratory depression, which is enhanced by the consumption of ethanol. {**True.**}

E. Buspirone has actions similar to the benzodiazepines. {**False: Buspirone lacks the anticonvulsant and muscle-relaxant properties of the benzodiazepines and causes only minimal sedation.**}

9.5 The correct answer is A.
Which of the following benzodiazepines shows the greatest potential for "rebound insomnia" after discontinuance of long-term treatment?

✔A. Triazolam. {**True: Triazolam and lorazepam are potent, short-acting agents, discontinuance of which often result in insomnia.**}

B. Flurazepam. {**False: Flurazepam and quazepam are low-potency, long-acting agents with little tendency to cause sleep problems on discontinuance of the drugs.**}

C. Alprazolam. {**False**}

D. Temazepam. {**False**}

E. Diazepam. {**False**}

9.6 The correct answer is E.
Which of the following statements is correct?

A. Ethanol at intoxicating levels shows first-order metabolism. {**False: Alcohol dehydrogenase is saturated at blood levels of alcohol observed during intoxication, and alchohol shows zero-order kinetics of elimination.**}

B. Respiratory depression induced by high doses of barbiturates can be treated by administration of ethanol. {**False: These are synergistic CNS depressants.**}

C. Disulfiram stimulates the oxidation of acetaldehyde. {**False: Disulfiram inhibits the conversion of acetaldehyde to acetate, leading to the toxic accumulation of acetaldehyde in individuals ingesting ethanol.**}

D. Benzodiazepines do not cause physical dependence. {**False: Physical dependence can develop as a result of long-term therapy.**}

✔E. Benzodiazepines can be used to treat the symptoms of withdrawal in the chronic alcoholic. {**True**}

Chapter 10: CNS STIMULANTS

10.1 The correct answer is D.
Which of the follow is NOT characteristic of cocaine overdosage?

A. Dilation of the pupil. {**Incorrect choice**}

B. Euphoria. {**Incorrect choice**}

C. Tachycardia. {**Incorrect choice**}

✔D. Peripheral vasodilation. {**False: Cocaine causes peripheral vasoconstriction.**}

E. Hallucinations. {**Incorrect choice**}

10.2 The correct answer is D.
Which of the following statements about amphetamine is INCORRECT?

A. Overdosage of amphetamine can be managed with chlorpromazine. {**Incorrect choice: Chlorpromazine relieves the CNS symptoms and the hypertension because of its α-blocking effects**}

✔B. Amphetamine is used as an adjunct with MAO inhibitors. {**Correct choice: Amphetamines should not be used in patients receiving MAO inhibitors, since amphetamine itself weakly inhibits MAO.**}

C. Amphetamine has a longer duration of action than cocaine. {**Incorrect choice: The euphoria caused by amphetamine lasts 4–6 hours, or four to eight times longer than the effects of cocaine.**}

D. Amphetamine depresses the hunger center in the hypothalamus. {**Incorrect choice.**}

E. Amphetamine acts on α- and β-adrenergic presynaptic terminals. {**Incorrect choice.**}

10.3 The correct answer is E.
Which of the following statements concerning tetrahydrocannabinol (THC) is correct?

A. THC decreases heart rate. {**False**}

B. THC increases muscle strength. {**False**}

C. THC decreases appetite. {**False**}

D. THC causes hypotension. {**False.**}

✔E. THC has antiemetic action. {**True: THC is sometimes used to treat the severe emesis caused by cancer chemotherapeutic agents.**}

10.4 The correct answer is A (1,2,3).
Phencyclidine

✔1. produces dissociative anesthesia. {**True**}
✔2. is an analog of ketamine. {**True**}
✔3. can cause hostile and bizarre behavior. {**True**}
   4. is nonaddicting. {**False**}

10.5 The correct answer is A (1,2,3).
Which of the follow drugs is/are correctly paired with their toxic effects?

✔1. Amphetamine: Paranoid psychosis. {**True: This state resembles schizophrenia.**}
✔2. Cocaine: Anxiety and depression. {**True.**}
✔3. LSD: Hallucinations. {**True.**}
   4. Nicotine (low doses): Decreased heart rate and blood pressure. {**False: Nicotine activates the sympathetic nervous system and causes hypertension and tachycardia.**}

Chapter 11: ANESTHETICS

11.1 The correct answer is E (1,2,3,4).
Which of the following statements is/are correct?

✔1. The more soluble the anesthetic gas, the slower it achieves equilibrium and the longer the induction time. {**True**}
✔2. Recovery is rapid from poorly soluble anesthetic gases and prolonged with agents having high blood solubility. {**True**}
✔3. Termination of anesthetic action of thiopental is primarily caused by redistribution of the drug from the brain to other tissues, particularly muscle. {**True**}
✔4. The more lipid soluble an anesthetic, the lower the concentration of anesthetic needed to produce anesthesia. {**True.**}

11.2 The correct answer is C (2,4).
Which of the following statements is/are correct?

   1. The potency of an anesthetic is proportional to the minimal anesthetic concentrations (MAC). {**False: The potency is inversely related to the MAC.**}
✔2. Induction and recovery are rapid with nitrous oxide. {**True: The solubility of nitrous oxide is low, which promotes a rapid entry and loss from the brain.**}
   3. Nitrous oxide is often used as a single agent in anesthesia. {**False: Nitrous oxide is most often used as a supplement to other anesthetics. In dental anesthesia, it is used alone.**}
✔4. Halothane with a MAC of 0.76% is more potent than nitrous oxide with MAC of 100%. {**True**}

11.3 The correct answer is A (1,2,3).
Which of the following statements concerning ketamine is/are correct?

✔1. Ketamine is used mainly for children and young adults for short diagnostic procedures. {**True**}
✔2. Ketamine produce analgesia without unconsciousness. {**True: Ketamine induces a dissociative state in which the patient appears awake but is unconscious and does not feel pain.**}
✔3. Ketamine produces a high incidence of post-anesthetic hallucinations. {**True**}
   4. Ketamine inhibits the central sympathetic outflow. {**False: Ketamine stimulates sympathetic outflow, causing stimulation of the heart and increased blood pressure and cardiac output.**}

11.4 The correct answer is E.
Which of the following anesthetics is most likely to require administration of a muscle relaxant?

   A. Ethyl ether. {**False: Ether produces good muscle relaxation.**}
   B. Halothane. {**False: Halothane produces moderate muscle relaxation.**}
   C. Methoxyflurane. {**False: Methoxyflurane produces good muscle relaxation.**}
   D. Benzodiazepines. {**False: Benzodiazepine produce good muscle relaxation.**}
✔E. Nitrous oxide. {**True: Nitrous oxide has virtually no muscle relaxing properties.**}

11.5 The correct answer is D.
Which of the following anesthetics exhibits the shortest induction time when each agent is administered at a concentration that ultimately produces surgical anesthesia?

   A. Ethyl ether. {**False**}
   B. Halothane. {**False**}
   C. Methoxyflurane. {**False**}
✔D. Nitrous oxide. {**True: Because of its low solubility, nitrous oxide rapidly saturates arterial blood reaching the brain.**}
   E. Benzodiazepine. {**False**}

11.6 The correct answer is C.
Which of the following statements is true?

   A. Halothane produces anesthesia within 1–2 minutes of administration. {**False: Halothane shows a slow onset of action because of its high solubility in blood.**}
   B. Thiopental is commonly used as single agent for anesthesia. {**False: Thiopental requires other agents for either neuromuscular paralysis or analgesia.**}

C. Halothane as well as thiopental produce depression of cardiovascular and respiratory system. {True}

D. Halothane is often hepatotoxic in pediatric patients. {False: Halothane is not extensively metabolized in pediatric patients, thus minimizing the potential for formation of toxic products.}

E. Halothane has less potential for hepatotoxicity than isoflurane. {False: Halothane shows more biotransformation than isoflurane and thus has greater potential for hepatotoxicity.}

Chapter 12: ANTIDEPRESSANT DRUGS

12.1 The correct answer is C.
Which one of following is an appropriate therapeutic use for imipramine?

A. Insomnia. {False: Benzodiazepines, such as flurazepam, are preferred.}

B. Epilepsy. {False.}

C. Bed-wetting in children. {True: Imipramine can be used with caution to contract the internal sphincter of the bladder.}

D. Glaucoma. {False.}

E. Mania. {False: Lithium is preferred.}

12.2 The correct answer is D.
MAO inhibitors are contraindicated with all of the following EXCEPT:

A. Indirect adrenergic agents, such as ephedrine. {Incorrect choice: Hypertensive crisis may result from use (concurrently or within 2 weeks) of MAO inhibitors and indirect sympathomimetic amines.}

B. Tricyclic antidepressants. {Incorrect choice: Mutual enhancement of effects with possibility of hyperpyrexia, hypertension, seizures, and death are possible.}

C. Beer and cheese. {Incorrect choice: Tyramine-containing foods, such as aged cheeses and beer, may precipitate a hypotensive crisis because of the accumulation and release of stored catecholamines from nerve terminals.}

D. Aspirin. {Correct choice: MAO inhibitors and aspirin can be take concurrently.}

E. Dopamine. {Incorrect choice: MAO inhibitors may lead to exaggerated response to dopamine.}

12.3 The correct answer is A.
Which of the following statements concerning tricyclic antidepressants is correct?

A. All the tricyclic antidepressants show similar therapeutic efficacy. {True: The choice of drug depends on the tolerance of side effects and the duration of action.}

B. Hypertension is a common adverse effect. {False: Orthostatic hypotension is a side effect.}

C. The tricyclic antidepressants selectively inhibit uptake of norepinephrine into the neuron. {False: Tricyclic antidepressants nonspecifically block the uptake of epinephrine and serotonin.}

D. These drugs show an immediate therapeutic effect. {False: The onset of the mood elevation is slow, requiring 2 weeks or longer.}

E. These drugs must be administered intramuscularly. {False: These drugs are usually given orally.}

Chapter 13 NEUROLEPTIC DRUGS

13.1 The correct answer is B.
The neuroleptic drugs

A. show a wide range of efficacy in treating schizophrenia. {False: Although the potency of the drugs vary, the efficacy of the antipsychotic agents are similar.}

B. all show the potential for causing tardive dyskinesia. {True: Tardive dyskinesia appears to be produced to the same degree and frequency by all the neuroleptic drugs when used in equieffective antipsychotic doses.}

C. bind selectively to D_2-dopaminergic receptors. {False: Most of the neuroleptic drugs block both D_1 and D_2 dopaminergic receptors.}

D. are useful in the treatment of epilepsy. {False: The neuroleptics can aggravate epilepsy.}

E. show antipsychotic effects immediately on administration. {False: The antipsychotic effects occurs after several weeks of administration.}

13.2 The correct answer is D (4).
The neuroleptic drugs

A. cause altered mental acuity. {False: The neuroleptics do not depress intellectual function of the patient.}

B. all cause similar extrapyramidal effects. {False: The tendency to produce motor disorders varies widely.}

C. are highly addictive. {False: The neuroleptic drugs produce some tolerance but little physical dependence.}

✔D. can produce orthostatic hypotension. {True: The neuroleptics block α-adrenergic receptors, resulting in low blood pressure.}

E. are excreted unchanged. {False: Most are metabolized by the cytochrome P-450 system.}

13.3 The correct answer is D.
All of the following are observed in patients taking neuroleptic agents EXCEPT:

A. Drowsiness. {Incorrect choice: Drowsiness is usually seen during the first 2 weeks of treatment.}

B. Hypotension. {Incorrect choice: Orthostatic hypotension is commonly observed.}

C. Altered endocrine function. {Incorrect choice: The neuroleptics depress the hypothalamus, causing amenorrhea, galactorrhea, infertility, and impotence.}

✔D. Diarrhea. {Correct choice: Anticholinergic actions of the neuroleptic drugs often produce constipation.}

E. Urinary retention. {Incorrect choice: This is commonly observed.}

13.4 The correct answer is A.
Which of the following is a therapeutic application of the neuroleptic agents?

✔A. Acute mania. {True: Neuroleptics are useful in psychotic disorders with acute agitation.}

B. Motion sickness. {False: Scopolamine is the drug of choice for treatment of motion sickness.}

C. Glaucoma. {False}

D. Insomnia. {False: Administration of the powerful antipsychotic drugs just for sleep problems is not good practice.}

E. Hypertension. {False}

Chapter 14: OPIOID ANALGESICS AND ANTAGONISTS

14.1 The correct answer is C (2,4).
Which of the following are actions of morphine that do not develop tolerance?

1. Respiratory depression. {False}
✔2. Pinpoint pupils. {True}
3. Euphoria. {False}
✔4. Constipation. {True}

14.2 The correct answer is B (1,3).
Codeine

✔1. is more effective than morphine in suppressing the cough reflex. {True}

2. is equivalent to morphine in producing euphoria. {False: Codeine produces less euphoria and rarely produces addiction.}

✔3. is a much less potent analgesic than morphine. {True}

4. is a synthetic opioid. {False: Codeine is obtained from the opium poppy.}

14.3 The correct answer is C (2,4).
Naloxone

1. produces respiratory depression in individuals who have not previously taken opioids. {False: Naloxone has no pharmacological effects in normal individuals.}

✔2. antagonizes the actions of morphine. {True: Naloxone is used to reverse the coma and respiratory depression of opioid overdose.}

3. has a short (10–15 minutes) duration of action. {False: The effects of naloxone last several hours}

✔4. can prompt the appearance of withdrawal symptoms in the heroin addict. {True: Naloxone blocks the effects of opioids and induces withdrawal.}

14.4 The correct answer is A.
All of the following statements concerning methadone are correct EXCEPT:

✔A. It has less potent analgesic activity than that of morphine. {Correct choice: Methadone shows an analgesic action similar to that of morphine.}

B. It has a longer duration of action than that of morphine. {Incorrect choice: Methadone is effective for 15–20 hours whereas morphine act for 4–6 hours.}

C. It is effective by oral administration. {Incorrect choice: This is one of the major advantages of using methadone in the controlled withdrawal of heroin and morphine abuser.}

D. Methadone causes a milder withdrawal syndrome than morphine. {Incorrect choice}

E. It has its greatest action on μ receptors. {**Incorrect choice**}

14.5 The correct answer is D.

Which of the following statements about pentazocine is INCORRECT?

A. It is a mixed agonist-antagonist. {**Incorrect choice: Pentazocine acts as an agonist on K receptors and μ receptors, but it is an antagonist at μ and δ receptors.**}

B. It may be administered orally or parenterally. {**Incorrect choice**}

C. It produces less euphoria than morphine. {**Incorrect choice**}

✓D. It is often combined with morphine for maximal analgesic effects. {**Correct choice: Pentazocine (a mixed agnonist-antagonist) should not be used with agonists, such as morphine, since it can block their actions.**}

E. High doses of pentazocine increase blood pressure. {**Incorrect choice.**}

14.6 The correct answer is A.

Which of the following statements about morphine is INCORRECT?

✓A. It is used therapeutically to relieve pain caused by severe head injury. {**Correct choice: Morphine cause increased the cerebrospinal fluid pressure secondary to dilation of cerebral vasculature.**}

B. Its withdrawal symptoms can be relieved by methadone. {**Incorrect choice: Opioid drugs show cross sensitivity.**}

C. It causes constipation. {**Incorrect choice**}

D. It is most effective by parenteral administration. {**Incorrect choice: Absorption from the gastrointestinal tract is unreliable.**}

E. It rapidly enters all body tissues, including the fetus of a pregnant woman. {**Incorrect choice**}

Chapter 15: DRUGS USED TO TREAT EPILEPSY

15.1 The correct answer is A (1,2,3).

Which of the following correctly pairs an antiepileptic drug with its therapeutic indication?

✓1. Ethosuximide: Absence seizures. {**True**}

✓2. Phenobarbital: Febrile seizures in children. {**True**}

✓3. Diazepam: Status epilepticus. {**True**}

4. Phenytoin: Absence seizures. {**False**}

15.2 The correct answer is E (1,2,3,4).

Which of the following statements concerning phenytoin is/are correct?

✓1. Phenytoin causes less sedation than phenobarbital. {**True**}

✓2. Phenytoin is not indicated for children under 5 years of age. {**True: Coarsening of facial features occurs in children.**}

✓3. Phenytoin is not effective for absence seizure. {**True: Phenytoin is not ineffective but may increase the severity of absence seizures.**}

✓4. The plasma half-life increased as the dose is increased. {**True: Saturation of hepatic metabolizing enzymes at high doses leads to a decrease in half-life.**}

15.3 The correct answer is B (1,3).

Which of the following drugs are useful in treating complex partial seizures?

✓1. Phenytoin. {**True**}

2. Phenobarbital. {**False**}

✓3. Carbamazepine. {**True**}

4. Valproic acid. {**False**}

Chapter 16: TREATMENT OF CONGESTIVE HEART FAILURE

16.1 The correct answer is A.

Which of the following most directly describes the mechanism of action of digitalis?

✓A. Inhibits sodium-potassium ATPase. {**True: The cardiac glycosides bind to and block the action of this energy-dependent pump.**}

B. Decreases intracellular sodium concentration. {**False: The cardiac glycosides inhibit the extrusion of sodium from the cell, leading to an increase in sodium levels within the cell.**}

C. Increases the intracellular level of ATP. {**False: The production of ATP is not significantly changed in the treated heart.**}

D. Stimulates the production of cAMP. {**False: This is the mechanism of action of the β-adrenergic agonists.**}

E. Decreases release of calcium from the sarcoplasmic reticulum. {**False: By increasing intracellular calcium, digitalis stimulates the SR to release additional calcium.**}

16.2 The correct answer is E.
All of the following are therapeutically useful in the treatment of congestive heart failure EXCEPT:

A. a vasodilator such as hydralazine. {**Incorrect choice: Hydralazine is a vasodilator and can reduce venous return (preload) to the heart.**}
B. a cardiac glycoside such as digoxin. {**Incorrect choice: Digoxin and other cardiac glycosides increase the contractility of the myocardium.**}
C. a β-adrenergic agonist such as norepinephrine. {**Incorrect choice: Norepinephrine acting through β₁ receptors of the heart exerts a positive inotropic effect.**}
D. a diuretic such as hydrochlorothiazide. {**Incorrect choice: Hydrochlorothiazide is a diuretic effective in reducing water retention associated with heart failure.**}
✔E. a β blocker like propranolol. {**Correct choice: Propranolol is a β blocker and would diminish the inotropic effects of intrinsic catecholamines.**}

16.3 The correct answer is E.
All of the following are useful in the treatment of digitalis overdose EXCEPT:

A. Digoxin immune FAB fragment. {**Incorrect choice: Purified fragments of antibodies specific for digoxin or digitoxin are used to treat potentially lethal toxicities.**}
B. Dietary potassium supplements for patients being treated concomitantly with diuretics. {**Incorrect choice: Hypokalemia is frequently encountered in individuals taking loop or thiazide diuretics and can predispose the patient to digitalis toxicity.**}
C. Lidocaine. {**Incorrect choice: Antiarrhythmic drugs are used for ventricular tachycardia.**}
D. Phenytoin. {**Incorrect choice: Antiarrhythmic drugs are used for ventricular tachycardia.**}
✔E. Quinidine. {**Correct choice: Quinidine may increase digitalis concentration by reducing renal clearance.**}

16.4 The correct answer is A (1,2,3).
Which of the following statements is/are correct?

✔1. Digoxin is more widely used than digitoxin because it has a shorter half-life. {**True**}
✔2. Serum levels of digoxin can be increased by quinidine. {**True**}
✔3. Digitoxin is used in patients with renal insufficiency. {**True**}

4. Digoxin is eliminated primarily in the bile. {**False: Digoxin is eliminated in the urine, whereas digitoxin is eliminated primarily in the bile.**}

16.5 The correct answer is C (2,4).
Which of the following aggravates a digitalis-induced arrhythmia?

1. Decreased serum calcium. {**False: Low levels of circulating calcium diminish the digitalis-stimulated calcium uptake into the cardiac cell.**}
✔2. Increasing heart rate with epinephrine. {**True: Agents that increase the heart rate enhance the toxicity of digitalis.**}
3. Decreased serum sodium. {**False: Low serum sodium enhances the efflux of sodium from the cardiac cell, leading to a diminished sodium-calcium exchange.**}
✔4. Decreased serum potassium. {**True: Low serum potassium further decreases the efflux of sodium from the cardiac cell, leading to an enhanced toxicity.**}

Chapter 17: ANTIARRHYTHMIC DRUGS

17.1 The correct answer is E.
All of the following pairs correctly match a drug with its action EXCEPT:

A. Quinidine: Blocks Na⁺ channels. {**Incorrect choice: All type I drugs interfere with sodium entry.**}
B. Bretylium: Blocks K⁺ channels. {**Incorrect choice**}
C. Verapamil: Blocks Ca⁺⁺ channels. {**Incorrect choice.**}
D. Propranolol: Blocks β adrenoceptors. {**Incorrect choice.**}
✔E. Procainamide: Blocks K⁺ channels. {**Correct choice: Procainamide blocks Na⁺ channels.**}

17.2 The correct answer is B.
Which one of the following statements is INCORRECT?

A. Lidocaine must be given parenterally. {**Incorrect choice: Lidocaine is given intravenously because of extensive first-pass transformation by the liver, which precludes oral administration.**}
✔B. Lidocaine is used mainly for atrial arrhythmias. {**Correct choice: Lidocaine is useful in treating ventricular arrhythmias.**}
C. Procainamide is associated with a reversible lupus phenomenon. {**Incorrect choice**}
D. Quinidine is active orally. {**Incorrect choice**}
E. All antiarrhythmic drugs can suppress cardiac contractions. {**Incorrect choice: All the antiarrhythmic drugs can exert a negative inotropic effect.**}

17.3 The correct answer is C.
Which one of the following statements is INCORRECT?

A. Quinidine prolongs repolarization and the effective refractory period. {**Incorrect choice**}
B. Mexiletine shortens repolarization and decreases the effective refractory period. {**Incorrect choice**}
✔C. Propranolol increases Phase 4 depolarization. {**Correct choice: Propranolol decreases Phase 4 depolarization.**}
D. Verapamil shortens the duration of the action potential. {**Incorrect choice**}
E. Amiodarone prolongs repolarization. {**Incorrect choice**}

17.4 The correct answer is A.
Antiarrhythmic drugs

✔A. may act by converting unidirectional block to a bidirectional block. {**True: A bidirectional block can decrease arrhythmias caused by reentry.**}
B. often cause an increase in cardiac output. {**False: All of the antiarrhythmic drugs exert some negative inotropic effect and decrease cardiac output.**}
C. as a group have mild side effects. {**False: the side effects are serious and include arrhythmias that can lead to sudden death.**}
D. all affect Na^+ channels in the cell membrane. {**False: Some antiarrhythmic drugs affect K^+ or Ca^{++} channels, or β adrenoreceptors.**}
E. are equally useful in atrial and ventricular arrhythmias. {**False: Although some antiarrhythmic drugs, such as quinidine, are useful in treating a wide variety of arrhythmias, most of these drugs have specific indications.**}

Chapter 18: ANTIANGINAL DRUGS

18.1 The correct answer is C.
The β adrenergic blockers, such as propranolol, are contraindicated as a treatment of angina in patients with all of the following conditions EXCEPT:

A. Congestive heart failure. {**Incorrect choice: β Blockers reduce cardiac output and may cause inadequate systemic perfusion.**}
B. Asthma. {**Incorrect choice: Nonspecific β blockers cause bronchoconstriction, which exacerbates the asthma.**}
✔C. Hypertension. {**Correct choice: β Blockers are among the several agents commonly used in treatment of hypertension.**}
D. Insulin-dependent diabetes. {**Incorrect choice: β Blocker can potentiate hypoglycemia following insulin injection because the normal catecholamine response to low blood sugar is inhibited by a β blocker.**}
E. Peripheral vascular disease. {**Incorrect choice**}

18.2 The correct answer is D.
All of the following statements concerning nitroglycerin are correct EXCEPT:

A. It causes an elevation of intracellular cGMP. {**Incorrect choice: The increased cGMP leads to vascular smooth muscle relaxation.**}
B. It undergoes significant first-pass metabolism in the liver. {**Incorrect choice: Nitroglycerin is commonly administered sublingually or transdermally to avoid hepatic inactivation.**}
C. It may cause significant reflex tachycardia. {**Incorrect choice: Increased heart rate results from the decrease in peripheral resistance and drop in blood pressure induced by nitroglycerin.**}
✔D. It significantly decreases AV conduction. {**Correct choice: In contrast to other antianginal drugs, such as Ca^{++}-channel blockers and β-adrenergic blockers, nitroglycerin does not block impulse conduction in the heart.**}
E. It can cause postural hypotension. {**Incorrect choice.**}

18.3 The correct answer is E.
Which one of the following is most effective in treating the ischemic pain of variant angina?

A. Propranolol. {**False**}
B. Sodium nitroprusside. {**False**}
C. Atropine. {**False**}
D. Isosorbide dinitrate. {**False**}
✔E. Nifedipine. {**True: Variant angina caused by spontaneous coronary spasm responds to the vasodilation effect of nifedipine.**}

18.4 The correct answer is B.
Which one of the following adverse effects is associated with nitroglycerin?

A. Hypertension. {**False: Nitroglycerin may cause postural hypotension.**}
✔B. Throbbing headache. {**True**}
C. Bradycardia. {**False**}
D. Sexual dysfunction. {**False**}
E. Anemia. {**False**}

Chapter 19: ANTIHYPERTENSIVE DRUGS

19.1 The correct answer is A (1,2,3).
Which of the following statements is/are correct?

✔1. Cerebral hemorrhage is a common complication of severe hypertension. {**True**}
✔2. Hypertension results from increased vascular smooth muscle tone, which leads to increased arteriolar resistance and reduced capacitance of the venules. {**True**}
✔3. Prazosin is likely to produce postural hypotension. {**True**}
   4. Antihypertensive therapy is designed to relieve the symptoms of high blood pressure. {**False: The hypertensive patient is usually asymptomatic until overt organ damage has occurred.**}

19.2 The correct answer is E (1,2,3, and 4).
Administration of ACE inhibitors leads to

✔1. decreased blood pressure. {**True: Captopril lowers peripheral vascular resistance by vasodilation causing a decrease in blood pressure.**}
✔2. decreased aldosterone levels. {**True: These drugs decrease circulating levels of aldosterone, causing decreased retention of sodium and fluid and increased retention of potassium.**}
✔3. increased bradykinin. {**True: Captopril increases levels of circulating bradykinin, causing vasodilation and elevated plasma concentrations of prostaglandins.**}
✔4. increased cardiac performance. {**True: As a result of the above changes, stroke and cardiac output are improved.**}

19.3 The correct answer is D.
Which of the following patients is most suited for primary therapy with hydrochlorothiazide?

A. Patients with gout. {**False: Thiazide diuretics cause hyperuricemia and can precipitate a gouty attack in susceptible individuals.**}
B. Patients with hyperlipidemia. {**False: Thiazide diuretics increase LDL cholesterol and may increase the risk of arthrosclerosis in patients with hyperlipidemia.**}
C. Young hypertensive patients with rapid resting heart rates. {**False: Patients with evidence of elevated catecholamine are best treated with β blockers.**}
✔D. Black patients and elderly patients. {**True: Among black patients, diuretics and calcium entry blockers are more effective than ACE inhibitors or β blockers. Diuretics are effective among the elderly.**}

E. Patients with impaired renal function. {**False: Thiazides cannot promote sodium excretion when renal function is severely impaired. The loop diuretics, such as furosemide, are used in patients with impaired renal function.**}

19.4 The correct answer is C.
All of the following produce a significant decrease in peripheral resistance EXCEPT:

A. Chronic administration of diuretics. {**Incorrect choice.**}
B. Hydralazine. {**Incorrect choice: Hydralazine causes direct vasodilation resulting in a decreased peripheral resistance, which in turn, prompts a reflex elevation in heart rate and cardiac output.**}
✔C. β blocker. {**Correct: β blockers act primarily by decreasing heart rate and cardiac output.**}
D. ACE inhibitors. {**Incorrect choice: ACE inhibitors decrease peripheral resistance with little effect on heart rate or cardiac output.**}
E. Clonidine. {**Incorrect choice: Clonidine acts mainly by decreasing peripheral resistance.**}

19.5 The correct answer is C.
Which one of the following acts at central presynaptic α_2 receptors?

A. Minoxidil. {**False: Minoxidil is a direct-acting vasodilator.**}
B. Verapamil. {**False: Verapamil causes vasodilation by inhibiting calcium ion flow into smooth muscle.**}
✔C. Clonidine. {**True: Clonidine reduces sympathetic outflow by stimulating α-adrenergic receptors.**}
D. Enalapril. {**False: Enalapril blocks the enzyme that converts angiotensin I to angiotensin II.**}
E. Hydrochlorothiazide. {**False: Hydrochlorothiazide acts by decreasing blood volume.**}

Chapter 20: DRUGS AFFECTING BLOOD

20.1 The correct answer is A.

The anticoagulant activity of warfarin can be potentiated by all of the following EXCEPT:

A. Rifampin. {**False: Rifampin induces the hepatic mixed function oxidases that metabolize warfarin.**}

B. Aspirin. {**True: Platelet inhibitors increase the anti-coagulant effect of warfarin.**}

C. Phenylbutazone. {**True: Phenylbutazone can transiently increase the level of the free drug by displacing it from its plasma albumin binding site.**}

D. Cimetidine. {**True: Cimetidine inhibits warfarin metabolism and causes potentiation of the anticoagulants.**}

E. Disulfiram. {**True: Disulfiram inhibits warfarin metabolism.**}

20.2 The correct answer is C.

Which of the following statements is/are correct?

1. Aspirin does not affect prostacyclin synthesis in endothelial cells. {**False: Endothelial cyclooxygenase is inactivated by aspirin; hence, prostacyclin synthesis is inhibited. However, at low doses, aspirin preferentially inhibits platelet cyclooxygenase.**}

2. Aspirin has been shown to decrease the probability of a second myocardial infarct. {**True**}

3. The anticoagulatory effect of heparin requires 12–24 hours to develop. {**False: The effects of heparin administered intravenously are immediate.**}

4. Heparin is a major antithrombotic drug for the treatment of deep vein thrombosis and pulmonary embolism. {**True**}

20.3 The correct answer is B.

Which of the following statements concerning warfarin is/are correct?

1. Warfarin treatment results in the production of inactive clotting factors that lack γ-carboxy-glutamyl side-chains necessary for calcium binding and subsequent activation. {**True: Warfarin inhibits the vitamin K-dependent carboxylation of glutamyl residues in several of the clotting factors.**}

2. Warfarin must be given intravenously. {**False: Warfarin is readily absorbed from the gastrointestinal tract.**}

3. The anticoagulant effects of warfarin can be overcome by the administration of vitamin K. {**True: High concentrations of vitamin K are able to overcome the effects of warfarin.**}

4. Warfarin can be used to prevent the clotting of blood drawn for chemical analysis. {**False: The anticoagulant effects of warfarin require 8–12 hours after drug administration** *in vivo*.}

20.4 The correct answer is B.

Which of the following statements concerning thrombolytic agents is/are correct?

1. Hemorrhage is a major side effect. {**True: The thrombolytic agents do not distinguish between the fibrin of an unwanted thrombus and the fibrin of a beneficial hemostatic plug.**}

2. Streptokinase is a proteolytic enzyme specific for fibrin-bound plasminogen. {**False: Streptokinase is an extracellular protein with no enzyme activity, but it forms an active complex with plasminogen, which then converts uncomplexed plasminogen to the active enzyme plasmin.**}

3. Clot dissolution occurs with a higher frequency when therapy is initiated rapidly after clots begin to form. {**True: Clots becomes more resistant to lysis as they age.**}

4. Streptokinase, urokinase, and tissue plasminogen activator (tPA) are equally specific for cleavage of plasminogen bound to fibrin.. {**False: tPA is relatively more specific for plasminogen bound to fibrin. This contrasts with urokinase and streptokinase, which are active with free plasminogen and induce a more pronounced thrombolytic state.**}

20.5 The correct answer is A (1,2, 3).

Which of the following compounds promotes platelet aggregation?

1. Thromboxane A_2. {**True: Thromboxane A_2 both inhibits the cAMP pathway and stimulates the release of inositol 1,4,5-triphosphate and diacylglycerol. The latter compounds promote platelet aggregation.**}

2. ADP. {**True**}

3. Collagen. {**True**}

4. Prostacyclin. {**False: Prostacyclin binds to platelet membrane receptors, leading to an increase in intracellular cAMP and an inhibition of aggregation.**}

Chapter 21: ANTIHYPERLIPIDEMIC DRUGS

21.1 The correct answer is B.

Which one of the following is the most common side effect of antihyperlipidemic drug therapy?

A. Elevated blood pressure. {**False**}

B. Gastrointestinal disturbance. {**True**}

C. Neurological problems. {**False**}

D. Heart palpitations. {**False**}

E. Migraine headaches. {**False**}

21.2 The correct answer is A.

Which one of the following hyperlipidemias is characterized by elevated plasma levels of chylomicrons and has no drug therapy available to lower the plasma lipoprotein levels?

✔A. Type I. {**True**}

B. Type II. {**False**}

C. Type III. {**False**}

D. Type IV. {**False**}

E. Type V. {**False**}

21.3 The correct answer is D.

Which one of the following drugs decreases *de novo* cholesterol synthesis by inhibiting the enzyme 3-hydroxy-3-methylglutaryl CoA reductase?

A. Clofibrate. {**False: Clofibrate increases the activity of lipoprotein lipase, thereby increasing the removal of VLDL from the plasma.**}

B. Niacin. {**False: Niacin inhibits lipolysis in adipose tissue and thus eliminates the building blocks needed by the liver to produce triacylglycerol and therefore VLDL.**}

C. Cholestyramine. {**False: Cholestyramine lowers the amount of bile acids returning to the liver via the enterohepatic circulation.**}

✔D. Lovastatin. {**True**}

E. Pyridoxal. {**False**}

QUESTIONS 21.4–21.7

DIRECTIONS: The group of questions below consists of five drugs (A–E) followed by a list of numbered statements. For each numbered statement, select the ONE drug from the list (A–E) that is most closely associated with it. Each drug may be selected once, more than once, or not at all.

Match each drug with the statement that best describes its mode of action:

A. Niacin.

B. Clofibrate.

C. Cholestyramine.

D. Probucol.

E. Mevastatin.

21.4 {**The correct answer is C: Cholestyramine.**}

Binds bile acids in the intestine, thus preventing their return to the liver via the enterohepatic circulation.

21.5 {**The correct answer is B: Clofibrate.**}

Causes a decrease in plasma triacylglycerol levels by increasing the activity of lipoprotein lipase.

21.6 {**The correct answer is A: Niacin.**}

Causes a decrease in liver triacylglycerol synthesis by limiting available free fatty acids needed as building blocks for this pathway.

21.7 {**The correct answer is E: Mevastatin**}

Inhibits 3-hydroxy-3-methylglutaryl CoA reductase, the rate-limiting step in cholesterol synthesis.

Chapter 22: DRUGS AFFECTING THE RESPIRATORY SYSTEM

22.1 The correct answer is D.

All of the following statements regarding the treatment of asthma are true EXCEPT:

A. β_2-Specific adrenergic agonist are most effective in treating asthma. {**Incorrect choice: Bronchodilation is mediated by β_2-adrenergic receptors; activation of α and β_1 receptors produce undesired side effects.**}

B. Corticosteroids aerosols are useful in the treatment of chronic asthma. {**Incorrect choice: Drugs such as beclomethasone act directly on the bronchial tree, reversing the edema, capillary permeability, and leukotriene synthesis of inflammation.**}

C. Ipratropium is useful in patients unable to take adrenergic agonists. {**Incorrect choice**}

✔D. Cromolyn is used in treating an acute asthmatic attack. {**Correct choice: Cromolyn is an effective prophylactic agent but is not useful in managing an acute asthmatic attack.**}

E. Cromolyn prevents the release of inflammatory mediators from mast cell. {**Incorrect choice: By blocking the release of inflammatory mediator cromolyn decreases the vasoconstriction, edema, and mucous formation of asthma.**}

22.2 The correct answer is D.

All of the following statements are true EXCEPT:

A. Propranolol is contraindicated in asthma. {**Incorrect choice: Blocking β_2 receptors in the lung cause contraction of the smooth muscle in the bronchioles precipitating a respiratory crisis in patients with chronic obstructive pulmonary disease, such as asthma.**}

B. Metaproterenol produces less tachycardia than isoproterenol when both drugs are given at doses producing equal bronchodilation. {**Incorrect choice: Metaproterenol is β_2-selective, whereas isoproterenol blocks both β_1 and β_2 receptors and therefore has a**} greater tendency for tachycardia, a typical response of β_1 blockade.}

C. H_1 Histamine receptor blockers, such a diphenhydramine, are useful in treating the symptoms of allergic rhinitis. {**Incorrect choice: Many of the symptoms of rhinitis are caused by histamine-mediated actions.**}

✔D. Dextromethorphan, being a derivative of morphine, has strong analgesic properties. {**Correct choice: This derivative does not relieve pain.**}

E. Rebound nasal congestion is a common adverse effect of prolonged use of α-adrenergic agonists. {**Incorrect choice: Rebound nasal congestion is particularly common if the α-adrenergic agonist is used for more than 2–3 days.**}

Chapter 23: DIURETIC DRUGS

23.1 The correct answer is C (2,4).
Which of the following diuretics can produce hypokalemia by continued use?

1. Spironolactone. {**False: This potassium-sparing diuretic decreases K^+ secretion and can cause hyperkalemia.**}

✔2. Acetazolamide. {**True: This carbonic anhydrase inhibitor diuretic increases K^+ loss in the urine and produces hypokalemia.**}

3. Amiloride. {**False: This potassium-sparing diuretic decreases K^+ secretion and can cause hyperkalemia.**}

✔4. Hydrochlorothiazide. {**True: This thiazide diuretic increases K^+ secretion into the urine and can lead to hypokalemia.**}

23.2 The correct answer is B (1,3).
Which of the following diuretics markedly increase(s) the excretion of calcium from the body?

✔1. Acetazolamide. {**True: Urine contains increased amounts of Ca^{++} in response to carbonic anhydrase inhibition.**}

2. Chlorothiazide. {**False: Thiazides reduce urinary secretion of Ca^{++}.**}

✔3. Furosemide. {**True: This loop diuretic promotes a large increase in urinary excretion of Ca^{++}.**}

4. Spironolactone. {**False: Spironolactone has little effect on excretion of Ca^{++}.**}

23.3 The correct answer if C (2,4).
Hydrochlorothiazide can produce which of the following actions?

1. Hyperkalemia. {**False: Hypokalemia is the most frequently encountered adverse effect of thiazide treatment.**}

✔2. Hyperuricemia. {**True: Thiazides decrease the excretion of uric acid by the acid secretory system.**}

3. Increase in blood pressure. {**False: The drug is used in the treatment of hypertension.**}

✔4. Hyperglycemia in diabetic patients. {**True: Thiazide diuretics may induce hyperglycemia in diabetic patients.**}

23.4 The correct answer is A (1,2,3).
In an addisonian patient, which of the following agents would have diuretic actions?

✔1. Amiloride. {**True: Amiloride does not depend on the presence of aldosterone for its action; thus one would observe the weak diuretic action characteristic of this drug.**}

✔2. Chlorothiazide. {**True: The usual effects of this drug would be observed.**}

✔3. Triamterene. {**True: Triamterene blocks K^+-Na^+ exchange by a mechanism that does not depend on the presence of aldosterone. Thus, triamterene, unlike spironolactone, is effective in Addison's disease, that is, primary adrenal insufficiency.**}

4. Spironolactone. {**False: Spironolactone competes for aldosterone and thus the drug would have no effect in the absence of endogenous hormone.**}

23.5 The correct answer is D (4).
Hyperkalemia is observed with which of the following diuretics?

1. Chlorothiazide. {**False: Chlorothiazide is a thiazide diuretic, which increases the secretion of K^+ into the urine.**}

2. Furosemide. {**False: Furosemide is a loop diuretic, which increases the secretion of K^+ into the urine.**}

3. Acetazolamide. {**False: Acetazolamide is a carbonic anhydrase inhibitor, which weakly increases the secretion of K^+ into the urine.**}

✔4. Spironolactone. {**True: Spironolactone is a potassium-sparing diuretic, which decreases the secretion of K^+ into the urine, resulting in hyperkalemia.**}

23.6 The correct answer is E (1,2,3,4).
Which of the following correctly pairs the diuretic drug with one of its adverse effects?

✔1. Furosemide: Ototoxicity. {**True**}
✔2. Chlorthalidone: Hyperuricemia. {**True**}
✔3. Spironolactone: Gynecomastia (development of enlarged breasts) in males. {**True**}
✔4. Acetazolamide: Metabolic acidosis. {**True**}

23.7 The correct answer is B (1,3).
Chlorothiazide increases the urinary excretion of

✔1. Sodium. {**True: Chlorothiazide is typical of the thiazide diuretics and inhibits Na⁺ resorption in the distal convoluted tubule.**}

2. Calcium. {**False: Calcium secretion is decreased, resulting in possible hypercalcemia.**}

✔3. Potassium. {**True: Chlorothiazide increases the Na⁺ concentration in the distal tubule. The Na⁺ ions may be exchanged for K⁺ leading to a loss of K⁺.**}

4. Uric acid. {**False: Thiazide diuretics decrease uric acid excretion. Thus, it usually prompts a symptomless hyperuricemia, but it may precipitate a gouty attack in susceptible individuals.**}

23.8 The correct answer is A (1,2,3).
Loop diuretics are useful in the treatment of which of the following conditions?

✔1. Congestive heart failure. {**True: Loop diuretics, such as furosemide, reduce the edema of congestive heart failure.**}

✔2. Acute pulmonary edema. {**True: Loop diuretics are particularly valuable in emergency situations, such as acute pulmonary edema, which require rapid, intense diuresis.**}

✔3. Ascites. {**True: Loop diuretics are useful in patients with ascites from hepatic cirrhosis.**}

4. Hypocalcemia. {**False: Loop diuretics are used in the treatment of hypercalcemia, since these drugs promote the increased secretion of Ca⁺⁺ in the urine.**}

23.9 The correct answer is E (1,2,3,4).
In which of the following patients would a loop diuretic be contraindicated or used with caution?

✔1. Diabetics. {**True: Hyperglycemia may develop.**}

✔2. Gouty patients. {**True: An acute gout attack may be triggered by a drug-induced hyperuricemia.**}

✔3. Patients with hypercalcemia. {**True: Loop diuretics increase secretion of Ca⁺⁺.**}

✔4. Patients being treated with aminoglycoside antibiotics. {**True: Hearing can be affected adversely by loop diuretics, particularly when used in conjunction with the aminoglycoside antibiotics.**}

Chapter 24: GASTROINTESTINAL DRUGS

24.1 The correct answer is C.
All of the following drugs are correctly matched to their actions EXCEPT:

A. Cimetidine: Blocks H₂ histamine receptors. {**Incorrect choice**}

B. Misoprostol: Inhibits adenylate cyclase. {**Incorrect choice**}

✔C. Omeprazole: Activates adenylate cyclase. {**Correct choice: Omeprazole inhibits the proton pump of the parietal cells.**}

D. Sucralfate: Protects ulcerated mucosa. {**Incorrect choice**}

E. Pirenzepine: Selectively blocks muscarinic receptors in stomach. {**Incorrect choice**}

24.2 The correct answer is B.
Which of the following is a bulk-forming laxative?

A. Castor oil. {**False: Castor oil is an intestinal irritant.**}

✔B. Psyllium. {**True**}

C. Colloidal bismuth. {**False: Colloidal bismuth is a mucosal protective agent.**}

D. Sucralfate. {**False: Sucralfate is a mucosal protective agent.**}

E. Phenolphthalein. {**False: Phenolphthalein is an intestinal stimulant.**}

24.3 The correct answer is A.
The use of a aluminum-containing antacid is most likely to cause?

✔A. Constipation. {**True**}

B. Diarrhea. {**False**}

C. Hypertension. {**False**}

D. Headache. {**False**}

E. Nausea. {**False**}

24.4 The correct answer is A.
Which one of the following statements is correct?

✔A. Histamine and prostaglandin E₂ have opposing actions on the secretion of gastric acid. {**True: Histamine stimulates HCl production, and prostacyclin inhibits gastric acid secretion.**}

B. Gastrin and acetylcholine induce a decrease in intracellular calcium levels. {**False: These agonists act through an increase in intracellular calcium levels.**}

C. Omeprazole blocks muscarinic receptors of the parietal cell. {**False: Omeprazole inhibits the proton pump of the parietal cell.**}

D. Pirenzepine is similar to atropine in its actions. {**False: Pirenzepine shows a greater specificity against the secretory function of the stomach, with less effect against salivary glands and smooth muscle.**}

E. Famotidine blocks the action of gastrin on the parietal cell. {**False: Famotidine competitively blocks the H₂ receptor.**}

Chapter 25: HORMONES OF THE PITUITARY AND THYROID

25.1 The correct answer is C.
Symptoms of hyperthyroidism include all of the following EXCEPT:

A. tachycardia. {**Incorrect choice**}
B. nervousness. {**Incorrect choice**}
✔C. poor resistance to cold. {**Correct choice: Individuals with hyperthyroidism often experience excess heat production.**}
D. body wasting. {**Incorrect choice**}
E. tremor. {**Incorrect choice**}

25.2 The correct answer is D.
Which of the following best describes the effect of propylthiouracil on thyroid hormone production?

A. It blocks the release of thyrotropin-releasing hormone. {**False: The thyroid hormones inhibit the secretion of thyroid-stimulating hormone from the anterior pituitary.**}
B. It inhibits uptake of iodide by thyroid cells. {**False**}
C. It prevents the release of thyroid hormone from thyroglobulin. {**False**}
✔D. It blocks iodination and coupling of tyrosines in thyroglobulin to form thyroid hormones. {**True**}
E. It blocks the release of hormones from the thyroid gland. {**False**}

25.3 The correct answer is A (1,2,3).
Drugs used in the treatment of hyperthyroidism include:

✔1. Propylthiouracil. {**True**}
✔2. Iodide. {**True**}
✔3. Methimazole. {**True**}
4. Triiodothyronine. {**False: This is a thyroid hormone which is overproduced in hyperthyroidism.**}

Chapter 26: INSULIN AND ORAL HYPOGLYCEMIC DRUGS

26.1 The correct answer is E.
Which one of the following series correctly ranks the insulin preparations from the agent with the most rapid onset of action to that with the slowest onset of action?

A. Ultralente insulin > isophane insulin > protamine insulin. {**False**}
B. Protamine insulin > zinc insulin > ultralente insulin. {**False**}
C. Isophane insulin > zinc insulin > protamine insulin. {**False**}
D. Zinc insulin > ultralente insulin > protamine insulin. {**False**}
✔E. Zinc insulin > Isophane insulin > ultralente insulin. {**True**}

26.2 The correct answer is C.
Which one of the following statements is correct?

A. Sulfonylureas decrease the secretion of insulin. {**False: Sulfonylureas increase the secretion of insulin.**}
B. Tolbutamide is effective in Type I diabetics. {**False: Type I diabetics have no β-cell function; therefore, sulfonylureas cannot act to increase insulin secretion.**}
✔C. Sulfonylureas increase release of insulin and increase insulin-sensitivity of target tissue. {**True**}
D. Glipizide increases glucagon secretion. {**False: The oral hypoglycemic agents often decrease glucagon release.**}
E. Chlorpropamide blocks insulin receptors. {**False.**}

26.3 The correct answer is C.
Which one of the following statements is correct?

A. Insulin can be administered orally. {**False: Insulin is administered intravenously, since the drug is destroyed in the GI tract.**}
B. Insulin is always required therapy in Type II diabetics. {**False: Diet therapy and/or sulfonylureas are often effective.**}
✔C. Protamine is added to insulin to decrease the rate of absorption of the hormone. {**True: Protamine complexes with insulin to form an insoluble complex that is slowly absorbed.**}
D. Sulfonylureas are useful in the treatment of ketoacidosis. {**False: Ketoacidosis is the most life-threatening consequence of Type I diabetes and requires adequate treatment with insulin.**}
E. Insulin acts by binding to receptors in the nucleus of target tissue. {**False: Insulin acts by binding to specific receptors in the cell membrane.**}

26.4 The correct answer is E.
All of the following are correct EXCEPT:

A. One of the most common side effects of oral hypoglycemic agents is gastrointestinal disturbances. {**Incorrect choice.**}
B. The most serious consequence of insulin overdose is hypoglycemia. {**Incorrect choice: Insulin facilitates glucose entry into the tissue, causing a decrease in blood glucose.**}
C. Weight reduction is often of therapeutic help in obese Type II diabetics. {**Incorrect choice**}
D. Sulfonylureas are contraindicated in patients with hepatic insufficiency. {**Incorrect choice**}

✔E. Insulin and glucagon have similar effects on metabolism. {**Correct choice: Insulin and glucagon have opposing actions on metabolism.**}

Chapter 27: STEROID HORMONES

27.1 The correct answer is E.

All of the following statements about glucocorticoids are correct EXCEPT:

A. They may produce peptic ulcers. {**Incorrect choice**}
B. They are useful in the treatment of refractory asthma. {**Incorrect choice**}
C. They are contraindicated in glaucoma. {**Incorrect choice**}
D. They are used in the treatment of Addison's disease. {**Incorrect choice**}
✔E. They exert their effect by binding to receptors in the cell membrane. {**Correct choice: All steroid hormones bind to receptors in the nucleus or the cytosol.**}

27.2 The correct answer is B.

Which of the following statements is true?

A. Diethylstibestrol enhances fertility by blocking the inhibitory effect of estrogen on the pituitary. {**False: Diethylstibestrol is a synthetic estrogen that acts directly on target tissues. Clomiphene inhibits the pituitary.**}
✔B. Tamoxifen is an estrogen antagonist. {**True**}
C. Dexamethasone has weak anti-inflammatory properties. {**False**}
D. Estrogens are mainly excreted unchanged in the urine. {**False: Estrogens are secreted as sulfated or glucuronidated metabolites.**}
E. Tamoxifen is used to treat infertility. {**False: Tamoxifen is used in the treatment of advanced breast cancer.**}

27.3 The correct answer is E.

All of the following are adverse effects associated with the used of oral contraceptive agents EXCEPT:

A. Edema. {**Incorrect choice**}
B. Breast tenderness. {**Incorrect choice**}
C. Nausea. {**Incorrect choice**}
D. Increased frequency of migraine headache. {**Incorrect choice**}
✔E. Increased risk of ovarian cancer. {**Correct choice: Oral contraceptive agents decrease the incidence of ovarian and endometrial cancers.**}

27.4 The correct answer is D.

Estrogen replacement therapy in menopausal women

A. restores bone loss accompanying osteoporosis. {**False: Estrogens decrease the age-related loss of bone, but these agent do not restore bone density once the bone has become demineralized.**}
B. may induce "hot flashes." {**False: Vasomotor symptoms of menopause, such as hot flashes, are decreased with estrogen replacement therapy.**}
C. may cause atrophic vaginitis. {**False: Symptoms of menopause, such as atrophic vaginitis, are decreased with estrogen replacement therapy.**}
✔D. is most effective if instituted at the first signs of menopause. {**True**}
E. requires higher doses of estrogen than are required with oral contraceptive therapy. {**False: Oral contraceptives contain higher doses of estrogen than those used with estrogen replacement therapy.**}

27.5 The correct answer is C.

Progestins

A. are not produced in males. {**False: Progesterone is synthesized by the testes in males.**}
B. increase HDL and decrease LDL. {**False: Progestins have the opposite effect.**}
✔C. attenuate the increased risk of endometrial cancer associated with estrogen-only oral contraceptive agents. {**True.**}
D. such as progesterone, are widely used in oral contraceptives. {**False: When orally administered, progesterone is largely inactivated by hepatic first-pass metabolism.**}
E. commonly induce weight loss. {**False: Weight gain is one of the side effects of progestins.**}

27.6 The correct answer is A.

Which one of the following is a synthetic estrogen used in oral contraceptives?

✔A. Mestranol. {**True**}
B. Norgestrel. {**False: Norgestrel is a progestin.**}
C. Clomiphene. {**False: Clomiphene is an antiestrogen.**}
D. Estradiol. {**False: Estradiol is largely inactivated by first-pass metabolism when administered orally.**}
E. Norethindrone. {**False: Norethindrone is a progestin.**}

Chapter 28: PRINCIPLES OF ANTIMICROBIAL THERAPY

28.1 The correct answer is D.

Which of the following statements is correct?

A. Isoniazid is a broad spectrum antibiotic. {**False: This** drug is effective only against <u>Mycobacteria</u> and therefore is a narrow spectrum antibiotic.}

B. Chloramphenicol is a narrow spectrum antibiotic. {**False: Chloramphenicol is effective against many bacteria and rickettsiae.**}

C. Ampicillin is a narrow spectrum antibiotic. {**False: Ampicillin is an extended spectrum penicillin that acts against both gram-positive staphylococci and gram-negative bacilli,e.g., <u>Haemophilus influenzae</u>.**}

✔D. Tetracycline is a broad spectrum antibiotic. {**True: Tetracycline is effective against bacteria and rickettsiae.**}

E. Initial treatment usually combines a broad spectrum and a narrow spectrum antibiotic. {**False: It is advisable to treat with the single agent that is most specific for the infecting organism.**}

28.2 The correct answer is E.

All of the following clinical indications require a combination of antibiotics (rather than a single agent) EXCEPT:

A. Mixed infections. {**Incorrect choice**}

B. Infections with clinical outcomes that depend on drug synergism. {**Incorrect choice**}

C. Infections that involve a risk of developing resistant organisms. {**Incorrect choice**}

D. Emergency situations involving an infection of unknown cause. {**Incorrect choice**}

✔E. Viral infections. {**Correct choice: Viral infections are not responsive to antibiotics.**}

28.3 The correct answer is D.

Which one of the following patients is least likely to require antimicrobial treatment tailored to the individual's condition?

A. Patient undergoing cancer chemotherapy. {**False: Anticancer drugs often suppress the immune function, and these patients require additional antibiotics to eradicate infections.**}

B. Patient with kidney disease. {**False: Impaired renal function may lead to the accumulation of toxic levels of antimicrobial drugs.**}

C. Elderly patient. {**False: Renal and hepatic function are often decreased among the elderly.**}

✔D. Patient with hypertension. {**True: Elevated blood pressure would not be expected to markedly influence the type of antimicrobial treatment employed.**}

E. Patient with liver disease. {**False: Impaired liver function may lead to the accumulation of toxic levels of antimicrobial drugs.**}

28.4 The correct answer is D.

In which one of the following clinical situations is

the prophylactic use of antibiotics NOT warranted?

A. Prevention of meningitis among individuals in close contact with infected patients. {**Incorrect choice: Meningitis is a sufficiently contagious and serious disease to warrant prophylactic use of antibiotics.**}

B. Patient with a heart prosthesis having a tooth removed. {**Incorrect choice: Following a tooth extraction bacteria of the oral cavity can readily enter the circulation and colonize on a prosthesis, causing a serious and often fatal infection.**}

C. Presurgical treatment for implantation of a hip prosthesis. {**Incorrect choice: Infection is such a serious complication that prophylactic antibiotics are warranted.**}

✔D. Patient who complains of frequent respiratory illness. {**Correct choice: Such illness may be of viral origin; further, consequences of chronic respiratory disorders may not warrant prophylactic use of antibiotics.**}

E. Presurgical treatment in gastrointestinal procedures. {**Incorrect choice: Infection is such a serious complication that prophylactic antibiotics are warranted.**}

28.5 The correct answer is A.
Broad spectrum antibiotics

✔A. increase the frequency of occurence of superinfections. {**True: Administration of broad spectrum antibiotics can alter the nature of normal bacterial flora and precipitate a superinfection that is normally kept in check by the presence of other microorganisms.**}

B. are appropriate for the ill patient requiring treatment before the sensitivity of the infective agent can be determined. {**False: This practice has led to the generation of resistant organisms. It is better to use a combination of a penicillin or cephalosporin with an aminoglycoside.**}

C. include isoniazid. {**False: Isoniazid is a narrow spectrum antibiotic.**}

D. are as effective against sensitive organisms in immunocompromised patients as they are against these organisms in immunocompetent individuals. {**False: Without assistance of the immune system, it is difficult to eliminate an infection with antimicrobial drugs, regardless of their spectrum.**}

E. have little effect on the nature of the normal intestinal flora. {**False: Broad spectrum antibiotics often markedly alter the kinds of microorganism growing in the gut.**}

28.6 The correct answer is B.
Which one of the following anti-infective agents is bactericidal?

A. Erythromycin. {**False: Erythromycin, tetracycline, clindamycin, and sulfonamides are bacteriostatic at therapeutic doses.**}
✔B. Penicillin. {**True**}
C. Tetracycline. {**False**}
D. Clindamycin. {**False**}
E. Sulfonamide. {**False**}

Chapter 29: FOLATE ANTAGONISTS

29.1   The correct answer is D.
Sulfonamides are useful in the treatment of which one of the following?

A. Influenza. {**False**}
B. Gonorrhea. {**False**}
C. Most streptococcal infections. {**False**}
✔D. Urinary tract infections. {**True: Sulfonamides at one time were the mainstay of the treatment of uncomplicated infections of the urinary tract.**}
E. Meningococcal infections. {**False**}

29.2   The correct answer is C.
Sulfonamides are agents of choice in the treatment of which one of the following?

A. Syphilis. {**False: Penicillin is the drug of first choice.**}
B. Cholera. {**False: Tetracycline is the drug of first choice.**}
✔C. Nocardiosis. {**True**}
D. Streptococcal pneumonia. {**False: Penicillin is the drug of first choice.**}
E. Rickettsial infections. {**False: Chloramphenicol or tetracycline is the drug of first choice.**}

29.3   The correct answer is C.
Trimethoprim

A. is less potent than sulfamethoxazole. {**False: Trimethoprim is 20 to 50 times more potent than sulfamethoxazole.**}
B. inhibits the enzyme dihydropteroate synthetase. {**False: Trimethoprim inhibits the enzyme dihydrofolate reductase.**}
✔C. causes adverse effects that can be lessened by simultaneous administration of folinic acid. {**True.**}
D. resistance has not been observed in microorganisms. {**False: Trimethoprim resistance has been observed in gram-negative bacteria caused by the presence of a plasmid, which codes for an altered**

dihydrofolate reductase with a lower affinity for the drug.}
E. stimulates purine synthesis. {**False: Trimethoprim inhibits both purine and pyrimidine synthesis.**}

29.4   The correct answer is D.
All of the following statements concerning sulfonamides are correct EXCEPT:

A. They require actively growing cultures for maximum antimicrobial activity. {**Incorrect choice: Sulfonamides are bacteriostatic and are most effective against growing microorganisms.**}
B. Allergic reactions are frequently seen adverse effects. {**Incorrect choice: Allergic reactions and crystalluria are the two most common adverse effects associated with sulfonamide treatment.**}
C. Treatment of patients with severe renal insufficiency may lead to crystalluria. {**Incorrect choice: The sulfonamides tend to have low solubilities and to form crystals in the kidney or bladder, particularly if urinary output is low.**}
✔D. They diminish activity of warfarin. {**Correct choice: Transient potentiation of the anticoagulant effect of vitamin K antagonists, such as warfarin or bis-hydroxycoumarin, results from their displacement from binding sites on serum albumin.**}
E. They compete with p-aminobenzoic acid for the enzyme dihydropteroate synthetase. {**Incorrect choice: The sulfonamides are competitive inhibitors of this enzyme.**}

29.5   The correct answer is D.
Sulfonamides increase the risk of neonatal kernicterus because they

A. diminish the production of plasma albumin. {**False**}
B. increase the turnover of red blood cells. {**False**}
C. inhibit the metabolism of bilirubin. {**False**}
✔D. compete for bilirubin binding sites on plasma albumin. {**True: Increased release of albumin-bound bilirubin increases the plasma concentration of free bilirubin, which can penetrate the CNS.**}
E. depress the bone marrow. {**False**}

Questions 29.6–29.9: For each numbered phrase, select the ONE drug (A–E) that is most closely associated with it. Each drug (A–E) may be selected once, more than once, or not at all.

A. Sulfasalazine.
B. Sulfadiazine.
C. Trimethoprim-sulfamethoxazole.

D. Mafenide acetate.

E. Sulfisoxazole.

29.6 The correct answer is D. {**Mafenide acetate.**}
It is used to prevent infections among burn patients. {**Creams containing mafenide acetate are used in burn units where they are used prophylactically to protect against infection with a variety of gram-negative and gram-positive micro-organisms.**}

29.7 The correct answer is A. {**Sulfasalazine.**}
It is used in the treatment of ulcerative colitis. {**Sulfasalazine is reserved for treatment of ulcerative colitis because the drug is not absorbed from the gut.**}

29.8 The correct answer is C. {**Trimethoprim-sulfamethoxazole.**}
It is effective in treating complicated or recurrent urinary infections.
{**Trimethoprim-sulfamethoxazole is effective in such infections.**}

29.9 The correct answer is B. {**Sulfadiazine.**}
It can cause crystalluria in patients with renal insufficiency. {**Sulfadiazine is one of the more insoluble of the sulfonamides and can form crystals in the kidney and bladder, particularly if urine volume is low or acidic.**}

29.10 The correct answer is A (1,2,3).
Which of the following statements is/are true for the combination of trimethoprim-sulfamethoxazole (co-trimoxazole)?

✔1. It has a broader spectrum of antimicrobial activity than either drug alone. {**True: The two drugs act synergistically to increase potency and to extend the antimicrobial spectrum.**}

✔2. It is used in the management of carriers of Salmonella typhi. {**True.**}

✔3. It is effective in the treatment of pneumonia caused by Pneumocystis carinii. {**True: It is currently the drug of choice, although high doses are required.**}

4. It is the drug of choice in treating enterococcal endocarditis. {**False: More potent bactericidal antibiotics are indicated in this severe infection.**}

29.11 The correct answer is C (2,4).
Sulfisoxazole

1. lowers the ratio of tetrahydrofolate to folate. {**False: Sulfisoxazole decreases the synthesis of folic**

acid, but it does not inhibit the subsequent reduction to tetrahydrofolate.}

✔2. is antagonized by p-aminobenzoic acid. {**True: Sulfonamides compete with p-aminobenzoic acid in the synthesis of folic acid. Thus, increased concentrations of PABA will reverse the effect of sulfonamides.**}

3. is bactericidal. {**False: Sulfonamides are bacteriostatic.**}

✔4. is useful in treating nocardiosis. {**True: Sulfisoxazole or sulfadiazine are effective in treating this fungal infection.**}

Chapter 30: INHIBITORS OF CELL WALL SYNTHESIS

30.1 Correct answer is D.
Which one of the following drugs is both penicillinase-resistant and effective by oral administration?

A. Methicillin. {**False: This antistaphylococcal penicillin is penicillinase resistant but is not stable in acid.**}

B. Carbenicillin. {**False: This antipseudomonal penicillin is neither penicillinase resistant nor stable in acid.**}

C. Penicillin V. {**False: This narrow spectrum penicillin is not penicillinase resistant but is stable in acid.**}

✔D. Amoxicillin plus clavulanic acid. {**True: This extended spectrum formulation is penicillinase resistant because of the presence of a β-lactamase inhibitor and is stable to acid.**}

E. Piperacillin. {**False: This antipseudomonal penicillin is neither penicillinase resistant nor acid stable.**}

30.2 Correct answer is A.
Which one of the following antibiotics is INCORRECTLY matched with an appropriate clinical indication?

✔A. Penicillin G: Pneumonia caused by Klebsiella pneumoniae. {**Correct choice: Cephalosporins are effective against Klebsiella.**}

B. Carbenicillin: Urinary tract infection caused by Pseudomonas aeruginosa. {**Incorrect choice: Indanyl carbenicillin is effective on oral administration.**}

C. Ampicillin: Bacterial meningitis caused by Haemophilus influenzae. {**Incorrect choice: However, resistance is now a problem.**}

D. Penicillin G: Syphilis caused by Treponema pallidum. {**Incorrect choice**}

E. Cefazolin: Osteomyelitis. {**Incorrect choice**}

30.3 Correct answer is C.

Piperacillin differs from ampicillin in all the following properties EXCEPT:

A. Stability in gastric acid. {**Incorrect choice: Piperacillin is not stable in acid, whereas ampicillin is suitable for oral administration.**}

B. Effectiveness as an antipseudomonal agent. {**Incorrect choice: Piperacillin is a far more potent antipseudomonal agent than is ampicillin.**}

✔C. Resistance to penicillinase. {**Correct choice: Both piperacillin and ampicillin are susceptible to the action of penicillinases.**}

D. Spectrum of antibacterial action. {**Incorrect choice: Piperacillin is active against** Pseudomonas aeruginosa **and ampicillin is not.**}

E. The broadness of the spectrum of susceptible bacteria. {**Incorrect choice: Ampicillin is an extended spectrum antibiotic, whereas piperacillin has a narrower spectrum.**}

30.4   Correct answer is A.
All of the following statements about penicillin G are correct EXCEPT:

✔A. It is excreted from the body primarily via the hepatobiliary route. {**Correct choice: The primary route of excretion of penicillin G is via the kidney.**}

B. Administered orally, it is variably absorbed because of its degradation by stomach acid. {**Incorrect choice: Oral administration of penicillin G is unreliable, in part because the β-lactam ring is cleaved in acid.**}

C. It is more effective in killing growing bacteria than microorganisms in the stationary phase. {**Incorrect choice: Penicillin G is bactericidal to growing microorganisms when they are actively making new cell wall material.**}

D. It can act synergistically with aminoglycosides. {**Incorrect choice: The effects of penicillins on cell wall synthesis facilitate the entry of the aminoglycosides into the cell leading to synergistic antimicrobial effects.**}

E. Levels in the blood can be increased by administration of probenecid. {**Incorrect choice: Administration of probenecid interferes with the secretion of penicillins and results in higher blood levels of penicillin and a prolonged half-life.**}

30.5   Correct answer is E.
Which one of the following statements about inhibitors of cell wall synthesis is INCORRECT?

A. The concentration of penicillin in the cerebrospinal fluid is higher when administered to patients with meningococcal meningitis than it is when given to normal patients. {**Incorrect choice: Inflammation increases penetration of penicillin into the CSF.**}

B. First generation cephalosporins are more effective against staphylococcal infections than are third generation cephalosporins. {**Incorrect choice**}

C. Cefoxitin is less likely to cause an allergic reaction in a patient that is hypersensitive to penicillin G than is penicillin V. {**Incorrect choice: All penicillin derivatives, including penicillin V, can potentially trigger an allergic reaction in patients sensitive to penicillin G. Cefoxitin can often be used in these patients. However, caution should be exercised, since there is about 15% cross-reactivity.**}

D. The half-life of procaine penicillin administered intramuscularly is greater than the half-life of penicillin G administered orally. {**Incorrect choice**}

✔E. Third-generation cephalosporins are susceptible to β-lactamase activity. {**Correct choice: Unlike the penicillins, cephalosporins are not sensitive to β-lactamase activity.**}

30.6   Correct answer is A (1,2,3).
Cephalosporins:

✔1. have the same mode of action as the penicillins. {**True: They both inhibit the synthesis of bacterial cell walls.**}

✔2. are more resistant to β-lactamases than are the penicillins. {**True**}

✔3. contain the β-lactam ring. {**True**}

4. as a group are all stable to stomach acid. {**False: Only cephalexin, cephradine, cefadroxil, cefaclor, and cefixime are stable to acid and can be administered orally.**}

30.7   Correct answer is E (1,2,3,4)
Third generation cephalosporins:

✔1. show greater activity than first generation cephalosporins against gram-negative bacilli. {**True**}

✔2. include agents that are active against Pseudomonas aeruginosa. {**True**}

✔3. include agents that are effective in treating Serratia marcescens infections. {**True**}

✔4. include agents that are effective in treating meningitis. {**True**}

30.8   Correct answer is A (1,2,3).
Vancomycin:

✔1. has an antibacterial spectrum similar to that of penicillin G. {**True**}

✔2. is effective against methicillin-resistant staphylococci. {**True**}

✔3. is given orally for the treatment of antibiotic-induced colitis. {**True**}

4. is inactivated by β-lactamases. {**False: Vancomycin is a complex glycopeptide.**}

Chapter 31: PROTEIN SYNTHESIS INHIBITORS

31.1 Correct answer is E.
Which one of the following diseases is NOT treated with a tetracycline derivative?

A. Cholera. {**Incorrect choice**}
B. Lyme disease. {**Incorrect choice**}
C. Rocky Mountain spotted fever. {**Incorrect choice**}
D. Mycoplasma pneumonia. {**Incorrect choice**}
✔E. Streptococcal infection. {**Correct choice: Most strains of streptococci are resistant.**}

31.2 Correct answer is A.
Which one of the following statements about tetracycline is INCORRECT?

✔A. Its use is rarely contraindicated because of resistant strains. {**Correct choice: Widespread resistance to tetracycline limits the clinical uses of this drug.**}
B. It is contraindicated in pregnancy. {**Incorrect choice: Deposition of tetracycline calcification in the fetus and growing children can occur. The drug has the potential for causing hepatic toxicity in the mother.**}
C. It is effective in treating infections caused by Chlamydiae. {**Incorrect choice**}
D. It can form poorly absorbable complexes with calcium ions. {**Incorrect choice: Dairy foods in the diet decrease absorption because of the formation of nonabsorbable chelates of tetracycline with calcium ions.**}
E. It can lead to discoloration of teeth if given to children. {**Incorrect choice**}

31.3 Correct answer is B.
Which one of the following statements about tetracyclines is INCORRECT?

A. Accumulation of tetracyclines by susceptible organisms is mediated by transport proteins located in the bacterial membrane. {**Incorrect choice**}
✔B. Tetracyclines, even at high concentrations, do not affect mammalian cell metabolism. {**Correct choice:**

At high concentrations, tetracycline enters mammalian cells by diffusion and interacts with mitochondrial ribosomes.}
C. Tetracyclines bind to the 30S subunit of the bacterial ribosome and block protein synthesis. {**Incorrect choice: Tetracyclines block access of the amino acyl-tRNA to the mRNA-ribosome complex at the acceptor site.**}
D. Phototoxicity is encountered most frequently with demeclocycline and doxycycline. {**Incorrect choice: Severe sunburn occurs when the patient receiving tetracyclines is exposed to sun or ultraviolet rays.**}
E. Doxycycline is the only tetracycline that may be used in treating patients with renal failure. {**Incorrect choice**}

31.4 Correct answer is C.
All of the following properties are exhibited by aminoglycosides EXCEPT:

A. They are poorly absorbed from the gastrointestinal tract. {**Incorrect choice: Aminoglycosides are given parenterally.**}
B. They have bactericidal properties. {**Incorrect choice: All aminoglycosides are rapidly bactericidal.**}
✔C. They can achieve adequate serum levels after oral administration. {**Correct choice: All are poorly absorbed from the gastrointestinal tract.**}
D. They bind to the 30S ribosomal subunit. {**Incorrect choice: They then interfere with assembly of the functional ribosomal apparatus or cause the 30S subunit of the complete ribosome to misread the genetic code.**}
E. They are not accumulated by anaerobic microorganisms. {**Incorrect choice: Anaerobes lack the oxygen-dependent system that is responsible for transporting the antibiotics across the cytoplasmic membrane, therefore, strictly anaerobic organisms are resistant.**}

31.5 Correct answer is A.
Which one of the following adverse effects is NOT observed with administration of aminoglycosides?

✔A. Anemia. {**Correct choice**
B. Nephrotoxicity. {**Incorrect choice: Kidney damage can range from mild renal impairment that is reversible to severe acute tubular necrosis.**}
C. Ototoxicity. {**Incorrect choice: Deafness may be irreversible.**}
D. Respiratory paralysis. {**Incorrect choice: Neuromuscular paralysis most often results after intraperitoneal or intrapleural application of large doses of aminoglycosides.**}

E. Allergic reactions. {**Incorrect choice: Contact dermatitis is a common reaction to topically-applied neomycin.**}

31.6 Correct answer is C.

All of the following statements about erythromycin are correct EXCEPT:

A. It is often used as a penicillin substitute. {**Incorrect choice**}

B. It binds to the 50S ribosomal subunit. {**Incorrect choice**}

✔C. It is contraindicated in patients with renal failure. {**Correct choice: Erythromycin is contraindicated in hepatic dysfunction.**}

D. Valid clinical uses include respiratory infections caused by Mycoplasma pneumoniae. {**Incorrect choice**}

E. It can cause epigastric distress. {**Incorrect choice**}

31.7 Correct answer is E (1,2,3,4).

Chloramphenicol possesses which of the following properties:

✔1. It is useful in treating infections caused by anaerobic organisms, such as Bacteroides fragilis. {**True**}

✔2. It exhibits a broad antimicrobial spectrum. {**True: Chloramphenicol is not only active against a wide range of gram-positive and gram-negative bacteria but also against other microorganisms such as rickettsiae.**}

✔3. It is reserved for well-defined indications in severely ill patients. {**True: Because of its toxicity, chloramphenicol is restricted to treatment of infections caused by salmonellae, Haemophilus influenzae, and organisms resistant to other drugs.**}

✔4. It may cause aplastic anemia, a usually fatal adverse effect. {**True**}

31.8 Correct answer is C (2,4).

Which of the following contribute(s) to the gray baby syndrome when chloramphenicol is administered to neonates?

1. Decreased intestinal absorption. {**False**}

✔2. Immature kidney function. {**True: Neonates have underdeveloped renal function and therefore accumulate the parent compound to levels that can interfere in the function of mitochondrial ribosomes.**}

3. Alteration of gastrointestinal flora. {**False**}

✔4. Low hepatic glucuronyl transferase activity. {**True: Neonates have a low capacity to glucuronidate the antibiotic and therefore accumulate the parent compound to levels that can interfere in the function of mitochondrial ribosomes.**}

31.9 The correct answer is C (2,4).

Which of the following statements is/are characteristic of clindamycin?

1. Antibacterial activity is destroyed by a β-lactamase. {**False**}

✔2. It may cause pseudomembranous colitis. {**True: Pseudomembranous colitis can be a serious or even fatal toxicity, which has limited the use of clindamycin.**}

3. Plasma levels must be controlled to avoid deafness. {**False**}

✔4. Effective against anaerobic bacteria. {**True: Including Bacteroides fragilis.**}

Questions 31.10–31.12: For each numbered phrase, select the ONE agent (A–E) that is most closely associated with it. Each agent (A–E) may be selected once, more than once, or not at all.

A. Minocycline
B. Gentamycin
C. Erythromycin
D. Doxycycline
E. Chloramphenicol

31.10 Correct answer is A. {**Minocycline.**}
This drug is effective in eradicating the meningococcal carrier state.

31.11 Correct answer is C. {**Erythromycin.**}
This drug can potentiate the effect of theophylline.

31.12 Correct answer is E. {**Chloramphenicol.**}
This drug can precipitate hemolytic anemia in patients deficient in glucose 6-phosphate dehydrogenase.

Chapter 32: QUINOLONES, URINARY TRACT, AND ANTITUBERCULAR AGENTS

Choose the ONE best answer.

32.1 Correct answer is B.

All of the following statements about methenamine are true EXCEPT:

A. It is used in chronic suppressive therapy of urinary tract infections. {**Incorrect choice**}

✔B. It has its major antibacterial effect at alkaline pH. {**Correct choice: Methenamine has its maximum effect at acidic pH—this is the reason the drug is often formulated with a weak acid such as mandelic acid.**}

C. It is contraindicated in renal insufficiency. {**Incorrect** choice: The formulation of methenamine with mandelic acid should not be administered to patients with kidney disease because the mandelic acid may precipitate.}

D. It may cause gastric disturbances. {Incorrect choice}

E. Its antimicrobial activity is confined to the urinary tract. {Incorrect choice: The acid pH of urine permits decomposition of methenamine to formaldehyde, which is toxic to all bacteria.}

32.2 Correct answer is D.

All of the following statements about nalidixic acid are true EXCEPT:

A. Nalidixic acid is only effective against infections located in the urinary tract. {Incorrect choice: Nalidixic acid does not achieve antibacterial levels in the circulation, but it is concentrated to effective levels in the urine.}

B. Children are more susceptible to nalidixic acid-induced CNS toxicities than are adults. {Incorrect choice}

C. Nalidixic acid interferes in the replication of bacterial DNA by interacting with DNA gyrase (topoisomerase II) during bacterial growth and reproduction. {Incorrect choice}

✔D. Nalidixic acid is more potent than ciprofloxacin. {Correct choice: Ciprofloxacin is more potent than nalidixic acid and has a similar antibacterial spectrum.}

E. Nalidixic acid should not be used in patients with compromised renal function. {Incorrect choice: Nalidixic acid concentrates in the urine.}

32.3 Correct answer is C.

All of the following statements about rifampin are true EXCEPT:

A. It is frequently used prophylactically for household members exposed to meningitis caused by meningococci or Haemophilus influenzae. {Incorrect choice}

B. It colors body secretions red. {Incorrect choice}

✔C. It disrupts bacterial lipid metabolism as its major mechanism of action. {Correct choice: Rifampin interacts with the β-subunit of bacterial DNA-dependent RNA polymerase and thereby inhibits RNA synthesis.}

D. Although rare, it can cause serious hepatotoxicity. {Incorrect choice}

E. When used alone, there is a high risk of the emergence of resistant strains of mycobacteria. {Incorrect choice: Because of the rapid emergence of resistant strains rifampin is never given as a single agent.}

32.4 Correct answer is D.

All of the following statements about isoniazid are true EXCEPT:

A. It produces age-dependent hepatotoxicity. {Incorrect choice}

B. It readily penetrates into infected cells. {Incorrect choice: It is therefore effective against bacilli growing intracellularly.}

C. It inhibits mycolic acid synthesis in susceptible mycobacteria. {Incorrect choice}

✔D. It may induce the symptoms of cyanocobalamin (vitamin B_{12}) deficiency. {Correct choice: Isoniazid reacts with pyridoxine (vitamin B_6), which can cause a deficiency of this vitamin.}

E. It potentiates the adverse effects of phenytoin when the patient receives both medications concurrently. {Incorrect choice: Isoniazid inhibits the metabolism of phenytoin.}

32.5 Correct answer is D.

Multiple-drug regimens are used for treatment of tuberculosis because:

A. administration of two drugs results in better penetration of cavitary lesions. {False}

B. lower doses may be used. {False}

C. multiple-drug regimens usually exhibit a potent synergistic effect. {False}

✔D. multiple-drug regimens markedly delay the appearance of drug-resistant organisms. {True: Because the organism grows slowly, resistant strains emerge during therapy. Multiple drug therapy is employed to delay the emergence of resistant strains.}

E. the organism grows rapidly and therefore must be treated aggressively over a short period of time. {False}

Chapter 33: ANTIFUNGAL DRUGS

Questions 33.1–33.3: For each numbered phrase, select the ONE drug (A–E) that is most closely associated with it. Each drug (A–E) may be selected once, more than once, or not at all.

A. Flucytosine
B. Griseofulvin
C. Penicillin G
D. Amphotericin-B
E. Ketoconazole

33.1 The correct answer is D. {Amphotericin-B.}

Binds to ergosterol present in cell membranes of sensitive fungal cells, thereby disrupting membrane function.

33.2 The correct answer is E. {Ketoconazole.}

Blocks lanosterol demethylation to ergosterol, thus disrupting fungal membrane integrity.

33.3 Correct answer is A. {Flucytosine.}
Is metabolized to a product that inhibits thymidylate synthetase and thus prevents DNA synthesis.

33.4 correct answer is D.
Which one of the following drugs is not used for the treatment of systemic fungal infections?

A. Amphotericin B. {Incorrect choice}
B. Flucytosine. {Incorrect choice}
C. Ketoconazole. {Incorrect choice}
✔D. Griseofulvin. {Correct choice: Griseofulvin use is restricted to the treatment of superficial mycotic infections.}
E. Fluconazole. {Incorrect choice}

33.5 The correct answer is D.
All of the following statements correctly describe ketoconazole EXCEPT:

A. It inhibits the conversion of lanosterol to ergosterol. {Incorrect choice}
B. It may produce gastrointestinal upsets. {Incorrect choice}
C. It can cause gynecomastia in males. {Incorrect choice}
✔D. It penetrates into the CSF. {Correct choice}
E. It should not be combined with amphotericin-B. {Incorrect choice}

33.6 Correct answer is E.
All of the following statements concerning griseofulvin are correct EXCEPT:

A. It is only effective against dermatophytic infections. {Incorrect choice}
B. It exacerbates acute intermittent porphyria. {Incorrect choice}
C. It induces the hepatic cytochrome P-450 system.. {Incorrect choice}
D. It enhances CNS depressant effects of ethanol.. {Incorrect choice}
✔E. Its use in therapy for superficial mycotic infections is usually short term (several days). {Correct choice: Griseofulvin accumulates in the infected, newly synthesized keratin-containing tissues making them unsuitable for the growth of the fungi. Therapy must be continued until normal tissue replaces infected tissue. This usually requires long term therapy.}

Chapter 34: ANTIPROTOZOAL DRUGS

Questions 34.1–34.3: For each numbered phrase, select the ONE drug (A–E) that is most closely associated with it. Each drug (A–E) may be selected once, more than once, or not at all.

A. Sodium stibogluconate
B. Diloxanide furoate
C. Pyrimethamine
D. Emetine
E. Metronidazole

34.1 The correct answer is D. {Emetine.}
A systemic amebicide.

34.2 The correct answer is C. {Pyrimethamine.}
Used in the treatment of toxoplasmosis.

34.3 The correct answer is A. {Sodium stibogluconate.}
Used in the treatment of leishmaniasis.

34.4 The correct answer is E.
All of the following statements about chloroquine are true EXCEPT:

A. It blocks protozoal DNA and RNA synthesis. {Incorrect choice: It thus prevents the parasite from replicating.}
B. Infected cells can concentrate the drug to a greater extent than can uninfected cells. {Incorrect choice}
C. It is the drug of choice for the treatment of an acute attack of falciparum or vivax malaria. {Incorrect choice}
D. Chronic administration may cause discoloration of nail beds and mucous membranes. {Incorrect choice}
✔E. Only exoerythrocytic forms of plasmodium are susceptible. {Correct choice: Only erythrocytic forms of the parasite are susceptible to chloroquine.}

34.5 Correct answer is A
All of the following statements about metronidazole are true EXCEPT:

✔A. It is administered intravenously because it is poorly absorbed after oral administration. {Correct choice: Metronidazole is rapidly and nearly completely absorbed after oral administration.}
B. It is effective against a wide variety of anaerobic bacteria. {Incorrect choice: These include anaerobic cocci and gram-negative and gram-positive bacilli.}
C. It produces a disulfiram-like effect on the ingestion of alcohol. {Incorrect choice}
D. Dosage should be reduced in patients with hepatic dysfunction. {Incorrect choice: Metabolism of the drug depends on hepatic oxidation by mixed function oxidase}
E. Therapeutic levels can be found in the cerebral spinal fluid. {Incorrect choice}

34.6 Correct answer is B.

All of the following statements about melarsoprol are true EXCEPT:

A. It reacts with sulfhydryl groups of various cellular substances, including enzymes. {Incorrect choice}

✔B. It is equally effective against African and American trypanosomiasis. {Correct choice: American trypanosomiasis, which is caused by T. cruzi, is not successfully treated with melarsoprol.}

C. Adequate trypanocidal concentrations of the drug appear in the cerebral spinal fluid. {Incorrect choice}

D. It can cause serious encephalopathy. {Incorrect choice}

E. It has a very short half-life in the body. {Incorrect choice}

34.7 Correct answer is C (2,4).
Which of the following statements about primaquine is/are correct?

1. It is effective against erythrocytic forms of malaria. {False: Primaquine eradicates the primary and secondary exoerythrocytic forms and the gametocytic forms of plasmodium.}

✔2. It is used to effect a cure of relapsing vivax malaria. {True: Primaquine is the only antimalarial agent that is effective in treating this disease.}

3. High (toxic) doses may produce corneal opacities. {False: Chloroquine, however, does produce optical problems}

✔4. Glucose 6-phosphate dehydrogenase deficient individuals are at risk for hemolytic anemia. {True}

34.8 Correct answer is A (1,2,3).
Metronidazole is effective against:

✔1. Trichomonas vaginalis. {True}
✔2. Entamoeba histolytica. {True}
✔3. Bacteroides fragilis. {True}
4. Aspergillus. {False}

Chapter 35: ANTHELMINTIC DRUGS

Questions 35.1–35.4: For each numbered phrase, select the ONE drug (A–E) that is most closely associated with it. Each drug (A–E) may be selected once, more than once, or not at all.

A. Mebendazole
B. Praziquantel
C. Niclosamide
D. Pyrantel pamoate
E. Thiabendazole

35.1 Correct answer is D. {Pyrantel pamoate.}

A drug of choice for the treatment of infections caused by roundworm, pinworm, and hookworm.

35.2 Correct answer is D. {Pyrantel pamoate.}
Acts as a depolarizing neuromuscular blocking agent.

35.3 Correct answer is B. {Praziquantel.}
A drug of choice for the treatment of all forms of schistosomiasis.

35.4 Correct answer is C. {Niclosamide.}
A drug of choice for the treatment of most tapeworm infections.

35.5 Correct answer is D.
All of the following statements about mebendazole are correct EXCEPT:

A. It is contraindicated in pregnant women. {Incorrect choice: Mebendazole has been shown to be embryotoxic and teratogenic in experimental animals.}

B. It is the drug of choice in the treatment of whipworm infections. {Incorrect choice}

C. It is effective by oral administration. {Incorrect choice}

✔D. It is active against cestodes. {Correct choice: Mebendazole is effective against nematodes.}

E. It interferes with glucose uptake by the parasite. {Incorrect choice: The drug thus causes the parasite to starve.}

Chapter 36: ANTIVIRAL DRUGS

36.1 Correct answer is A.
All of the following statements about acyclovir are correct EXCEPT:

✔A. It is the treatment of choice for influenza infections. {Correct choice: Amantadine is the drug of choice.}

B. It is incorporated into the viral DNA causing premature DNA chain termination. {Incorrect choice}

C. It is the treatment of choice in herpes simplex encephalitis. {Incorrect choice}

D. It reduces the duration of lesions associated with genital herpes infections. {Incorrect choice}

E. It inhibits only actively replicating viruses, not latent ones. {Incorrect choice}

36.2 Correct answer is D.
All of the following statements about amantadine are correct EXCEPT:

A. It is effective in the prophylaxis of influenza A infections. {Incorrect choice: However, administration

of amantadine must begin before exposure to influenza A infection.}

B. It causes CNS disturbances at high doses. {**Incorrect choice**}

C. It reduces the duration and severity of systemic symptoms of influenza A. {**Incorrect choice: However, amantadine must be started within 48 hours after the onset of the disease.**}

✔D. It is extensively metabolized. {**Correct choice**}

E. It is effective in the treatment of some cases of Parkinson's disease. {**Incorrect choice**}

36.3 Correct answer is C.

Which one of the following antiviral agents exhibits the greatest selective toxicity?

A. Idoxuridine. {**False**}

B. Amantadine. {**False**}

✔C. Acyclovir. {**True: Acyclovir is monophosphorylated in the cell by the herpes virus-coded enzyme, thymidine kinase. Thus, uninfected cells show little activation of the drug, and the toxicity is therefore highly selective for herpes virus-infected cells.**}

D. Zidovudine. {**False**}

E. Ribavirin. {**False**}

36.4 Correct answer is C.

All of the following statements about zidovudine (AZT) are correct EXCEPT:

A. It must be converted to the nucleotide form to express its antiviral activity. {**Incorrect choice. This is done by mammalian thymidine kinase.**}

B. It is incorporated into growing viral but not mammalian nuclear DNA. {**Incorrect choice: The viral reverse transcriptase favors introduction of AZT into DNA; cellular DNA polymerases are more selective.**}

✔C. It is currently used to treat severe herpes virus and respiratory syncytial virus infections as well as AIDS. {**Correct choice: Zidovudine is currently used only in the treatment of HIV infections.**}

D. It is toxic to bone marrow and causes adverse hematological effects. {**Incorrect choice**}

E. It penetrates the CNS. {**Incorrect choice**}

Questions 36.5–36.8: For each numbered phrase, select the ONE drug (A–E) that is most closely associated with it. Each drug (A–E) may be selected once, more than once, or not at all.

A. Amantadine
B. Zidovudine (AZT)
C. Idoxuridine
D. Vidarabine
E. Ganciclovir

36.5 The correct answer is C. {**Idoxuridine.**}
It is restricted to the topical treatment of herpes simplex keratitis.

36.6 The correct answer is A. {**Amantadine.**}
It is used solely in the treatment of influenza A infections.

36.7 The correct answer is D. {**Vidarabine.**}
It is an adenosine analog that is active against all members of the herpes virus group that infects humans.

36.8 The correct answer is E. {**Ganciclovir.**}
It is used in the treatment of cytomegalovirus infections in immunocompromised patients.

Chapter 37: ANTICANCER DRUGS

37.1 The correct answer is B (1,3).
Which of the following agents show(s) cytotoxicity that is cell cycle specific?

✔1. Methotrexate. {**True: Methotrexate shows maximal cytotoxic effects in the S phase.**}

2. Dactinomycin. {**False: With the exception of bleomycin, all the antibiotic anticancer agents are cell cycle nonspecific, but they tend to have a greater effect in cycling cells.**}

✔3. Bleomycin. {**True**}

4. Mechlorethamine. {**False: Mechlorethamine is toxic in both cycling and resting cells, but proliferating cells are more sensitive.**}

37.2 The correct answer is B (1,3).
Which of the following drugs is/are metabolized to a cytotoxic product?

✔1. 6-Mercaptopurine. {**True: In order to exert its antileukemic effect, 6-mercaptopurine must be converted to the corresponding nucleotide.**}

2. Dactinomycin. {**False: Dactinomycin directly interferes with DNA-dependent RNA polymerase.**}

✔3. 5-Fluorouracil. {**True: 5-Fluorouracil is devoid of antineoplastic activity and must be converted to the corresponding deoxynucleotide.**}

4. Lomustine. {**False: Lomustine directly exerts cytotoxic effects by inhibiting DNA replication.**}

37.3 The correct answer is B.
All of the following agents cause their cytotoxic effects by interference in DNA transcription EXCEPT:

A. Doxorubicin. {**Incorrect choice**}

✔B. Tamoxifen. {**Correct choice**}

C. Cyclophosphamide. {Incorrect choice}

D. Mechlorethamine. {Incorrect choice}

E. Cisplatin. {Incorrect choice}

37.4 The correct answer is E.
Myelosuppression is a particularly serious toxicity with all of the following EXCEPT:

A. Vinblastine. {Incorrect choice}

B. Cyclophosphamide. {Incorrect choice}

C. Cytarabine. {Incorrect choice}

D. Mechlorethamine. {Incorrect choice}

✔E. L-Asparaginase. {Correct choice}

37.5 The correct answer is A.
Cells resistant to methotrexate may

✔A. have higher than normal levels of dihydrofolate reductase. {True: Resistant cells may have elevated levels of dihydrofolate reductase.}

B. have higher levels of formyl tetrahydrofolate. {False: Methotrexate inhibits dihydrofolate reductase and, therefore, leads to lower than normal levels of the reduced tetrahydrofolate derivatives.}

C. metabolize the drug to inactive products. {False: Methotrexate does undergo metabolism by the host, but this is not a factor in resistance.}

D. have a decreased metabolic need for folate. {False: The metabolic need for folate is high in all rapidly dividing cells.}

E. show an increased uptake of methotrexate. {False: A decrease in influx may be associated with resistance.}

37.6 The correct answer is E.
All of the following statements are true EXCEPT:

A. Patients with Hodgkin's disease being treated with procarbazine should be cautioned against ingesting food derived from fermentative sources. {Incorrect choice: Procarbazine inhibits monoamine oxidase, an enzyme required to metabolize tyramine found in fermentative sources, such as cheese and some wines.}

B. Vincristine is effective in inducing remission in childhood ALL. {Incorrect choice}

C. X-irradiation of the craniospinal axis is an effective adjuvant therapy in the treatment of acute lymphocytic leukemia. {Incorrect choice}

D. Treatment with alkylating agents can induce secondary tumors. {Incorrect choice: Most antineoplastic agents are mutagens and can induce tumors that may arise after the original cancer was cured.}

✔E. Tamoxifen complexes with DNA to inhibit RNA synthesis. {Correct choice: Tamoxifen forms a complex with the estrogen receptor.}

Chapter 38: ANTI-INFLAMMATORY DRUGS

38.1 The correct answer is C.
In which of the following conditions would aspirin be contraindicated?

A. Myalgia. {False: Aspirin is effective in reducing muscle pain.}

B. Fever. {False: Aspirin has antipyretic actions and is used to treat fever.}

✔C. Peptic ulcer. {True: Among the NSAIDs, aspirin is among the worst for causing gastric irritation.}

D. Rheumatoid arthritis. {False: Because of its anti-inflammatory properties, aspirin is used to treat pain related to the inflammatory process, for example, in the treatment of rheumatoid arthritis.}

E. Unstable angina. {False: Low doses of aspirin decrease the incidence of transient ischemic attacks in men.}

38.2 The correct answer is E.
Overdoses of salicylates lead to all of the following EXCEPT:

A. Nausea and vomiting. {Incorrect choice}

B. Tinnitus (ringing or roaring in the ears). {Incorrect choice}

C. Marked hyperventilation. {Incorrect choice}

D. Increased metabolic rate. {Incorrect choice}

✔E. Increase in blood pH. {Correct choice: Overdose of salicylates cause acidosis.}

38.3 The correct answer is D.
Acetaminophen has all of the following properties EXCEPT:

A. It is a weaker anti-inflammatory agent than aspirin. {Incorrect choice: Acetaminophen has little anti-inflammatory effects, but it has analgesic and antipyretic activities equal to those of aspirin.}

B. It reduces fever of viral infections in children. {Incorrect choice: Acetaminophen is the analgesic-antipyretic of choice for children with viral infections; aspirin can increase the risk for Reye's syndrome in children.}

C. It is an aspirin substitute in patients with peptic ulcer. {Incorrect choice: Acetaminophen is a suitable substitute for the analgesic and antipyretic effects of aspirin in those patients with gastric complaints.}

✔D. It exacerbates gout. {Correct choice: Acetaminophen does not antagonize the uricosuric agent probenecid and therefore may be used in patients with gout.}

E. It causes hepatotoxic effects at high doses. {Incorrect choice}

38.4 The correct answer is C.
Which of the following statements concerning gold salts is correct?

   A. They may provide immediate relief of arthritic pain. {**False: Gold salts may not provide clinical improvement until after several weeks of administration.**}

   B. They act by inhibiting prostaglandin synthesis. {**False: Gold salts are thought to suppress phagocytosis and lysosomal enzyme activity in macrophages.**}

✔C. They frequently cause dermatitis of the skin or mucous membranes. {**True.**}

   D. They are drugs of first choice in treating arthritis. {**False: Gold salts are used in rheumatoid arthritis that does not respond to NSAIDs.**}

   E. They must all be given intramuscularly. {**False: Auranofin can be taken by mouth.**}

38.5 The correct answer is A (1,2,3).
Which of the following are correctly paired?

✔1. Indomethacin: Causes frontal headaches. {**True**}

✔2. Sulindac: Long half-life permits daily or twice daily dosing. {**True**}

✔3. Naproxen: Better tolerated than aspirin in some patients. {**True**}

   4. Phenylbutazone: Less toxic than aspirin. {**False: phenylbutazone should be used only after less toxic agents have proved ineffective.**}

38.6 The correct answer is A (1,2,3).
Colchicine:

✔1. is used prophylactically to reduce the number of acute gouty attacks. {**True**}

✔2. can cause serious GI problems. {**True: The cells of the intestinal epithelium show a rapid turnover, making them particularly susceptible to mitotic blockage by colchicine.**}

✔3. inhibits microtubule function. {**True: Mobility of granulocytes is impaired, decreasing their migration into the affected area.**}

   4. has general use as an anti-inflammatory drug. {**False: The anti-inflammatory activity of colchicine is specific for gout and is only rarely effective in other inflammatory diseases.**}

38.7 The correct answer is B (1,3).
Allopurinol:

✔1. decreases uric acid in the blood. {**True: Allopurinol reduces the production of uric acid by competitively inhibiting uric acid biosynthesis.**}

   2. increases excretion of uric acid. {**False**}

✔3. produces increased excretion of xanthine. {**True: Inhibition of xanthine oxidase by allopurinol results in accumulation of xanthine.**}

   4. is a toxic compound with a high frequency of adverse effects. {**False: Allopurinol is well tolerated by most patients.**}

Chapter 39: AUTACOIDS

39.1 The correct answer is D.
Which of the following are major effects of angiotensin II?

   A. Inhibition of the sympathetic nervous system. {**False: The sympathetic nervous system is activated by angiotensin II.**}

   B. Vasodilation. {**False: Angiotensin II causes direct contraction of vascular smooth muscle, especially that of the arterioles.**}

   C. Decreased blood pressure. {**False: Vasoconstriction and increased water retention result in an increase in blood pressure.**}

✔D. Promotes sodium and water retention and potassium wasting. {**True: These actions are mediated by an increased release of aldosterone from the adrenal gland.**}

   E. Hypotension. {**False: The actions of angiotensin on the vascular system lead to an increase in blood pressure.**}

39.2 The correct answer is E.
Angiotensin converting enzyme (ACE) has all of the following properties EXCEPT:

   A. converts bradykinin to inactive fragments. {**Incorrect choice**}

   B. is localized in the endothelium of the blood vessels of the lungs, kidney, and other organs. {**Incorrect choice**}

   C. is also known as peptidyl dipeptidase. {**Incorrect choice**}

   D. Is a dipeptidase. {**Incorrect choice: ACE is also known as peptidyl dipeptidase.**}

✔E. is inhibited by saralasin. {**Correct choice: Saralasin is an angiotensin receptor blocker, not an ACE inhibitor.**}

39.3 The correct answer is A .
All of the following statements are true EXCEPT:

✔A. Serotonin acts through the same receptors that bind histamine. {**Correct choice: The actions of serotonin are mediated by cell-surface receptors that are different from those that bind histamine.**}

   B. At high blood levels of angiotensin II, saralasin lowers arterial blood pressure, whereas at low blood levels of angiotensin II, saralasin increases arterial blood pressure. {**Incorrect choice: In the** presence of high blood levels of angiotensin II, saralasin functions as a competitive antagonist by blocking tissue receptors, and thus lowering arterial blood pressure. However, at low angiotensin II levels, saralasin acts as an agonist, increasing blood pressure.}

C. Phenelzine inhibits serotonin degradation. {**Incorrect choice: Phenelzine inhibits monoamine oxidase inhibitor which is a major degradative enzyme for serotonin.**}

D. Tricyclic antidepressants, such as imipramine, increase serotonin levels in the synapse. {**Incorrect choice: Imipramine inhibits the membrane uptake of serotonin.**}

E. Reserpine depletes the store of serotonin in the neurons and may precipitate a depressive episode. {**Incorrect choice**}

39.4 The correct answer is C.
Ergot alkaloids:

A. cause vasodilation. {**False: Vasoconstriction leading to tissue ischemia is one of the toxic complications associated with an overdose of these drugs.**}

B. exert their actions by binding to specific ergot amine receptors. {**False: The ergot alkaloids interact with adrenergic, dopaminergic, and serotonin receptors.**}

✔C. are useful in treating acute migraine headache. {**True: Ergotamine acts to counteract cerebral vasodilation that plays a role in migraine headaches.**}

D. are useful to maintain uterine muscle tone during pregnancy. {**False: The ergot alkaloids are contraindicated in pregnancy because of their ability to cause uterine contraction and abortion.**}

E. have actions similar to those of nitroprusside. {**False: Nitroprusside is a powerful vasodilator that is used to treat vasoconstriction that is characteristic of an overdose with ergot alkaloids.**}

39.5 The correct answer is A (1,2,3).
Histamine H_1 receptor blockers are useful in the treatment of

✔1. urticaria. {**True**}

✔2. seasonal rhinitis. {**True**}

✔3. drug reactions. {**True**}

4. bronchial asthma. {**False: H_1-histamine receptor blockers are not effective in bronchial asthma.**}

39.6 The correct answer is C (2,4).
Which of the following statements regarding histamine H_2 receptor blockers is/are correct?

1. Cimetidine is more potent and longer acting than ranitidine. {**False: Ranitidine is the more potent and longer acting drug.**}

✔2. Cimetidine shows little or no effect because of interactions with H_1 histamine receptor. {**True: Cimetidine has low affinity for H_1 receptors.**}

3. Ranitidine has endocrine effects, including gynecomastia, galactorrhea, and reduced sperm count. {**False: The antiandrogen effects described are characteristic of cimetidine, not ranitidine.**}

✔4. Cimetidine binds to hepatic mixed function oxidase and, therefore, inhibits the microsomal metabolism of certain drugs. {**True**}

39.7 The correct answer is B (1,3).
Which of the following statements regarding the effects of histamine is/are true?

✔1. The cardiovascular effects of histamine are mediated by both H_1 and H_2 receptors. {**True: Histamine causes positive chronotropism (H_1 effect) and positive inotropism (H_1 and H_2 effects).**}

2. Stimulation of histamine H_1 receptors results in smooth muscle relaxation. {**False: Stimulation of H_1 receptors causes smooth muscle constriction.**}

✔3. Combination of histamine with H_2 receptors causes stimulation of gastric acid secretion. {**True**}

4. The effect of histamine on the skin is a result of the stimulation of H_1 receptors. {**False: Stimulation of both H_1 and H_2 receptors result in the classical "triple response" in the skin.**}

Information contained in this index

FREQUENTLY PRESCRIBED DRUGS
Drug names marked with asterisk (*) are among the top 30 prescription drugs in the United States. These drugs often deserve special attention because of their wide spread use.

MAJOR CITATION
Page number shown in **bold** indicates location of the most extensive discussion of the drug or topic

Diazepam*, **93-95**, *93*
(VALIUM)

TRADE NAMES
Trade name(s) for the drug are shown in CAPITAL LETTERS

PRONOUNCIATION
Page number in *italics* indicates location of pronounciation of drug.

Index

Figure Sources

Figure 2.5 modified from H.P. Range and M.M. Dale, Pharmacology, Churchill Livingstone (1987)

Figures 6.9, 6.10 and 6.11 modified from Allwood, Cobbold and Ginsburg, British Medical Bulletin 19:132 (1963)

Figure 9.6 modified from A. Kales, Excertpa Medical Congress Series 899:149 (1989)

Figure 10.4 modified from N.L. Benowitz, Science 319:1318 (1988)

Figure 17.3 modified from J.A. Beven and J.H. Thompson, Essentials of Pharmacology, Harper and Row (1983)

Figure 19.5 modified from B.J.Materson, Drug Therapy, November p.157 (1985)

Figures 21.4 and 21.8 modified from R.H. Knopp, Hospital Practice 23:22 (1988)

Figures 25.2 and 26.5 modified from B.G. Katzun, Basic and Clinical Pharmacology, Appleton and Lange (1987)

Figures 27.5 and 27.6 modified from D.R. Mishell, Jr., New England Journal of Medicine 320:777 (1989)

Figure 32.5 from data of U.S. Public Health Service

Figure 32.6 modified from data of D.A. Evans, K.A. Maley and V.A. McRusick, British Medical Journal 2:485 (1960)

Figure 36.2 modified from R. Dolin, Science 227:1296 (1985)